ALLE ZEIT WACH 1842

E. Faist, J. Ninnemann, D. Green (Eds.)

Immune Consequences of Trauma, Shock, and Sepsis

Mechanisms and Therapeutic Approaches

With 185 Figures and 92 Tables

Springer-Verlag Berlin Heidelberg New York
London Paris Tokyo Hong Kong

Editor:

Priv.-Doz. Dr. med. Eugen Faist
Dept. of Surgery
LM University Munich
Klinikum Großhadern
Marchioninistr. 15
8000 Munich 70, FRG

John L. Ninnemann, Ph. D.
Associate Adjunct Professor of Surgery
University of California
San Diego, California 92103, USA

Douglas R. Green, Ph. D.
Associate Professor of Immunology
University of Alberta Edmonton
Alberta T6G 2H7, Canada

ISBN-13:978-3-642-73470-0 e-ISBN-13:978-3-642-73468-7
DOI: 10.1007/978-3-642-73468-7

Library of Congress Cataloging in Publication Data.
Immune consequences of trauma, shock, and sepsis: mechanisms and therapeutic approaches/E. Faist, J. Ninnemann, D. Green, eds.
Includes index.
ISBN-13:978-3-642-73470-0 (alk. paper: U.S.)
1. Wounds and injuries – Immunological aspects. 2. Traumatic shock – Immunological aspects. 3. Septicemia – Immunological aspects. 4. Immunosuppressions – Pathogenesis. I. Faist, E. (Eugen). II. Ninnemann, John L. III. Green, Doug, R. (Douglas R.) RD93.I53 1989 617'.1–dc19 89-4066

Softcover reprint of the hardcover 1st edition 1989

Typesetting: Brühlsche Universitätsdruckerei, Giessen

2124/3020-543210 – Printed on acid-free paper

Preface

Six hundred clinicians and basic researchers from all over the world have participated in the 1st International Congress on The Immune Consequences of Trauma, Shock and Sepsis – Mechanisms and Therapeutic Approaches, which was held in Munich March 3–5, 1988. The discussions centered on our major concern, namely that despite careful hygiene and vigorous antibiotic therapy, the infection rate in patients with severe injuries or in those who undergo major surgery remains high and is often accompanied by late death due to sepsis.

During the Munich meeting, these experts demonstrated the importance of applied immunology as a promising biological approach for understanding sepsis and ultimately preventing its development. The nature, causes, and potential therapy of trauma-associated immunological defects were the subjects of a wide array of scientific work presented. This book contains the most valuable papers on essential immunologic mechanisms and the latest knowledge of pathophysiologic alterations. This volume, thus, presents an overview of the scientific state of the art with regard to alterations of host defense following trauma shock, and sepsis.

Munich, February 1989

G. Heberer, M. D.
Professor of Surgery
and Chairman
Ludwig-Maximilians-
University Munich
Klinikum Großhadern

Preface

It is generally recognized and increasingly well documented that trauma-associated changes in the immune response are highly complex and ripe for dissection with modern immunologic tools.

The most topical key issues and research trends were exhaustively discussed by basic researchers, clinical immunologists and clinicians during the 1st International Congress on the Immune Consequences of Trauma, Shock and Sepsis – Mechanisms and Therapeutic Approaches.

This volume is derived from the vast amount of information presented during this conference. It represents an inventory of current knowledge in seven sections and, as a whole, it is an up to date survey of almost all significant data on altered host defense mechanisms in states of trauma, shock, and sepsis.

Besides general aspects of the development of trauma induced immunodeficiency and the neuroendocrine response to severe injury and sepsis, the effect of trauma on specific and nonspecific immune mechanisms is described in detail. The mediator regulated monocyte/T-cell interaction, B-cell function, pathobiochemical mechanisms in inflammation, oxygen radical responses, complement activity and acute-phase protein production are central points of interest and are described from various points of view.

An important question addressed in a large number of chapters concerns the triggers of immunodeficiency after trauma. We know that there is a clear association between the severity and extent of trauma and the degree of the immune deficiency. Stress hormones, products of the cyclooxygenase and lipoxygenase pathways, denatured proteins, and bacterial endotoxins are closely examined regarding their role within the armada of active suppressor substances.

In a further section, the immunology of the skin as well as the immune regulation of wound healing and compensatory organ growth are scrutinized. This is followed by the discussion of the impact of a number of therapeutic regimens like blood transfusion, nutrition, anesthesia, or special surgical procedures.

Any or all of the immune deficiences that accompany severe trauma may contribute greatly to the ensuing high risk of sepsis. Without knowing the precise nature and cause of the deficiency, however, the design of appropriate therapy is difficult. Nevertheless, some success has been achieved towards restoring the immune status and improving the chances of survival in severely injured individuals. The final section of this book considers these therapeutic approaches.

As in other disease states, e.g., cancer or AIDS-related complex, it is a very long way from experimental results to clinical application of immunomodulation. A number of authors have evaluated and related the experimental and clinical observations in order to develop strategies for the therapeutic use of immunomodulators. In many in vitro and in vivo trauma models, biological response modifiers, including thymic hormones, interferons, interleukins, or cyclooxygenase inhibitors and many synthetic substances, have been extensively studied over recent years. Besides immunoglobulin substitution in immunocompromised hosts, more specific therapies are also under investigation like the use of polymyxin B or monoclonal and polyclonal antibodies to lipopolysaccharides to neutralize endotoxin.

Clearly, much more information will be needed before the best strategies of immunotherapy can be designed. One major problem area in research into immunodeficiency disease, that of trauma-associated immunological failure, may prove to be tractable using current techniques. The Munich Conference and this volume serve to provide the immune consequences of trauma and highlight up to date information and understanding about this subject.

We believe that this book will be an invaluable reference work to researchers, clinicians, and those working in related fields and would like to record our thanks to all contributors for sharing their knowledge with us.

The authors are very much indebted to the editorial staff of Springer Verlag for their willingness and terrific support in publishing this book.

They would also like to thank Mrs. R. Maier for invaluable secretarial assistance, Mrs. E. Hanesch for the cover design, and Drs. W. Ertel and M. Storck for correcting the proofs and preparing the subject index.

Munich, February 1989

E. Faist
J. Ninnemann
D. Green

List of Contributors

Alexander, W. J., MD, Prof. of Surgery
Dept. of Surgery, Univ. of Cincinnati, Medical Center, Cincinnati, Ohio 45229, USA

Antonacci, A. C., MD, Assoc. Prof. of Surgery
The New York Hospital-Cornell, Medical Center, Dept. of Surgery, 525 East 68th Street, F-1920 New York, New York 10021, USA

August, D. A., MD, Assoc. Prof. of Surgery
Dept. of Surgery, Yale University, School of Medicine, New Haven, Connecticut 06510, USA

Baker, C. C., MD, FACS Assoc. Prof. of Surgery
Yale University, Dept. of Surgery, 333 Cedar Street, New Haven, Connecticut 06510, USA

Barbul, A., MD, Assoc. Prof. of Surgery
Dept. of Surgery, Sinai Hospital of Baltimore, Hoffberger Bldg., 2433 W. Belvedere Avenue, Suite 12, Baltimore, Maryland 21215, USA

Baue, A. E., MD, Prof. of Surgery
St. Louis University, 1325 S. Grand Blvd., St. Louis, Missouri 63104, USA

Bolla, K., MD.
Cilag Ltd., Hochstr. 201–209, 8200 Schaffhausen, Switzerland

Bottomly, K., MD
Section of Immunobiology and Department of Pathology, Howard Hughes Medical Institute, Yale University, School of Medicine, New Haven, Connecticut 06510, USA

Border, J. R., MD, Prof. of Surgery
Dept. of Surgery, 462 Grider Street, Buffalo, New York 14215, USA

Braquet, P., Ph. D
Institut Henri Beaufour Research Labs, 72, avenue des Tropiques, 91940 Les Ulis, France

Brown, G. E., MD
Dept. of Surgery, Beth Israel Hospital, 330 Brookline Avenue, Boston, Massachusetts 02215, USA

Chaudry, I. H., Ph. D, Prof. of Surgery
Michigan State University, Dept. of Surgery, B424 Clinical Center, East Lansing, Michigan 48824–1315, USA

Cheadle, G., MD
550 South Jackson Street, Dept. of Surgery, University of Louisville, Louisville, Kentucky 40292, USA

Christou, N. V., MD, PhD, Assoc. Prof. of Surgery
Dept. of Surgery, Room S10–30, Royal Victoria Hospital, 687 Pine Avenue, West, Montreal, Quebec, H3A 1A1, Canada

Čolić, M., MD
Inst. for Experimental Medicine, Military Medical Academy, Crnotravska 17, Belgrade 11002, Yugoslavia

Deitch, E. A., MD, Assoc. Prof. of Surgery
Louisiana State University, Medical Center, 1501 Kings Highway, Shreveport, Louisiana 71130–3932, USA

DeMarinis, J., MD
51 Blossom St., Shriners Burns Institute, Boston, Massachusetts 02114, USA

Di Padova, F. E., MD
Preclinical Research, Bld. 386, Room 143, Sandoz Ltd., Basle 4002, Switzerland

Durum, S. K., MD
Laboratory of Molecular, Immunoregulation, National Cancer Institute, Frederick Cancer Research Facility, Frederick, Maryland 21701, USA

Dwenger, A., MD
Klinische Biochemie und Unfallchirurgie, Med. Hochschule, 3000 Hannover 61, FRG

Ertel, W., MD
Dept. of Surgery, Klinikum Grosshadern, LMU Munich, Marchioninistr. 15, 8000 Munich 70, FRG

Faist, E., PD Dr. med.
Dept. of Surgery, Klinikum Grosshadern, LMU Munich, Marchioninistr. 15, 8000 Munich 70, FRG

Flegel, W. A., MD
DRK-Blutspendezentrale und Abt. Transfusionsmedizin der Universität Ulm, Ob. Eselsberg, 7900 Ulm/Donau, FRG

Friedman, H., PhD, Prof. of Surgery
Dept. of Medical Microbiology and Immunology, Box 10, 12901 North 30th Street, Tampa, Florida 33612, USA

Fritz, H., Prof. Dr. rer. nat.
Leiter des Institutes für Klin. Chemie und Klin. Biochemie, Chirurgische Klinik Innenstadt der Universität München, Nußbaumstr. 20, 8000 Munich 2, FRG

Gadd, M. A., MD
Univ. of California at San Diego H640B, 225 Dickinson St., San Diego, California 92130, USA

Gemmell, C. G., MD
Depts. of Bacteriology, Respiratory Medicine and Anaesthesia and Regional Burns Unit, Glasgow Royal Infirmary, 86 Castle Street, Glasgow G4 OSF, UK

Gibbons, R., PhD
U.C.S.F. – Immunogenetics Lab., Rm. HSE 520, 3rd & Parnassus Aves. San Francisco, California 94143, USA

Green, D., PhD, Assoc. Prof. of Surgery
Dept. of Immunology, 8–63 Med. SCI Building, Univ. of Alberta, Edmonton, Alberta T66 2H7, Canada

Guilbert, L., MD, Assoc. Prof. of Surgery
Dept. of Immunology, 8–63 Med. SCI Building, Univ. of Alberta, Edmonton, Alberta, Canada

Hadden, J. W., MD, Prof.
Univ. of South Florida, Dept. of Internal Medicine, Program of Immunpharmacology, Box 19, 12901 North Street, Tampa, Florida 33612, USA

Hansbrough, J. F., MD, FACS, Assoc. Prof. of Surgery
Dept. of Surgery/Div. of Trauma, Univ. of California, Medical Center San Diego, 225 Dickinson Street H-640-B, San Diego, California 92103–1990, USA

Heberer, G., Prof. Dr. med., Dr. h. c.
Dept. of Surgery, Klinikum Großhadern, LMU Munich, Marchioninistr. 15, 8000 Munich 70, FRG

Heideman, M., MD, PhD, Assoc. Prof. of Surgery
Gothenburg University, Dept. of Surgery I, Sahlgren's Hospital,
41345 Gothenburg, Sweden

Hosford, D., MD
Institut Henri Beaufour, 17 avenue Descartes, 92350 Le Plessis-Robinson,
France

Hoyt, D. B., MD
UCSD Medical Center, 225 Dickinson Street, H-640-B, San Diego,
California 92103, USA

Hufnagel, B., MD
Abteilung für Verbrennungs- und Plastische Wiederherstellungschirurgie,
Klinikum der RWTH Aachen, Pauwelsstr., 5100 Aachen, FRG

Janeway, A., MD, Prof. of Pathology
Yale University, School of Medicine, New Haven, Connecticut 06510, USA

Jochum, M., PD Dr. med.
Abt. f. Klin. Chemie und Klin. Biochemie, Chirurgische Klinik Innenstadt der
Universität München, Nußbaumstr. 20, 8000 Munich 2, FRG

Kinnaert, P., MD
Hôpital Erasme, 808 Route de Lennik, 1070 Brussels, Belgium

Köller, M., MD
Med. Mikrobiol. und Immunol., AG Infektabwehr, Ruhr-Universität,
4630 Bochum 1, FRG

Kupper, T. S., MD, Assoc. Prof. of Surgery
Yale University, School of Medicine, Dept. of Dermatology, 333 Cedar Street,
New Haven, Connecticut 06510, USA

Lanser, M. E., MD, Assoc. Prof. of Surgery
Harvard Medical School, Beth Israel Hospital, 330 Brookline Avenue, Boston,
Massachusetts 02215, USA

Livingston, D. H., MD
University of Louisville, Dept. of Surgery, 550 S. Jackson St., Louisville,
Kentucky 40292, USA

Malangoni, M. A., MD
Dept. of Surgery, Univ. of Louisville, Louisville, Kentucky 40292, USA

Mannick, J., MD, Prof. of Surgery
Brigham & Women's Hospital, 75 Francis Street, Boston, Massachusetts 02115,
USA

Meakins, J. L., MD, DSc, FRCSC, FACS, Prof. of Surgery McGill University
Royal Victoria Hospital, 687 Pine Avenue, Montreal, Canada

Miller-Graziano, L., PhD, Assoc. Prof. of Surgery
University of Massachusetts, Medical Center, Dept. of Surgery, 55 Lake Avenue North, Worcester, Massachusetts 01605, USA

Müller, P. K., MD
GBF, Gesellschaft für Biotechnologische Forschung, 3300 Braunschweig, FRG

Muhrer, K. H., PhD
Center of Surgery, Justus-Liebig-University, Klinikstr. 29, 6300 Giessen, FRG

Nelson, D., PhD
Univ. of Minnesota, Box 124, Mayo Building, Minneapolis, Minnesota 55455, USA

Ninnemann, J. L., PhD, Assoc. Prof. of Surgery
Surgical Immunology Laboratory, Dept. of Surgery H-890A, UCSD Medical Center, 225 Dickinson Street, San Diego, California 92103, USA

Olszewski, L., MD, Prof. of Surgery
Polish Academy of Sciences, Medical Research Center, Dept. for Surgical Research and Transplantology, 5 Chalubinskiego, 02-004 Warsaw, Poland

Ozkan, N., MD,
Surgical Immunology Laboratory, Dept. of Surgery, H-890A, UCSD Medical Center, 225 Dickinson Street, San Diego, California 92103, USA

Pignol, B., MD
I.H.B. Research Labs, 72 avenue des Tropiques, 91952 Les Ulis, France

Radosevic-Stasic, B., PhD,
Medical Faculty, University of Rijeka, Olge Ban 20, 5100 Rijeka, Yugoslavia

Redl, H., MD, Univ.-Doz.
Ludwig Boltzmann Institute for Experimental Traumatology, Donaueschinger Str. 13, 1200 Vienna, Austria

Rodrick, L., PhD Assoc. Prof. of Surgery
Dept. of Surgery, Brighman & Women's Hospital, 75 Francis Street, Boston, Massachusetts 02115, USA

Rothe, G., MD
Mildred-Scheel-Labor für Krebszellforschung, Max-Planck-Institut für Biochemie, 8033 Martinsried, FRG

Sagawa, T., MD
2nd Dept. of Surgery, Ehime Univ. School of Med., 791-02 Shigenobu-cho, Onsen-gun, Japan

Schmucker, P., Prof. Dr. med.
Deutsches Herzzentrum, Berlin, Augustenburger Platz 1, 1000 Berlin 45, FRG

Stephan, W., MD
Biotest Pharma GmbH, Research Department, Flughafenstr. 4, 6000 Frankfurt (Main) 73, FRG

Teodorczyk-Injeyan, J. A., Ph. D
The Ross Tilley Burn Centre, Wellesley Hospital, 160 Wellesley Str. E., Toronto, Ontario M4Y 1J3, Canada

Udovic-Sirola, M. MD
Dept. of Anaesthesiology, Medical Falculty,
Clinical Hospital Center, Rijeka, University of Rijeka
Olge Ban 20, 51000 Rijeka, Yugoslavia

Walz, A., MD
Theodor Kocher Institut, University of Bern, 3012 Bern, Switzerland

Ward, P. A., MD, Prof. of Surgery
The University of Michigan, Medical School, Dept. of Pathology, Medical Science, I M5240/0602, 1301 Catherine Rd., Ann Arbor, Michigan 48109-0602, USA

Warden, G. D., MD, Prof. of Surgery
Shriners Burns Institute, 202 Goodman Street, Cincinnati, Ohio 45219, USA

Waymack, J. P., MD, Ass. Prof. of Surgery
U.S. Army Institute of Surgical Research, Brooke Army Medical Center, Ft. Sam Houston, San Antonio, Texas 78234, USA

Winchurch, R. A., PhD
F. S. Key Medical Center, 4940 Eastern Ave., Baltimore, Maryland 21224, USA

Contents

Section 1

General Aspects

Section 2

Trauma and Specific Immune Mechanisms

2.1 Monocyte T-Cell Interaction and Its Mediators

Section 1

General Aspects

The Immune Consequences of Trauma: An Overview

J. L. Ninnemann

Introduction

Trauma, considered as a whole, remains the greatest single killer of the US adult population. A significant component of mortality after injury is due to an induced immunological deficiency, a defect responsible for septic death. While discussion of immune deficiency states usually brings to mind AIDS, or well defined congenital diseases, there has been increasing interest in and concern for immunological depression acquired as a result of accidental or operative injury in an otherwise normal host. An excellent recent sampling of the literature, for example, can be found in the November/December 1987 issue of the *Journal of Burn Care and Rehabilitation,* which contains papers from a recent conference on the subject. The material for this review, in fact, is taken from one of the papers in this volume (Ninnemann 1987). In the case of major injuries, immunological changes can be precipitous and leave the host vulnerable to life-threatening sepsis. Fortunately, however, injury induced immune depression is completely reversible, and with an understanding of its causes has come the hope of controlling immunity in favor of the host.

Unfortunately, the immune deficiency which results from injury is a unique entity that is very difficult to study, mainly because of the great variety in the extent and combination of injuries, each of which may make a unique contribution to the immunological mosaic. Most of the information currently available has been obtained through the study of thermal injuries. The immunological changes which occur as a result of burns appear to be similar to the changes induced by other types of tissue injury.

Immune Depression in Burn Patients

It is clear that major thermal injuries often precipitate a profound, multicentric immunological depression which is thought to predispose patients to sepsis. Impairment of immune function is almost universal in patients with greater than 40% body surface area burns, and in very young or very old patients with far smaller burns. Briefly, the immunological changes which occur in these patients include the following:

1. Totally eliminated skin test reactivity and recall antigen responses
2. The release of endotoxin, tissue degradation products, hormones, cytokines and lymphokines with immunosuppressive properties into the general circulation

Immune Consequences of
Trauma, Shock and Sepsis
Eds. Faist/Ninnemann/Green

3. Activation of the complement system (both classical and alternate pathways) with the production of complement split products with immunoregulatory capabilities
4. Reduced monocyte/macrophage function with increased suppressor macrophage function, increased immunosuppressive prostaglandin E production, and depressed phagocytosis
5. A transcient depression in B-cell numbers and immunoglobulin production (both primary and secondary responses are affected)
6. Depression of neutrophil functions including chemotaxis, phagocytosis, chemiluminescence, and intracellular killing
7. Depletion of fibronectin and serum opsonic activity
8. Decreased natural-killer (NK) cell and lymphokine activated killer (LAK) cell function
9. Long-term and profound depression of T lymphocyte response with increased T suppressor cell activity
10. A reported reversal of T lymphocyte helper cell/suppressor cell ratios

The acute-burn-care period is a period of particularly diminished macrophage and lymphocyte function, vigorous suppressor T cell activity and reduced help, the circulation and activity of characterized and uncharacterized immunosuppressive mediators, the presence of leukopenia/lymphopenia, and a deficiency in IL-2 production and IL-2-dependent T cell activation. The immunological alterations in burn patients have been reviewed in greater detail elsewhere (Ninnemann 1981, 1982, 1983). Two clinical manipulations seem critical to reversing burn induced immune changes: removal of the dead or injured tissue and restoration of the surface barrier to wound colonization through wound closure. Immunological perturbations will persist in burn patients as long as these two conditions are not met. With closure of the burn wound often comes rapid restoration of immunological competence and, frequently, full recovery of the patient. The earlier these clinical manipulations can be accomplished, the earlier immunological restoration will be achieved, thereby decreasing septic threat and increasing patient chances for survival. In addition, experiments aimed at boosting immune responsiveness in burned animals also show a reduction of sepsis, which suggests that similar clinical manipulation of human burns, while not yet attempted, might be useful (Hansbrough et al. 1985).

Trauma-Associated Immunodeficiency

It is widely held that burns represent a model by which the immunological changes which occur following other types of traumatic injury, and following major surgery (a type of controlled trauma), can be better understood. Indeed, many of the changes which occur in burn patients also occur following blunt or penetrating trauma (Howard 1979); however, relatively few attempts have been made to study patients with such injuries. While research is hampered by the difficulty in grouping patients for study, there is clearly a correlation between a high injury severity score (ISS) and the development of immune depression (O'Mahoney et al. 1984; Keane et al. 1982). The exact threshold of injury which results in loss of immune competence, however, has not been established as it has for burn patients.

As with the burn patient, the most important clinical evidence of immune depression in the trauma patient is the dramatic increase of septic complications which accompanies increasing injury severity. For example, Baker et al. (1980) studied 437 accidental deaths in San Francisco during 1977 and it was found that 78% of late deaths were due to sepsis. Polk (1979) has noted a similar incidence for septic death (75%) in patients with major thermal injuries. Most of the trauma patients in Baker's study who died from sepsis had multiple injuries, and it was hypothesized that many of the deaths could have been prevented by extensive early debridement. As noted above, this procedure has been shown to help restore immunological competence in burn patients (reviewed in Ninnemann 1987).

Patients with major traumatic injuries are frequently anergic. In a study of 176 trauma patients (129 with blunt injuries, 27 with thermal injuries, and 20 with penetrating injuries), Christou and Yurt (1983) found that such a lack of skin test reactivity (anergy), detected upon patient admission was indicative of frequent sepsis and later patient death. In addition, a decrease in neutrophil function has been reported to accompany anergy following blunt trauma. In a study of 31 blunt trauma patients, it was found that six patients had normal skin test reactions with no sepsis or death, while 25 demonstrated skin test anergy with 20% sepsis and 16% mortality rates (Christou and Meakins 1982). Abnormalities of polymorphonuclear leukocyte (PMN) chemotaxis and adherence were detectable within 2 h of injury, and appeared to be related to both anergy and the occurrence of circulating immunosuppressive factors in the blood. No major abnormalities in serum immunoglobulin levels or in complement levels were detected. Keane et al. (1983) showed that trauma patient lymphocytes displayed a reduced response to mitogens and alloantigens proportional to the extent of injury, infectious sequelae, and prognosis. Keane et al. (1982) also reported an increase in suppressor cell activity following multiple trauma in three of the group of four patients studied.

In 1984, O'Mahoney et al. compared the T cell mitogen response, percentage of putative suppressor (OKT8+) and helper (OKT4+) lymphocytes, circulating suppressor-cell activity, and serum suppression of lymphocyte activation in 31 multiple trauma patients with ten normal controls. They found significant suppression in lymphocyte response to mitogens 1–5 days after injury in 12 of the patients, and a shift in the normal OKT4+/OKT8+ T cell ratio, followed by the appearance of serum suppressive activity in 6 of the 12 patients. Circulating suppressor cell activity (measured by functional assays) was seen early after injury in three of 12 patients. O'Mahoney concluded that impaired T lymphocyte function commonly follows severe multiple injury, and that this was a major factor predisposing patients to sepsis.

Immunological Changes Following Surgery

In light of the immunological changes which occur following injury, it is disturbing, though perhaps not surprising, that patients undergoing major surgical procedures are also prone to develop immunological depression. The first careful study demonstrating this fact was carried out by Slade et al. (1975) who measured in vivo and in vitro immune function following nephrectomy in 12 normal renal transplant donors. All were normal individuals with normal immune responsiveness prior to surgery. Total lymphocyte, B cell, and T cell numbers, mitogen and mixed lymphocyte responses decreased upon induction of anesthesia and continued to fall during (and after) operation. The in vivo delayed hypersensitivity response to cutaneous antigen challenge declined more gradually and was still falling at the fifth postoperative day. While these findings clearly indicated immunological compromise in these patients, Slade et al. reported no clinically significant problems with sepsis.

Contrary to Slade, however, there is evidence that immune depression in surgical patients can have clinical consequences. Again using a standard skin testing procedure, Christou et al. (1982), in a prospective study of 503 skin test-positive surgical patients, found that 6.4% developed a long lasting anergy in the postoperative period. This anergy group had a 41% rate of sepsis and a 22% mortality rate, compared to 5% sepsis and 3% mortality in the reactive group. Christou concluded that only major surgical procedures (esophagogastrectomy, colectomy, aortic resection, etc.) resulted in anergy, however the extent of surgery required to produce immunological depression and anergy is still in question. Fabricius et al. (1980) recently studied patients who underwent simple surgery for inguinal hernia, and found a profound suppression of T lymphocyte function as measured by T cell colony formation, while conventional tests such as phytohemaglutinin (PHA) stimulation showed no significant change.

Greco et al. (1978) reported immune depression in 85% of the normal elective surgery patients they studied via a leukocyte migration inhibition assay. Abnormalities persisted for 60 days or longer in half of the patients studied. Christou and Meakins (1979) reported a larger series of patients in whom skin test anergy and neutrophil chemotactic response were measured, and they concluded that the worst combination for a surgical patient was cutaneous anergy coupled with decreased neutrophil chemotaxis. When they occurred together, these two tests were predictors of a high rate of sepsis and frequent mortality. Christou and Meakins also showed that the serum of anergic patients contained circulating mediators which were responsible for the depressed neutrophil response. Subsequent attempts to characterize the serum-borne inhibitor of neutrophil chemotaxis showed that it was of low molecular weight (Christou and Meakins 1983).

Lymphocyte response is also altered by surgery, an effect primarily confined to T cell responses (measured in vitro via mitogen or antigen stimulation) and mediated by suppressor cell activation (Wang et al. 1980; Salo 1978). In addition, the induction of a primary, cellular immune response to DNCB appeared to be profoundly impaired in cancer patients as a result of surgery (Tarpley et al. 1977), also indicating lymphocyte response abnormality.

Immunotherapy in Surgical Patients

Specific attempts to modify the depressed response in trauma patients have included application of a variety of nonspecific immunomodulators. It should be noted, however, that none of these approaches has proven completely satisfactory. The use of adjuvants, for example, can be harmful when administration is at a temporal distance for exposure to antigen. *Corynebacturium parvum* usage is known to correlate with a high lymphoma rate. Bacille Calmette-Guérin (BCG), *C. parvum,* and levamisole are all allergens, and may be effective only under special circumstances (BCG, for example, is thought to be effective in melanoma because of shared antigens). There is also a clear indication that nutritional status is related to immune deficiency, and that special attention to restoring nutritional balance in surgical/trauma patients is also critical to restoring immunological competence. But again, there is controversy concerning the effects of specific supplements such as protein, carbohydrate, fat, or single nutrients. Clearly there is a need for further work in this area.

Summary and Conclusions

Recent research has shown that burn patients, multiple trauma patients, and patients undergoing major surgical operations all suffer an acquired immunological deficit, a deficit which predisposes such surgical patients to life-threatening sepsis. Patients with thermal injuries have been best studied, to date, and it is thought that patients with other types of injury, whether accidental or surgically induced, suffer similar changes in immune responsiveness. All burn patients experience a severe, multicentric immunological depression when injuries exceed a threshold of approximately 40% body surface area. Macrophage and T cell deficits top the list of clinically important changes in these patients. While the threshold of injury producing such changes has not been clearly established in multiple trauma and surgical patients, it is clear that immune depression is also common following major injury or operation. To date, attempts to pharmacologically restore immunological competence in these patients have been disappointing. The best results have been achieved through early excision of damaged tissue and vigorous nutritional support.

References

Baker CC, Oppenheimer L, Stephens B, Lewis FR, Trunkey DD (1980) Epidemiology of trauma deaths. Am J Surg 140:144–150

Christou NV, Meakins JL (1979) Neutrophil function in surgical patients: two inhibitors of granulocyte chemotaxis associated with sepsis. J Surg Res 26:355–364

Christou NV, Meakins JL (1982) Phagocytic and bactericidal functions of polymorphonuclear neutrophils from anergic surgical patients. Can J Surg 25:444–448

Christou NV, Meakins JL (1983) Partial analysis and purification of polymorphonuclear neutrophil chemotactic inhibitors in serum from anergic patients. Arch Surg 18:156–160

Christou NV, Yurt RW (1983) Anergy testing in surgical patients. Infect Surg Oct:692–700
Christou NV, Superina R, Broadhead M, Meakins JL (1982) Postoperative depression of host resistance: determinants and effect of peripheral protein-sparing therapy. Surgery 92:786–792
Fabricius E, Stahn R, Fabricius HA (1980) Funktionsstörungen des thymusabhängigen Immunsystems nach operativen Eingriffen. Fortschr Med 98:7630–7633
Greco RS, Dick L, Duckenfeld J (1978) Perioperative suppression of the leukocyte migration inhibition assay in patients undergoing elective operations. Surg Gynecol Obstet 147:717–720
Hansbrough JF, Zapata-Sirvent R, Peterssen V, Bender EM, Claman HN (1985) Modulation of suppressor cell activity and improved resistance to infection in the burned mouse. J Burn Care Rehabil 6:270–274
Howard RJ (1979) Effect of burn injury, mechanical trauma, and operation on immune defenses. Surg Clin North Am 59:199–211
Keane RM, Munster AM, Birmingham W (1982) Suppressor cell activity after major injury: indirect and direct functional assays. J Trauma 22:770–773
Keane RM, Birmingham W, Shatney CM, Winchurch RA, Munster AM (1983) Prediction of sepsis in the multi-traumatic patient by assays of lymphocyte dysfunction. Surg Gynecol Obstet 156:163–167
Ninnemann JL (ed) (1981) The immune consequences of thermal injury. Williams and Wilkins, Baltimore
Ninnemann JL (1982) Immunologic defenses against infection: alterations following thermal injuries. J Burn Care Rehabil 3:355–366
Ninnemann JL (ed) (1983) Traumatic injury: infection and other immunologic sequelae. University Park Press, Baltimore
Ninnemann JL (1987) Trauma, sepsis, and the immune response. J Burn Care Rehabil 8:462–468
O'Mahoney JB, Palder SB, Wood JJ, McIrvine A, Rodrick ML, Demling RH, Mannick JA (1984) Depression of cellular immunity after multiple trauma in the absence of sepsis. J Trauma 24:869–875
Polk HC (1979) Consensus summary on infection. J Trauma 19 [Suppl]:894–896
Salo M (1978) Effect of anaesthesia and open heart surgery on lymphocyte responses to phytohemagglutinin and concanavalin A. Acta Anasthesiol Scand 22:471–439
Slade MS, Simmons RL, Yunis E, Greenburg LJ (1975) Immunodepression after major surgery in normal patients. Surgery 78:363–372
Tarpley JL, Twomey PL, Catalona WJ, Chretien PB (1977) Suppression of cellular immunity by anesthesia and operation. J Surg Res 22:195–201
Wang BS, Heacock EH, Wu AVO, Mannick JA (1980) Generation of suppressor cells in mice after surgical trauma. J Clin Invest 66:200–209

Trauma: Immune Deficiency, Immune Suppression, or Just Immune Cell Redistribution?

W. L. Olszewski and I. Grzelak

The term "post-traumatic immunodepression" is being frequently used in the contemporary surgical literature. Is there, however, enough scientific evidence for such a term to be used whenever the human body is suffering from trauma? Trauma is a complex set of events comprising acute neurohormonal regulation, reaction to "self" uncovered antigens and subsequently, but not immediately, reaction against invading pathogens. The mechanisms behind the trauma related changes in immune competence are not yet elucidated, but it would be difficult to accept, from an evolutionary point of view, the notion that immune reactions were depressed after trauma when tissue reparative processes develop actively. Our suggestion would be that the changes observed in the early post-traumatic stage (initial 3 days) are not due to the depressed responsiveness of blood mononuclear cells but rather to their depletion from circulation possibly due to redistribution from the blood to the tissues.

We studied the immune responsiveness in patients without evident inflammatory processes undergoing major range elective abdominal surgery which seems to be the best model of a "programmed" trauma. We found that the events observed in the peripheral-blood mononuclear (PBM) cells are most likely due to the depletion of this circulating population of certain subsets which either transiently settled in bone marrow or were involved locally in the immune processes.

The influence of operative trauma on the quantity and proportion of cooperating mononuclear cells was studied using monoclonal antibodies in the peripheral blood of patients with stage 0 uterine cancer who underwent hysterectomy (Grzelak et al. 1984). The percentage of $OKM1^+$ cells (monocytes) had increased on day 1 by 12.4%, on day 3 by 24.8%, and had returned to normal by day 7 (Fig. 1). The percentage of large $OKIa1^+$ cells (expressing Ia antigen) on day 1 was increased by 186.9%, while on day 3 it had returned to a normal level. There was a decrease on day 1 of the number and percentage of $OKT3^+$ cells (all T lymphocytes) by 17.4%, $OKT4^+$ cells (helper/inducer cells) by 27.9%, $OKT8^+$ cells (suppressor/cytotoxic cells) by 24.6%, and small $OKIa1^+$ cells by 49.4%. The number and percentage of T lymphocytes remained below the preoperative level throughout the observation period. However, the number of helper cells had increased significantly on day 5, while suppressor cells remained below the preoperative level during the entire observation period. The rising ratio of $OKT4^+$/$OKT8^+$ cells reflected the kinetics of recovery of the helper over the suppressor cell population.

Based on the observed changes in blood cell numbers and proportions of populations, a subsequent decrease in responsiveness of PBM subsets would be ex-

Immune Consequences of
Trauma, Shock and Sepsis
Eds. Faist/Ninnemann/Green

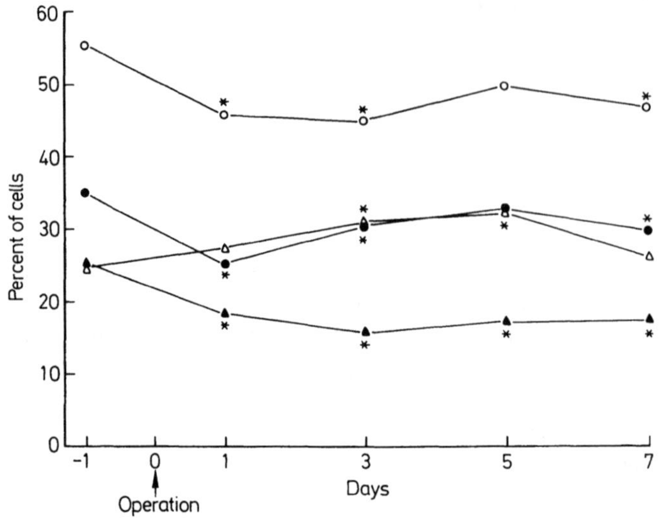

Fig. 1. PBM cells characterized using monoclonal antibodies in patients who underwent surgery: OKM1$^+$ (–△–), OKT3$^+$ (–○–), OKT4$^+$ (–●–), OKT8$^+$ (–▲–). Values from patients; *values on consecutive postoperative days vs. day −1 ($P<0.05$) [3]

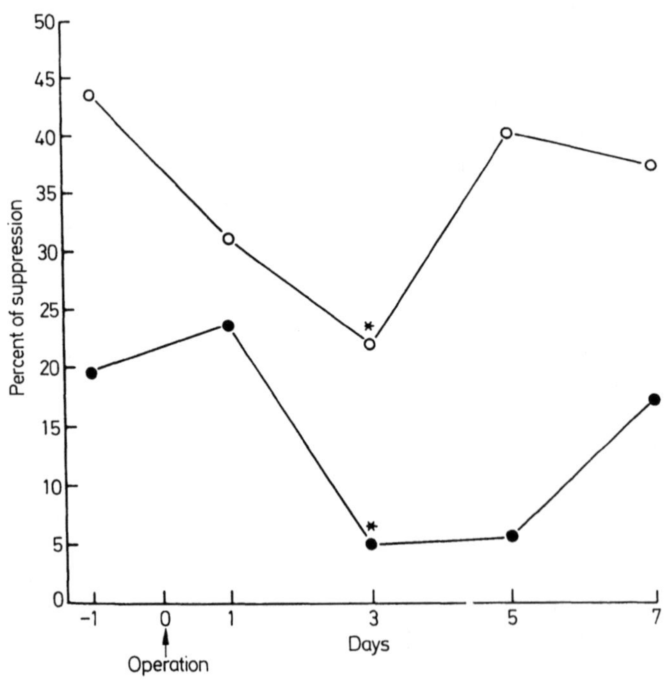

Fig. 2. Suppressor-cell activity directed toward autologous PBM stimulated with PHA at concentrations of 4.5 µg/ml (–○–) and 18 µg/ml (–●–). Freshly obtained PBM were cultured with Con A for 20 h and after treatment with mitomycin added to fresh PBM. *Values on day +3 vs. preoperative, $P<0.05$ [2]

pected in various in vitro assays. We found (Grzelak et al. 1983) that the operation brought about a decrease on the second postoperative day in the responsiveness of PBM to various concentrations of phytohemagglutinin (PHA) by 19.2% –28.8% and to concanavalin A (Con A) by 31.2%–41.8%, concomitantly with a decline in Con A SC (suppressor cells) activity from 43.7%–22.0% (Fig. 2). When the Con A SC were tested against RC (responder cells) obtained from blood samples drawn prior to surgery and stored at −196 °C, an increase in the postoperative SC activity from 41.6%–52.2% was observed which might indicate a postoperative stimulation of SC. However, when Con A SC were raised from PBM drawn before surgery and tested against RC obtained postoperatively, they displayed a decreased suppressive activity from 27.2%–2.7%. This might be due to the pre- and postoperative stimulation of RC masking the effectiveness of SC.

Consequently, the next step was to investigate whether the decreased postoperative SC activity was due to a concomitant drop in the number of circulating SC with OKT8 phenotype. The effect of surgery on SC activity was assessed in a Con A assay and in parallel with the concentration of OKT8$^+$ cells in peripheral blood (Grzelak et al. 1985). An evident decrease in the number of freshly obtained OKT8$^+$ and cocultured for 20 h with Con A OKT8$^+$ cells and subsequently a drop in whole blood suppressor activity was found in the immediate postoperative period (Fig. 3). The recovery of the SC activity but not of the OKT8$^+$ cell levels was observed on day 5. A nonsignificant decrease in erythrocyte rosette-forming cell (E-RFC) suppressor activity compared with that of whole blood SC suggests that function of T suppressors had not been affected. The non-T cells did

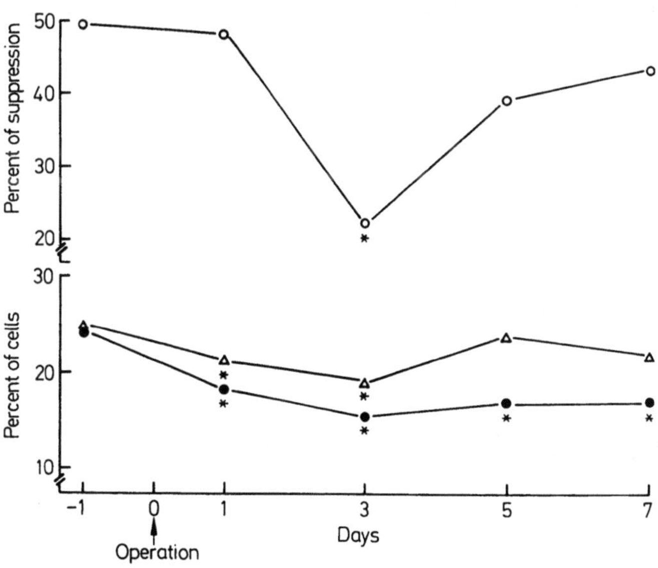

Fig. 3. The PBM Con A SC activity towards autologous PBM cells stimulated with PHA at 4.5 µg/ml (–o–) and percentage of freshly obtained PBM OKT8 cells (–●–) and OKT8$^+$ cells after 20 h culture with 10 µg/ml Con A (–△–). *Postoperative vs. day −1, $P<0.05$ [4]

not produce any suppressive effect. These results indicate that the postoperative drop in the blood SC activity was due to the temporary depletion and not to the depressed function of SC.

Autologous mixed lymphocyte reaction (AMLR) is a reaction in which T cells with the inducer/helper phenotype proliferate when cultured with irradiated or mitomycin C-treated non-T cells from the same individual. Postoperative depletion of the circulating T-cell pool could be reflected in a decreased AMLR. Changes in AMLR were studied in 23 patients undergoing cholecystectomy (Grzelak et al. 1987). The preoperative level of AMLR in patients was 6098 ± 3506 cpm, and remained within the range of healthy volunteers, 5616 ± 3122 cpm. Following surgery AMLR decreased to 1960 ± 1738 cpm ($P<0.01$) on day 1, to 2394 ± 2026 cpm ($P<0.02$) on day 3, and to 3343 ± 2802 cpm ($P<0.05$) on day 5. A concomitant decrease in peripheral blood OKT4$^+$ cells was seen, from 34.9 ± 3.9% on day −1 to 24.1 ± 5.4% on day 1 ($P<0.01$; Fig. 4). A return of AMLR to the preoperative level was observed on day 7 and of OKT4$^+$ cells percentage on day 5. When cultures were supplemented with interleukin 2 (IL2) from the MLA144 cell line, a postoperative increase in AMLR was observed in all patients by an average of 206% (from 1960 ± 1738 to 5988 ± 5460 cpm) on day 1, 277% (from 2394 ± 2026 to 9017 ± 8834 cpm) on day 3, and 74% (from 3343–2802 to 5806 ± 4816 cpm) on day 5. Simultaneous study of endogenous IL2 activity in supernatants of patients lymphocytes stimulated with PHA, using the CTLL-2 cell line, showed a decrease in IL2 production by a mean 30%–40% on day 3 after surgery, and normalization on days 5 and 7. It was concluded that surgical trauma caused a decrease of AMLR in the early postoperative period. This decrease seems to be due to the putative sequestration of circulating cells producing IL2 to the traumatized tissues and later also to the decline in IL2 production by circulating T4$^+$ cells.

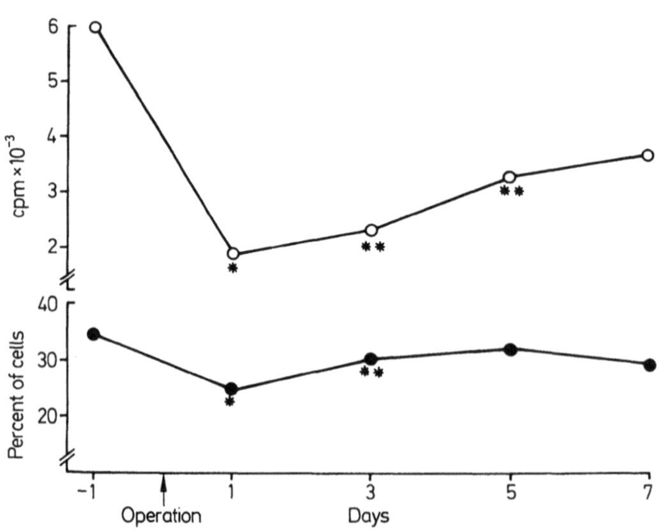

Fig. 4. The AMLR response in a 7 day culture (–o–) and percentage of OKT4$^+$ cells (–●–) in patients after cholecystectomy. *Postoperative vs. day −1, $P<0.01$, **$P<0.05$ [5]

The most convincing indirect proof for the diminished concentration of circulating mature T cells as a cause of low responsiveness of PBM was provided by the results of studies on patients with advanced cancer. The effects of surgery on peripheral blood mononuclear cell responsiveness to mitogens and on SC activity assessed in a Con A assay were studied in patients with stage 0 and stage III–IV cancer (Grzelak et al. 1988). Patients were exposed to a similar surgical trauma, the same type of anesthesia and to no pre- and early postoperative radio- or chemotherapy. A more pronounced postoperative decrease in the lymphocyte count, responsiveness to PHA (Fig. 5) and Con A, and SC activity was found in the nonadvanced than in the advanced cancer group. These findings indicate an impaired mobilization and distribution capacity of circulating lymphocytes in patients with advanced neoplastic disease.

A common finding in all quoted studies was a drop in the number of circulating T cells in blood in the early postoperative period with a subsequent decrease of reactivity of this subset when the whole PBM population was cultured. Changes in the proportions of functional subsets were also observed. Less helper cells were, as expected, accompanied by lower production of IL2. Interestingly, when a pure T cell population was used for functional studies the level of responsiveness was almost normal. This indicates that operative trauma first of all brings about regulatory changes in circulating immune-cell distribution. The functional

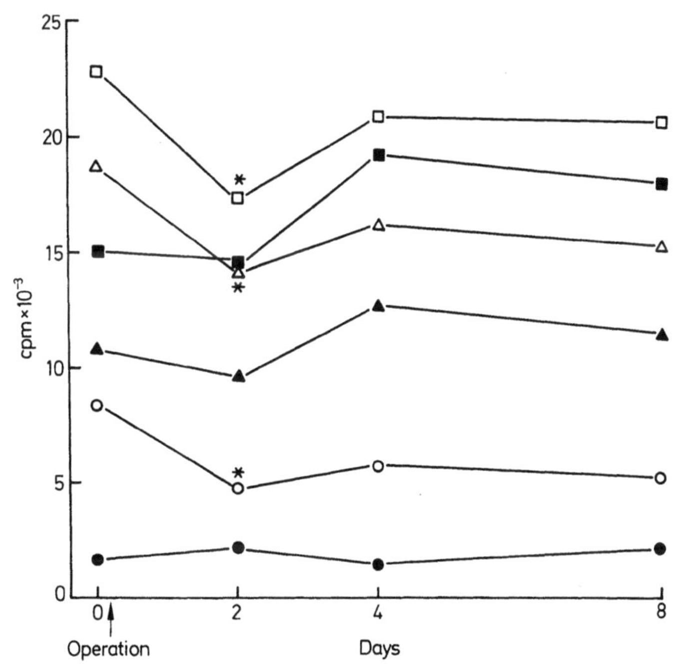

Fig. 5. The responsiveness of PBM to PHA in the nonadvanced (*open signs*) and advanced (*filled signs*) cancer groups. (–□–) 90 μg/ml, (–△–) 18 μg/ml, (–○–) 4.5 μg/ml PHA. *Postoperative vs. day −2, $P<0.05$. Note a fall in the responsiveness in the nonadvanced group but no changes in the advanced group [6]

assessment of the quantitatively deficient population may at that time be falsely read as depression of reactivity. In protracted shock, fulminant infection, and large denuded and colonized surfaces, the immunodeficiency might be more or less a true interpretation as the equilibrium between the invading pathogens and the defense capacity of the organism becomes distorted. However, in the initial stages of shock or infection all of the observed changes in the immune system should rather be interpreted as regulatory processes aimed at elimination of "non-self" antigens and preservation of self-integrity.

The phenomenon of redistribution of circulating lymphocytes, monocytes and granulocytes during hypothalamus-pituitary-adrenal axis activation is well known in man and animals (for review see Olszewski 1987). However, its mechanism and place in the adjustment processes remains unclear. Circulating lymphocytes leave blood and lymph nodes and settle temporarily in the bone marrow and partly in the skin and gut. Bilateral adrenalectomy abolishes this effect which indicates that steroids are responsible for the changes in lymphocyte recirculation. Experimental studies have shown (Cox and Ford 1982) an increase in the rate of entry of lymphocytes to bone marrow, the retarding effect of prednisolone on lymphocyte traffic through the bone marrow and spleen, and impaired influx into the lymph nodes. On the other hand, increased release of steroids is accompanied by circulating neutrophilia and accelerated release of neutrophils from the bone marrow. Taken together, the complex mechanism of immune-cell migration (Fig. 6) integrated with the hormonal regulation should be taken into consideration when the results of in vitro functional tests of PBM are to be interpreted in shock states. The changed traffic and distribution of lymphoid cells, appearance in blood of immature populations, changes in circulating hormone levels, volume of cells accumulating at the site of injury, their local proliferation, and the biological activity of released lymphokines all affect the peripheral blood population, the only cells available for rapid clinical evaluation.

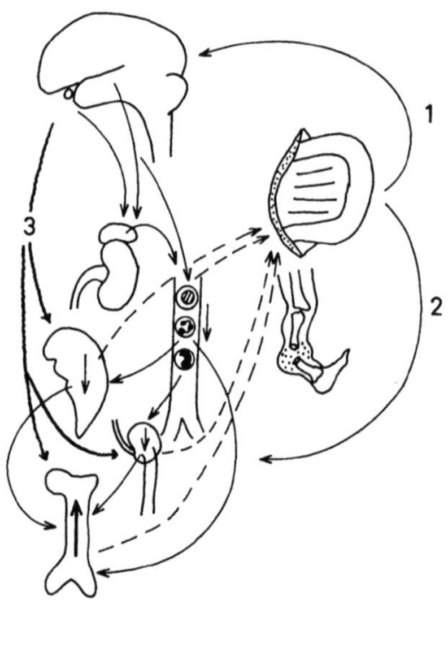

Fig. 6. Schematic drawing indicating the pathways of signals from the injured tissue (laparotomy, broken leg) to the neurohormonal system and lymphoid organs. *1*, signal to the CNS; *2*, signal to the lymphoid organs; *3*, signal from CNS to lymphoid organs. *Arrows* show functional relationships between organs. *Arrows* in the spleen, bone, lymph node, and blood show direction of quantitative changes in the initial phases of shock. A sample of blood cells cannot give insight into the complex regulatory immune events

The results of our studies clearly indicate that the only factor affecting the results of a functional test of PBM might be temporary depletion of blood of certain subsets. No active inflammatory processes, evident infection or medication would rule out the reasons for immune deficiency.

References

Cox JH, Ford WL (1982) The migration of lymphocytes across specialized vascular endothelium. IV. Prednisolone acts at several points on the recirculation pathways of lymphocytes. Cell Immunol 66:407

Grzelak I, Olszewski WL (1988) The influence of surgery on the responsiveness of blood lymphocytes in patients with advanced cancer. J Surg Oncol (submitted)

Grzelak I, Olszewski WL, Engeset A (1983) Suppressor cell activity in peripheral blood in cancer patients after surgery. Clin Exp Immunol 51:149

Grzelak I, Olszewski WL, Engeset A (1984) Influence of operative trauma on circulating blood mononuclear cells: analysis using monoclonal antibodies. Eur Surg Res 16:105

Grzelak I, Olszewski WL, Engeset A (1985) Decreased suppressor cell activity after surgery. J Clin Lab Immunol 16:201

Grzelak I, Olszewski WL, Rowinski W (1987) Blood mononuclear cell production of IL1 and IL2 following moderate surgical trauma. Eur Surg Res (in press)

Olszewski WL (1987) Immune cell migration in vivo. CRC, Boca Raton, p 125

Neuroendocrine Response to Severe Trauma and Sepsis

A. E. Baue

Introduction

The metabolic and neuroendocrine responses to injury are important parts of the stress reaction. They teleologically provide a better opportunity for a biologic organism to survive under adverse circumstances or when injured. John Hunter nearly two centuries ago described the reactions to injury as inducing "both the disposition and the means of cure." This suggested that injury initiates a sequence of responses that are both the result of the injury as well as mechanisms by which the biologic organism can survive and heal the injury. The objective of this complex coordinated sequence of responses is maintenance of blood flow, oxygen delivery, organ perfusion, and mobilization and utilization of substrates for healing and recovery.

Claude Bernard emphasized the importance of maintaining the "milieu interne" for survival (Bernard 1878–1879). The ability of a biologic organism to respond or adapt to a noxious stimulus and preserve its internal environment was originally called the "emergency theory" by Walter Cannon (1914). He developed the concept of homeostasis and emphasized the role of the sympathetic nervous system. Ferdinand Hoff described such a chain of reactions with the term *vegetative Gesamtumschaltung* (translated as "autonomic shift" or "total alteration of the internal environment") and emphasized the importance of the hypothalamus (Hoff 1930). Leriche referred to it as a "maladie post operatoire" (cited in Lambret and Driessens 1937). Hans Selye initially used the term "general alarm reaction." His concept of the "general adaptation syndrome" emphasized the importance of the pituitary-adrenocortical system in this reaction (Selye 1946). Detailed studies of the response to injury began in good part with Sir David Cuthbertson, who pioneered work on the response of individuals with long-bone fractures. He recognized that there is a response of the entire organism to a local injury (Cutherbertson 1936). Other outstanding contributions have been made by John E. Howard, William B. Abbott, and Francis D. Moore. In a detailed series of metabolic studies, Moore traced the response from injury to recovery. Significant contributions in this field have also been made by Pope, Elkington, Ellman, Fox, Rhoads, Levinson, Lockwood, and Meyer; and more recently by Kinney and Gump, Shires, Wilmore, and Pruitt (Baue et al. 1984).

An injury is followed by an acute phase of neuroendocrine stimulation that Moore called the "injury phase" (Table 1). Corticotropin (ACTH) and cortisol secretions increase, antidiuretic hormone is released, catecholamines and glucagon are increased, and aldosterone secretion increases in correspondence with ac-

Immune Consequences of
Trauma, Shock and Sepsis
Eds. Faist/Ninnemann/Green

Table 1. The stages following injury

I.	The injury phase – lasts 2–5 or more days – length is related to the magnitude or dose of injury and presence or absence of complications
II.	The turning point – the neuroendocrine response turns off
III.	The anabolic phase – gain in muscular strength – the phase of positive nitrogen balance
IV.	Late anabolism – gain in weight and body fat – the phase of positive caloric balance – months to years

tivation of the renin-angiotensin system. Insulin levels do not rise appropriately for the level of circulating blood sugar. Estrogens, androgens, and 17-ketosteroids are depressed (Moore 1952, 1959). There may be some increase in growth hormone, and it has been thought that there was little change in thyroid function. These acute responses involve those rapidly acting hormonal or neuroendocrine changes that produce quick and finely tuned adjustments to altered circumstances in order to preserve the internal environment. In contrast, the long-term regulators (growth hormone, thyroid hormones, estrogens, and androgens) either show small increases or may actually decrease during stress reactions. The neuropeptide hormones of the central nervous system, particularly in the hypothalamus (somatostatin, beta-endorphins, and enkephalins), have recently been described. These hormones probably play a role in the stress reaction, although their exact participation is as yet not well documented. The beta-endorphins stimulating morphine-like receptors may be responsible for the sedative effect of severe injury.

When an individual survives the injury phase and begins a normal convalescence without complications, there occurs what Moore called the "turning point" – the neuroendocrine response shuts down and returns to normal regulation. If, however, the injury phase continues because of the severity of the injury, multiple systems injury, or complications such as infection, then the injury phase, the abnormal hormonal response, and catabolism continue. If the individual does not then respond, this may result in multiple organ failure, the final common pathway after severe injury or complications of an operation (Baue 1975; Faist 1983).

An injury and a major operation are similar in that they provide a threat to a biologic organism. Throughout this discussion, I will use the term "injury" synonymously with either a traumatic event (such as a motor vehicle accident) or a planned traumatic event in the operating room (such as an abdominal perineal resection for a carcinoma of the rectum). Although the extent of injuries, magnitude of the response, number of organs involved, suddenness of the event, and the unplanned experience of trauma will differ, the biologic response to the injury is similar. A clean elective operation produces a level of stress beyond the fasting, resting state; stress produced by a multisystem injury, however, is much greater.

The Normal Response: Endocrine Correlates (Efferent Pathways)

The injury phase begins with the stress response and normal neuroendocrine alterations and activation. This activation begins in the hypothalamus. A complicated series of reactions occurs in the hypothalamic-pituitary-adrenal axis. There are a variety of mediators and modulators. Hypothalamic activation leads to arginine vasopressin (antidiuretic hormone, ADH) release from the neurohypophysis, to epinephrine secretion from the adrenal medulla and norepinephrine release from sympathetic nerve endings (Table 2). Specialized endocrine neurons in the hypothalamus secrete corticotropin releasing hormone (CRH), which goes to the adenohypophysis (pituitary) and is the main stimulant to the chromophobe cells for corticotropin (ACTH) production. CRH is a complex polypeptide with many components and synergistic relationships. The roles, if any, of other hypothalamic releasing hormones – thyrotropin releasing hormone (TRH), luteinizing hormone releasing hormone (LHRH), and somatostatin (growth hormone) releasing inhibitory factor (SRIF) – in injury are unknown.

The endocrine correlates, beginning with the pituitary, are increases in ACTH secretion and circulating levels (Table 3). Although the primary stimulant to ACTH secretion is CRH, ADH and angiotensin-2 from the kidneys also stimulate ACTH with injury. ACTH acts on the adrenal zona fasciculata by way of adenylate cyclase and cAMP to produce cortisol (glucocorticoid). Within minutes cortisol is released and circulates, either freely or bound to cortisol binding globulin. Free cortisol freely enters cells and is bound to receptors that interact with DNA in the nucleus to modulate messenger RNA transcription. Thus cortisol has

Table 2. Hormonal changes with injury: hypothalamus-neural control

Increased corticotrophin releasing hormone-stimulates ACTH release	
No thyrotropin releasing hormone	No recognized role
No luteinizing hormone releasing hormone	No recognized role
No somatostatin	No recognized role
Increased arginine vasopression (ADH) – increased production in hypothalamus and release from posterior pituitary	
Increased secretion of adrenaline from adrenal medulla	
Increased secretion of noradrenaline from sympathetic nerve endings	

Table 3. Hormonal changes with injury: pituitary neural and hormonal control

ACTH – increased
Endorphins – increased
Growth hormone – increased
Prolactin – increased
FSH-LH – decreased
Alpha-melanocyte stimulating hormone – no change
Beta-lipotropin hormone – no change
TSH – no change or decrease
Arginine vasopressin – increased

many profound effects including restitution of blood volume after hemorrhage, inhibiting extrahepatic protein synthesis, potentiating glucose production, and inhibiting immune responses. There may be other direct stimulants for cortisol secretion with injury other than ACTH, such as angiotensin-2 and aldosterone.

The immunosuppressive and antiinflammatory properties of glucocorticoids include inhibition of activity or production of prostaglandins, histamine, kinins, lymphokines, and T-cell growth factor. Thus they suppress the body's normal defense mechanisms. This has led to the suggestion that they prevent the normal responses to trauma from proceeding to a stage of producing tissue damage and threatening homeostasis.

Endorphins are endogenous peptides with opiate-like biological activity. They are found in the brain in identical secretory granules of pituitary corticotropic cells along with ACTH and also elsewhere in the brain, pancreas, and gastrointestinal (GI) tract. The system is complex with at least three classes of opiate receptors and a number of endogenous peptides including methionine- and leucine-enkephalin and alpha- and beta-endorphins.

Endorphin (opiate peptide) secretion from the pituitary is parallel to that of ACTH and it is probably released by the same stimuli of stress and trauma. Circulating levels rise after operation for as long as 72 h with loss of circadian rhythm. Its physiologic role remains unclear but may produce some analgesia and a calming effect along with other receptor interactions. Pharmacologic infusions of beta-endorphin produce analgesia. The opiate peptides seem to reduce the release of substance P, an excitatory neurotransmitter. Thus the endogenous opiate system may have a modulating effect on noxious stimuli and the sympathetic response. The circulating endorphins may have some cardiodepressant effects on blood pressure and cardiac function. They may also participate in the regulation of glucose metabolism. Severe alterations have been associated with postoperative delirium (Levine 1984).

Pain modification after injury may involve other hormones (i.e., norepinephrine and serotonin) and ion channel control by the central nervous system.

The other pituitary hormones do not seem to have great importance with injury other than to decrease if activity is not necessary for survival. Growth hormone is increased, but how or why is not understood. It does not seem to play a major role with injury. Alpha-melanocyte stimulating hormone and beta-lipotropin hormone responses to injury are not known. It has been established in burn patients that prolactin levels are increased in both men and women. The reasons for this are not known. Follicle stimulating hormone (FSH) and luteinizing hormone (LH) increased on day 1, and then decreased significantly and remained low for about 2 weeks and are often normal or low normal. They are also decreased after operation in burn patients. This is consistent with depression of reproductive capability (menses and libido) after injury. All of the hormones from the anterior pituitary gland were found to have an altered circadian rhythm. Thyroid stimulating hormone (TSH) levels do not change appreciably. The effects of growth hormone and prolactin after injury are probably metabolic, such as inhibiting insulin action on muscle and increasing lipolysis. Growth hormone acts either directly or through a family of polypeptide hormones called somatomedins. Their site of synthesis is not known, but values can be measured in plasma and they have insulin-like anabolic activity. With injury somatomedin levels are low and return to normal on the third day or so. Thus they parallel insulin levels rather than growth hormone.

The gut-brain peptides, including vasoactive intestinal polypeptides (VIP), cholecystokinin octapeptides (CCK-8), substance P, neurotensin, methionine enkephalin, and leucine enkephalin, have uncertain roles. The role of other agents is also uncertain. Angiotensin-2 and vasopressin levels increase as described. Bradykinin, oxytocin, carnosine, and bombesin activities are not known.

ADH secretion increases greatly with injury. During normal homeostasis, the primary stimulant to ADH secretion is an increase in plasma osmolality, which is measured in the osmoreceptors in the hypothalamus. With injury, other factors become more important in ADH release. Fear, pain, hemorrhage, decreased atrial, arterial, and portal pressures, and certain drugs (including morphine, barbiturates, and anesthetic agents) all stimulate ADH through the hypothalamus, leading to conservation of water. The primary stimulant after injury is decreased effective blood volume. Angiotensin-2 may also affect ADH release. Vasopressin acts on the renal collecting system to control free water clearance. It has vascular pressor effects and may also have metabolic effects on hepatic glycogenolysis.

Aldosterone secretion increases greatly with injury (Table 4). Its production is controlled in normal homeostasis by the renin-angiotensin system. Stimulation of the myoepithelial cells of the juxtaglomerular apparatus by the sympathetic system or locally results in production of renin, an enzyme that circulates and cleaves an alpha-1-globulin produced in the liver to form angiotensin-1. Angiotensin-1 is converted to the active form angiotensin-2 by a converting enzyme in the lung, kidney, or blood. Angiotensin-2 has a very short half-life and is a potent general vasoconstrictor that has a direct chronotropic and inotropic effect on the heart. It seems also to have an endocrine effect, increasing vasopressin secretion and sympathetic and adrenal medullary activity. It is the prime stimulus for aldosterone secretion from the zona glomerulosa of the adrenal cortex. Aldosterone acts on the distal nephron of the kidney to increase reabsorption of sodium with chloride and water in exchange for potassium and hydrogen. This allows the injured individual to deal with increased potassium and acidosis with injury.

This plays a major role in hemorrhage in man, composing a regulatory volume-dependent feedback mechanism. ACTH, which has a minor role in stimulating aldosterone secretion in normal individuals, plays a more important role after injury or operation. Aldosterone secretion, with its effects on sodium conservation, seems to occur with injury whether or not there is an alteration in renal blood flow, vascular volume, and renin production.

Table 4. Hormonal changes with injury: adrenal cortex-hormonal control; medulla-autonomic control

Cortisol – increased
Aldosterone – increased
Adrenal estrogens and androgens – no change or decrease
Catecholamines – increased

With injury, anxiety, and many anesthetic agents, catecholamine production and release both from the adrenal medulla as epinephrine and norepinephrine and from sympathetic nerve endings only as norepinephrine. The adrenal medulla is stimulated from the brain stem through the splanchnic sympathetic nerves by a number of stimuli including arterial hypotension and cerebral hypoglycemia. Catecholamines stimulate adrenergic receptors of the $alpha_1$ and $alpha_2$ and $beta_1$ and $beta_2$ types for cardiovascular effects. They seem to be the primary agents producing the hypermetabolism of burns and other injuries. Catecholamines also have many direct metabolic effects including increased hepatic glycogenolysis and gluconeogenesis from lactate and increased peripheral glycogenolysis from muscle and lipolysis of fat. They act also in other tissues by stimulation of hormones to increase renin release and decrease insulin and to increase glucagon secretion from the pancreas. Plasma dopamine levels increase after injury, presumably from sympathetic terminals. Concentrations are low, and nothing is known about its effect. The levels parallel those of norepinephrine.

Thyroid activity decreases with injury. Initially TSH levels remain the same or decrease somewhat as does thyroxine (T_4). However, triiodothyronine (T_3) levels decrease quickly after an injury or operation with a general anesthetic. Reverse T_3 (rT_3) levels increase, indicating a shift from an active form of circulating thyroid hormone to an inactive form. Thus the activity of thyroid hormone seems to be minimal at a time when the individual has maximum catabolic stress. If the injury is very severe and prolonged, then both TSH and T_4 may decrease to very low levels. The same changes seem to occur with any severe illness. This has been called the "euthyroid sick syndrome."

From the pancreas, glucagon secretion and circulating levels are increased, particularly in the portal system. Insulin levels remain normal or increase slightly but do not respond appropriately or proportionate to the hyperglycemia that occurs with injury. In addition suppression of the action of insulin on peripheral tissues by catecholamines, growth hormone, and cortisol limits substrate utilization. Thus the anabolic hormone insulin is depressed. The catabolic (counterregulatory or stress) hormones – catecholamines, cortisol, and glucagon – are increased. Sympathetic innervation to the pancreas and cathecholamines both result in release of glucagon and inhibition of insulin. Glucagon stimulates glycogen breakdown in the liver, amino acid uptake, deamination, and gluconeogenesis. Insulin antagonizes the hepatic effects of glucagon.

Gonadal function is decreased, with both testosterone and estrogen decreasing. There is prolonged reduction of 17-ketosteroids in the urine. Erythropoietin production is increased, particularly with blood loss and the renin-angiotensin system is activated.

Local tissue factors produce major effects, and this information is now unfolding. Interleukin-1 (IL-1) seems to be the wound hormone produced by white cells and macrophages that has profound metabolic effects along with temperature elevation and immune stimulation (Filkins et al. 1985; Dinarello 1984; Duff et al. 1982). Amongst the many and profound effects of IL-1 on acute phase protein production, IL-2 production and temperature elevation are its potential effects on other hormone levels and activity such as in the pituitary (Bernton 1987). There are many other monokines (Table 5). The prostaglandins are important tis-

Table 5. Mediators changing following injury

Prostaglandins	Prostacyclins Thromboxanes
Leukotrienes Histamine Serotonin	
Kallikreins	Bradykinin
Monokines (cytokines)	Interleukin-1 (monocytes) Hepatocyte stimulating factor Cachectin – tumor necrosis factor (macrophages)
Lymphotoxin	Tumorolytic protein from lymphocytes
Interferons	
Granulocyte-macrophage colony Stimulating factor	
Epidermal growth factor	

sue mediators for some of the effects of IL-1 and other activities, as are the leukotrienes. Histamine, serotonin, and bradykinin from platelets, white cells, and cells at the site of injury all add to the local tissue effects with injury through these enzyme cascades.

The magnitude of the neuroendocrine response is proportional to the severity of injury or operation. When hormone levels were studied in patients having inguinal hernia repair or laparoscopy, there were no significant changes. Patients having cholecystectomy or appendectomy had increases in plasma cortisol, norepinephrine, and epinephrine at 1 and 24 h (Chernow et al. 1987). These levels returned to normal before 5 days. Samples were not taken between 1 and 5 days. Stoner and his group (1979) found positive relationships between concentrations of epinephrine, norepinephrine, and dopamine and the Injury Severity Score (ISS) of a patient. However, ACTH and cortisol responses are more variable with maximal early responses of both found at an ISS of 12. We found that patients with multiple system injury or severe sepsis admitted to an intensive care unit (ICU) often had low normal levels of ACTH and cortisol, which increased only with recovery. These patients had extremely high levels of catecholamines, particularly norepinephrine.

Severe Injury and Sepsis

This neuroendocrine response is an important part of homeostasis and preservation of the internal environment. It is geared to allow an individual to survive an insult without treatment. With modern surgical therapy, the neuroendocrine response helps modulate excesses or inadequacies of treatment. With severe overwhelming injury and with sepsis, this response may be excessive, deleterious, or interfere with therapy (Neugebauer et al. 1987).

An example of this would be an injured patient with liver disease in which the secondary hyperaldosteronism of the liver disease is added to the increased aldosterone secretion that occurs with injury and volume changes. The damaged liver cannot break down aldosterone; thus it continues to circulate with higher activity for a longer period of time. In such a patient, fluid resuscitation with crystalloid solutions containing sodium is necessary. However, such fluid, instead of promoting urine output, may simply be kept in the body because of the hyperaldosteronism; thus fluid overload would easily be produced. This could quickly lead to the hepatorenal syndrome unless a diuretic is given to promote urine output in the face of this phenomenon.

Failure of parts or all of this system have not been considered. Until recently, there have been few studies of endocrine function beyond the first few days of injury. This has been particularly true in very sick patients who are deteriorating and who will eventually die.

The potential importance of altered hormonal activity that may occur or continue late after an injury is not totally clear. A patient treated in an ICU for a severe injury or for complications may have continuing manifestations of an overwhelming stress response. However, it has become apparent more recently that other hormonal abnormalities may occur as the injury phase continues or as complications develop. Extensive thermal trauma has been associated with a prolonged increase in the metabolic rate, compared with a short but transient increase in the metabolic rate of patients with perforated ulcers. Cope et al. (1953), however, found that in such patients suffering from thermal trauma, protein-bound iodine and iodine-131 uptake in the thyroid gland were normal. They concluded that the thyroid gland plays no part in elevating the metabolic rate in such circumstances. It was only later that specific thyroid hormone levels could be measured.

More recently, Portnay et al. (1974) determined that prolonged chronic starvation for as long as 4 weeks could produce a decrease in circulating T_3 levels and an increase in reverse (r) T_3 levels (an inactive form). As this occurred, T_4 levels remained fairly normal. Other researchers found that such changes occurred in patients who had chronic illness, diabetes, severe liver disease, or various acute illnesses including myocardial infarction and uremia. This was called the "low T_3 syndrome." It has generally been thought that this syndrome does not produce hypothyroidism, but rather is an adaptation in patients who are euthyroid (Zaloga 1985). In summarizing a low T_3 syndrome symposium in 1981, Hesch stated: "Low T_3 is an epiphenomenon occurring without exception as a secondary consequence to other disturbances in the sick individual." Thus, the basic question concerning this syndrome was and still is: Are low T_3 and increased rT_3 levels a concomitant of clinical deterioration and acute and chronic illness and of no clinical significance, or does this represent or produce a metabolic advantage or problem?

Wilmore et al. (1974) described the predominant role of catecholamines in patients who underwent severe and prolonged stress. High concentrations of catecholamines seems to mediate the hypermetabolic response to injury and infection. A reciprocal relationship between thyroid hormone and catecholamine levels was reported in burn patients. On the other hand, Tevaarwek et al. (1978) found that catecholamines stimulated the conversion of T_3 to T_4, especially in thyrotoxic crisis. The pressure of infection adds another level of stimulus to the stress response with increased IL-1 and production of cachectin (tumor necrosis factor) from macrophages as well (Beutler 1986).

Burn and Traumatized Patients Who Survive

In a recent study in the surgical ICU at Yale, Robert Gelfand compared six burned or multiply injured patients with five controls. The clinical data are shown in Table 6, indicating that all six of the patients survived. The basal endocrine data shown in Table 7 indicate that all the patients had the low T_3 syndrome and were returning toward normal by day 5. Other values were within fairly normal levels. Note that both cortisol and ACTH levels were low normal. Epinephrine and norepinephrine were appropriately elevated. When these patients received

Table 6. Clinical data

Patient	Age	Sex	Admitting diagnosis	Days in SICU	Outcome
MA	16	M	Burns (60% BSA)	15	Survived
RM	38	M	Burns (30% BSA), inhalation injury	8	Survived
JC	46	M	Burns (50% BSA)	7	Survived
PR	36	M	Multiple trauma (pelvic and leg compound fractures, retroperitoneal hematoma)	7	Survived
BV	70	F	Burns (35% BSA)	5	Survived
NS	36	M	Burns (70% BSA)	12	Survived

SICU, Surgical intensive care unit; BSA, body surface area.

Table 7. Basal endocrine data

Measurement (normal range)	Day 2	Day 5
Circulating hormone levels		
T_4 (4.6–9.2 μg/100 ml	3.6 ± 0.9	5.2 ± 0.9
TBC (16.8–25.7 μg/100 ml)	11.8 ± 2.0	16 ± 1.7
FT_4 (1.0–2.1 ng/100 ml)	1.5 ± 0.3	1.6 ± 0.3
T_3 (800–200 ng/100 ml)	48 ± 13	68 ± 16
TSH (<7 μU/ml)	2.8 ± 0.7	4.0 ± 0.4
Prolactin (≦20 ng/ml)	16.2 ± 6.7	
Growth hormone (<5 ng/ml)	5.7 ± 1.5	
Somatomedin C (0.34–1.9 U/ml)	0.55 ± 0.07	
ACTH (<80 pg/dl)	24 ± 6	
Cortisol (12–24 μg/dl)	24 ± 6	17 ± 2
24-h urinary excretion		
Epinephrine (<20 μg/24 h)	23 ± 5	
Norepinephrine (<80 μg/24 h)	145 ± 41	
Free cortisol (20–90 μg/24 h		296 ± 61

Specimens were obtained during the first week of hospitalization in the Surgical ICU (generally the 2nd and 5th days after admission).

Table 8. Plasma cortisol response to synthetic ACTH[a]

Patients	Time		
	0	30 min	60 min
MA	13	24	28
RM	15	26	34
JC	31	43	41
PR	18	32	33
BV	50	65	93
NS	16	28	35
Mean	24	36	44
SEM	6	6	10
Normal controls (research personnel aged 26–32)			
RG	10	22	28
RL	9	23	29
MC	12	26	34
KZ	9	53	62
PC	9	33	38
Mean	10	31	38
SEM	1	6	6

[a] Cortrosyn, 250 μg injected intravenously at time 0 together with TRH, 500 μg. Cortisol results in μg/100 ml.

Table 9. Serum TSH and prolactin response to TRH[a]

Patients	TSH (μU/ml)			Prolactin (ng/ml)		
	0	30 min	60 min	0	30 min	60 min
MA	3	20	23	4	65	49
RM	1	19	16	6	80	45
JC	3	23	22	25	74	55
PR	3	13	11	45	100	53
BV	5	37	29	3	120	65
NS	3	18	17	14	53	40
Mean	3	22	20	16	82	51
SEM	1	3	3	7	10	4
Controls						
RG	3	14	11	8	34	22
RL	1	9	8	8	44	32
MC	4	63	47	11	92	80
KZ	1	14	10	26	160	79
PC	1	8	7	18	34	31
Mean	2	22	17	14	73	49
SEM	1	10	8	3	24	13

[a] Thyrotropin releasing hormone, 500 μg, administered intravenously at time 0 together with cortrosyn, 250 μg.

Table 10. Serum growth hormone response to TRH plus cortrosyn

Patients	Time		
	0	30 min	60 min
MA	2	20	5
RM	12	26	18
JC	2	10	3
PR	5	34	28
BV	7	18	12
NS	6	8	6
Mean	6	19	12
SEM	2	4	4
Controls			
RG	6	3	5
RL	2	10	4
MC	3	10	30
KZ	11	40	21
PC	3	4	2
Mean	5	13	12
SEM	2	7	6

[a] TRH, 500 µg, and cortrosyn, 250 µg, administered intravenously at time 0. Growth hormone results in ng/ml.

cortrosyn (250 µg injected intravenously) along with TRH of 500 µg, there was a prompt response in cortisol in all patients, which seemed quite appropriate and normal (Table 8). Table 9 indicates the response of TSH to TRH injection, showing a prompt and brisk response at 30 min, leveling off at 60 min. The controls are shown below. Prolactin also responded appropriately to TRH injection, as did growth hormone (Table 10). Thus, in these patients there was quite a normal and vigorous response to both ACTH and TRH in contrast to our previous group of patients. The contrast, however, is not in this group. None of these patients deteriorated and died. All recovered and left the ICU by the fifth or sixth day. The response to ACTH and TRH was measured, however, on the first day, when all the responses would be intact. If these patients had deteriorated, the responses 2 weeks later might have been quite different.

The Hormonal Milieu in Very Sick ICU Patients

Recently we studied the hormonal milieu and possibility of altered thyroid function in 25 patients in the surgical intensive care unit who had severe, life-threatening illnesses (Baue et al. 1984). Sixteen patients had septic complications and nine had multiple system injuries. On admission to the ICU, serial measurements were begun of T_4, T_3, T_4-binding globulin, TSH, ACTH, cortisol, prolactin, human growth hormone, catecholamine, insulin and glucose, lactate, retinol-binding protein, prealbumin, and transferrin levels. All patients initially had low normal levels of T_4 (4.5 ± 2 µg/100 ml) and T_3 (55 ± 26 ng/100 ml), with normal TSH

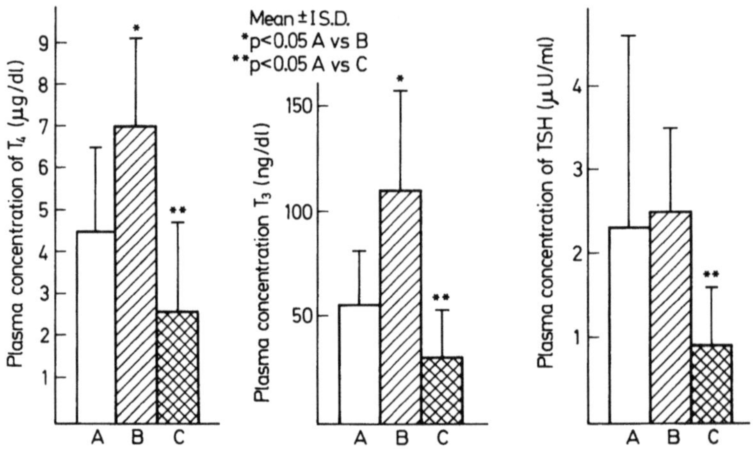

Fig. 1. T_4, T_3, and TSH levels in patients admitted to the ICU. *A*, On admission to the ICU; *B*, on discharge from the ICU (those who recovered); *C*, patients who died (values a day or so before death); $*P<0.05$ (*A* vs. *B*); $**P<0.05$ (*A* vs. *C*)

Table 11. ACTH, cortisol, prolactin, and growth hormone levels during the study

	Initial	Survival	Death
ACTH	14.0± 18.5 pg/ml	42.3± 32.6 (p<0.05)	31.3± 41.2
Cortisol	13.8± 9.6 µg/ml	15.2± 4.3	18.4± 10.7
Prolactin	308.0±281 µE/ml	505.0±436.0	166.0±100.0
Growth hormone	2.3± 1.6 ng/ml	1.0± 0.8	1.5± 1.6

levels (2.3±2.3 µU/ml) (the "low T_3 syndrome"). The 11 surviving patients had their levels increase to normal before leaving the ICU (T_4, 7.0±2.1 µg/100 ml; T_3, 110±48 ng/100 ml; and TSH, no change). The 14 patients who died showed further decreases before death (T_4, 2.6±2.1 µg/100 ml; T_3, 30.6±23.5 ng/100 ml; and TSH, 0.9±0.7 µU/ml) (Fig. 1). The corticotropin, cortisol, prolactin, and growth hormone levels were normal throughout the study (Table 11). Catecholamine levels were high initially and decreased in surviving patients. Epinephrine levels increased greatly in nonsurvivors before death, and the norepinephrine-epinephrine ratio decreased from 5.7:1 to 2:1 (Table 12). After protirelin (TRH) stimulation, the TSH level increased either minimally or not at all in six patients who eventually died (Table 13). Other values did not change or show trends.

In this study, all of the patients had a low T_3 level when they entered the ICU; the T_4 levels were also low normal in many patients. The decrease of both T_3 and T_4 levels in those patients who eventually died also indicates an alteration of the peripheral handling and/or release of T_4. There was no relationship of the corticotropin or cortisol levels to the thyroid hormone level in this study.

Why the thyrotropin level does not increase in the presence of low T_3 levels remains unexplained. The high catecholamine levels and a decreased norepineph-

Table 12. Epinephrine and norepinephrine levels the study

	Initial	Survival	Death
Epinephrine (E)	162.0±159.0 pg/ml	89.0± 31.0 p<0.05	531.0±482.0 p<0.05
Norepinephrine (NE)	925.0±691.0 pg/ml	690.0±305.0	1070.0±660.0
Ratio NE/E	5.7	7.8	2.0

Table 13. TRH administration (200 µg i.v.)

	TSH before TRH (µU/ml)	TSH after TRH[a] (µU/ml)	Catecholamines[b]
S	1.0	2.3	–
D	0.9	1.1	+
D	2.0	3.1	–
D	0.7	1.4	–
D	1.9	3.7	+
D	0.7	2.5	+
D	0.7	0.7	+

S, Survived; D, died; [a] sample obtained 30 min after trh; [b] patients recieving catecholamines (+) and none (ü).

rine to epinephrine ratio in patients who died suggest the possibility that the catecholamines attempted to compensate for the depression of the thyroid axis – or perhaps they produced it. There was an inverse relationship of thyroid hormone levels to catecholamine levels, which was particularly striking for epinephrine. As thyroid hormone levels improved, catecholamine levels returned toward normal. This inverse relationship of norepinephrine and epinephrine with the thyroid hormone levels may be a regulatory mechanism of severe sepsis or may be overwhelming stress with the drive of catecholamines and the disappearance of thyroid hormone.

The effects that the extremely low T_3, T_4, and TSH levels found in this study might have had on the functioning of these patients and on their particular organ or cell functions cannot presently be determined. The ability to measure the effectiveness of thyroid hormones on an individual patient is difficult. A few studies have been carried out that attempted to restore thyroid hormones in such patients with potential depletion. Such an investigation was conducted by Becker et al. (1982) in the United States Army Surgical Research Laboratories in San Antonio. Becker concluded that burn patients had reduced thyroid hormone levels that were possibly related to reduced TSH stimulation; however, replacement of T_3 did not alter the metabolic rate or mortality in these seriously ill burn patients. Beneficial results have been reported using T_3 in the treatment of severe dopamine-dependent septic shock. Protirelin or TRH has been used in a number of shock models with improvement after experimental endotoxin hemorrhagic shock and spinal trauma. The mechanism of this is very unclear.

Our study therefore indicates hypothalamic and pituitary dysregulation or suppression and altered release and/or peripheral metabolism of T_4 and T_3. Whether this represents a deficiency of thyroid hormone for cell and organ function remains to be established (Hasselgren 1987). The inverse relationship of catecholamines and thyroid hormone levels is again noted.

Thus we can conclude that there is hypothalamic-pituitary dysregulation or suppression in patients who eventually die in a surgical ICU. Whether this represents hormonal insufficiency for cell and organ function that is detrimental to the individual, inability to synthesize neuropeptides and other hormones, the down regulation of a dying organism, or suppression by catecholamines remains to be determined.

Adrenal Insufficiency

It has also been observed that some patients undergoing severe and prolonged stress have cortisol levels that are lower than would be predicted. There may be a wide variation among individuals and their adrenal corticol response to severe stress. Sibbald et al. (1987) measured hormonal levels in 26 injured septic patients. Plasma cortisol levels and their response to cortrosyn were measured. Four of these patients had greatly increased adrenal corticol activity with plasma cortisol levels very high; all four died within 5 days. Seventeen of the 26 patients had an appropriate response to infection and plasma cortisol levels increased following synthetic ACTH. However, five patients had some impairment of adrenal corticol function. Their plasma cortisol levels were low (13 μg/100 ml), and the response to cortrosyn was much less than would be expected. Thus there seem to be some septic patients who cannot mount an adrenal response, and this may indicate a lack of adrenal reserve or impending adrenal failure. More recently, Finlay and McKee (1982) found that low absolute levels and falling serial levels of cortisol were associated with a significantly higher mortality in severely stressed patients. They found that critically ill patients in an ICU had loss of their circadian rhythm. In such patients they found that many had low normal levels of cortisol; in a number of them, no positive response was retained. This suggested adrenal corticol insufficiency. In patients who survived, clinical improvement was accompanied by a spontaneous rise in morning cortisol and a return to a positive response to ACTH. In some, steroid therapy was given; but those numbers were too small to determine whether it affected mortality. Patients who showed progressive falls in morning cortisol levels had a markedly increased mortality when compared with those whose levels remained high. This suggests again the possibility that in severely stressed septic patients adrenal deficiency, lack of adrenal reserve, or other problems may develop.

Endocrine insufficiency of the adrenal or elsewhere can occur because of spontaneous hemorrhage or anticoagulation. It can be an idiopathic autoimmune abnormality of the gland, or metastatic carcinoma can be involved. It may also be possible that there can be endocrine exhaustion, suppression with overwhelming stress, or binding problems.

Summary

Other abnormalities of central endocrine function, particularly of the pituitary, have been described. Functional alterations have been described after spontaneous infarction of the pituitary gland, including hypothyroidism, defective TSH augmentation by protirelin, and relative corticotropin-adrenal insufficiency. Pituitary abnormalities have been found at autopsy in patients who died of comdepasse (respirator brain). Pituitary apoplexy and Sheehan's syndrome is well known, as is Friderichsen syndrome of acute adrenal hemorrhage in patients with meningitis. Thus there may be other endocrine abnormalities in such patients, and these should be sought in those dying after injury in an ICU. Further information is needed to help determine whether neuroendocrine dysfunction and exhaustion may be a part of the multiple system or organ failure seen in injured and operated patients. Exhaustion could result from a failure of protein synthesis. Suppression could occur from overwhelming stress, particularly pathologically high levels of catecholamines, or there could be binding problems with various circulating inhibitors that develop with severe tissue injury or consumption with such injury. Many of these changes set the stage for immunosuppression and immunoalteration with injury.

References

Baue AE (1975) Multiple, progressive or sequential failure – a syndrome of the 70s. Arch Surg 110:779–781

Baue AE, Guenther B, Hartl W, Ackenheil M, Heberer G (1984) Altered hormonal activity in severely ill patients after injury or sepsis. Arch Surg 119:1125–1132

Becker RA, Vaughan GM, Ziegler MG, Seraile LG, Goldfarb IW, Mansour EH, McManus WF, Pruitt BA (1982) Hypermetabolic low triiodothyronine syndrome of burn injury. Crit Care Med 10:870–875

Bernard C (1878–1879) Lecons sur les phenomenes de la vie communs aux animaux et aux vegetaux. Balliere, Paris

Bernton EW, Beach JE, Holaday JW, Smallridge RC, Fein HG (1987) Release of multiple hormones by a direct action of interleukin-1 on pituitary cells. Science 238:519–521

Beutler B, Cerami A (1986) Cachectin and tumour necrosis factor as two sides of the same biological coin. Nature 320:584–588

Cannon WB (1914) The emergency function of the adrenal medulla in pain and the major emotions. Am J Physiol 33:356

Chernow B, Alexander HR, Smallridge RC, Thompson WR, Cook D, Beardsley D, Fink MP, Lake CR, Fletcher JR (1987) Hormonal responses to graded surgical stress. Arch Intern Med 147:1273–1278

Cope O, Nardi GL, Quijano M, et al. (1953) Metabolic rate and thyroid function following acute thermal trauma in man. Ann Surg 137:165–174

Cutherbertson DP (1936) Further observations on the disturbance of metabolism caused by injury, with particular reference to the dietary requirements of fracture cases. Br J Surg 23:505–520

Dinarello CA (1984) Interleukin-1 and the pathogenesis of the acute-phase response. N Engl J Med 311:1413–1418

Duff GW, Durum SK (1982) Fever and immunoregulation: hyperthermia, interleukins 1 and 2, and T-cell proliferation. Yale J Biol Med 55:437–442

Faist E, Baue AE, Dittmer H, Heberer G (1983) Multiple organ failure in polytrauma patients. J Trauma 23:775–787

Filkins JP (1985) Monokines and the metabolic pathophysiology of septic shock. In: Mediator mechanisms in shock. Fed Proc 44:300–304
Finlay WEI, McKee JI (1982) Serum cortisol levels in severely stressed patients. Lancet I:1414–1415
Hasselgren P-O, Chen I-W, James JH, Sperling M, Warner BW, Fischer JE (1987) Studies on the possible role of thyroid hormone in altered muscle protein turnover during sepsis. Ann Surg 206:18–24
Hesch R-D (1981) The "low T_3 syndrome". Serono Symposia. Academic, London, vol 40
Hoff F (1930) Unspezifische Therapie und natürliche Abwehrvorgänge. Springer, Berlin
Lambret O, Driessens J (1937) Les modifications humorales post-operatoires: pathogenie-traitement: recherches personnelles. J Int Chir 2:223–265
Levine J (1984) What are the functions of endorphins following thermal injury? J Trauma 24:S168–176
Moore FD (1959) Metabolic care of the surgical patient. Saunders, Philadelphia
Moore FD, Ball MR (1952) The metabolic response to injury. Thomas, Springfield
Neugebauer E, Lorenz W, Maroske D, Barthlen W, Ennis M (1987) The role of mediators in septic/endotoxic shock: a meta-analysis evaluating the current status of histamine. Theoret Surg 2:1–28
Portnay GI, O'Brien JT, Bush J, et al. (1974) The effect of starvation on the concentration and binding of thyroxine and triiodothyronine in serum and on the response to TRH. J Clin Endocrinol Metab 39:191–194
Selye H (1946) The general adaptation syndrome and the alarm reaction. J Clin Endocrinol Metab 6:117–230
Sibbald WJ, Short A, Cohen MP, Wilson RF (1977) Variations in adrenocortical responsiveness during severe bacterial infections. Ann Surg 186:29–33
Stoner HB, Frayn KN, Barton RN, et al. (1979) The relationships between plasma substrates and hormones and the severity of injury in 277 recently injured patients. Clin Sci 56:563
Tevaarwerk GJM, Malik MH, Boyd D (1978) Preliminary report on the use of propranolol in thyrotoxicosis: I. Effect on serum throxine, triiodothyronine and reverse triiodothyronine concentrations. Can Med Assoc J 119:350–360
Wilmore DW, Long JM, Mason AD, et al. (1974) Catecholamines: mediator of the hypercatabolic response to thermal injury. Ann Surg 180:653–669
Zaloga GP, Chernow B, Smallridge RC, et al. (1985) A longitudinal evaluation of thyroid function in critically ill surgical patients. Ann Surg 201:456–464

Section 2

Trauma and Specific Immune Mechanisms

2.1 Monocyte T-Cell Interaction and Its Mediators

Regulation of Hematopoiesis by Growth Factors: Proliferation of the Murine Macrophage as a Model for Stimulatory and Inhibitory Effects

L. J. Guilbert and D. R. Branch

Introduction

Sepsis is the major cause of late deaths after thermal or traumatic injury (Miller et al. 1982). Central to host resistance to sepsis is maintenance of the levels and functions of immune cells: granulocytes, monocytes, and lymphocytes, all of which are of hematopoietic origin. Among the many documented alterations in the function and levels of blood cells following thermal injury are anemia (Wallner and Vantrin 1986), loss of neutrophil chemotaxis (Nelson et al. 1986), immediate neutrophil leukocytosis (McIver 1933) and delayed granulocytopenia (Asko-Seljavaara 1986). Many of the elements that regulate function of blood cells also regulate production (Warren and Ralph 1986). Thus, sepsis following trauma can be viewed, in part, as a consequence of dysfunction in the regulation of hematopoiesis.

It is the purpose of this article to introduce and review hematopoiesis from the point of view of control by soluble (humoral) factors and then to illustrate the complex and interacting nature of humoral control with results from our laboratory that examine a well-defined experimental model. The review is focused on the myeloid arm of blood-cell formation which includes production of erythrocytes, the granulocytes (neutrophilic, eosinophilic, basophilic), monocytes, and platelets. The experimental data presented is focused even further in examining the regulation of the growth of macrophages in culture.

Hematopoiesis

Blood cells, both myeloid and lymphoid, all derive from a common class of self renewing, pluripotent stem cells (reviewed in Metcalf 1984, see Fig. 1). These cells give rise to myeloid hematopoietic stem cells which also have large replicative ability but which have lost the potential to produce lymphocytes. Maturation at this very immature cell stage proceeds with continued loss of potential, both in terms of the numbers and types of cells that individual progenitor cells can produce. Eventually, progenitor cells restricted to producing a single blood-cell type arise, marking the origin of specific differentiation lineages. These unipotent progenitor cells continue to mature, giving rise to the morphologically identifiable hematopoietic cells and finally to nongrowing, functional blood cells. Regulated proliferation accompanies differentiation at all stages.

Immune Consequences of
Trauma, Shock and Sepsis
Eds. Faist/Ninnemann/Green

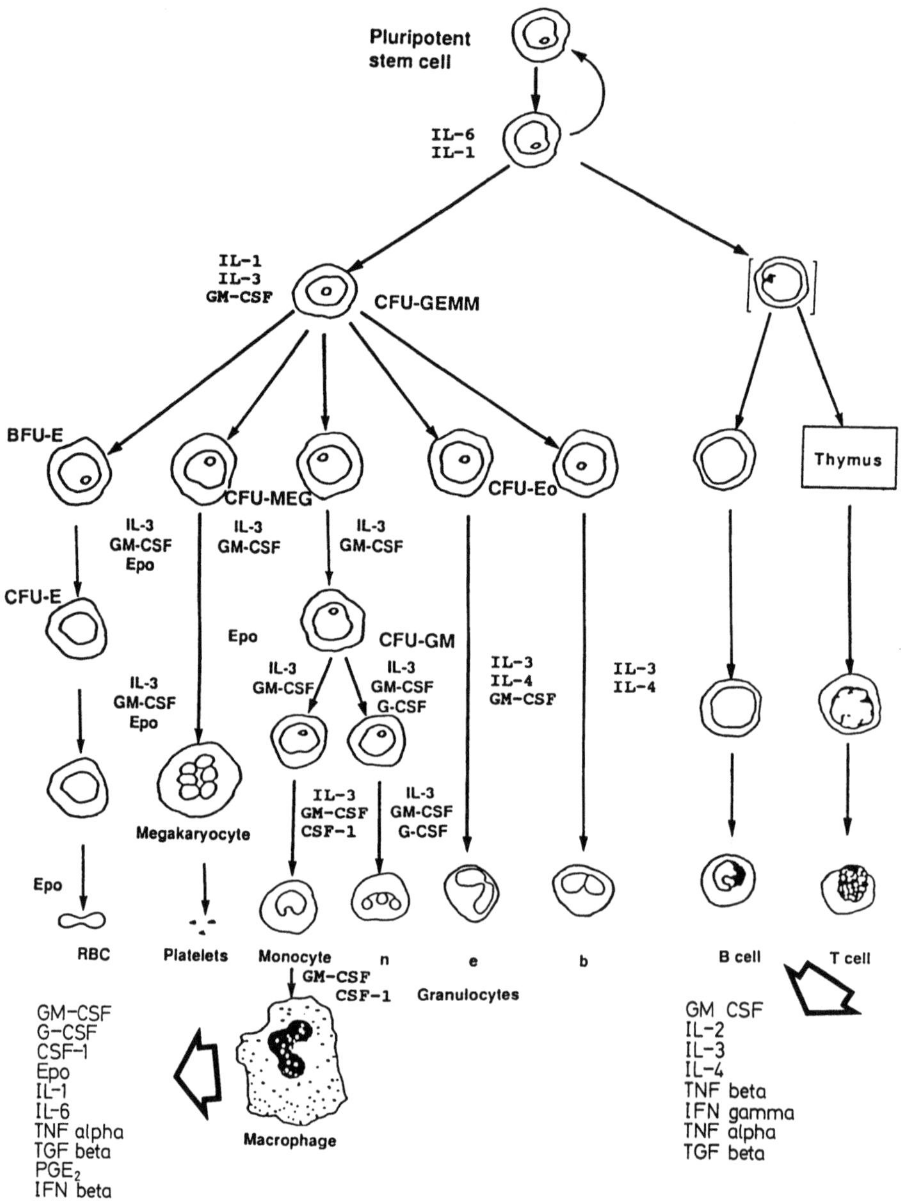

Fig. 1. Regulation of hematopoiesis by hematopoietic growth factors. Scheme modified from Clark and Kamen (1987). Progenitor cells denoted in *large letters,* factors in *small letters.* Factor production by macrophages and T lymphocytes denoted in *boldface*

Table 1. Soluble factors inhibiting hematopoiesis

Factor	Progenitor target[a]	Source[b]	Range
PGE_2	Late[c]	Monocytes	Short/long
IFN alpha/beta	Intermediate	Ex/monocytes	Short
IFN gamma	Intermediate	T cells	Short
TNF alpha	Intermediate	Monocytes/T cells	Short
TNF beta	Intermediate	T cells	Short
TGF beta	Early	Ex/monocytes/T cells	Short

[a] Maturity of hematopoietic progenitor cells in cell lineages, referring to Fig. 1: late, CFU-E, CFU-GM, etc., or more mature; early, CFU-GEMM or less mature; intermediate, progenitors between early and late.
[b] Ex, Outside lymphohematopoiesis.
[c] Monocyte progenitors are especially sensitive.
IFN, Interferon; TNF, tumor necrosis factor; TGF, transterming growth factor; CFU, colony-forming unit, where -E, erythroid; -GM, granulocyte, macrophage; -GEMM, granulocyte, erythroid, macrophage, mega karyocyte.

Table 2. Soluble factors stimulating hematopoiesis

Factor	Target	Sourcc[a]	Range
Erythropoietin	Erythroid[b]	Ex/monocytes	Long
G-CSF	Neutrophil[b]	Ex/monocytes	Short
CSF-1	Monocytic[b]	Ex/monocytes	Long/Short
GM-CSF	Hematopoietic	Ex/monocytes/T cells	Short
IL-1	Hematopoietic	Ex/monocytes/T cells	Long/short
IL-2	Hematopoietic	T cells	Short
IL-3	Hematopoietic	T cells	Short
IL-4	Hematopoietic	T cells	Short
IL-6	Hematopoietic	Ex/monocytes	?

[a] Ex, Outside lymphohematopoiesis.
[b] Differentiation lineage specific.

Regulation of Hematopoiesis

Proliferation is regulated at multiple levels. There is both positive and negative control, the control elements can operate over long range (greater that 10 cell diameters, endocrine) or short range (cell-cell contact, paracrine or autocrine), and the elements can target cells of widely differing maturities (Tables 1, 2).

Inhibitors of Hematopoiesis

Although maintenance of stem cells in a quiescent state by inhibitors or cell-cell contact (reviewed in Toksoez et al. 1980) has long been an accepted dogma, little is known of the mechanism of inhibition of stem-cell proliferation. Recently, however, transforming growth factor beta (TGF beta), has been shown to be a selective and potent inhibitor of the development of only the very immature progenitor cells such as the colony-forming unit – granulocyte, erythroid, macrophage, mega karyocyte (CFU-GEMM; Keller et al. 1988). Other well defined molecules, such as tumor necrosis factor (TNF alpha; reviewed in Le and Vilcek 1987), prostaglandin E_2 (PGE_2; Williams 1979), or immune interferon (IFN gamma; Zoumbos et al. 1984), have been shown to inhibit hematopoiesis at other levels (see Table 1 for summary). Although there are nonhematopoietic source cells for inhibitors such as TNF, TGF beta, and PGE_2, it is noteworthy that activated macrophages and T lymphocytes, both hematopoietic in origin, and immune cells, are potent producers of these known inhibitory molecules (reviewed in Le and Vilcek 1987; Moses et al. 1987; Broxmeyer 1984; see Fig. 1). Therefore, it is not surprising that these cells should be the focus of research on the suppression of lymphohematopoiesis associated with postburn trauma.

Stimulators of Hematopoiesis

Hematopoietic cells not only do not proliferate and mature in the absence of hematopoietic growth factors, they die (Metcalf 1970; Tushinski et al. 1982). Thus, hematopoietic growth factors influence the survival, growth, maturation and function of blood, and blood forming cells. Table 2 lists the eight well characterized growth factors arrayed in Fig. 1. All are glycoproteins, are encoded by different genes and bind distinct cell-surface receptors at physiologic concentrations (reviewed in Metcalf 1986). The factors fall into two major categories according to their specificity of action: lineage specific factors and hematopoietins.

All of the factors in Table 2 have been purified, characterized, cloned and are available in recombinant form. Several recent reviews and articles detail the physiochemical properties, chromosomal location and mechanism of expression of the human factors: granulocyte colony stimulating factor (G-CSF), colony-stimulating factor 1 (CSF-1), granulocyte-macrophage colony stimulating factor (GM-CSF), interleukin-3 (IL-3; Clark and Kamen 1987), IL-1 (Le and Vilcek 1987), IL-4 (Paul and Ohara 1987), and IL-6 (Ikebuchi et al. 1987). All except IL-1 are encoded by single genes. IL-1 exists at least in the alpha and beta forms, of which the alpha form has been documented to have effects on hematopoiesis (Stanley et al. 1986; Mochizuki et al. 1987). All except CSF-1 are single polypeptide chains. The transcript for CSF-1 can be spliced into two messages, one encoding a 145 amino acid chain and the other a 233 amino acid chain (Wong et al. 1987). Homodimers (and probably heterodimers) of either of these chains are biologically active and bind to the same receptor (Wong et al. 1987; L. J. Guilbert unpublished). Production of most of the factors is inducible (not yet known for IL-6) with regulation at the transcriptional and mRNA turnover levels (Shaw and Kamen 1987). Receptors to the factors have all been described (reviewed in Metcalf 1986; Clark and Kamen 1987; Le and Vilcek 1987; Ohara and Paul 1987). Genes encoding receptors to IL-2 (Cosman et al. 1984), CSF-1 (Sherr et al. 1985) and IL-1 (Simm et al. 1988) have been cloned. The best characterized are those for IL-2 and CSF-1, the latter of which is the product of the proto-oncogene c-*fms* (Sherr et al. 1985), a transmembrane tyrosine kinase. With the exception of the CSF-1 receptor, which can be present at over 100000 copies per cell (Guilbert and Stanley 1986), fewer than 10000 high-affinity receptors per cell appear to be the norm for the other factors (reviewed in Clark and Kamen 1987).

The lineage specific factors erythropoietin, G-CSF, and CSF-1 exert their dominant, although not exclusive, action on the production of a single blood-cell type. Erythropoietin is a classical endocrine hormone. Its production is predominantly in the kidney, serum levels correlate with the degree of hypoxia, and nothing else can replace it in stimulating the later stages of erythrocyte production (Eaves and Eaves 1985). In contrast, G-CSF and CSF-1, although their actions within hematopoiesis are relatively limited to neutrophil and monocyte production, respectively, do not appear to be the only factors able to carry out these functions (see Fig. 1). In addition, CSF-1 appears to have an important function outside hematopoiesis on the placental trophoblast, a tissue of epithelial origin (Athanassakis, Vassiliadis, Guilbert, and Wegmann, submitted for publication). However, all three lineage-specific factors strongly stimulate both the proliferation of the more mature progenitor cells of their respective lineages and the function of the mature cells (reviewed in Clark and Kamen 1987). Extrapolation places a lineage-specific factor at this level for all six lineages. The recent and very intense interest in hematopoietic growth factors should lead to the rapid characterization of growth factors, inhibitors, or conditions that uniquely specify levels of basophiles, eosinophiles, and platelets.

Hematopoietins are growth factors that stimulate production of several blood-cell types (Fig. 1, Table 2). Of these, IL-1 alpha and IL-6 appear to act in a complementary fashion (complete synergy) on very immature progenitor cells with the other hematopoietic growth factors to stimulate production (Stanley et al. 1986; Mochizuki et al. 1987; Ikebuchi et al. 1988). In cultures of unfractionated marrow cells, the other hematopoietins, IL-3, GM-CSF and IL-4, appear able to stimulate proliferation of both mature and immature progenitor cells (Ihle 1985; Metcalf 1986; Rennick et al. 1987). However, as pure preparations of recombinant factors and better methods for enriching hematopoietic cells have become available, there is increasing evidence that at least two growth factors are required for complete mitogenic stimulation of individual subclasses of all hematopoietic cells (Williams et al. 1987). For example, macrophage colony formation from murine progenitor cells in serum-free medium requires the lineage-specific factor CSF-1 plus either of the hematopoietins GM-CSF or IL-3 (Guilbert 1985).

The mechanism of hematopoietic growth factor complementation is largely unexplored although specificity has been observed in the ability of hematopoietins to down-regulate receptors for lineage-specific factors (Walker et al. 1985). Other, not entirely mutually exclusive, possibilities are that receptors for hematopoietins send qualitatively different signals than do the receptors for lineage-specific factors. However, syngergy between inducible factors which are undetectable in normal biological fluids (such as IL-1, IL-3 and GM-CSF) and lineage-specific factors which are present in relatively high concentrations in normal fluids (such as erythropoietin and CSF-1) makes biological sense. Thus, immunologic induction of either macrophages or T cells would be able, with great leverage, to stimulate several hematopoietic lineages simultaneously.

Homeostasis

Normal steady-state hematopoiesis therefore represents a homeostasis between stimulation and inhibition in which inducible, short-range factors may have a minimal role. Gross immunologic perturbation resulting from bacterial invasion can be predicted to lead to rapid release of factors that both stimulate and inhibit hematopoiesis. It makes biologic sense to stimulate production of monocytes and granulocytes, but it also makes sense to protect the system from potential exhaustion by inhibiting the cycling of stem cells. At present too little of a quantitative nature is known of the balancing effects of stimulators and inhibitors on hematopoiesis to be able to effectively model responses to trauma. However, enough of a qualitative nature is known to picture such responses as complex and interactive.

Noteworthy in this regard is the plasticity of the response of a single cell, the monocyte/macrophage, to stimulation potentially arising from burn. Bacterial cell wall lipopolysaccharide can induce production of tumour necrosis factor (TNF), an inhibitor of hematopoiesis, and G- and GM-CSFs, stimulators of hematopoiesis from monocytes (Warren and Ralph 1986). Both TNF and GM-CSF can induce production of CSF-1, the growth stimulator specific to the monocyte differentiation lineage, from monocytes (Oster et al. 1987; Horiguchi et al. 1987). In turn, CSF-1 can induce production of TNF from monocytes (Warren and Ralph 1986) suggesting an autocrine-amplification loop. Thus, activation of macrophage/monocytes can lead to the production of both stimulators and inhibitors of hematopoiesis and the production of such regulatory elements by monocytes is part of a highly interactive, even an autoreactive, network. The interaction of a homogeneous population of macrophages to some of the elements of this network is examined below.

Regulation of Murine Macrophage Proliferation

Individual subclasses of progenitor cells constitute less than 0.1% of total marrow cells, and thus cannot be readily studied in isolation or in number. We have found that murine bone marrow derived macrophages (BMM), which can be obtained as relatively homogeneous populations, respond to the same growth factors as macrophage progenitors; i.e., CSF-1, GM-CSF and IL-3 (Guilbert 1985). However, unlike the progenitors, which required two factors for proliferation, BMM responded to each factor alone, albeit to differing degrees. We therefore asked whether the above growth factors cooperatively stimulated BMM proliferation. Preliminary studies indicated only marginal cooperation between the factors (data not shown).

Reasoning that perhaps larger cooperative effects might be masked by the heterogeneity of primary cells, we have reexamined the question using a repeatedly cloned, growth-factor dependent cell line, S1, derived from BMM as previously described (Branch and Guilbert 1986). Like BMM, S1 cells come rapidly to quiescence in the absence of growth factors and proliferate to differing degrees in response to maximally stimulating levels of the three macrophage growth factors

Table 3. Stimulation of S1-cell proliferation by CSF-1, GM-CSF, and IL-3

Colony-stimulating factor	Maximal response[a] (cpm)
None	955 ± 420
CSF-1	31 844 ± 8 162
GM-CSF	37 426 ± 2 029
IL-3	5 158 ± 653

[a] Proliferation assessed as uptake of ^{3}HTdR as described in the legend to Fig. 2. Levels of growth factors are maximally stimulatory for S1 cells: CSF-1 = 5×10^3 U/ml; rGM-CSF = 250 ng/ml; IL-3 = 1000 U/ml.

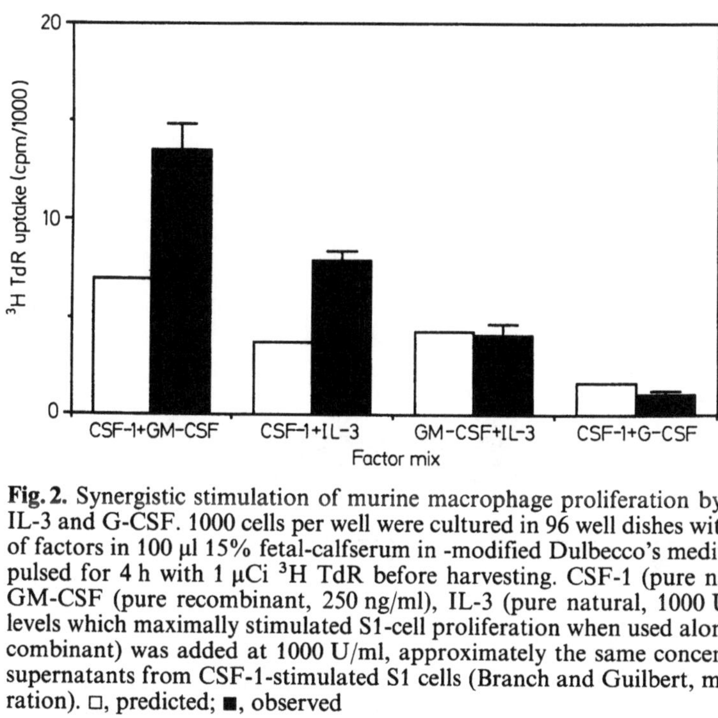

Fig. 2. Synergistic stimulation of murine macrophage proliferation by CSF-1, GM-CSF, IL-3 and G-CSF. 1000 cells per well were cultured in 96 well dishes with the combinations of factors in 100 µl 15% fetal-calfserum in -modified Dulbecco's medium for 3 days, then pulsed for 4 h with 1 µCi ^{3}H TdR before harvesting. CSF-1 (pure natural, 3000 U/ml), GM-CSF (pure recombinant, 250 ng/ml), IL-3 (pure natural, 1000 U/ml) were used at levels which maximally stimulated S1-cell proliferation when used alone. G-CSF (pure recombinant) was added at 1000 U/ml, approximately the same concentration detected in supernatants from CSF-1-stimulated S1 cells (Branch and Guilbert, manuscript in preparation). □, predicted; ■, observed

(Table 3). However, unlike BMM, these cells respond to combinations of CSF-1 and the hematopoietins synergistically (Fig. 2). In contrast, combinations of GM-CSF and IL-3 appear unable to act synergistically. The ability of low levels of CSF-1 to enhance the mitogenic effects of GM-CSF is illustrated in Fig. 3. Synergy between IL-1 and CSF-1 is also observed in a similar experiment (Fig. 4). Surprisingly, G-CSF, a factor assigned specifically to the neutrophil lineage (Walker et al. 1985), inhibits S1-cell proliferation stimulated by CSF-1 (Fig. 2).

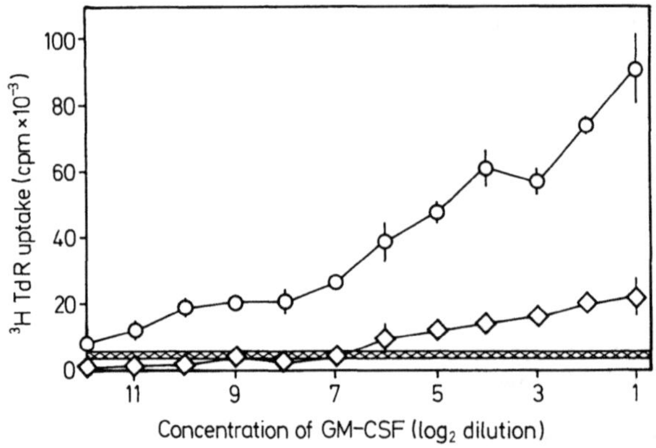

Fig. 3. Stimulation of S1-cell growth by GM-CSF with (○) and without (◇) suboptimal concentrations of CSF-1 (200 U/ml). For materials and methods, see legend Fig. 2. *Hatched area* depicts uptake stimulated by CSF-1 alone ±1 SD. *Abscissa,* doubling dilutions of GM-CSF in the cultures expressed as $\log_2$ dilution of a stock containing 100 ng/ml

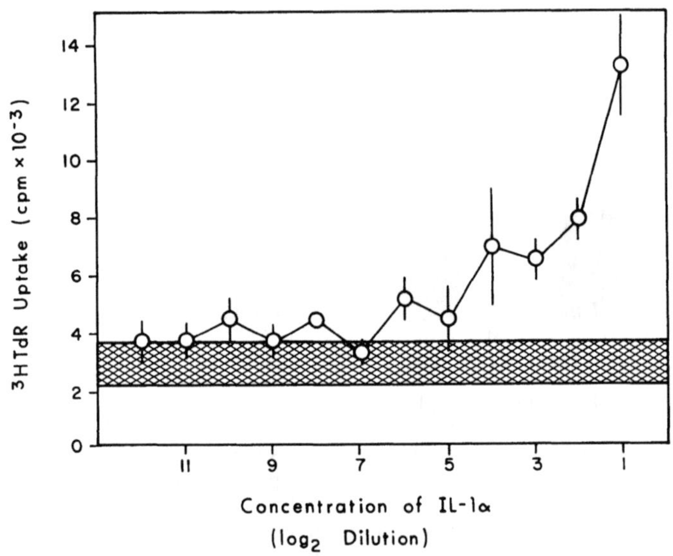

Fig. 4. Stimulation of S1-cell growth by IL-1 alpha with (○) and without (—) suboptimal levels of CSF-1 (500 U/ml). For materials and methods, see legend Fig. 2. *Hatched area* depicts ^{3}HT TdR uptake stimulated by CSF-1 alone ±1 SD. *Abscissa,* doubling dilutions of IL-1 alpha (pure recombinant) in the cultures expressed as $\log_2$ dilution of a stock containing 4000 U/ml

These results indicate that CSF-1 synergistically cooperates with GM-CSF, IL-3 and IL-1 to stimulate the growth of murine macrophages and negatively cooperates with G-CSF. The observation that GM-CSF and IL-3 do not act synergistically indicates certain specificity in the complementation. It is of interest that CSF-1, GM-CSF, IL-1 and G-CSF, but not IL-3, are macrophage products subject to induction (see above, Fig. 1). These observations suggest that macrophages, like other hematopoietic cells, require at least two growth factors for full mitogenic stimulation, and that one factor is supplied by the target cell in response to the other. The results also indicate that CSF-1-induced release of monokines such as G-CSF (and PGE_2, data not shown) inhibits CSF-1 stimulated proliferation. How much autocrine synergy contributes to the proliferation stimulated by CSF-1, GM-CSF and IL-3, and autoinhibition modulates that stimulation, remains to be determined.

References

Asko-Seljavaara S (1986) Granulocyte kinetics in burns. J Burn Care Rehabil 8:492–495
Branch DR, Guilbert LJ (1986) Practical in vitro assay systems for the measurement of hematopoietic growth factors. J Tissue Culture Methods 10:101–108
Broxmeyer HE (1984) Negative regulators of hematopoiesis. In: Wright D, Greenberger J (eds) Long-term bone marrow. Liss, New York, p 363
Clark SC, Kamen R (1987) The human hematopoietic colony stimulating factors. Science 236:1229–1237
Cosman D, Cerrette DP, Larsen A, Park L, Marach C, Dower S, Gillis S, Urdal D (1984) Cloning, sequence and expression of human interleukin-2 receptor. Nature 312:768–771
Eaves AC, Eaves CJ (1985) Erythropoiesis in culture. In: McCulloch EA (ed) Clinics in hematology. Saunders, Toronto, p 371
Guilbert LJ (1985) Mononuclear phagocytes and progenitors. In: van Furth R (ed) Mononuclear phagocytes, functional aspects. Nijhoff, The Hague, pp 233–244
Guilbert LJ, Stanley ER (1986) The interaction of ^{125}I-colony stimulating factor-1 with bone marrow-derived macrophages. J Biol Chem 261:4024–4032
Horiguchi J, Warren MK, Kufe D (1987) Expression of the macrophage-specific colony-stimulating factor in human monocytes treated with granulocyte-macrophage colony-stimulating factor. Blood 69:1259–1261
Ihle JN (1985) Biochemical and biological properties of IL-3. Contemp Top Mol Immunol 10:93
Ikebuchi K, Wong GG, Clark SC, Ihle JN, Hirai Y, Ogawa M (1988) Interleukin-6 enhancement of interleukin-3-dependent proliferation of multipotential hematopoietic progenitors. Proc Natl Acad Sci USA (in press)
Keller JR, Sing GK, Ellingsworth L, McNiece IK, Quesenberry PJ, Ruscetti FW (1988) The effect of transforming growth factor beta 1 on early hematopoietic cell growth. J Cell Biochem [Suppl] 12A:133
Le J, Vilcek J (1987) Tumor necrosis factor and interleukin 1: cytokines with multiple overlapping biological activities. Lab Invest 56:234–248
McIver MA (1933) A study in extensive cutaneous burns. Ann Surg 97:670–682
Metcalf D (1970) Studies on colony formation in vitro by mouse bone marrow cells. II. Action of colony stimulating factor. J Cell Physiol 76:89–99
Metcalf D (1984) The hemopoietic colony stimulating factors. Elsevier, Amsterdam
Metcalf D (1986) The molecular biology and functions of the granulocyte-macrophage colony stimulating factors. Blood 67:257–267
Miller SE, Miller CL, Trunkey DD (1982) The immune consequences of trauma. Surg Clin North Am 62:167–182
Mochizuki DY, Eisenman JR, Conlon PJ, Larsen AD, Tushinski RJ (1987) Interleukin 1 regulates hematopoietic activity, a role previously ascribed to hemopoietin 1. Proc Natl Acad Sci USA 84:5267
Moses HL, Coffey RJ Jr, Loef EB, Lyons RM, Keski-Oja J (1987) Transforming growth factor beta regulation of cell proliferation. J Cell Physiol [Suppl] 5:1–7

Nelson RD, Hasslen SR, Ahrenholz DH, Solem LD (1986) Mechanisms of loss of human neutrophil chemotaxis following thermal injury. J Burn Care Rehabil 8:496–502

Ohara J, Paul WE (1987) High affinity receptors for B cell stimulatory factor a (interleukin 4) expressed on lymphocytes and other cells of the hematopoietic lineage. Nature 325:537

Oster W, Lindemann A, Horn S, Mertelsmann R, Hermann F (1987) Tumor necrosis factor (TNF)-alpha but not TNF-beta induces secretion of colony stimulating factor for macrophages (CSF-1) by human monocytes. Blood 70:1700–1703

Paul WE, Ohara J (1987) B cell stimulatory factor 1/interleukin 4. Annu Rev Immunol 5:429

Rennick D, Gemmell L, Yang G, Muller-Sieburg C, Arai N, Smith G, Lee F (1987) Interleukin 4/B cell stimulatory factor 1: a bifunctional regulator of hematopoietic progenitor cell growth. Proc Natl Acad Sci USA 84:6884

Shaw G, Kamen R (1987) A conserved AU sequence from the 3′ untranslated region of GM-CSF mRNA mediates selective mRNA degradation. Cell 46:659–667

Sherr CJ, Rettenmier CW, Sacca R, Roussel MF, Look AT, Stanley ER (1985) The c-fms proto-oncogene product is related to the receptor for the mononuclear phagocyte growth factor, CSF-1. Cell 41:665–676

Simm J et al. (1988) Presented at the UCLA Symposia on Quantitative Biology: growth factors and their receptors. Keystone, Colorado, 24–28 January 1988

Stanley ER, Bartocci A, Patinkin D, Rosendaal M, Bradley TR (1986) Regulation of very primitive, multipotent, hemopoietic cells by hemopoietin-1. Cell 45:667–674

Toksoez D, Dexter TM, Lord BI, Wright EG, Lajtha LG (1980) The regulation of hematopoiesis in long-term bone marrow cultures. II. Stimulation and inhibition of stem cell proliferation. Blood 55:931–936

Tushinski RJ, Oliver IT, Guilbert LJ, Tynan PW, Warner JR, Stanley ER (1982) Survival of mononuclear phagocytes depends on a lineage-specific growth factor that differentiated cells destroy. Cell 28:71–81

Walker F, Nicola NA, Metcalf D, Burgess AW (1985) Hierarchical down-modulation of hemopoietic growth factor receptors. Cell 43:269–276

Wallner SF, Vautrin R (1986) The anemia of thermal injury: mechanism of inhibition of erythropoiesis. Proc Soc Exp Biol Med 181:144–150

Warren MK, Ralph P (1986) Macrophage growth factor CSF-1 stimulates human monocyte production of interferon, tumor necrosis factor, and colony stimulating activity. J Immunol 137:2281–2285

Williams N (1979) Preferential inhibition of murine macrophage colony formation by prostaglandin E. Blood 53:1089–1094

Williams DE, Hangoc G, Cooper S, Boswell HS, Shadduck RK, Gillis S, Waheed, Urdal D, Broxmeyer HE (1987) The effects of purified recombinant murine interleukin-3 and/or purified natural murine CSF-1 in vivo on the proliferation of murine high- and low-proliferative potential colony-forming cells: demonstration of in vivo synergism. Blood 70:401

Wong GG et al. (1987) Human CSF-1: molecular cloning and expression of 4kb cDNA encoding the human urinary protein. Science 235:1504

Zoumbos NC, Djeu JY, Young NS (1984) Interferon is the suppresser of hematopoiesis generated by lymphocytes in vitro. J Immunol 133:769

The Activation of Immune Effector Cells: Role of Helper and Inflammatory CD4 T Cell Subsets *

K. Bottomly and C. A. Janeway, Jr.

The overwhelming infection that so frequently undoes the best efforts of surgeons dealing with major trauma, burns, and shock is believed to result from a failure of normal immunological responsiveness. In attempting to understand the immune compromise that attends major trauma, one must first understand the workings of the normal immune system. This paper will briefly review data that have led us to propose that the immune system is divided into effector compartments, and that each effector compartment is under the control of a T-cell-bearing CD4 on its cell surface, with distinct CD4 T cells activating different effector mechanisms (for a more extensive review, see Janeway et al. 1988).

The Immune System Has Evolved to Combat Infection

A central postulate of this model is that the immune system has evolved to allow the vertebrate host to resist infection by pathogenic microorganisms. This view is widely held, and needs no further defense here. However, it is as well to mention in an era in which the antigens used most commonly in experimental immunology are soluble proteins that the most biologically relevant antigens are particulate, living microorganisms of a nearly infinite variety.

Different Classes of Microorganisms Proliferate in Different Microenvironments

Different microorganisms inhabit distinct parts of the body. In particular, one can divide bacteria into those that proliferate outside cells, and are inactivated by

Table 1. Major categories of pathogens

Pathogen category	Examples of microorganisms
Extracellular	*Diplococcus pneumoniae, Streptococcus*
Intracellular	*Mycobacterium tuberculosis, Listeria monocytogenes, Pneumocystis carinii*
Viruses	All species

* Supported by NIH grant CA-29606 and the Howard Hughes Medical Institute.

Immune Consequences of
Trauma, Shock and Sepsis
Eds. Faist/Ninnemann/Green

being engulfed by phagocytes, and those that preferentially grow in cellular vesicles. Viruses occupy a third niche, namely the cellular cytoplasm. These are summarized in Table 1.

The Immune System Is Compartmentalized to Respond to Distinct Challenges in Distinct Microenvironments

Vertebrates survive despite exposure to a variety of pathogenic microorganisms, provided immune function is not compromised. Thus, effective defenses against each class of pathogen listed in Table 1 must exist. It is the central hypothesis of our work that mature, protective responses to distinct classes of microorganisms reflect the activation of distinct sets of T-lymphocytes, as summarized in Table 2. Before detailing these distinct subsets and their unique roles, it is important to point out that not all immune effector responses are in fact T cell dependent; indeed, T-independent immune effector responses clearly play an important role in immune homeostasis.

Table 2. How could MHC allele determine CD4 T-cell subset activated?

Model	Implication
Different ligand	Distinct receptor repertoire
Ligand density	Different signaling requirement
Different APC	Different accessory signals

Both T-Dependent and T-Independent Immune Effector Responses Are Important in Resistance to Infection

A T-cell immune response takes several days to generate; for helper T cells, priming requires at least 4 days in vivo. However, antibody can be produced much earlier than this in some responses that do not require specific T-cell help. Likewise, it takes days to generate effective specific cell-mediated immunity, but T-independent macrophage responses occur rapidly. As soon as macrophages encounter certain microorganisms, they start to produce interleukin-1 (IL-1), IL-6, and tumor necrosis factor (TNF), which serve to raise body temperature, to call forth

Table 3. T-independent and T-dependent responses to different classes of microorganism

Type of microorganism	T-independent response	T-dependent response
Extracellular	T-I B-cell response	T-D B-cell response
Intracellular bacteria	T-I macrophage response (IL-1, IL-6, TNF)	T-D macrophage activation (interferon γ)
Virus	NK cells, interferons-α, β	Cytolytic T cells

acute-phase proteins, and to cause local changes that may contribute to containment and clearance of the infection, such as recruitment of phagocytic cells and local hemostasis. Finally, while generation of specific cytolytic T cells in response to viral infection takes about 5–7 days, early production of interferon-α activates natural killer (NK) cells, which play an important role in nonspecific resistance to viral infection. These two types of response are summarized in Table 3.

Most T-Independent Immune Responses Are Rapid, Have Little Specificity, Contain but Do Not Clear Infection, and Do Not Provide Long-Lasting Protection

Each of the T-independent responses listed above can contribute to immune defense. It is clear that defects in these low-specificity immediate responses can be of major consequence to the host, and the evaluation of early host immune dysfunction should clearly include an evaluation of such cells. However, the major theme of this report is the role of T cells in the activation of immune effector cells, and it is such responses that complete the protective immune response. This can be seen from the consequences of defective immune responses in individuals who fail properly to activate their T cells. Furthermore, as detailed below, these T-independent responses function best in local containment of infection, and may cause pathology when they become systemic.

Systemic T-Independent Responses Can Cause Pathology

Certain components of T-independent immune responses almost certainly play a role in local immune defense, but cause pathology when their production becomes systemic, or when their local production is not regulated. For instance, local production of TNF probably serves a critical role in the containment of infection before specific immunity can mediate clearance. Thus, TNF can cause local margination and influx of polymorphonuclear leukocytes, local alterations in metabolism, and local hemostasis, all of which can contribute to containment of an infection. However, systemic TNF causes fever, shock, disseminated intravascular coagulopathy, and cachexia. These opposing faces of the same response strongly suggest that the physiological role of TNF is in containment of infection in local sites, and experimental studies support this construction. It is when TNF is released into the systemic circulation that pathological effects appear.

T-Dependent Responses Follow a Significant Lag Phase, but Are Highly Specific, Serve to Eliminate Infection, and Provide Long-Lasting Protection

Unlike the T-independent immune responses, which while inducible do not generate immunological memory, and which generally cannot totally eliminate infection, T-dependent immune responses can provide these functions. A failure to mount a T-dependent response will almost always lead to eventual disseminated infection, since the T-independent host defense system in most cases contains, but does not eliminate, the pathogen. Thus, it is essential to understand the nature of the T-dependent immune response. In the subsequent sections, the role of CD4 T cells of distinct functional phenotypes will be examined, and will be shown to play a critical role in the activation of distinct immune effector cell populations. It is interesting to note that either the same or very similar final effector cells eventually mediate protection against infection in both T-independent and T-dependent modes of function.

CD4 T Cells Exist in Two Distinct Functional Sets, Termed Helper and Inflammatory

Work over the past few years has shown that cloned CD4 T-cell lines in the mouse can be subdivided into two distinct sets of cells. Working with functional assays, we have shown that some CD4 T cells will help B cells for specific antibody responses, while others will not. In two other assays systems, those cloned lines that would not help were shown to be cytolytic, and to be capable of mediating delayed-type hypersensitivity by local passive transfer of cells, while the cloned lines that could not mediate these functions were helper T cells. Based on this distinction in function, we named these cloned T-cell lines helper T cells and inflammatory T cells, respectively.

Because effector T cells are believed to mediate their effects mainly by the induced release of antigen-non-specific effector molecules, such as lymphokines and cytotoxins, we have evaluated the production of these molecules by our cloned T-cell lines. It was observed that cloned T-cell lines that help, release different lymphokines than those released by cloned T-cell lines that do not help, as summarized in Table 4. It can be seen that IL-4 appears to be a unique helper-T-cell lymphokine, while IL-2, IFN-γ, and lymphotoxin are distinct inflammatory T-cell lymphokines. As IL-4 is a B-cell-activating lymphokine, while IFN-γ is a prominent macrophage activator, the selective production of these lymphokines agrees well with the functional phenotype of the clones producing them.

Studies using cloned T-cell lines are always open to the criticism that long-term in vitro culture may lead to phenotypes not found in vivo due to terminal differentiation of cells. In order to determine if this functional dichotomy exists in freshly isolated T cells, three approaches have been taken. First, in vivo systems dominated by humoral or cell-mediated immunity, thought to be consequences of selective activation of helper or inflammatory CD4 T cells respectively, were examined for production of distinctive lymphokines. In the murine immune response to human collagen type IV, certain MHC haplotypes are associated with activation of helper T cells and production of antibody, while others are associated with activation of inflammatory T cells and cell-mediated immunity. Second, monoclonal antibodies have been generated that distinguished subsets of CD4 T cells, and also subdivided cloned T-cell lines into the helper and the inflammatory set. Normal CD4 T cells fractionated by these antibodies were then analyzed for lymphokine production upon short-term activation. It was shown that one anti-

Table 4. Cloned T-cell lines can be divided into two types on the basis of functional phenotype and lymphokines released

Function measured	Cloned T-cell type		Ref.
	Helper	Inflammatory	
B-cell proliferation	Yes	Yes	Bottomly et al. (1983) Tite and Janeway (1984) Tite et al. (1984)
Polyclonal Ig secretion	Yes	Yes/No	Bottomly et al. (1983) Tite and Janeway (1984) Tite et al. (1984)
Help for specific antibody	Yes	No	Kim et al. (1985)
Cytotoxicity	No	Yes	Tite and Janeway (1984) Tite et al. (1985)
Suppression of specific B-cell response	No	Yes	Bottomly et al. (1983)
DTH responses	No	Yes	Cher and Mosmann (1987)
Lymphokine released			
IL-2	No	Yes	Mosmann et al. (1986) Woods et al. (1987)
IL-3	Yes	Yes	Mosmann et al. (1986) Woods et al. (1987)
Il-4	Yes	No	Mosmann et al. (1986) Killar et al. (1987)
IL-5	Yes	Yes	West et al. (1987)
GM-CSF	Yes	Yes	Woods et al. (1987) Mosmann et al. (1986)
IFN-γ	No	Yes	Tite et al. (1985) Mosmann et al. (1986)
LT	No	Yes	Tite et al. (1985)

body, specific for a subset of CD45 molecules (called CD45R), could indeed subdivide CD4 T cells into those that produce IL-4 and those that produce IL-2 and IFN-γ. Production of other lymphokines remains to be determined. The IL-4-producing subset provides helper function in B-cell activation assays, while the IL-2-producing subset does not. While a more extensive analysis of these two systems is required, it is likely from these results that CD4 T cells in the mouse belong to two distinct subsets, and that these are equivalent to those observed earlier using cloned T cells.

The most important conclusion from these results is that some T cells will contribute to humoral immunity, while others will contribute to cell-mediated immunity. Thus, one CD4 T-cell subset, the helper T cells, will activate B cells to provide humoral immunity to extracellular pathogens, while the other will activate macrophages for immunity to intracellular parasites. After describing the functional activity of these cells in more detail, the distinctive activation conditions required by each of these two subsets of CD4 T cells will be discussed. Understanding these activation conditions is an essential precondition to directing the immune response properly to one or another type of protective immunity.

CD4 Helper T Cells Are Responsible for B-Cell Activation to Antibody Production Required in Protection Against Extracellular Parasites

CD4 helper T cells, which produce a variety of B-cell-activating lymphokines, are the major cell responsible for activation of resting B cells to antibody production. Cloned lines of helper T cells are able to help B cells make specific antibody responses. These cells secrete the B-cell-activating lymphokines IL-4, IL-5, and IL-6 upon activation. In addition, they produce IL-3 and GM-CSF. This cluster of lymphokines enables helper T cells to activate B cells to produce IgM antibody early in the response, and to switch to IgG1 and IgE synthesis through the action of IL-4, and to IgA synthesis through the action of IL-5. IL-6 appears to be involved in terminal differentiation of antibody-secreting cells. In addition to these B-cell-activating properties, IL-4 is a cofactor for mast cell growth, while IL-5 is a cofactor for eosinophil differentiation. IL-3 and GM-CSF help in the production of large numbers of phagocytic cells, both macrophages and polymorphonuclear leukocytes. IL-6 is a lymphokine with pleiotropic effects.

The action of helper T-cell lymphokines is to produce antibodies of many different isotypes, which interact with Fc receptors on a variety of different effector cell types. IgM antibody is largely confined to vascular spaces; through complement fixation it is both a lytic and an opsonic antibody. IgG1 is an excellent opsonin, and plays a major role in protection of extracellular spaces. IgE associates with mast cell receptors, and leads to mast cell activation upon encountering antigen. Thus, this antibody provides for ready access of immune reactants to sites of antigen deposition, especially just below lining and surface epithelia. And IgA binds the poly Ig receptor on the basolateral face of various epithelial cells, thus being transported to the luminal face and providing surface protection. In this way, antibodies induced by helper T cells are targeted to virtually every site in the body, and perform the necessary function of keeping bacteria and their products out of the extracellular spaces.

CD4 Inflammatory T Cells Activate Macrophages to Destroy Intracellular Bacteria

Inflammatory T cells are poor B-cell activators, although the IFN-γ they release probably plays a critical role in switching B cells activated by helper T cells to the production of IgG2a antibody. This antibody is particularly important in some forms of immunity, and helper T cells appear to be inefficient in inducing its production. However, it seems likely that the major function for inflammatory T cells is to activate macrophages, allowing them to destroy any intracellular bacteria living in their vesicles. This function is well mediated by IFN-γ. In addition, inflammatory T cells are also cytotoxic. While killing macrophages would appear to be counterproductive in immune defense, it may be necessary for those parasites that must remain within macrophages in order to grow. In these cases, the cytolytic effect of inflammatory T cells may help in removing the pathogen from its essential microenvironment.

In addition to producing IFN-γ and lymphotoxin, involved in cell killing, inflammatory T cells also produce IL-2, required both for their own clonal expansion and for the activation of cytolytic T cells. Finally, like helper T cells, inflammatory T cells produce IL-3 and GM-CSF, allowing them to recruit the phagocytic effector cells required for their function in cell-mediated immunity.

CD4 T Inflammatory T Cells Also Contribute to the Activation of CD8 Killer T Cells Required for Immunity to Viruses

Viruses differ from bacteria in not synthesizing their own proteins; rather, they use the biosynthetic machinery of their host cell to produce the products encoded in their genomes. Because of this, peptide fragments of viral proteins are presented by class I MHC antigens, and the complexes are recognized by CD8 T cells rather than by CD4 T cells. However, activation of CD8 T cells by virus peptides associated with class I MHC molecules appears to require or to be greatly enhanced by the action of CD4 inflammatory T cells, which produce IL-2, a major growth factor for cytolytic T cells. Thus, although again in this case the final effector cell is not a CD4 T cell, CD4 T cells are probably important in contributing to the activation of such cells.

T Cells in Epithelia Bear Unique T-Cell Receptors and Play as yet Undetermined Roles in Host Defense

Recently, it has become apparent that there is a second type of T-cell receptor, consisting of CD3 associated with a $\gamma:\delta$ heterodimer. Such cells are found in a highly enriched form in skin and the lining epithelia of the gut in mice (Janeway, unpublished results); they are very infrequent in normal peripheral lymphoid tissue. There are too little data at present to state what such cells are doing in these locations. However, as trauma, especially burn trauma, affects skin in a massive fashion, it is well to be aware of the presence of these cells. Their activation and/or destruction by trauma may be of importance. Furthermore, their great enrichment in epithelia suggests an important role in defense of the body surfaces, surely a critical factor in preventing systemic infection. The influence of CD4 T cells and their products on the functioning of these cells has not been examined.

The Priming of Suitable CD4 T Cells Is a Critical Step in the Establishment of Host Immunity

In the course of an immune response, probably no event is as important as the priming of virgin T cells. In particular, the priming of CD4 T cells is of the utmost importance, since these cells activate most of the effector cells in the immune response as described above. However, before they can do so, they must themselves be activated by encountering antigen: class II MHC complexes on the surface of a suitable antigen-presenting cell.

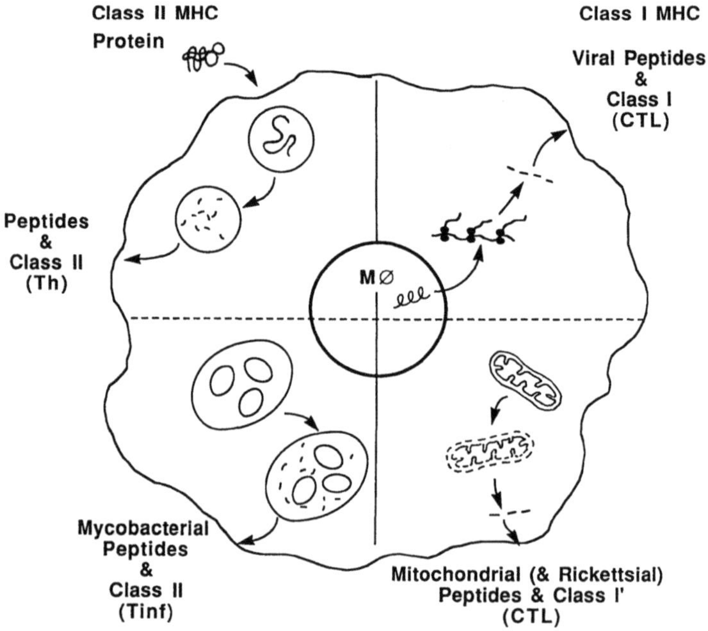

Fig. 1. A hypothetical macrophage presenting antigens derived from different categories of microbe. Antigens are presented as peptide fragments associated with class I major histocompatibility complex (MHC) proteins (*right*) or class II MHC proteins (*left*). The MHC molecule that presents peptides depends on the origin of the peptide. Those peptides, deriving from proteins synthesized outside the cell, or in the cellular vesicles, are presented with class II MHC, while those derived from proteins synthesized in the cell's cytoplasm are presented by class I MHC molecules.
Proteins taken up by phagocytosis or endocytosis will be degraded in endosomes and/or lysosomes and presented with class II MHC molecules. In most cases, these antigen: class II MHC complexes will be presented at low density, and are predicted to prime CD4 helper T cells in conjunction with IL-1. Proteins produced by intracellular bacteria will be presented by class II MHC molecules at a much higher ligand density, since they are synthesized within the cell, and are predicted to prime CD4 inflammatory T cells. Those T cells can then active infected macrophages to kill the intracellular bacteria.
Viruses utilize the cell's own protein synthetic machinery to produce their proteins. Intracellular degradation of these viral proteins generates peptides that are carried to the cell surface by class I MHC molecules, where they activate CD8 cytotoxic T cells. These T cells can kill the infected cell, halting the infection. Finally, a unique class I-like molecule presents peptides derived from mitochondrial genes to cytotoxic T cells. It is proposed that this pathway of presentation is also utilized by the cytoplasmic bacterial genera Chlamydia and Rickettsia, allowing cytolytic T cells to kill the infected cells in which such microbes must exist

The existence of two separate classes of CD4 T cells further complicates this step in immunity, since it is now relevant to ask which subset of CD4 T cell is primed in a given experimental situation. We have examined several experimental situations to determine what might control this process. These studies suggest at least two aspects to the control of this step in the response.

First, CD4 helper T cells require IL-1 for clonal expansion, while CD4 inflammatory T cells do not. This reflects the use of IL-4 as an autocrine growth factor for helper T cells, and the finding that IL-4 is only a growth factor for helper T cells when IL-1 is also present. By contrast, CD4 inflammatory T cells use IL-2 as their autocrine growth factor, and do not utilize IL-1 in any aspect of their growth cycle. Thus, antigen-presenting cells, such as macrophages, which produce abundant IL-1, may play a more important role in CD4 helper T-cell priming and clonal expansion than they do in priming of inflammatory CD4 T cells.

Second, we have discovered an Ir gene control of priming of helper and inflammatory T cells in the immune response of mice to human type IV collagen. This suggests that some aspect of the ligand, of which the Ir gene product is an essential component, in some way controls the priming of T-cell subsets. A hint as to how this may occur comes from studying T-cell subset priming in B-cell-deprived mice. Such mice, primed with protein antigens, generate normal helper T cells but are lacking CD4 inflammatory cells. For protein antigens, B cells differ from macrophages in two ways: they do not produce significant IL-1, and they can concentrate antigen to a very high level.

These findings taken together suggest that helper T cells are normally primed by antigen presented at low ligand density on macrophage surfaces, while inflammatory T cells are primed on cells that present a high density of ligand. We believe that the normal course of inflammatory T-cell priming involves a response to macrophages in which intracellular bacteria are actively proliferating. This situation is analogous to that of the antigen-specific B-cell-concentrating protein antigen by means of the Ig receptor. In this case, the intracellular bacteria synthesize their proteins in the lysosomes of the macrophage, and thus the macrophage presents a very high ligand density to the T cells (Fig. 1).

Summary and Conclusions

The analysis of the normal immune response to infectious agents needs to take account of the type of microorganism, its microenvironment, and emerging concepts of immune surveillance. T-independent immune responses provide a front line for resisting infection; however, T-dependent responses play the critical role in elimination of infection and in long-term protection of the host. It appears that CD4 T cells control this process, and fall into functional subsets. These subsets provide protection against different classes of pathogens, and have different activation and growth requirements. Understanding these requirements may better allow us to control the immune response in a variety of clinical situations including trauma, shock, and sepsis in the future.

References

Bottomly K, Kaye J, Jones F III, Jones B, Janeway CA Jr (1983) A cloned, antigen-specific, Ia-restricted Lyt-1$^+$, 2$^-$ T cell with suppressive activity. J Mol Cell Immunol 1:42

Cher D, Mosmann TR (1987) Two types of murine helper T cell clone. II. Delayed-type hypersensitivity is mediated by Th1 clones. J Immunol 138:3688

Killar L, MacDonald G, West J, Woods A, Bottomly K (1987) Cloned, Ia restricted T cells that do not produce interleukin 4 (IL-4)/B cell stimulatory factor 1 (BSF-1) fail to help antigen-specific B cell. J Immunol 138:1674

Kim J, Woods A, Becker-Dunn E, Bottomly K (1985) Distinct functional phenotypes of cloned Ia restricted helper T cells. J Exp Med 162:188

Mosmann T, Cherwinski H, Bond MW, Giedlin M, Coffman RL (1986) Two types of murine T helper cell clones. I. Definition according to profile of lymphokine activities. J Immunol 136:2348

Tite JP, Janeway CA Jr (1984) Cloned helper T cells can kill B-lymphoma cells in the presence of specific antigen: Ia-restriction and cognate vs non-cognate interactions in cytolysis. Eur J Immunol 14:878

Tite JP, Kaye J, Jones B (1984) The role of major histocompatibility complex determinant recognition at the B-cell surface by T-cells in the triggering of B-cells: analysis of the interaction of cloned helper T-cells with normal B-cells in differing states of activation and with B-cells expressing the xid defect. Eur J Immunol 14:553

Tite JP, Powell MB, Ruddle NH (1985) Protein-antigen specific Ia-restricted cytolytic T cells: analysis of frequency, target cell susceptibility, and mechanisms of cytolysis. J Immunol 135:25

West J, Carding S, Honjo T, Rasmussen R, Takatsu K, Woods A, Kinashi T, Bottomly K (1987) $CD4^+$ T cell clones of distinct functional phenotypes all induce polyclonal B cell responses and produce interleukin-5 (IL-5). Submitted for publication

Woods A, West J, Rasmussen R, Bottomly K (1987) Granulocyte-macrophage colony stimulating factor produced by cloned $L3T4a^+$, class II-restricted T cells induces HT-2 cells to proliferate. J Immunol 138:4293

The Role of Inhibitory Cells in Burn Trauma-Associated Immunodeficiency

D. R. Green, R. Marcotte, and N. Wang

The Appearance of Immune Defects and Inhibitory T Cells Following Severe Burn

Burn trauma is associated with an array of immunologic defects which strikingly increase the risk of sepsis and death (Bjornson and Bjornson 1984; Munster 1984; Moran and Munster 1987). One goal of research in this area is to identify the nature and/or causes of these defects as a first step towards diagnosis and therapy. Defects in T-lymphocyte function (Teodorczyk-Injeyan et al. 1986) and in the function of myeloid cells (Alexander and Wixson 1970; Altman et al. 1977) have been analyzed in severely burned patients. Further, serum immunosuppressive factors from burned patients can produce such defects in normal cells (Ozkan and Ninnemann 1985). This suggests that the immunodeficiency which follows thermal trauma is "active," that is, it is imposed on the cells of the immune system. This is, of course, not surprising, given that the immunodeficiency is environmentally acquired.

It is difficult, in a burned patient, to distinguish between effects of the burn and iatrogenic effects of therapy. Therefore, animal models of thermal trauma have proven extremely useful in the analysis of burn-associated immune defects. Using such animal models, immunologic defects similar to those described for burn patients have been described and can be attributed to an effect of the thermal trauma.

Active immunosuppression has been documented both in burn patients and in the animal models of thermal trauma, implicating both suppressor macrophages (Baker et al. 1979) and suppressor T cells (Munster 1976; Miller and Clandy 1979) as important mediators of the immunodeficiency. In other models of immune regulation, macrophages have been shown to play a critical role in the generation of suppressor T cells (Rogers et al. 1980; El Masry et al. 1986) suggesting that these activities may be interrelated. It should be noted, however, that the term "suppressor," whether applied to a macrophage or a T cell, is meant only as a description of its *functional* activity, without implying anything about its cell surface phenotype or its uniqueness as a cellular entity. That is, the cell might function to depress immune responses under one set of conditions but have other functions under other conditions. Because of the confusion surrounding the definition of suppressor T cells, we have opted to employ the term "inhibitory T cell" to mean any T cell which functions to down regulate immune responses. The use of this term is not meant to distinguish these cells from the suppressor T cells described by ourselves and others.

Immune Consequences of
Trauma, Shock and Sepsis
Eds. Faist/Ninnemann/Green

A Time Course of Immune Regulation after Thermal Trauma in Mice

Because the immune system is highly dynamic, it is useful to consider how it performs over time (as opposed to its behavior at a single time point). Using a mouse model of 30% trinitrobenzene sulfonic acid (TBSA) scald burn, it was observed that splenic antigen presenting cell (APC) function (assessed by antigen presentation to T cell clones) was defective 24 h postburn and returned after 4 days (Kupper et al. 1985 b). Similar defects in APC function have been observed following ultraviolet irradiation of the skin (Letvin et al. 1980), which, like burns, also promotes the generation of inhibitory T cells (Fisher and Kripke 1982). T cell function, assessed by mixed lymphocyte response, was impaired by 3 days postburn, and shortly thereafter (4–6 days postburn) cells capable of inducing suppression of immune responses were detected (Kupper and Green 1984; Green et al. 1987). These T cells were found to be Ly-1^{high}, L3T4^+, Ly-2^-, and required the presence of Ly-2^+ T cells in the assay cultures to manifest suppression (Kupper and Green 1984; Green et al. 1987). By day 7–8 postburn, potent inhibitory Ly-2^+ T cells were active in the spleen, and persisted to about day 15, with immune responses returning to near normal by day 21 (Kupper and Green 1984). Between days 4 and 8 postburn, removal of the inhibitory T cells restored normal function of the remaining T cells, as assessed in the mixed lymphocyte response (Kupper and Green 1984; Kupper et al. 1985 a).

Given the numerous immunologic defects which follow thermal trauma, one strategy for the identification of those which are of primary importance is to relate a particular defect to the increased sensitivity to sepsis associated with the trauma. Seven days postburn, mice do not display an increased sensitivity to sepsis following injection of*Pseudomonas aeruginosa* (Stieritz and Holder 1975), but do show a loss of resistance to sepsis induced by caecal ligation and puncture (CLP) (Zapata-Sirvent et al. 1986). Interestingly then, inhibitory T cells taken from animals 7 days postburn have the ability, when injected into normal animals, of rendering the recipients extremely susceptible to sepsis induced by CLP (Kupper et al. 1985 a). These T cells, and the immune responses they inhibit in vivo, therefore, appear to have a central role in the burn-associated immunodeficiency which increases susceptibility to sepsis 7 days postburn.

Generation of an Inhibitory T Cell Hybridoma Using T Cells from Thermally Traumatized Mice

We observed previously that T cells from thermally traumatized mice release soluble inhibitory substances into culture supernatants (Green et al. 1987). It was likely, then, that T cell hybridomas, produced from such cells, would constitutively produce these soluble inhibitors in large quantity. We therefore purified T cells from the spleen of mice 7 days postburn and fused them with BW5147 thymoma cells using polyethylene glycol. The cells were selected in hypoxanthine aminopterin, and thymidine (HAT) and supernatants tested for their ability to inhibit a primary, in vitro, antisheep red blood cell plaque-forming cell (anti-SRBC PFC) response. Cells displaying such inhibitory activity in the supernatants were

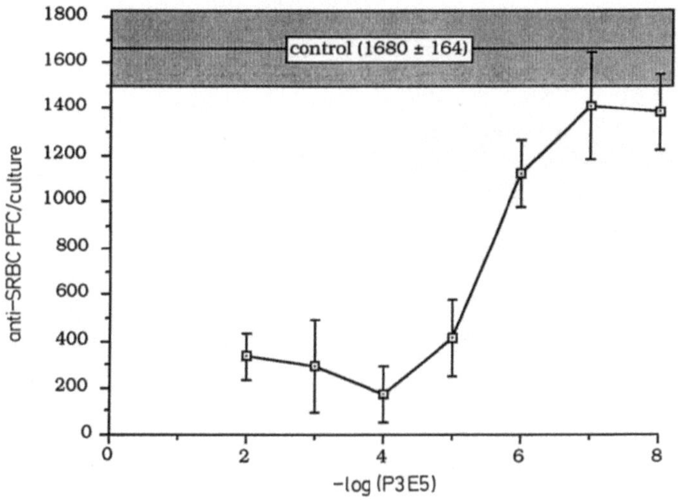

Fig. 1. Titration of P3E5-derived inhibitory activity. The T cell hybridoma P3E5 was cultured in serum-free medium and 48 h supernatants collected. These supernatants were added at the dilutions shown to triplicate cultures of C57BL/6 spleen cells with sheep red blood cells (*SRBC*) as antigen. After 5 days, the anti-SRBC PFC response was assessed

extensively subcloned. One such cell has been named P3E5 (Wang et al., manuscript in preparation).

The supernatants of P3E5 contain a potent activity capable of inhibiting anti-SRBC responses and mixed lymphocyte cultures in vitro (see Fig. 1). This activity is precipitated with 40% saturated ammonium sulfate, nondialyzable (10000 mol.wt. cut-off), and is destroyed by boiling (10 min), although it is stable at 56 °C (1 h). Further, it is sensitive to digestion with proteases, and rapidly loses activity at $pH \leq 4$ or $pH \geq 10$. Taken together, these data suggest that the activity is due to a protein, which we have called an "inhibitory lymphokine."

On the other hand, the inhibitory lymphokine from P3E5 produces no effects in lymphocyte responses to lipopolysaccharides (LPS) or conconavalin A, nor does it affect (stimulate or inhibit) cell lines responsive to granulocyte-macrophage colony stimulating factor (GM-CSF), IL-3, or tumor necrosis factor α/β (TNF α/β) (data not shown).

To examine the effects of the P3E5-derived inhibitory lymphokine in vivo, cell supernatants were precipitated with ammonium sulfate and dialyzed against normal saline. Animals were injected, i.v. with approximately 10^4 units of activity (1 unit equals the amount required to inhibit the PFC response 50%) and suffered no overt effects. Picryl chloride was applied 3 days later to the shaved abdomen in order to sensitize the animals for a contact hypersensitive response. The ears were challenged 7 days later with the sensitizing agent, and ear swelling assessed at 24 h. As shown in Fig. 2, animals injected with the inhibitory lymphokine failed to generate a contact hypersensitive response, while animals injected with an equivalent amount of material prepared from the supernatants of BW5147 cells (the fusion partner) generated normal responses.

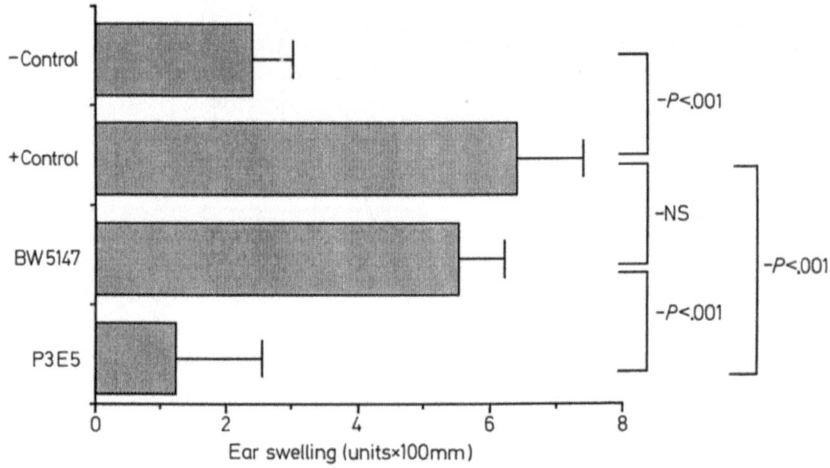

Fig. 2. Effect of P3E5-derived inhibitory lymphokine on induction of contact hypersensitivity responses in vivo. C57BL/10 mice (6 per group) were injected, i.v., with approximately 10^4 units of P3E5-derived inhibitor (0.2 ml), or an equivalent amount of material prepared from supernatants of BW5147. Picryl chloride was applied 3 days later to the shaved abdomen of these animals, and to an additional group of untreated animals (+ control). Picryl chloride was applied 7 days later to the ears, including one group of unsensitized mice (− control). Ear swelling was assessed using engineer's callipers after 24 h

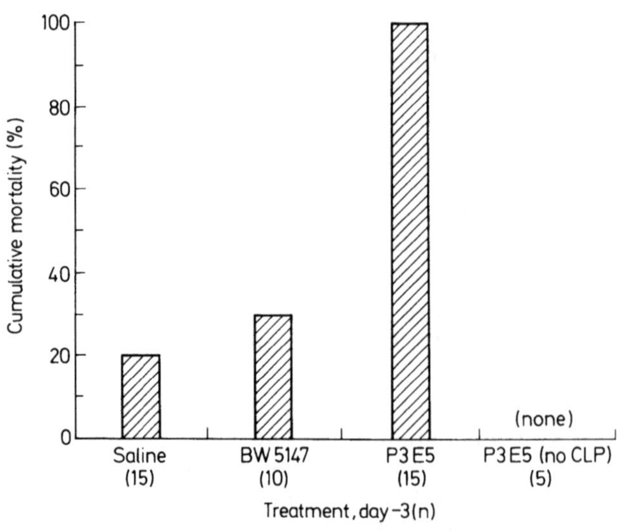

Fig. 3. Effect of P3E5-derived inhibitory lymphokine on resistance to lethal sepsis after caecal ligation and puncture (CLP). C57BL/6 mice were injected, i.v., with 0.2 ml saline, BW5147-derived material, or P3E5-derived inhibitor (approximately 10^4 units). Three days later, animals were subjected to CLP and mortality was assessed over 12 days. One group of animals were injected with the P3E5-derived inhibitor but were not subjected to CLP. Results shown are from two experiments. No mortality was observed beyond day 6 in either experiment

The critical test, however, of the relevance of the immune defects produced by the P3E5-derived inhibitory lymphokine is its effects on induction of sepsis. Therefore, animals were injected, i.v., with approximately 10^4 units of inhibitor, or an equivalent amount of material from BW5147 cells. Three days later, animals were subjected to CLP using a 26 g needle. Mortality was assessed over the next 12 days. As can be seen in Fig. 3, prior exposure to the P3E5-derived inhibitory lymphokine resulted in a markedly increased mortality after CLP. Thus, by these criteria, the inhibitory lymphokine mimics those burn-associated immune defects which are most relevant to the control of sepsis.

We are currently working to purify and identify this inhibitory lymphokine. It remains to be demonstrated that this substance is produced by T cells from burned animals (although it is highly likely). It will also be useful to determine whether this inhibitor is one of those found in serum following burn. Characterization of this inhibitor will therefore offer new routes to diagnosis and therapy of burn-associated immunodeficiency.

A number of T cell-derived, antigen-nonspecific inhibitory proteins have been described in immunoregulatory systems. These include γ-interferon (Trinchieri and Perussia 1985), transforming growth factor-β (Kehrl et al. 1986), lymphotoxin (Leopardi and Rosenau 1984), soluble immune-response suppressor (Aune et al. 1983), and monoclonal nonspecific suppressor factor (Nakamura et al. 1986). The relationship of P3E5-derived inhibitory lymphokine to any of these other substances is unknown, although the biological and physiochemical characteristics of our inhibitor appear to set it apart from those listed here. This, of course, in no way precludes potential roles for these inhibitors in the immunodeficiency which follows severe burn.

If, indeed, T cells in severely burned individuals release a substance related to the P3E5-derived inhibitory lymphokine, our studies will have important implications for our understanding of the role of inhibitory T cells in thermal trauma-associated immunodeficiency and the mechanisms by which it occurs. Even if this is true, however, we will be no closer to understanding why severe burn injury activates T cells to produce this substance. We turn now to this question.

Why Does Thermal Trauma Induce Immunodeficiency?

It is paradoxical that the immune system dysfunctions at a time when it is most needed, such as following severe traumatic injury. Many of the researchers in this field, including ourselves, are interested in ascertaining how this happens. For example, mediators such as prostaglandins, released shortly after injury, may act upon other cells (such as T lymphocytes) to produce lasting effects. Other scenarios are, of course, also possible. Given, however, that biological processes evolve through natural selection, where is the logic in this disastrous immunodeficiency?

One problem with teleological reasoning in evolutionary theory is that we often fail to demonstrate that natural selection is capable of acting upon a biological phenomenon of interest. Severe burn is an excellent case in point. In the absence of care (fluid resuscitation, etc.) it is extremely unlikely that a severely burned (or otherwise traumatized) individual will survive to become septic. It is likely, then, that natural selection never had anything to "say" about immune defects following severe trauma. This would suggest that the immunodeficiency which accompanies thermal trauma is a result of properties of the immune system which behave inappropriately under these severe conditions.

A second problem with such reasoning, which bears on the first, comes from the fact that natural selection only operates within the constraints of development. The result is that biological systems are often not optimal, because they are often "designed" based on other functions (Gould 1980). This view would also support the idea that trauma-induced immunodeficiency is an accident of the way in which the immune system is "put together," rather than a biological phenomenon which was selected because it somehow optimized fitness.

We are left, then, to determine why the immune system has a structure such that trauma-induced immunodeficiency occurs. Based, in part, on the observation that immunodepression accompanies all examined cases of organ generation and regeneration in mature mammals, we recently proposed a novel theory for the evolution of the immune system (Green and Wegmann 1986). A primitive function of the immune system, not concerned with immune protection, may have been a surveillance mechanism for the detection of damaged autologous tissue and the release of growth factors for accelerated repair. When this process was exploited by parasites (in order to increase the number of target cells for invasion) a strong pressure was placed on the generation of a mechanism to distinguish damaged self tissue from parasitized tissue. Eventually this became an immune mechanism for the elimination of the parasites. However, the ancestral function, that of auxillary repair, was maintained (as evidenced in a number of organ generation and regeneration systems in which T lymphocytes enhance growth of the nonlymphoid tissue). We have termed this "immunotrophism." There was, therefore, a constraint on the system due to the different functions of immune destruction and immunotrophism: growth factors, released for the purposes of tissue repair, could now stimulate the destructive mechanisms normally employed for parasite clearance, and thus, autoimmunity became an unwanted outcome. We proposed that immunosuppressive mechanisms, activated during the immunotrophic process, developed to prevent the autoimmune destruction which could ensue. Thus, following tissue damage, there is a local immunosuppression accompanying the release of growth factors into the target tissue. Presumably, the loss of resistence to potential pathogens is off-set, under these conditions, by the benefit of preventing autoimmunity.

Burns and other severe traumatic injury, then, might represent an extreme (and inappropriate) version of this basic mechanism, which was not corrected through selection for the reasons discussed above. Autoreactivity has been described following severe burn (Dobke et al. 1981), and subsequent immunosuppression down regulates this response (Kupper and Green unpublished observations). By our argument, this immunosuppression, due to the severity of the thermal injury and the proposed properties of the immune system, is excessive (and does not contribute to fitness). The prevention of potential autoimmune reactivity becomes irrelevant as compared to the increase in the risk of sepsis due to the immunodepression. Therefore, while reversal of the immune suppression (say, by blocking inhibitory lymphokines) could increase autoreactivity, this is likely to be a relatively minor concern, while the benefits of such reversal will be substantial.

Conclusions

Herein, we have discussed the role of inhibitory T cells in the immunodeficiency which accompanies severe burn injury. While it is inappropriate (and probably incorrect) to conclude that such T cells are the central cause of all of the immune defects which follow thermal trauma, our evidence supports the view that these cells are extremely important in producing those immune defects which increase risk of sepsis after the first week post- burn. Other immune defects, occurring early post-burn, might contribute to the activation of these cells (e.g., prostaglandin production, APC dysfunction, etc.) or may work in parallel to depress immunity.

To investigate the mechanisms by which such inhibitory T cells depress immunity, we generated a T cell hybridoma from murine T cells taken 7 days post-burn, and found that it produced a potent inhibitory lymphokine. This inhibitory lymphokine was capable of suppressing immune responses both in vitro and in vivo, and when injected into normal animals, rendered the recipients sensitive to the induction of lethal sepsis. We are currently addressing the purification and characterization of this inhibitor in order to learn more about its role in thermally-induced immunodeficiency.

We concluded our discussion by addressing a question somewhat off the central theme, and considered why the immune system should be suppressed at a time when it is most needed. These ruminations lead into some interesting areas which may shed light on a number of properties of the immune system which have been somewhat ignored until recently.

The immune system is highly complex, involving many interacting elements and regulatory signals. By focusing on one element, the inhibitory T cell, we hope to gain insight into one small piece of the puzzle of burn-induced immunodeficiency. With enough insight, some of the other pieces may fall into place.

Acknowledgements. This work was supported by MA9950 from the Medical Research Council of Canada. DRG is an Alberta Heritage Scholar.

References

Alexander JW, Wixson D (1970) Neutrophil dysfunction and sepsis in burn injury. Surg Gynecol Obstet 130:431

Altman LC, Furukawa CT, Klebanoff SJ (1977) Depressed mononuclear leukocyte chemotaxis in thermally injured patients. J Immunol 119:199

Aune TM, Webb DR, Pierce CW (1983) Purification and initial characterization of the lymphokine soluble immune response suppressor. J Immunol 131:2848

Baker CC, Miller CL, Trunkey DD (1979) Identity of mononuclear cells which compromise the resistance of trauma patients. J Surg Res 26:478

Bjornson AB, Bjornson HS (1984) Theoretical interrelationships among immunologic and hematologic sequelae of thermal injury. Rev Infect Dis 6:704

Dobke M, Grzybowski J, Zoltowska A, Danowska A (1981) Autoimmune effects of thermal injury. In: Ninneman JL (ed) The immune consequences of thermal injury. Williams and Wilkins, Baltimore, p 150
El Masry MN, Fox EJ, Rich RR (1986) Opposing immunoregulatory functions of $CD8^+$ lymphocytes: a requirement for monocytes in suppressor cell induction. J Immunol 137:2468
Fisher MS, Kripke ML (1982) Suppressor T lymphocytes control the development of primary skin cancers in ultraviolet irradiated mice. Science 216:1133
Gould SJ (1980) The panda's thumb. Norton, New York, pp 19–44
Green DR, Wegmann TG (1986) Beyond the immune system: the immunotrophic role of T cells in organ generation and regulation. Prog Immunol 6:1100
Green DR, Wang N, Zheng H (1987) A suppressor-inducer factor produced by burn trauma-associated T cells. J Burn Care Rehabil 8:521
Kehrl JH, Wakefield LM, Roberts AB, Jakowew S, Alvarez-Mon M, Derynck R, Sporn MB, Fauci AS (1986) The production of TGF-β by human T lymphocytes and its potential role in the regulation of T cell growth. J Exp Med 163:1037
Kupper TS, Green DR (1984) Immunoregulation after thermal injury. J Immunol 133:3047
Kupper TS, Baker CC, Ferguson TA, Green DR (1985a) A burn induced Ly-2 suppressor T cell lowers resistance to bacterial infection. J Surg Res 38:606
Kupper TS, Green DR, Durum SK, Baker CC (1985b) Defective antigen presentation to a cloned T helper cell by macrophages from burned mice can be restored with interleukin-1. Surgery 98:199
Leopardi E, Rosenau W (1984) Production of α-lymphotoxin by human T cell subsets. Cell Immunol 83:73
Letvin NL, Fox IJ, Greene MI, Benacerraf B, Germain RN (1980) Immunologic effects of whole body ultraviolet (UV) irradiation. II. Defect in splenic adherent cell antigen presentation for stimulation of T cell proliferation. J Immunol 125:1402
Miller CL, Clandy BJ (1979) Suppressor T cell activity induced as a result of thermal injury. Cell Immunol 44:201
Munster AM (1976) Post-traumatic immunosuppression is due to activation of T suppressor cells. Lancet I:1329
Munster AM (1984) Immunologic response of trauma and burns, an overview. Am J Med 76:142
Moran K, Munster AM (1987) Alterations of the host defence mechanisms in burned patients. Surg Clin North Am 67:47
Nakamura M, Ogawa H, Tsunematsu T (1986) Isolation and characterization of a monoclonal nonspecific suppressor factor (MNSF) produced by a T cell hybridoma. J Immunol 136:2904
Ozkan AN, Ninnemann JL (1985) Suppression of in vitro lymphocyte and neutrophil responses by a low-molecular wight suppressor active peptide from burn patient sera. J Clin Immunol 5:172
Rogers TJ, Nowowiekjski I, Webb DR (1980) Partial characterization of a prostaglandin-induced suppressor factor. Cell Immunol 50:82
Stieritz DD, Holder IA (1975) Experimental studies of the pathogenesis of infections due to *Pseudomonas aeruginosa*: description of a burned mouse model. J Infect Dis 131:688
Teodorczyk-Injeyan JA, Sparkes BG, Mills GB, Peters WJ, Falk RE (1986) Impairment of T cell activation in burn patients: a possible mechanism of thermal injury-induced immunosuppression. Clin Exp Immunol 65:570
Trinchieri G, Perussia B (1985) Immune interferon: a pleiotropic lymphokine with multiple effects. Immunol Today 6:131
Wolfe JHN, Wu AYO, O'Connor NE, Sapiroschetz I, Mannick JA (1982) Anergy, immunosuppressive serum, and impaired lymphocyte blastogenesis in burn patients. Arch Surg 117:1266
Zapata-Sirvent RL, Hansbrough JF, Bender EM, Bartle EJ, Mansour MA, Carter WH (1986) Postburn immunosuppression in an animal model. IV. Improved resistance to septic challenge with immunomodulating drugs. Surgery 99:53

Macrophage – T-Cell Interactions in Surgical Sepsis

C. C. Baker

Introduction

As surgical and anesthetic management of patients with multiple injuries or those requiring major surgery have improved, the types of problems facing clinicians have changed. A chronicle of this evolution is provided by the various military conflicts in this century. In World Wars I and II, most deaths occurred due to irreversible hemorrhagic shock. In the Korean War, many casualties survived the initial period of shock but developed acute renal failure (ARF) with a mortality of 50% [1]. More rapid transport of injured patients, better management of shock, and the use of dialysis in Vietnam led to a lower incidence of ARF [2]. However, a new complication appeared in the form of adult respiratory distress syndrome (ARDS). Respiratory failure often occurred in patients without thoracic injuries and was associated with a mortality of 50%–60% [3]. Although early aggressive resuscitation of patients in shock and utilization of positive pressure ventilation have decreased the incidence of ARF and ARDS, the mortality for these complications has not changed appreciably in the last ten years [4].

Unfortunately, trauma and major elective surgical patients who now usually survive the early complications of shock, ARF, and ARDS often go on to develop systemic sepsis 3–4 weeks following injury or operation [5]. Sepsis in this setting is often associated with multiple organ failure, carrying a mortality of 65%–75% [6]. While neurologic injury leads to 50% of early deaths following trauma, 75% of the late deaths are secondary to sepsis [7]. Deaths from surgical sepsis are usually related to a breakdown in the patient's immune system that occur for unknown reasons. Since host resistance in early sepsis depends on recognition of antigen (i.e., bacteria) by cells of the monocyte-macrophage lineage, we have recently examined the early phases of sepsis to ascertain the aberrations in macrophage function that lead to subsequent immunosuppression and to follow the time course of these abnormalities.

In recent years there has been an explosion in information regarding the specific immune system – namely bursa equivalent cells (B cells), thymus-derived cells (T cells) and macrophages. It has become increasingly clear that these cells have critical cellular functions [7], that they produce monokines and lymphokines [8], and that they have a critical role in reciprocal regulation by way of these soluble mediators [9]. Some of the studies outlined below were designed to examine these complex interactions as they relate to the problem of surgical sepsis.

Immune Consequences of
Trauma, Shock and Sepsis
Eds. Faist/Ninnemann/Green

The Model

Although antibiotics are of obvious importance in treating systemic sepsis, they are often inadequate in immunocompromised surgical patients after major surgery or trauma. Efforts to predict which patients will develop sepsis have met with variable results. Although work is in progress to evaluate the immunologic abnormalities in trauma patients [4, 10, 11], most of the work on immunosuppression after injury has been performed in animals [12, 13]. Most animal studies of sepsis, including injection of live bacteria [14] or endotoxin [15], are not adequate analogs of human sepsis. Accordingly, the research described in this paper utilizes cecal ligation and puncture (CLP), a clinically relevant animal model of sepsis [16, 17] that may have close parallels to sepsis in humans.

The early phase of sepsis represents a potentially reversible situation; in the late phase of sepsis, however, profound immunosuppression occurs and the host generally dies regardless of therapy. The cardiovascular-hemodynamic patterns of sepsis have been well described in man by MacLean et al. [18] and in the animal model of CLP by Wichterman [17]. In man during the early phases of sepsis, the patient is often in a *hyperdynamic* phase with tachycardia, elevated cardiac output, warm extremities, and decreased peripheral vascular resistance. In the rat and mouse model of CLP, these same findings have been observed [16, 17] and are also associated with piloerection and bacteremia in the 4–6 h period after CLP. During the later phase of sepsis and septic shock in man, there is a *hypodynamic* phase associated with decreased cardiac output, cool extremities, and often increased peripheral vascular resistance [18]. There is a similar cardiovascular response in the rodents we have studied at 18–24 h after CLP, at which time they exhibit apathy, lack of preening and failure to eat or drink [16, 17]. The close correlation between the response patterns to sepsis in man and CLP in the mouse suggests that the latter is a clinically relevant model for studying the various immune abnormalities in sepsis.

Since control of multiple clinical variables is more difficult in humans than in experimental animals, our recent studies in this area have been done in a murine model of CLP [16]. Because endotoxin has been implicated as having a possible role in sepsis, we have chosen to study endotoxin-resistant (C_3H/HeJ) and endotoxin-sensitive (C_3H/HeN) mice with intra-abdominal sepsis produced by CLP. Initial mortality studies are depicted at 24 h (Table 1) and 96 h following CLP (Table 2). These data show a substantially lower mortality for both needle sizes at 96 h in the endotoxin-resistant C_2H/HeJ mice [19].

Table 1. Mortality at 24 h after CLP

Strain	Needle size	
	25 gauge	19 gauge
C_3H/HeN	0%	70% [a]
C_3H/HeJ	0%	10%

[a] Significantly increased versus C_3H/HeJ ($P<0.05$).

Table 2. Mortality at 96 h after CLP

Strain	Needle size	
	25 gauge	19 gauge
C_3H/HeN	45% [a]	100% [a]
C_3H/HeJ	0%	15%

[a] Significantly increased versus C_3H/HeJ ($P<0.05$).

Immunologic Studies

After these initial results, studies were designed to evaluate the successive steps in antigen recognition including macrophage interleukin-1 (IL-1) production, macrophage antigen presentation, and macrophage–T-cell interaction will be assayed using the antigen-specific T cell clone D10.G4.1 as described by Kaye and Janeway [20]. This T helper cell clone allows dissection of the specific steps of antigen recognition and processing and the presentation of antigen to T cells by macrophages. This T helper cell clone will recognize conalbumin as an antigen in the context of I-A^k when the antigen has been properly processed by macrophages which recognize the H-2^k major histocompatibility locus. The various steps involved in this process are complex and have been outlined in detail [21, 22].

The antigen presenting cells (APC) recognize antigen in the presence of Ia on the surface of the macrophage. This complex of Ia plus antigen on the macrophage surface is one of the critical steps in antigen processing and requires recognition of antigen and proper expression of Ia on the surface of the macrophage. The second critical step is the elaboration of IL-1 which, in combination with the Ia-antigen complex, will lead to release of IL-2 by helper T cells. IL-2 production triggers proliferation of the helper T cells that are required for T cell cooperation in antibody production by B cells. Initially, we have attempted to analyze IL-1 production and antigen presentation in the two different mouse strains after CLP. Subsequent studies will be designed to evaluate the various aspects of antigen recognitions.

First, by using fragments of conalbumin digested by cyanogen bromide, the antigen processing step on the surface of the macrophage can be identified as a specific component of antigen recognition. Secondly, measurements of IL-1 levels can be performed easily in this system thereby allowing better understanding of the IL-1 changes in sepsis. Thirdly, utilization of the 3D3 anti-D10 antibody, which replaces the need for expression of Ia on the surface of the macrophage in the T cell activation process, can identify the importance of Ia in this process [21].

Initially, basic immunologic studies were performed in CBA/J mice after CLP. At 17 h after CLP, the animals had a depressed mixed lymphocyte response (32902 versus 85892 for control, $P<0.01$) and antibody forming cell response (864 versus 1600 for control, $P<0.01$) [20].

Recently, we have examined IL-1 production and antigen presentation following CLP in the endotoxin-sensitive C_3H/HeN mice. Macrophage production of

IL-1 was markedly increased to 300% of control 1 h after CLP, fell toward normal by 16 h, peaked again (370% of control) at day 6 after CLP, and then returned to baseline by day 16 after CLP. Antigen presentation paralleled IL-1 for the first 6 days (although in a more tightly restricted fashion). By day 8 after CLP, however, the antigen presentation assay fell to 60% of normal (a significant depression), following the second peak of IL-1. By day 16, antigen presentation had also returned to normal [20].

Discussion

Numerous investigators [23, 24] have pointed out that host resistance to sepsis, especially gram-negative sepsis, is primarily regulated by polymorphonuclear leukocytes and is relatively independent of the specific immune system. Recently, however, Braley-Mullen has suggested that suppressor T cells can regulate the antibody response to bacterial antigen [25]. We have recently shown that suppressor T cells in vivo can even lower host resistance to bacterial infection [26]. It is becoming increasingly clear, from these and other studies, that recognition of bacteria by antigen presenting cells along with the cooperation of T cells in antibody production by B cells are critical to host defense against bacteria. Therefore, a close examination of the immune system may lead to important new insights in our understanding of sepsis.

Since the key initial step in host resistance to sepsis is antigen or bacterial recognition by macrophages, it seems reasonable to study this cell and its function in the early phases of sepsis. Since T cell proliferation is critical to B cell activation and antibody production, it seemed reasonable to hypothesize that macrophage dysfunction or alterations in macrophage–T-cell interaction could be related to the immunosuppression seen after trauma and/or sepsis.

The studies outlined above provide some insight into these areas. First of all, the CLP studies in the C_3H/HeJ and C_3H/HeN mice suggest endotoxin plays a role in the mortality from sepsis in this model since the endotoxin-resistant animals (C_3H/HeJ) had a significantly lower mortality. Interestingly, Rosenstreich has recently shown that C_3H/HeJ animals do not respond to endotoxin, partly because their macrophages fail to produce prostaglandin E_2 (PGE_2) [27]. This finding may correlate with trauma in man since Faist et al. have demonstrated that an increase in macrophage PGE_3 is correlated with a decrease in T cell IL-2 production and IL-2 receptor expression after major trauma [28].

The initial studies of CBA/J mice after CLP suggested major defects in T cell function [MLC) as well as the more global function of antigen processing (APC). It is interesting that CBA/J and C_3H/HeN mice have essentially the same mortality after CLP [16, 19]. When the data on IL-1 and antigen presentation are analyzed for the C_3H/HeN mice, it appears that excessive production of IL-1 by macrophages is followed by a decrease in antigen presentation. Although these data are preliminary and certainly do not prove causality, the possibilities are intriguing. It is possible that excessive levels of IL-1 could down regulate macrophage antigen presenting function. Kupper and Green have previously raised this possibility in some elegant experiments [29], and it has been suggested that defective antigen presentation after thermal injury could lead to the generation of suppressor T cells. Certainly thermal injury, with its destruction of skin and keratinocytes, could lead to a massive outpouring of IL-1 that would fit with this hypothesis. Many more studies will need to be done before these complex issues can be clarified.

Summary

Sepsis has emerged as one of the major challenges to clinicians caring for critically ill and injured patients in the 1980s. Obviously, the factors leading to the syndromes of sepsis and multiple organ failure are complex and multifactorial. Nonetheless, host defenses and the specific immune system appear to play an important role in this scenario. This paper has described the value of using the model of cecal ligation and puncture (CLP) in studying surgical sepsis. Initial studies suggest that endotoxin plays a role in the sepsis following CLP. Immunologic studies have demonstrated defects in T cell and antigen presenting cell function. The latter may be due to excessive production of interleukin 1 (IL-1). Further studies designed to dissect the specific immune response must be performed before definite statements can be made regarding thc pathophysiology of surgical sepsis. Careful studies will be needed before therapeutic maneuvers can be attempted in humans.

References

1. Baxter CR, Zedlitz WH, Shires GT (1964) High output acute renal failure complicating traumatic injury. J Trauma 4:567–572
2. Hardaway RM (1978) Vietnam wound analysis. J Trauma 18:635–643
3. Blaisdell FW, Lewis FR Jr (1977) Recognition of the respiratory distress syndrome of shock and trauma: historical aspects. In: Blaisdell FW, Lewis FR Jr (eds) Respiratory distress syndrome of shock and trauma. Saunders, Philadelphia, pp 1–8
4. O'Mahoney JB, Palder S, Rodrick M et al. (1984) Depression of cellular immunity after multiple trauma in the absence of sepsis. J Trauma 24:869–875
5. Miller SE, Miller CL, Trunkey DD (1982) The immune consequences of trauma. Surg Clin North Am 62:167–182
6. Baker CC, Degutis LC, DeSantis JG, Baue AE (1985) The impact of a trauma service in a university hospital. Am J Surg 149:453–458
7. Bendtzen K, Petersen J (1984) Role of interleukin-1 in antigen induced lymphokine production. Cell Immunol 83:101–106
8. Dinarello CA (1984) Interleukin-1. Rev Infect Dis 6:51–95
9. Beller DI, Unanue ER (1982) Reciprocal regulation of macrophage and T cell function by way of soluble mediators. In: Pick E, Mizel S (eds) Lymphokines, vol 6, pp 25–36
10. Baker CC, Miller CL, Trunkey DD (1979) Identity of mononuclear cells which compromise the resistance of trauma patients. J Surg Res 26:478–487
11. Antonacci AC, Calvano SE, Reaves LE, Prajapati A, Bockman R, Walte K, Mertelsman R, Gupta S, Good RA, Shires GT (1984) Autologous and allogeneic mixed lymphocyte responses following thermal injury in man: the immunomodulatory effects of Interleukin 1, Interleukin 2, and a prostaglandin inhibitor. Clin Immunol Immunopathol 30:304–320

12. Kupper TS, Green DR, Chaudry IH et al. (1984) A cyclophosphamide sensitive suppressor T cell circuit induced by thermal injury. Surgery 95:679–706
13. Wang BS, Heacock EH, Wu AVO, Mannick JA (1980) Generation of suppressor cells in mice after surgical trauma. J Clin Invest 66:200–209
14. Hinshaw LB, Beller BK, Archer LT, Flourney DJ, White GL, Phillips RW (1974) Recovery from lethal *Escherichia coli* shock in dogs. Surg Gynecol Obstet 139:851–856
15. Hardaway RM III (1980) Endotoxemic shock. Dis Colon Rectum 24:597–604
16. Baker CC, Chaudry IH, Gaines HO, Baue AE (1983) Evaluation of factors affecting mortality following sepsis in a murine cecal ligation and puncture model. Surgery 94:331–335
17. Wichterman KA, Baue AE, Chaudry IH (1980) Sepsis and septic shock – a review of laboratory models and a proposal. J Surg Res 29:189–201
18. MacLean RD, Mulligan WG, McLean APH, Duff JW (1967) Patterns of systemic shock in man – a detailed study of 56 patients. Ann Surg 166:543–562
19. Baker CC, Kupper TS (1985) Clarification of the role of endotoxin in intra-abdominal and systemic sepsis. Surg Forum 36:68–70
20. Baker CC, Yamada AH, Faist E, Kupper TS (1987) Interleukin-1 and T cell function following injury. J Burn Care Rehabil 8:503–508
21. Kaye J, Porcelli JT, Jones B, Janeway CA Jr (1983) Both a monoclonal antibody and antisera specific for determinants unique to individual cloned helper T cells can substitute for antigen and antigen presenting cells in the activation of T cells. J Exp Med 158:836–856
22. Kaye J, Gillis S, Mizel SB, Shevark EM, Malek TR, Dinarello CA, Lachman LB, Janeway CA (1984) Growth of a cloned T cell line induced by monoclonal antibody specific for the antigen receptor: Interleukin 1 is required for the expression of receptors to Interleukin 2. J Immunol 133:1339–1345
23. Alexander JW (1972) Host defense mechanisms against infection. Surg Clin North Am 52:1367–1378
24. Meakins JL et al. (1978) Delayed hypersensitivity and neutrophil chemotaxis: effect of trauma. J Trauma 18:240–247
25. Braley-Mullen H (1983) Activation of type III pneumococcal polysaccharide specific suppressor T cells in mice. J Immunol 131:2190–2198
26. Kupper TS, Baker CC, Ferguson TA, Green DR (1985) Burn induced Ly-2 suppressor T cell lower resistance to bacterial infection. J Surg Res 38:606–612
27. Rosenstreich DL, Globe LM, Wahl LM et al. (1977) Analysis of the cellular defects of endotoxin-unresponsive C_3H/HeJ mice. In: Schlessinger D (ed) Microbiology. American Society of Microbiology, Washington DC, pp 314–320
28. Faist E, Mewes A, Baker CC, Strasser T, Alkan SS, Rieber P, Heberer G (1987) Prostaglandin E_2 (PGE_2) dependent suppression of IL-2 production in patients with major trauma. J Trauma 27:837–848
29. Kupper TS, Green DR (1985) In vivo exposure to IL-1 or ETAF causes loss of antigen-presenting cell function. Br J Rheumatol 24 [Suppl 1]:98–101

The Relationship Between T Cells and Interleukin 1

S. K. Durum, K. Muegge, F. Aiello, and L. Takacs

Introduction

Interleukin 1 (IL1) has a broad range of effects on a variety of target cells, such that it has been rediscovered a number of times (reviewed in Durum et al. 1985). The immunological discovery of IL1 (Gery et al. 1972) was based on its ability to induce proliferation of T cells, namely thymocytes, in the presence of a co-mitogenic stimulus. This review will focus on the relationship between T cells and IL1.

Is IL1 Really Required for T-cell Activation?

It would seem that the effect of IL1 on T cells would be well understood by now, nearly twenty years after the thymocyte effect of IL1 was observed. Some of the most dramatic IL1 effects, in fact the standard bioassays for IL1, involve effects on T cells: thymocyte comitogenesis, comitogenesis of the D10 line, and IL2 induction in the LBRM33-1A5 thymoma.

Several years ago, various groups proposed that during physiological immune responses, IL1 played a role in the activation of T cells: antigen-presenting cells (APC) provide IL1 to T cells, along with processed antigen and Ia on the APC surface (Smith et al. 1980; Shaw et al. 1980; Larsson et al. 1980). There are a number of subsequent studies that support this model (deFreitas et al. 1983; Scala and Oppenheim 1983; Williams et al. 1985; Kurt-Jones et al. 1985; Chu et al. 1985). Our own studies on this subject have used murine T-cell clones; the surprising result was that many of these clones produced their own IL1 and utilized it as an autocrine growth factor (Tartakovsky et al. 1986; Durum et al. 1987, 1988), and this will be discussed further. But there are also studies that fail to find any requirement for IL1 in T-cell activation (Malek et al. 1985). In a recent commentary Dr. Steven Mizel, who has made many contributions to IL1 research, directly challenged the theory that IL1 was required for T-cell activation (Mizel 1987). In this study, anti-IL1 antiserum failed to block normal T-cell proliferation. However, this failure could be due to IL1 being inaccessible to the antibodies, for example at the synapse between T cell and APC – a comparable failure is usually experienced in trying to block T-cell recognition of antigenic peptides. It is clear that the T-cell recognizes these peptides but, nevertheless, it is very difficult to block recognition with antibodies. Therefore, blocking IL1 production with antisense oligonucleotides may inhibit T-cell activation when antibodies fail. In sum-

Immune Consequences of
Trauma, Shock and Sepsis
Eds. Faist/Ninnemann/Green

mary, there is evidence for and against IL1 performing essential functions during antigen presentation.

Why is this a significant question? The AIDS epidemic has reminded us all that the ability of T cells to initiate immune responses is essential to life. Toward the understanding of T-cell activation, immense effort has been focused on the antigen-receptor apparatus, and at the later event of IL2 action, while little is understood of other signals that T cells require from APC. In the ensuing discussion, we will outline our own studies concerning the relationship of IL1 to T cell clones, hybrids, and normal T cells.

Clones

T-cell clones are nontransformed cells maintained in vitro by continuous restimulation with antigen and APC. We tested whether T-cell clones needed IL1 from APC. We began the analysis with the murine T-cell clone D10. It seemed likely that D10 would require IL1 from APC, since D10 unequivocally recognized IL1 as a comitogenic signal along with antigen receptor cross-linking by antibody. We tested whether D10 required IL1 from an APC while the latter presented the appropriate nominal antigen or alloantigen. We concluded that the APC did not have to provide IL1 to D10, because, surprisingly, D10 produced its own IL1 during this interaction (Tartakovsky et al. 1986).

We then tested a large panel of murine T-cell clones and concluded that most of them produced IL1. IL1-alpha mRNA was detected in T-cell clones by northern analysis and by in-situ hybridization. Mosmann et al. (1986) have grouped T-cell clones into type I or II, depending on the lymphokines produced; however, in collaboration with T. Mosmann, we detected IL1 mRNA in both groups. The IL1 produced by T-cell clones reacted with antimurine IL1-alpha antiserum. Most importantly, anti-IL1-alpha antiserum blocked proliferation of several T-cell clones when stimulated by a type of APC that did not produce IL1 (B cells). We concluded therefore that IL1 was produced by T-cell clones and served an autocrine role (Tartakovsky et al. 1986; Durum et al. 1987; Durum et al. 1988; Ozaki et al. 1988; Tartakovsky et al., submitted; Muegge et al., submitted).

T-cell Hybrids

In addition to T-cell clones, discussed above, the other type of homogeneous antigen-specific T cell is the hybrid, created by fusing in vivo primed T cells with BW5147, a hypoxanthine aminopterin thymidine (HAT)-sensitive thymoma. T-cell hybrids produce IL2 following antigen presentation; however it was already clear that T-cell hybrids could not require exogenous IL1 from an APC, since artificial membranes containing Ia and antigen were a sufficient stimulus (Watts et al. 1984).

We tested the possibility that T-cell hybrids produced their own IL1 as do T-cell clones (discussed above). Initially, a panel of four hybrids were obtained from R. Chesnut and H. Grey: two were specific for ovalbumin plus IA^d, one for allo-IE^d, and one for auto-IA^d. None produced detectable IL1 biological activity when stimulated either with APC or with ConA, and thus these hybrids were different from most clones. Then, S. Ozaki and J. Berzofsky developed a technique for producing T-cell hybrids from T-cell clones; they produced two such hybrids and demonstrated that they preserved the antigen specificities (myoglobin plus IA^d) of the parent clones. We therefore had the opportunity to compare IL1 production by hybrids with that of their parent clones. In both cases, the parent clone produced IL1 activity, but the hybrid did not. We tested the possibility that the IL1 gene, active in the parent clones, was suppressed in hybrids; the hybrid "C7" was analyzed for the production of IL1 mRNA. The surprising result was that hybrid C7 produced IL1-alpha mRNA but apparently did not translate it, since we could not detect IL1 protein by immunoprecipitation and SDS-PAGE (or by biological activity as noted above). The presence of IL1 mRNA, without protein, is provocative and could indicate a potentially important control of IL1 production at the translational level. However, it is equally possible that the IL1 mRNA present in hybrid C7 is defective. We conclude that T-cell hybrids neither acquire IL1 from APC, nor do they produce active IL1 [Ozaki et al. 1988; Muegge et al., submitted).

Normal T Cells

Since many T-cell clones produce IL1, and clones are generally taken to be representative of normal T cells, it seems likely that normal T cells can produce IL1. However, from our studies, the frequency must be very low, since we could not detect IL1 in T cells stimulated for a short-term in a variety of ways in vivo or in vitro. However, T cells from antigen-primed lymphnodes began to produce detectable IL1 activity after 3 days of antigen restimulation in vitro, and this was quite strong by 2 weeks. The most likely explanation is that antigen stimulation induces proliferation of infrequent T cells that are capable of continuous growth in vitro, and that many such T cells produce IL1.

To determine how frequent IL1-producing T cells are in vivo, we developed an in situ hybridization technique for tissue sections to visualize cells producing IL1 mRNA. Histologically, the results show that the highest concentration of IL1 mRNA producing cells is contained in the same general location as T cells in spleen, lymphnodes and thymus (Takacs et al., submitted); whether some of these cells are actually T cells remains to be determined and awaits our developing a technique for antibody staining of these sections that is compatible with in situ hybridization. Do normal T cells require IL1, either from APC or as an autocrine? Unfortunately, the supply of antimurine IL1 antisera has been too limited for us to test this. In the future new antibodies and other techniques will be used to approach this important question.

We have preliminary data on one such technique: use of antisense-IL1 oligonucleotides to block IL1 production. In collaboration with W. Farrar and A. Bellan, we have constructed antisense oligonucleotides against several of the cytokines, including murine IL1-alpha, and tested the ability of these oligonucleotides to block production of the relevant cytokine. An antisense-IL1-alpha, 20mer in length, appears to block the majority of new IL1 production by murine macrophages, whereas a nonsense 20mer does not block; this technique is therefore promising as a means of answering whether IL1 is essential to T-cell activation. We conclude that normal T cells producing IL1, though rare, probably exist in vivo, since they appear fairly rapidly in culture; whether IL1 is required for normal T-cell activation remains to be tested.

What Does IL1 Do to the T Cell?

As an extension of the first question (whether IL1 is really required for T-cell activation), it is quite unclear *how* IL1 acts on those types of T cells that show unequivocal IL1 effects. It is generally observed that IL1 acts as a second signal on T cells, i.e., together with PHA on thymocytes or LBRM (model T cells), and with antigen-receptor cross-linking on D10. Based on this "costimulator" property, there are two broad possible mechanisms: first, that IL1 simply amplifies a signal from the T-cell antigen receptor complex; second, that IL1 delivers its own unique second signal. There are very few published data on the subject of how IL1 acts on model T cells. The first step involves binding to membrane receptors. Some model T cells have as many as 20000 binding sites (Bron and MacDonald 1987), but it is clear that a very low number of sites is sufficient: we estimated less than 100 sites were present on D10, an extremely IL1-sensitive T cell (Akahoshi and Durum, unpublished).

It was initially proposed that IL1 induces IL2 production in normal T cells (Smith et al. 1980; Shaw et al. 1980; Larsson et al. 1980); this is no longer considered a general mechanism, although two model T cells, LBRM and EL4, react in this way. Further, some data have appeared, suggesting that IL1 induces receptors for IL2 on D10 (Kaye and Janeway 1984) (although this is now known to be unrelated to proliferation of this cell which uses IL4 rather than IL2), and on thymocytes (Mannel et al. 1985).

Postreceptor events have been sought, but little positive data have been published. Abraham et al. (1987) failed to detect effects on phospoinositide metabolism or intracelllar Ca^{2+}. We have failed to observe IL1 effects on cAMP levels in D10 (Elliot and Durum, unpublished). P. Simon has also failed to detect typical second messengers in EL4, but has recently observed a very early release of linoleic acid from EL4 membranes, suggesting that IL1 activates a phospholipase (Simon et al. 1987). Some reports have also implicated arachidonate metabolites in IL1-induced comitogenesis of thymocytes (Dinarello et al. 1983; Farrar and Humes 1985). We observed a sharp increase in ornithine decarboxylase (ODC) activity 18 h following the action of IL1 on D10; however the same increase was observed following IL2 treatment of this cell line, meaning that ODC activation is a late event common to mitogenic stimuli of this cell, rather than being a unique IL1 signal (Endo and Durum, unpublished). Mizel observed that IL1 was internalized by T cells and moved to the nucleus (Mizel 1987). Considering this nuclear localization together with our observation that D10 produced high levels of intracellular IL1, we tested a possible intracellular role for internalized IL1 in T cells. We have microinjected IL1 into D10, but have thus far failed to detect a mitogenic action (Smith and Durum, unpublished).

At the mRNA level, IL1 was observed to induce c-myc expression in D10 (Kovacs et al. 1986). However, it is not clear whether myc proteins are necessary or sufficient for the IL1 proliferative effect in D10. In LBRM, IL1 increased mRNA levels of several species either alone or together with PHA (Hagiwara et al. 1987).

How Does IL1 Affect the APC?

The effects of IL1 on APC are just beginning to be evaluated. It was reported that in vivo injections of relatively crude IL1 preparations caused a down-regulation of APC function (Kupper et al. 1985). However, Koide et al. (1987) have recently made the provocative observation that pure IL1 is able to induce dendritic cells, which are already efficient APC, to become even more effective in stimulating T-cell proliferation. This effect appeared to be mediated through more efficient binding of T cells to dendritic cells. Perhaps the binding of T cells was enhanced by IL1 because cell adhesion molecules were induced on dendritic cells; indeed, IL1 has been reported to induce ICAM-1 on endothelial cells (Dustin et al. 1986), and ICAM-1 is an adhesion molecule on non-T cells that bridges to LFA-1 on T cells (Makgoba et al. 1988).

Our own studies indicate powerful positive effects of IL1 on APC. Our studies developed from the recent observation of others that treating APC with the cross-linking agent carbodiimide (ECDI) changed their properties: ECDI-fixed APC did not induce proliferation of T-cell clones, but rather, they induced tolerance (Jenkins and Schwartz 1987). While these results appeared to indicate that ECDI was destroying some essential property of the APC, our data suggest that the actual effect of ECDI is to prevent essential new structures from appearing on the APC during the interaction with T cells. Our evidence for this is that ECDI-fixed APC are perfectly capable of presenting antigen to a T-cell clone if the APC have been previously treated with IL1; we interpret this to mean that IL1 induces the appearance of new membrane structures on the APC. We observed that for both the nominal and alloantigens. ECDI treatment completely abolished APC function, whereas treating the APC with IL1 prior to ECDI fixation apparently induced the appearance of structures that are essential for presenting antigen to this T cell clone (D10, G4.1). For the purposes of discussion, we have coined the term "inducible membrane accessory structures" or "IMAS."

IMAS induction by recombinant murine IL1 (10 μ/ml) occurs within 6 h of incubation and is dependent on temperature (37 °C but not 4 °C) and protein synthesis (blocked by cycloheximide). IMAS was not replaced by any soluble mediators we have tried, including IL1 itself, IL2, IL4 or crude conditioned media. The failure of IL1 itself to replace the IL1-induced structures argues against membrane IL1 being the minimal IMAS and, moreover, we failed to detect membrane IL1 following treatment of APC with soluble IL1. Increased density of Ia on APC could not be detected following IL1-treatment (Aiello et al., submitted). Thus, we do not feel that IMAS is either membrane IL1 or increased Ia. Good candidates for IMAS would be cell adhesion molecules. ICAM-1 is one such adhesion molecule which is present on some types of APC and it binds to its ligand, LFA-1 on T cells. ICAM-1 is induced by IL1 in endothelial cells (Dustin et al. 1986) and is a reasonable candidate for IMAS, the IL-induced structure on APC in our system. But IMAS could also be a novel membrane adhesion molecule, or possibly a stimulating structure (rather than an adhesion molecule) present on APC.

The significance of the preceding observations is that IL1 may perform an essential role in preparing APC to interact with T cells. Our objective is to identify IL1-induced structures on APC, and in doing so, we would hope to generate strategies for controlling T-cell activation and immune tolerance. For example, since IL1-induced structures are essential to activating our model T-cell clone, antibodies blocking these structures should block T-cell activation, and may induce tolerance in vivo.

How Is IL1 Induced during an Immune Response?

It is important to determine the mechanism of IL1 induction during immune responses. IL1 is not a constitutive product of macrophages, or probably of most other cells. Thus, for IL1 to serve its various roles in immune responses, it would need to be induced. We have recently analyzed a large number of murine tissues for IL1 gene expression by in situ hybridization; we concluded that the highest levels in the body occur in lymphoid organs at sites that contain T cells (Takacs et al., submitted). The mechanism of IL1-induction should be investigated as a facet of understanding and potentially regulating the immune response. An important pathological aspect of the IL1-induction process is the etiology of chronic inflammatory diseases, especially rheumatoid arthritis. In this disease, IL1 is present in synovial fluid, and widely believed to contribute to many of the pathological features, including bone erosion and growth of pannus. This is a disease with an autoimmune component, and it is therefore possible that a local immune reaction continually induces IL1.

Two mechanisms have been described for T-cell induction of IL1 production by accessory cells. One mechanism involves cell contact, is restricted by class II molecules, and anti-class II antibodies block the induction (Farr et al. 1977; Durum and Gershon 1982; Durum et al. 1984). A second mechanism involves a soluble mediator produced by the T cell, which then activates macrophages to produce IL1. Our efforts will focus on the latter mechanism involving a lymphokine. This possibility was probably first suggested by Atkins et al. (1972) as a mechanism for inducing "endogenous pyrogen," one of the activities of IL1, and was also observed by others over the years (Meltzer and Oppenheim 1977) and a biochemical characterization was initiated (Dinarello and Kent 1985).

Recently, our laboratory (Takacs et al. 1987) and another (Weaver and Unanue 1986) described soluble factors produced by murine T-cell clones that induced IL1 production by macrophages. Our laboratory, in collaboration with that of J. Bersofsky, analyzed a panel of nine murine T-cell clones specific for various myoglobin peptides. Two clones induced exceptionally high levels of IL1 from a heterogeneous splenic APC population. These two clones were unusual, and distinct from others in the panel, in that they were restricted to myoglobin in association with a low responder type Ia (IE^k). One of the clones, abbreviated "3.2," was selected for further study as to mechanism of IL1 induction. Clone 3.2 induced detectable levels of IL1 after 4 h of contact with splenic APC. This induction process was antigen dependent, MHC restricted, and radioresistant on the part of both T-cell and IL1-producing cell. IL1-induction was attributable to a soluble mediator produced by the activated T-cell clone, this mediator then subsequently induced IL1-production by macrophages.

This IL1-inducing lymphokine produced by clone 3.2 was distinct from interferon-gamma, colony stimulating factor 1 (CSF-1), IL1, and tumor necrosis factor (TNF) as described by Takacs et al. (1987), and IL2 and IL3 were later tested and showed no activity in this system. Biochemical characterization of the activity showed the major activity was approximately 5 kd witha pI of 8. We aimed to characterize this lymphokine further. Clone 3.2, though it stably produced the lymphokine, could not be grown in large quantities, since, typical of T-cell clones, it replicated slowly and required antigen presenting cells. We therefore produced T-cell hybridomas, which grow rapidly and require no feeders. Hybridomas were produced by fusing with HAT-sensitive, mycoplasma-free BW5147. Fusions were performed with clone 3.2. A second group of hybrids was produced with lymph-node cells from (C3H × BALB/c)F_1 mice primed seven days in vivo with sperm whale myoglobin, and restimulated two days in vitro. From a group of ten hybrids made from clone 3.2 and 52 hybrids made from lymph node cells, one lymph node hybrid was selected for further study because it produced the highest titers of IL1-inducing factor. This hybrid was designated "LN420." Current efforts are directed at cDNA cloning the lymphokine.

References

Abraham RT, Ho SN, Barna TJ, McKean DJ (1987) Transmembrane signalling during interleukin-1 dependent T cell activation. Interaction of signal 1- and signal 2-type mediators with the phosphoinositide-dependent signal transduction mechanism. J Biol Chem 262:2719

Atkins E, Feldman JD, Francis L, Hursh E (1972) Studies on the mechanisms of fever accompaying delayed hypersensitivity: the role of the sensitized lymphocyte. J Exp Med 135:1113

Bron C, MacDonald HR (1987) Identification of the plasma membrane receptor for interleukin 1 on mouse thymoma cells. FEBS Lett 219:365–368

Chu ET, Lareau M, Rosenwasser LJ, Dinarello CA, Geha RS (1985) Antigen presentation by EBV-B cells to resting and activated T cells: role of interleukin 1. J Immunol 134:1676–1681

deFreitas EC, Chesnut RW, Grey HM, Chiller JM (1983) Macrophage-dependent activation of antigen-specific T cells requires antigen and a soluble monokine. J Immunol 131:23–29

Dinarello CA, Kent EF (1985) Chemical characterization of an interleukin 1-inducing substance derived from human mixed leukocyte reactions: IL1 inducing substance is not gamma interferon. Yale J Biol Med 58:101

Dinarello CA, Marnoy SO, Rosenwasser LJ (1983) Role of arachidonate metabolism in the immunoregulatory function of human leukocyte pyrogen/lymphocyte-activating factor/interleukin 1. J Immunol 130:890

Durum SK, Gershon RK (1982) Interleukin 1 can replace the requirement for I-A-positive cells in the proliferation of antigen-primed T cells. Proc Natl Acad Sci USA 79:4747

Durum SK, Higuchi CA, Ron Y (1984) Accessory cells and T cell activation. The relationship between two components of accessory cell function: Ia and IL1. Immunobiology 168:123

Durum SK, Schmidt JA, Oppenheim JJ (1985) Interleukin 1: an immunological perspective. Annu Rev Immunol 3:263
Durum SK, Brody DT, Tartakovsky B (1987) IL1 as a selfserving principle in T cell clones. In: Cavaillon JM, Haeffner-Cavaillon N (eds) Forum on interleukin-1. Ann Pasteur Inst 38:469–472
Durum SK, Finnegan A, Brody DT, Kovacs EJ, Smith MR, Berzofsky JA, Young HA, Tartakovsky B (1988) T cell interleukin 1. In: Webb DR, Pierce CW, Cohen S (eds) Molecular basis of lymphokine action. Humana, Clifton, pp 117–122
Dustin ML, Rothlein R, Bhan AK, Dinarello CA, Springer TA (1986) Induction by IL1 and interferon-gamma: tissue distribution, biochemistry, and function of a natural adherence molecule (ICAM-1). J Immunol 137:245
Farr AG, Dorf ME, Unanue ER (1977) Secretion of mediators following T lymphocyte-macrophage interaction is regulated by the major histocompatibility complex. Proc Natl Acad Sci USA 72:3542
Farrar WL, Humes JL (1985) The role of arachidonic acid metabolism in the activities of interleukin 1 and 2. J Immunol 135:1153–1159
Gery I, Gershon RK, Waksman BH (1972) Potentiation of the T lymphocyte response to mitogens. I. The responding cell. J Exp Med 136:128–138
Hagiwara J, Huang JS, Arai N, Herzenbeng LA, Arai K, Zlotnik A (1987) Interleukin 1 modulates messenger RNA levels of lymphokines and of other molecules associated with T cell activation in the T cell lymphoma LBRM33-1A5. J Immunol 138:2514–2519
Jenkins MK, Schwartz RH (1987) Antigen presentation by chemically modified splenocytes induces antigen-specific T cell unresponsiveness in vitro and vivo. J Exp Med 165:302
Kaye J, Janeway CA (1984) Induction of receptors for interleukin 2 requires T cell Ag: Ia receptor crosslinking and interleukin 1. Lymphokine Res 3:175–182
Koide SL, Inaba K, Steinman RM (1987) Interleukin 1 enhances T-dependent immune responses by amplifying the function of dendritic cells. J Exp Med 165:515
Kovacs EJ, Oppenheim JJ, Young HA (1986) Induction of c-fos and c-myc expression in T lymphocytes after treatment with redombinant interleukin 1-alpha. J Immunol 137:3649
Kupper TS, Green DR, Durum SK, Baker CC (1985) Defective antigen presentation to a cloned T helper cell by macrophages from burned mice can be restored with interleukin 1. Surgery 98:199–206
Kurt-Jones EA, Beller DI, Mizel SB, Unanue ER (1985) Identification of a membrane-associated interleukin 1 in macrophages. Proc Natl Acad Sci USA 82:1204–1208
Larsson E, Iscove NN, Coutinho A (1980) Two distinct factors are required for induction of T cell growth. Nature 283:664
Makgoba MW, Sanders ME, Ginther Luce GE, Dustin ML, Springer TA, Clark EA, Mannoni P, Shaw S (1988) ICAM-1 a ligand for LFA-1-dependent adhesion of B, T and myeloid cells. Nature 331:86–88
Malek TR, Schmidt JA, Shevach EM (1985) The murine IL2 receptor. III. Cellular requirements for the induction of IL2 receptor expression on T cell subpopulations. J Immunol 136:2405
Mannel DN, Mizel SB, Diamanstein T, Falk W (1985) Induction of interleukin 2 responsiveness in thymocytes by synergistic action of interleukin 1 and interleukin 2. J Immunol 134:3108
Meltzer M, Oppenheim JJ (1977) Bidirectional amplification of macrophage-lymphocyte interactions: enhanced lymphocyte activation factor production by activated mouse peritoneal cells. J Immunol 118:77
Mizel SB (1987) Interleukin 1 and T cell activation. Immunol Today 8:330–332
Mosmann TR, Cherwinsky H, Bond MW, Giedlin MA, Coffman RL (1986) Two types of murine helper T cell clone. I. Definition according to profiles of lymphokine activities and secreted proteins. J Immunol 136:2348–2357
Ozaki S, York-Jolley J, Durum SK, Muegge K, Berzofsky JA (1988) Production of T-T hybrids from T cell clones: direct comparison between cloned T cells and T hybridoma cells derived from them. J Immunol (In press)

Scala G, Oppenheim JJ (1983) Antigen presentation by human monocytes: evidence for stimulant processing and requirement for interleukin 1. J Immunol 131:1160–1166
Shaw J, Caplan B, Paetkau V, Pilarski LM, Delovitch TL, McKenzie FC (1980) Cellular origins of co-stimulator (IL2) and its activity in cytotoxic T lymphocyte responses. J Immunol 124:2231
Simon PL, Clark MC, Henderson LS, Kassis S (1987) Interleukin-1-stimulated EL-4 cells release linoleic acid, which augments translocation of protein kinase C and production of interleukin-2. (abstract) J Leukocyte Biol 42:580
Smith KA, Lachman LB, Oppenheim JJ, Favata MF (1980) The functional relationship of the interleukins. J Exp Med 151:1551
Takacs L, Berzofsky JA, York-Jolley J, Akahoshi T, Blasi E, Durum SK (1987) IL-1 induction by murine T cell clones: detection of an IL-1 inducing lymphokine. J Immunol 138:2124
Tartakovsky B, Kovacs EJ, Takacs L, Durum SK (1986) T cell clone producing an IL1-like activity after stimulation by antigen-presenting B cells. J Immunol 137:160–166
Watts TA, Brian AA, Kappler JW, Marrack P, McConnell JM (1984) Antigen-presentation by supported planar membranes containing affinity-purified I-A^d. Proc Natl Acad Sci USA 81:7564
Weaver KC, Unanue ER (1986) T cell induction of membrane IL-1 on macrophages. J Immunol 137:3868
Williams JM, deLoria D, Hansen JA, Dinarello CA, Loertscher R, Shapiro HM, Strom TB (1985) The events of primary T cell activation can be staged by use of sepharose-bound anti-T3 (64.1) monoclonal antibody and purified interleukin 1. J Immunol 135:2249–2255

Trauma-Induced Alterations of the Lymphokine Cascade

E. Faist, W. Ertel, A. Mewes, S. Alkan, A. Walz, and T. Strasser

Introduction

With increasing knowledge about the fundamental importance of cytokines for the regulation of almost all immune responses, new avenues for the better understanding of trauma-induced alterations of cell-mediated immune response mechanisms have been made accessible. The biochemical and biological characterization of mediators and the resulting possibilities for their species-specific recombination were preconditions for the availability and the feasibility of reproducible studies of mediator behavior in pathological states of hemorrhagic shock and trauma.

Mainly because of the above reasons, the amount of work dealing with trauma-induced quantitive and qualitative alterations of immunomediators has been rather limited until recently. Wood et al. were the first investigators to report in 1984 about the altered in vitro synthesis of interleukins 1 and 2 (IL-1, IL-2) in patients with burn trauma [37]. In the supernatants of peripheral blood mononuclear cell (PBMC) cultures they found a persistent reduction of measurable IL-2, the degree of which was proportional to the severity of the burn trauma sustained.

Among the multitude of defects in cell-mediated immunity (CMI) induced by mechanical and burn trauma, the depression of IL-2 synthesis is a major and consistently reported dysfunction [1, 2, 9, 37]. A lymphokine released by T lymphocytes after appropriate stimulation, IL-2 is essential for the development of proliferative T cell responses to antigenic and mitogenic stimuli. Inability to synthesize adequate amounts of IL-2 has been suggested to be the basis of defective T cell function following major trauma with the subsequent development of sepsis [3].

The Lymphokine Cascade

Studies on the mechanism of IL-2 production have shown that the monocyte/T cell interaction via the monokine IL-1 is an absolute requirement for IL-2 synthesis [12].

The initiation of cellular and humoral immune responses following antigen contact involves the interaction of the monocyte (Mø) as an antigen-presenting and antigen-processing cell with the T helper (T_H) cell as the pacemaker of T- and B-effector lymphocytes. This process involves a specific sequence of cellular ac-

Immune Consequences of
Trauma, Shock and Sepsis
Eds. Faist/Ninnemann/Green

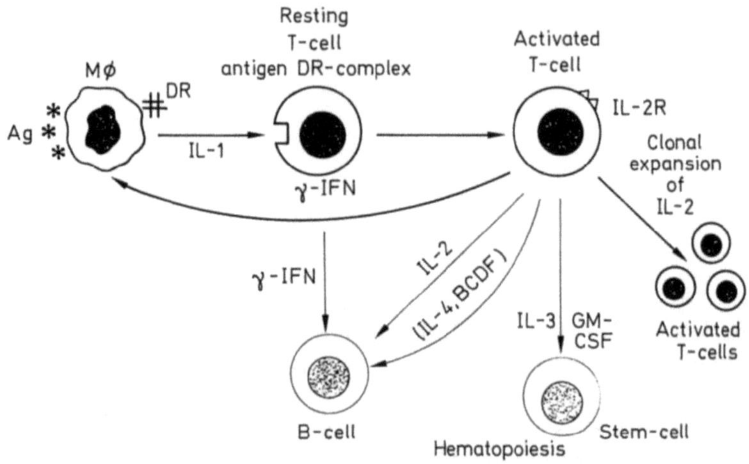

Fig. 1. A model of the lymphokine-induced interactions of antigen-presenting monocytes and lymphocytes

tions and functionally different unspecific cytokine mediators. Several levels of control are necessary for the successful development of an immune response of that kind (Fig. 1).

1. Synthesis and release of IL-1 from Mø [24].
2. The interaction of IL-1- with IL-2-synthetizing cells. This step, as mentioned above, is the precondition for IL-2 release and requires intact Mø function.
3. IL-2 synthesis from T_H cells. Adequate IL-2 release is dependent on the presence of a sufficient number of functionally intact T_H cells.
4. The interaction of IL-2- with IL-2-sensitive responder cells. During this phase, an equivalent number of intact T-effector cells, cell function and capacity of IL-2 receptors, or TAC is required.

Within this cascade-like circuit of forward regulation of specific immune response mechanisms, continuous macrophage participation can only be sustained via lymphokine production by activated T cells, predominantly by interferon-γ (IFN-γ), which is identical to macrophage-activating factor (MAF). Besides its feedback effect on the Mø, synergistically with IL-2, IFN-γ is also an important factor in inducing proliferation and maturation of active cytotoxic T cells [35].

There are also synergistic interactions directed towards adequate B-cell function between IL-2 and other lymphokines like B-cell growth factor (BCGF), B-cell stimulating factor (IL-4) or T-cell replacing factor (TRF) [16, 19, 20, 33, 34].

Macrophages play a central role in CMI [30], exercising powerful regulatory influences over immune responses in the form of both help and suppression. Antigen-presenting cells mediate antigen processing, expression of cell surface class II glycoprotein (Ia antigen), and elaboration of IL-1 [21]. Each of these processes is required for successful antigen-specific activation of the T_H cells and subsequent release of IL-2, which is central to so many immune functions. Green and coworkers have shown that defective antigen presentation by macrophages may preferentially activate the T-suppressor cell pathways [18].

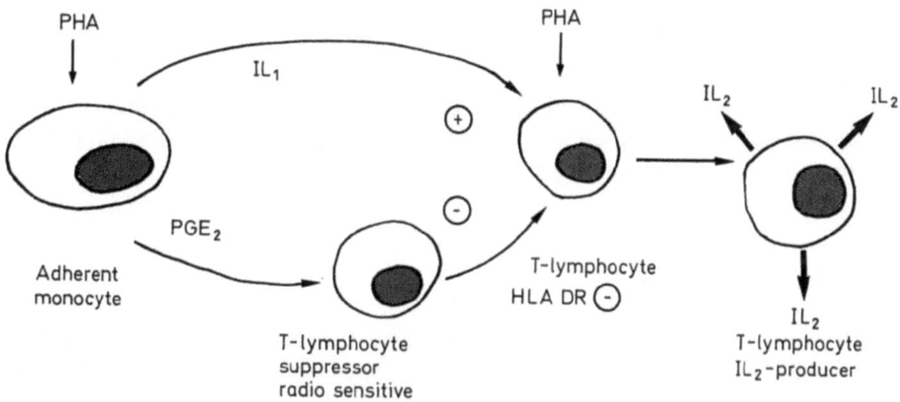

Fig. 2. A model of the regulatory pathways of IL-2 production in humans

The macrophage exerts its inhibitory function on the immune response via secretion of prostaglandins (PG) of the E series [14, 29]. Chouhaib and colleagues developed a most interesting model describing the negative control of human IL-2 production [7, 8]. Their hypothesis was that IL-2 synthesis is regulated through the release of inhibitory mediators from the monocyte, one of which is PGE_2. They postulated that these inhibitory monokines do not interact directly with IL-2-producing T cells, but rather activate a radiosensitive subset of T cells, with some of these precursors expressing CD8+ and others the CD4+ antigen. When the radiosensitive T cell has been activated by PGE_2 it becomes radioresistant and expresses the CD4+ phenotype exclusively. IL-2-producing T cells are then inhibited by direct cell to cell contact (Fig. 2).

This model seemed to be most intriguing to us, not only as a way of understanding the mechanisms that may modulate IL-2 production in a state of immunological homeostasis, but also as a way of explaining the crucial role that PGE_2 plays within the complex disturbances of specific immunocompetence following trauma.

Down-Regulation of CMI via the Monokine PGE_2

In vitro studies have shown that PGE_2, as a regulatory monokine released from inhibitory Mø, augments the proliferation of T suppressor cells, inhibits T_H- and B-cell proliferation, interferes with facilitatory Mø/T_H interaction, and decreases facilitatory Mø activity (antigen presentation, expression of the immune response antigen, and IL-1 synthesis) [4, 13, 25, 28, 31]. As a direct consequence of human burn injuries, the release of large amounts of PGE_2 from macrophages in vitro and high PGE_2 concentrations (increased over 30-fold) have been found [26]. Prostaglandins of the E series, after binding to the lymphocyte on special binding sites [15], exert their influence on the cell through membrane-bound cyclic nucleotides. These stimulate cyclic AMP (cAMP), and a rise in cAMP is associated with inhibition of mitogenesis, reduced production of lymphokines, inhibition of lymphocyte-mediated cytolysis, and inhibition of T-lymphocyte rosette formation. Administration of cyclooxygenase inhibitors such as indomethacin or ibuprofen to phytohemagglutinin (PHA)-stimulated cultures of PBMCs of normals as well as of trauma and tumor patients decreases prostaglandin synthesis and results in an increase in the proliferative responses [10, 15].

Materials and Methods

In a series of studies our laboratory scrutinized the mediator-dependent alterations of cell-mediated immune function following major mechanical trauma. We investigated the time course and extent of depressed IL-2 synthesis and wanted to elucidate which putative inhibiting factors play a key role in the deficiency of IL-2 production [9]. In these experiments IL-2 was generated from four different PHA-stimulated PBMC cultures (Fig. 3) on post-trauma days 1, 3, 5, 7, 10, 14, and 21 as follows:

1. Untreated cells (C)
2. Cells incubated with the cyclooxygenase inhibitor indomethacin (C+Indo)
3. A cell suspension depleted of adherent cells (C-AC)
4. A PBMC suspension that was preincubated with low-dose 4-hydroperoxycyclophosphamide (C+400H-CYP), which is known to be selectively inhibitory for T suppressor lymphocytes (TS) [27]; this was used to study the role of TS in the regulation of IL-2 synthesis.

A second lymphokine, IFN-γ was measured in order to understand its possible role in control of CMI, especially given its identity with MAF, following trauma. Furthermore, we scrutinized macrophage activity following trauma by obtaining serial measurements of the monokines IL-1 and PGE_2 [11]. PBMC phenotyping for T lymphocytes and Mø was also carried out over an observation period of 21 days after trauma.

The ultimate objective of our studies was to answer the following questions:

- Are altered control mechanisms in terms of changed monokine synthesis and/or elevated T-suppressor activity responsible for a change CMI?
- Do quantitative and/or functional alterations of the lymphokine-producing cells represent an essential deficit? And finally, could we restore suppressed lymphokine synthesis with immunomodulatory interventions?

Results

Phenotyping of PBMC Subpopulations

There was a highly significant reduction of CD3+ and CD4+ T lymphocytes in PBMC cultures. There was only a very slight tendency towards normalization up to day 21. In parallel to these subpopulations, the mitogen-induced suppression of IL-2R was also considerably impaired (Fig. 4).

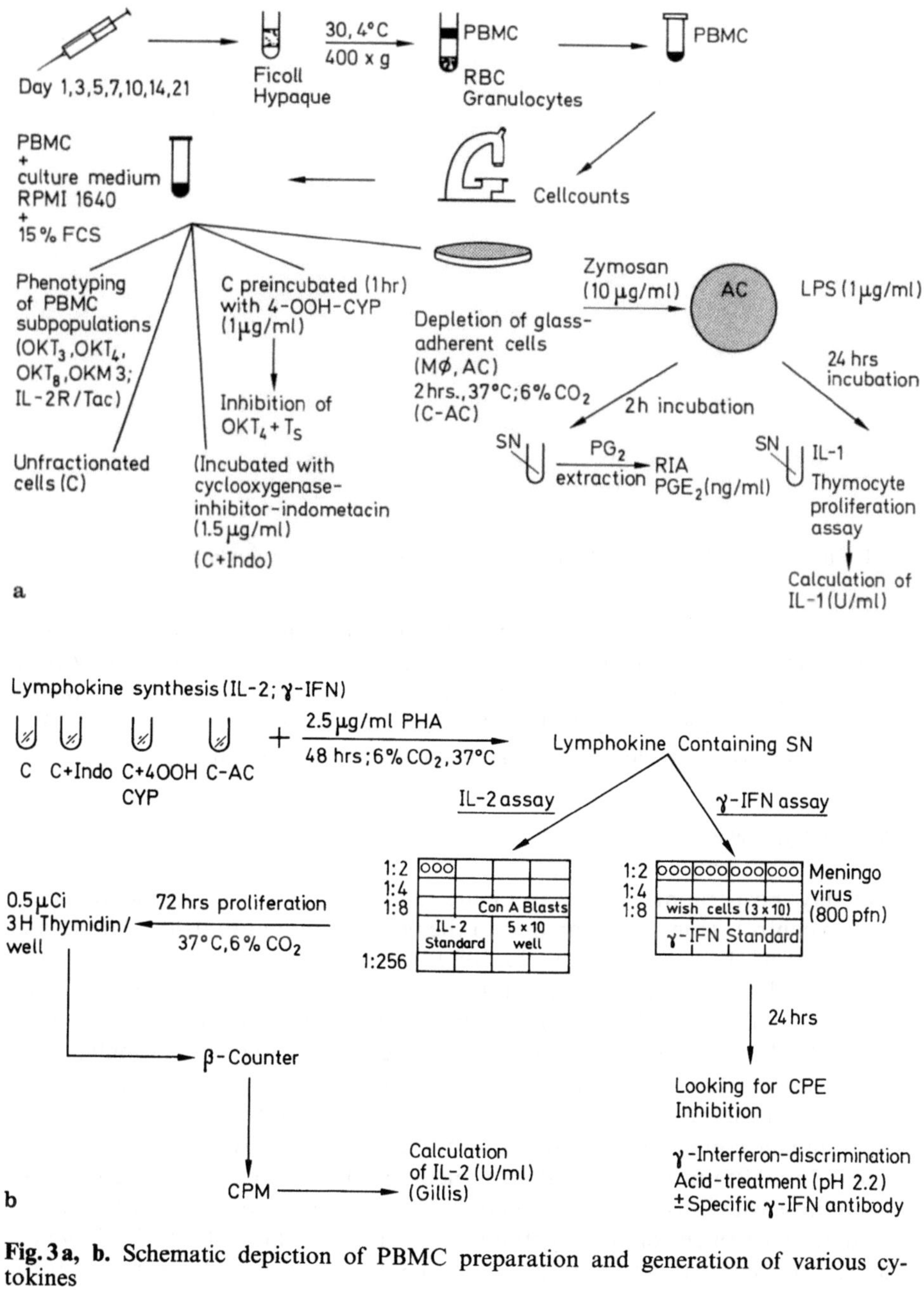

Fig. 3 a, b. Schematic depiction of PBMC preparation and generation of various cytokines

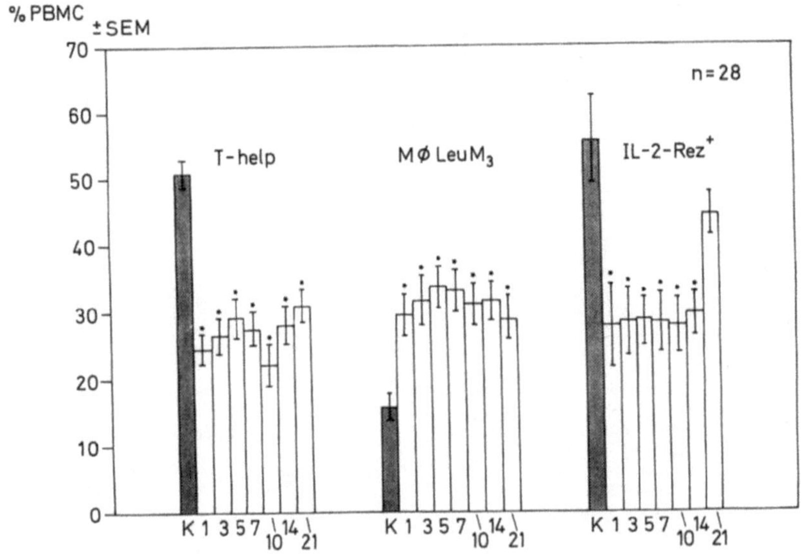

Fig. 4. Changes in PBMC phenotypes compared to control (*K*) following trauma

In contrast to the severe reduction of the T-cell population, the phenotyping of Mø showed a significant elevation of LeuM3+ mononuclear phagocytes, starting immediately after the onset of trauma and staying at this level for 3 weeks and longer. Compared with 15% LeuM3+ cells in normal subjects, the LeuM3+ cells always showed an elevation of $\geqq$100% above normal values.

Cytokine Synthesis

On all days post-trauma there was a marked reduction of IL-2 production compared to controls (Fig. 5). Compared to the normal amount of 0.90 ± 0.05 U/ml, the amount of IL-2 generated by 2×10^6 PBMCs decreased by more than 60% ($p<0.01$), following a slight initial recovery. We saw a nadir between day 5 and day 7 and only very slow recovery until day 21 with an average value of 0.49 ± 0.08 U/ml, a value associated with severe suppression. Interestingly, there is a parallel profile of IL-2 synthesis and IL-2 receptor expression (Fig. 6). When we compared the profile of in vitro IL-2 synthesis of individuals with different post-traumatic courses, we found less severe suppression of IL-2 synthesis on day 5 and 7 ($p<0.05$) in patients with an uncomplicated post-traumatic course (I) than in those with infectious complications (II) (Fig. 7). In group I patients we observed an impairment of IL-2 synthesis to an average value of 0.6 U/ml, which is a reduction compared to normal values of 33%. In patients that survived their infectious complications, we saw a nadir of IL-2 synthesis on day 5 with a value of 0.19 ± 0.04 U/ml, equal to a reduction of 80% from normal values. On day 21 post-trauma IL-2 synthesis was equal in both patient groups. Only in 4 (13%) of 30 patients was IL-2 synthesis following major trauma within normal ranges over the complete post-traumatic course.

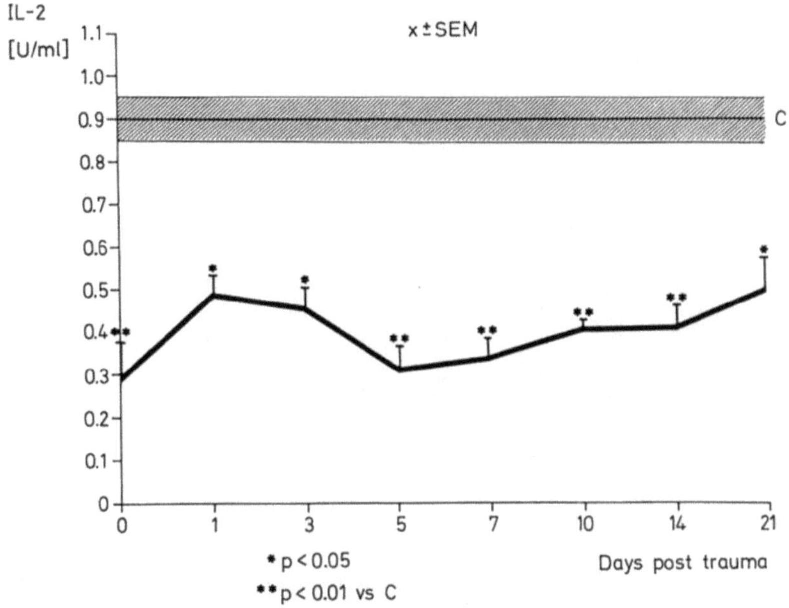

Fig. 5. IL-2 synthesis on various days following trauma. *C*, control value

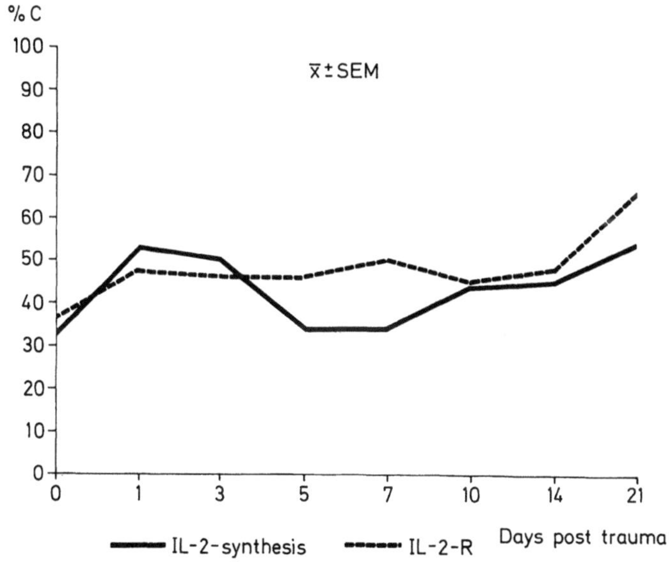

Fig. 6. Comparison of profiles of IL-2 synthesis and IL-2 receptor (*IL-2R*) expression following trauma

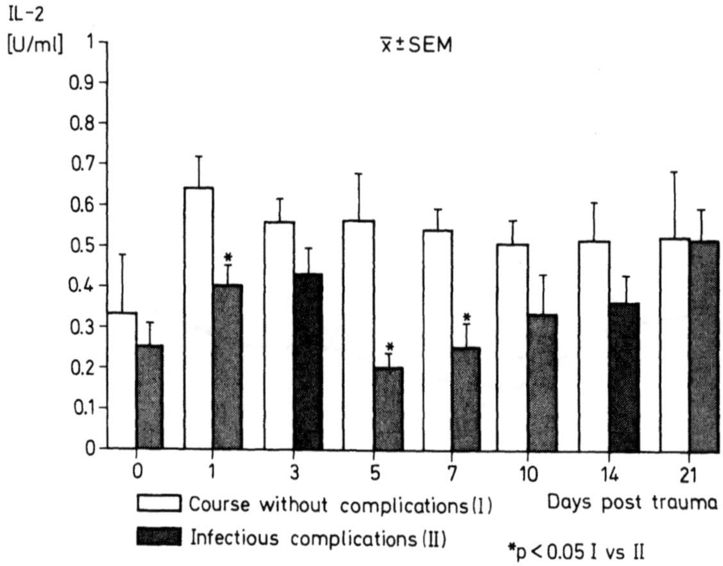

Fig. 7. Comparison of in vitro IL-2 synthesis following trauma of patients with uneventful course and those with infectious complications

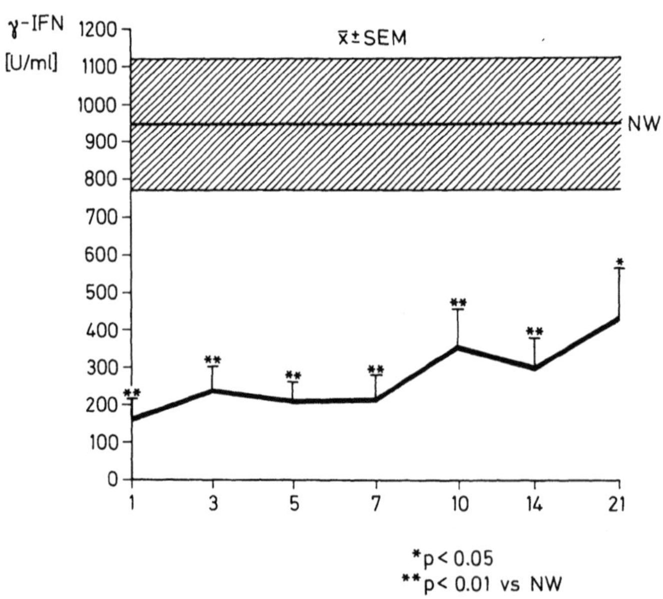

Fig. 8. IFN-γ synthesis on various days following trauma. *NW*, Control values

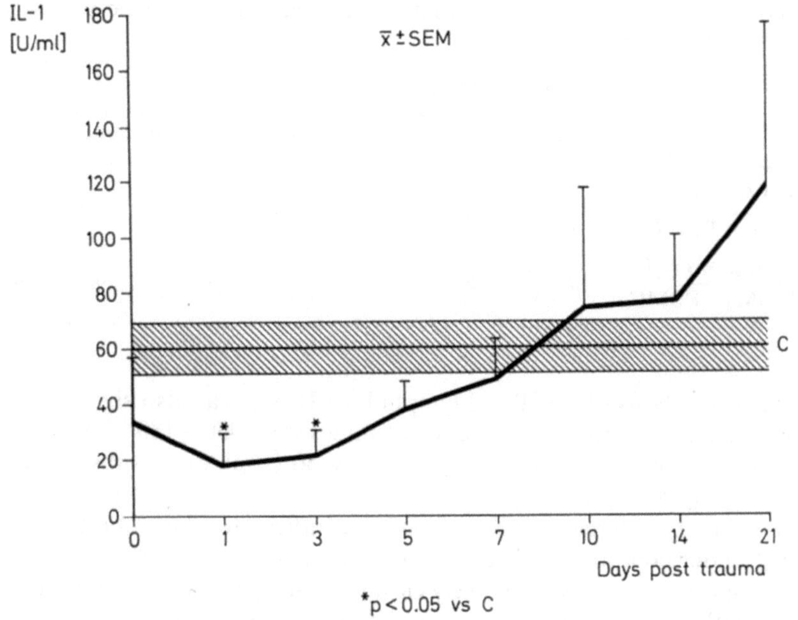

Fig. 9. Macrophage interleukin (IL-1) synthesis on different days following trauma. *C*, Control value

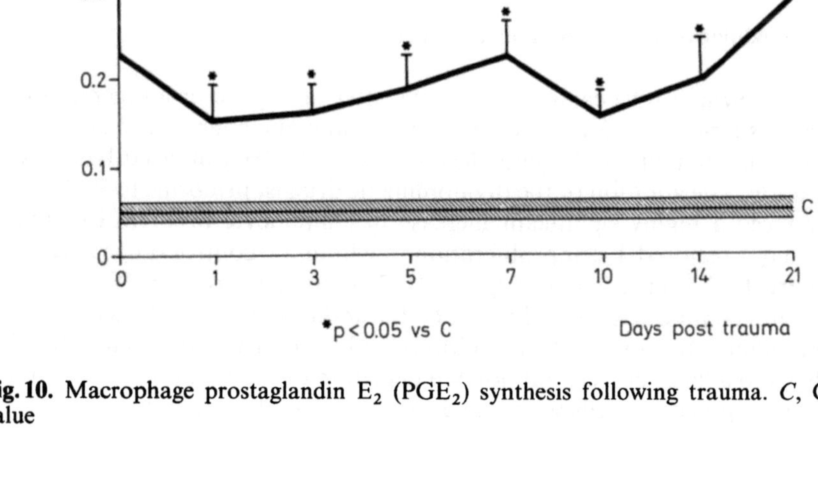

Fig. 10. Macrophage prostaglandin E_2 (PGE_2) synthesis following trauma. *C*, Control value

Table 1. Monocyte in vitro IL-1 and PGE_2 synthesis. f IL-1 and f PGE_2 are the monokine synthesis factors for a single macrophage

	Days after trauma								
	Control	0	1	3	5	7	10	14	21
f IL-1 $\frac{\text{IL-1 (U/ml)}}{\text{\% LeuM}_3+\text{PBMC}}$	4.6	1.4	0.6	0.7	1.1	1.5	2.6	2.4	4.2
f PGE_2 $\frac{\text{PGE}_2\text{ (ng/ml)} \times 10^3}{\text{\% LeuM}_3+\text{PBMC}}$	3.8	8.8	5.4	5.2	5.3	6.9	5.2	6.0	10.0

The in vitro synthesis of the T-cell lymphokine IFN-γ was also significantly reduced on all days post-trauma. The control values were 950 ± 180 U/ml. Until day 7 synthesis was reduced to an average of 200 ± 50 U/ml, but it subsequently recovered slowly up to day 21 (Fig. 8).

There were highly different profiles of in vitro synthesis for the monokines IL-1 and PGE_2, under conditions of persisting monocytosis. While the amount of PGE_2 in the supernatants was excessively elevated during the whole observation period, IL-1 synthesis was massively impaired between days 1 and 3 post-trauma, returning after that rather rapidly to within the normal range (60 ± 9 U/ml) (Fig. 9). Compared to the normal levels of PGE_2 (0.054 ± 0.01 ng/ml), even on the day of the trauma the PGE_2 output in monocyte cultures was increased up to four-fold (0.22 ± 0.08 ng/ml). Between day 1 and day 7 we saw a continuous elevation, with a drop in lower values until day 14 and a rise to 0.28 ± 0.08 ng/ml on day 21 (Fig. 10).

In order to determine approximately the amount of monokine synthesized by individual macrophages, in one study the macrophage cytokine synthesis was expressed as the monokine output divided by the percentage of macrophages in the individual patient. We calculated a monokine synthesis factor and saw that there is a clear shift of monokine synthesis in favor of elevated PGE_2 output and suppressed IL-1 synthesis (Table 1).

In Vitro Modulation of T-Lymphocyte Function

The lymphoproliferative capacity of T cells after mitogenic or antigenic stimuli was clearly suppressed during the whole post-traumatic course. The addition of highly purified human IL-2 could elevate or restore PHA-induced lymphocyte proliferation. The addition of the thymomimetic drug isoprinosine to PBMC cultures induced a highly significant increase in lymphocyte proliferation and as early as day 1 restored T-cell proliferation to within the control range (Fig. 11).

In vitro IL-2 synthesis (Fig. 12) and IL-2 receptor expression (Fig. 13) of T lymphocytes could be clearly enhanced by the addition of the cyclooxygenase inhibitor indomethacin to the PBMC cultures. Only indomethacin could restore IL-2 synthesis to a large degree, but not Mø depletion or the blockage of functional T-suppressor precursor cells with 4-hydroperoxycyclophosphamide.

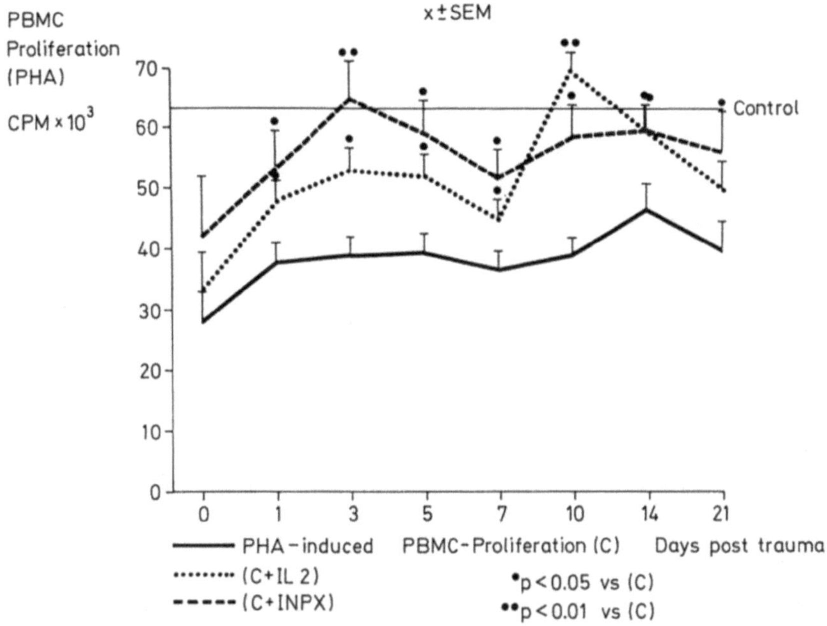

Fig. 11. Augmentation of PHA-induced PBMC proliferation (*C*) following trauma with addition of human IL-2 (*C+IL-2*) and the synthetic immunomodulator isoprinosine (*INPX*)

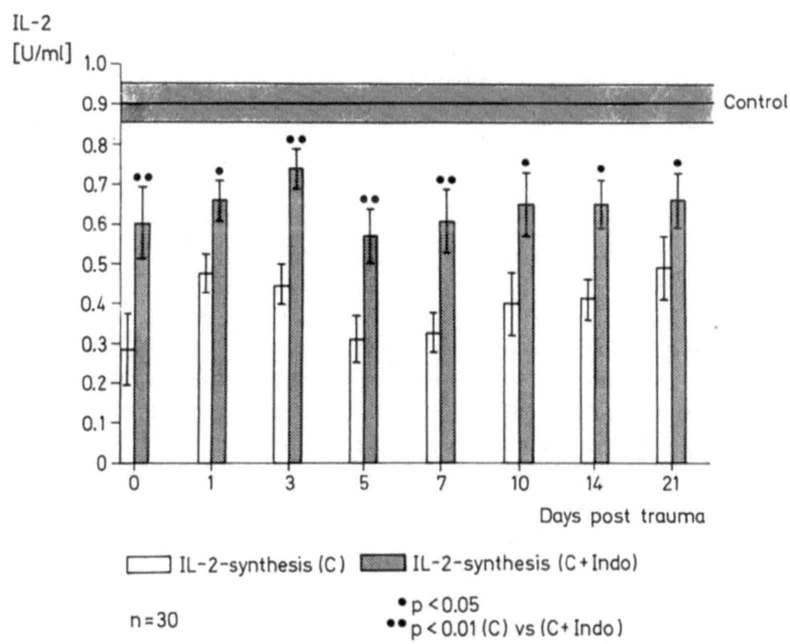

Fig. 12. IL-2 synthesis on various days following trauma. *C* refers to patients PMBCs, *C+Indo* refers to patients' PBMCs cultured with indomethacin at 1 mg/ml. *Asterisks* denote values of *C+Indo* that are statistically different from *C* values

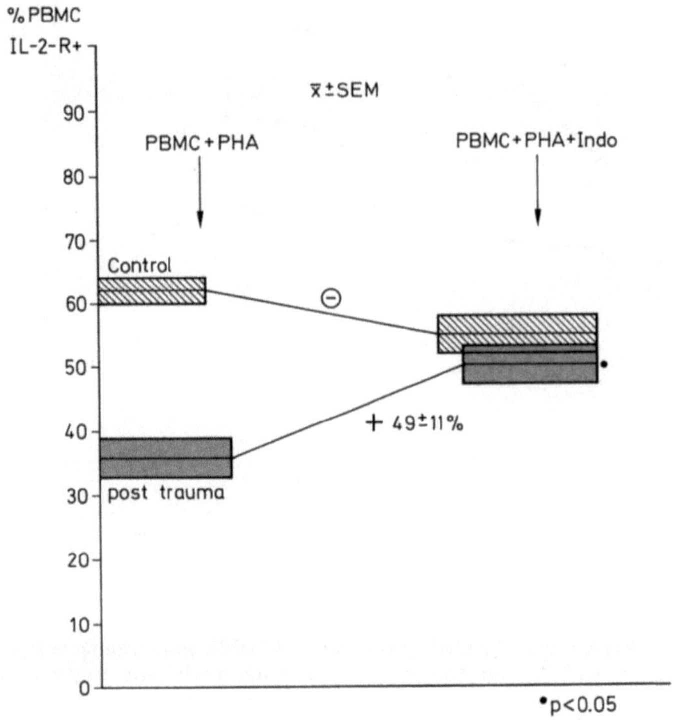

Fig. 13. Influence of cyclooxygenase inhibition on IL-2R expression of patient and control PBMCs in PHA-stimulated cell cultures. *Asterisks* denote statistically significant values between PBMC+PHA and PBMC+PHA+Indomethacin

Discussion

From a wide array of in vitro studies of PBMCs and multiply injured patients, we concluded that there is a far-reaching disruption of Mø/T-cell interaction, based on suppressed synthesis of the positive regulatory mediators IL-1, IL-2, and IFN-γ and a simultaneous clear increase in the negative regulatory monokine PGE_2 (Fig. 14). The cellular factor in the disturbance of the IL-1/IL-2 cascade has been identified as a lack of CD4+ helper/inducer lymphocytes and the massive elevation of negative regulatory Mø. The immunorestorative effect of cyclooxygenase inhibition gave strong evidence for the negative regulatory impact of PGE_2 on IL-2 synthesis and IL-2 receptor expression. These studies indicated that the sensitivity of T-lymphocytes in injured humans to the negative regulatory influence of PGE_2 is considerably raised [17].

The complete dissociation of Mø/T-cell interaction must also lead to a defect of specific antibody synthesis following major injury in spite of the potentially intact B-cell function. We also showed a defect of terminal B-cell maturation and a switch from IgM to IgG production that can also be attributed very closely to Mø-induced immunosuppression [36]. Our findings indicate a severe depression of CMI, leading to down-regulation of the immune response caused by the release

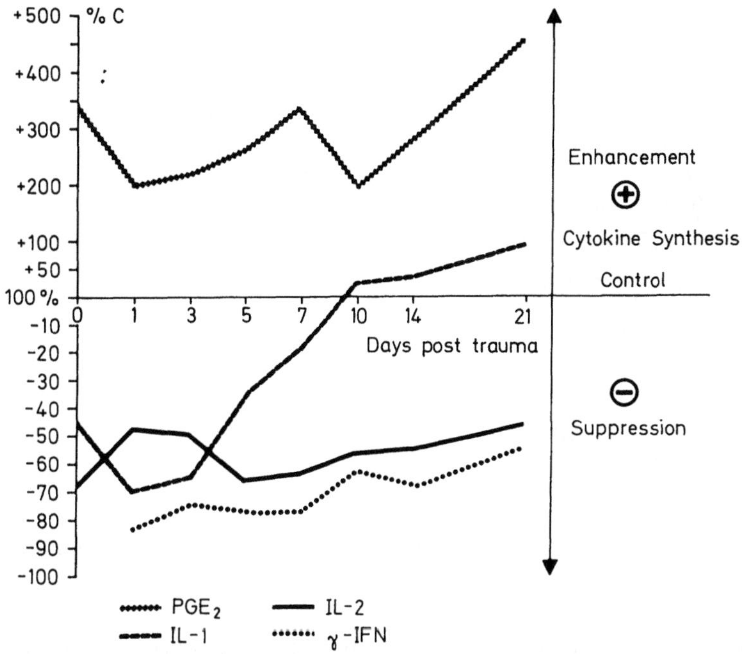

Fig. 14. Overview of different profiles of cytokine synthesis on consecutive days following major trauma. The 100% mark expresses the control value

of suppressive molecules, predominantly PGE_2. This deleterious process may be maintained or even partially induced by deficient IFN-γ synthesis, since IFN-γ has been demonstrated to promote IL-1 synthesis and to reduce macrophage suppressor activity by inhibiting PGE_2 release [5]. Our findings of severely impaired synthesis of IFN-γ following major trauma correspond closely to those of Suzuki and Pollard, who found suppressed production of this lymphokine in burned mice until day 7 after injury [32]. IFN-γ showed a comparable profile of inhibition to that of IL-2.

Suzuki and Pollard postulated that the splenic adherent cells suppressed production of IFN-γ in burned animals. In our studies, however, we were unable to enhance depressed IFN-γ synthesis by depleting adherent cells using indomethacin or by blocking T-suppressor precursor cells with C-400H-CYP (data not shown here). It is unclear what factors induced macrophages to be predominantly active as inhibitory cells following injury (Fig. 15). The macrophage is a captive of its environment, with its function being triggered by several serum factors. Ninnemann and Stockland have identified excessive PGE_2 release in patients with major thermal injury leading to immunosuppression [26]. The presence of excessive amounts of immune complexes or complement factors following injury may initiate negative regulatory immune responses by stimulating macrophages to secrete PGE_2. Our observations that a shift from help to suppression may take place within macrophages following major trauma compare well with observations by Cahill and Hopper, who described differential secretion of PGE and IL-1 in sensitized and unsensitized mice following infection with *Salmonella enteriditis*

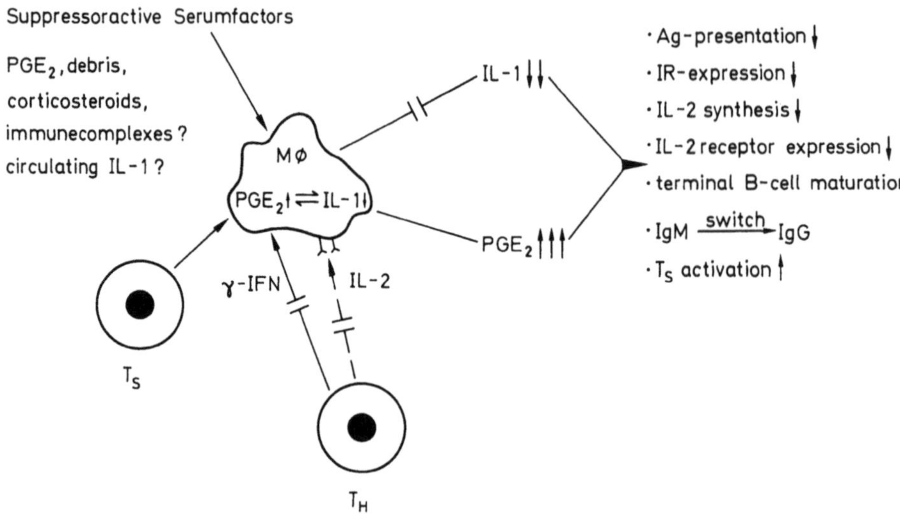

Fig. 15. A model of factors and functional consequences of altered monocyte behavior following trauma

[6]. Elevated macrophage production of PGE_2 in burn trauma was originally reported by Miller et al., who also found that increased macrophage PGE_2 synthesis in multiply injured patients was induced through T-suppressor cells in parallel with a reduction of plasminogen activator in identical cells [22, 23].

To elucidate further the crucial role of peripheral blood macrophages in post-traumatic immunosuppression, more differentiated characterization of these cells must be carried out. It remains unclear whether trauma induces a certain behavior in a distinct macrophage subpopulation, whether there is a qualitative shift from up- to down-regulatory macrophages, whether these changes may be due to newly recruited cells that are less differentiated, and finally, whether these changes are reversible. In a number of studies it was shown that there are multiple disturbances of CMI following major trauma. The macrophage suppressor function and the significantly reduced numbers of CD4+ T cells result in a considerable reduction of IL-2 and IFN-γ synthesis. The IL-2 deficiency leads to a lack of terminal T-cell expansion and T-cell proliferation. IFN-γ deficiency results in a lack of feedback macrophage activation with reduced capacity of antigen presentation and inadequate IL-1 synthesis. Competent CMI is further reduced by the impaired IL-2 receptor expression, which is also caused at least in part via PGE_2 and can be reversed by the addition of cyclooxygenase inhibitors. In our study, T-suppressor activity did not play any essential role in blocking cellular immune responses.

There are a variety of immunological disorders after severe trauma and there is evidence that the negative regulatory macrophages may be the initial point of post-traumatic immunosuppression. If immunomodulatory therapy is to succeed, it should be aimed primarily at the restoration of the impaired Mø/T-cell interaction. Any therapy model should optimally combine several interventions. Selective chemotherapeutic immunomodulation would probably be most effective after the serum has been cleared of circulating immunosuppressive agents. Blockage of PGE_2 synthesis through the administration of cyclooxygenase inhibitors and/or PGE_2-specific antibodies should reduce the inhibitory potential of macrophages. The substitution of IFN-γ in low, nontoxic doses could possibly restore adequate facilitory macrophage activity by inducing IL-1 synthesis and improving antigen presentation. The administration of thymomimetic T-cell activators (TP-5, isoprinosine) or low-dose recombinant IL-2 might be useful to accelerate the induction of receptor sites on T-cells and to a low additional recruitment of immunocompentent cells from the circulating pool.

More complete understanding of altered immune function after trauma, on a cellular level, as well as increasing experience in human immunomodulatory interventions, must be gained to determine a basic model of in vivo immune response modification. However, as our understanding of the complex mechanisms of the lymphokine cascade develops, we will probably become more selective and hesitatant about challenging this circuit in vivo, in order not to burden the immunocompromised patient further by bypassing defective immune mechanisms, the consequences of which are hard to predict.

References

1. Abraham E, Regan RF (1985) The effects of hemorrhage and trauma on interleukin 2 production. Arch Surg 120:1341–1344
2. Akiyoshi T, Koba F, Arinaga S et al. (1985) Impaired production of interleukin-2 after surgery. Clin Exp Immunol 59:45–49
3. Antonacci AC (1984) How do immunomodulators affect host defense in the burn patient? J Trauma 24:101–105
4. Bonney RJ, Davies P (1984) Possible autoregulatory functions of the secretory products on mononuclear phagocytes. In: Adams DO, Hanna MG Jr (eds) Contemporary topics in immunology, vol 13. Plenum, New York, p 199
5. Boraschi D, Censini S, Tagliabue A (1984) Interferon reduces macrophage-suppressive activity by inhibiting prostaglandin E_2 release and inducing interleukin 1 production. J Immunol 133:764–768
6. Cahill J, Hopper KE (1982) Immunoregulation by macrophages: differential secretion of prostaglandin E and interleukin during infection with *Salmonella enteritidis*. Cell Immunol 67:229–240
7. Chouaib S, Fradelizi D (1982) The mechanism of inhibition of human IL-2 production. J Immunol 129:2463–2468
8. Chouaib S, Chateroud L, Klatzman D et al. (1984) The mechanisms of inhibition of human IL-2 production. II PGE_2 induction of suppressor T-lymphocytes. J Immunol 132:1851–1852
9. Faist E, Mewes A, Baker CC et al. (1987) Prostaglandin E_2 (PGE_2)-dependent suppression of interleukin 2 (IL-2) production in patients with major trauma. J Trauma 27:837
10. Faist E, Kupper T, Baker CC et al. (1986) Depression of cellular immunity after major injury: its association with posttraumatic complications and its reversal with immunomodulation. Arch Surg 121:1000–1005
11. Faist E, Mewes A, Strasser Th, Alkan S et al. (1988) Alteration of monocyte (Mø) function following major injury. Arch Surg 123,3:287
12. Farrar JJ, Benjamin WR, Hilfiker M et al. (1982) The biochemistry, biology and role of Interleukin-2 in the induction of cytotoxic T-cell and antibody forming B-cell responses. Immunol Rev 62:129

13. Fischer A, Dupandy A, Griscelli C (1981) Role of prostaglandin E_2 in the induction of nonspecific T lymphocyte suppressor activity. J Immunol 126:1452–1455
14. Goodwin JS, Bankhurst AD, Messner RP (1977) Suppression of human T-cell mitogenesis by prostaglandin: existence of a prostaglandin producing suppressor cell. J Exp Med 146:1719
15. Goodwin JS, Webb DR (1980) Regulation of the immune response by prostaglandins. Clin Immunol Immunopathol 15:106–122
16. Grabstein K, Eisenman J, Mochizaki D et al. (1985) Purification to homogeneity of a B-cell stimulating factor. J Exp Med 163:1405
17. Grbic JT, Wood JJ, Jordan AJ et al. (1985) Lymphocytes from burn patients are more sensitive to suppression by prostaglandin E_2. Surg Forum 108
18. Greene DR, Chue B, Ferguson TA et al. (1985) Production of an antigenspecific component of suppressor inducer factor by a helper T-cell clone: possible role for IL-1 at the interface of immunity and tolerance. Br J Rheumatol 26:74–79
19. Howard M, Nakanishi K, Paul WE (1984) B-cell growth and differentiation factors. Immunol Rev 78:185
20. Howard M, Farrar J, Hilfiker M et al. (1982) Identification of T-cell derived B-cell growth factor distinct from interleukin-2. J Exp Med 55:914
21. Kupper TS, Green DR, Durum SK et al. (1985) Defective antigen presentation to a cloned T-helper cell by macrophages from burned mice can be restored with interleukin 1. Surgery 98:199–206
22. Miller CL, Fink MP et al. (1988) Mechanisms of altered monocyte prostaglandin E_2 production in severely injured patients. Arch Surg 123:293
23. Miller CL (1981) Secondary immunodeficiency in burns and after surgical trauma. Clin Immunol Allergy 1:641–667
24. Neef JR, Curl GR, Woody JN (1981) Absolute requirements for adherent cells in the production of human IL-2. Cell Immunol 3:142–150
25. Ninnemann JL (1984) Prostaglandins and immunity: prostaglandins in inflammation and disease. Immunol Today 5:170
26. Ninnemann JL, Stockland AE (1984) Participation of prostaglandin E_2 in immunosuppression following thermal injury. J Trauma 24:201–207
27. Ozer H, Cowens JW, Calvin M et al. (1982) In vitro effects of hydroperoxy-cyclophosphamide on human immunoregulatory subset function. J Exp Med 155:276
28. Picker LJ, Raff HV, Goldyne ME, Stabo JD (1980) Metabolic heterrogeneity among human monocytes and its modulation by PGE_2. J Immunol 124:2557
29. Rice LA, Laughter AU, Twomey JJ (1979) Three suppressor systems in human blood that modulate lymphoproliferation. J Immunol 122:991
30. Rosenberg S, Lipsky PE (1981) Macrophage-lymphocyte cooperation in human immune responses. In: Dingle JT, Gordon JL (eds) Cellular interactions. Elsevier, Amsterdam
31. Schrör K (1984) Prostaglandine und verwandte Verbindungen; Bildung, Funktion und pharmakologische Beeinflussung, Vol 2. Thieme, Stuttgart, p 138
32. Suzuki R, Pollard RB (1982) Mechanism for the suppression of gamma interferon responsiveness in mice after thermal injury. J Immunol 129:1811–1816
33. Swain SL, Dennert G, Warner JF (1982) Culture supernatants of a stimulated T-cell line have helper activity that acts synergistically with interleukin-2 in the response of B-cells to antigen. Proc Natl Acad Sci USA 78:2517
34. Takatsu K, Tanaka K, Tominaga A et al. (1980) Antigen-induced T-cell replacing factor (TRF): III. Establishment of a T-cell hybrid clone continously producing TRF and functional analysis or released TRF. J Immunol 25:2646
35. Trinchieri G, Perussia B (1985) Immune interferon: a pleiotropic lymphokine with multiple effects. Immunol Today 6:131
36. Twomey JJ (1982) Disorders of macrophages: excessive immunosuppression. In: Twomey JJ (ed) The pathophysiology of human immunologic disorders. Urban and Schwarzenberg, Munich, pp 29–50, 125–147
37. Wood JJ, Rodrick ML, O'Mahony JB, Rodrick L et al. (1984) Inadequate interleukin 2 production: a fundamental immunological deficiency in patients with major burns. Ann Surg 200:311–320

Alterations of Monocyte Function Following Major Injury *

C. L. Miller-Graziano, G. Szabo, T. Takayama, and Jia-yan Wu

Alteration in monocyte/macrophage (MØ) functions post-trauma increasingly appears to be related to the development of post-trauma immunoincompetence and metabolic derangement [1–11]. These inimical post-trauma alterations in monocytes can be categorized into three types: (1) depression in antigen-presenting function due to alterations in antigen processing or presentation, (2) alterations in monokine secretion, and (3) stimulation of inhibitory MØ factor production. Our hypothesis is that a post-trauma shift in the ratio of MØ subsets may be causal in all three of these types of monocyte defects.

One indication of a post-trauma defect in antigen presentation and/or processing is the detection of defective MØ phagocytosis [12]. Phagocytosis is an important first step in antigen processing [13, 14]. Alterations in monocyte antigen-presenting function have been repeatedly reported in animal models postinjury [4]. This reduced ability of monocytes to induce T-lymphocyte proliferation has been examined in a murine model using the D10.G4.1 T-cell line as a proliferative indicator [15]. This murine T-cell line is somewhat unique in that it requires the monokine interleukin 1 (Il-1) for proliferation and does not elaborate the lymphokine interleukin 2 (Il-2) but rather Il-4 [16, 17]. Consequently, a defect in the D10 assay in the postinjury animal model may not necessarily be the result of depressed antigen presentation-processing but rather a decrease in monocyte Il-1 production. The D10 type of murine T-helper lymphocyte (TH2) is not initially generated by immune stimulation, is primarily involved in B-lymphocyte activation, and is responsive to the Il-2 secreted by TH1 cells [18]. In addition, the TH2-lymphocyte may primarily be stimulated by a B-lymphocyte as an antigen-presenting cell. In contrast, the TH1 cell's interaction with the monocyte/macrophage appears to be more dependent on cell-cell contact and the expression of immune response antigens [16]. In human T cells, this distinction between TH1 and TH2 on the basis of their lymphokine production has not been demonstrated [19]. The initial antigen-induced TH_1 – MØ interactions may not directly require Il-1 but rather another monokine such as Il-6, which is elaborated by fibroblasts and monocytes in response to Il-1 [20–23]. Consequently, the demonstration that MØs from burned animals do not stimulate the D10 cell line must be interpreted with caution because the D10 (TH2) assay may not provide an actual analogy to the MØ antigen presentation and processing required for stimulation of TH1 cells. A defect in the D10 assay may not be indicative of an initial defect in MØ-T cell interaction or in antigen presentation-processing.

* This study was supported by grants GM36214 and DAMD 17-86-C-6091 from the U.S. Public Health Service.

Immune Consequences of
Trauma, Shock and Sepsis
Eds. Faist/Ninnemann/Green

Another line of evidence for an MØ antigen-presenting defect comes from studies on generations of primary antibody-forming cells in vitro [24]. MØs isolated from burned mice are not able to trigger induction of the primary anti-sheep erythrocyte response when added to normal syngeneic splenocytes from which MØs have been depleted. However, these data again do not distinguish whether the MØs from the thermally injured animals have a defect in antigen presentation and processing or whether the problem is defective mediator production. Increased MØ inhibitory action could also be the cause of the depressed antibody-forming cell response. In fact, Kupper and Duriem reported that defective burned MØ induction of D10 proliferation could be reversed by an addition of Il-1 [25]. These data can be interpreted as demonstrating a defect in Il-1 production or excessive MØ suppressive activity which is overcome by exogenous Il-1 addition rather than an antigen presentation defect. A post-trauma defect in the tetanus toxoid presentation of antigen to T cells was recently described [26]. However, this depressed proliferation could be due to suppressor T cells (T_s) or to excessive PGE_2 production by MØ. No definitive experiments have been performed directly to examine post-trauma human MØ antigen-presenting capacity in the absence of competing T_s or inhibitory MØ.

One of the approaches that we have taken to examine post-trauma MØ alterations is to segregate MØ into inhibitory and facilitory subsets by rosetting the MØ with a high-affinity receptor for human IgG1. It has been repeatedly reported that MØ-producing prostaglandin E_2 could be segregated from Il-1-producing or antigen-presenting MØ subsets [27–29]. Our approach was twofold. First, if the inhibitory MØ could be segregated from antigen-presenting MØ, then the patient's MØ antigen-presenting function could be examined without complicating concurrent inhibitory responses. Second, if some MØ surface marker could be definitely associated with a particular MØ function, then complex bioassays for monitoring patient immune status could be eliminated in favor of assessment of alterations in MØ phenotype. In our initial studies, we confirmed that antigen-presenting MØ appeared not to bear high densities of the FcRI (high-affinity receptor for mouse immunoglobulin G2a and human IgGI and IgG3) (Table 1) [30]. When we began to segregate the $FcRI^+$ and $FcRI^-$ MØ subsets of the patients in order to develop a protocol for examining antigen presentation, we were surprised to find that immunosuppressed patients had a shift in the proportion

Table 1. FcRI-negative MØs are the primary antigen-presenting population

T cell+	Exp 4	Exp 9	Exp 11
Ag[a]	193	758	676
MØp[b]	6983	15492	10306
Fc^+MØp	2253	2578	2639
Fc^+MØp+Ag	474	4387	2262
Fc^-MØp	19428	15492	10979
Fc^-MØp+Ag	23454	26445	21308
MØ	486	2578	2743

[a] 10 µg tetanus toxoid.
[b] Monocyte/macrophages incubated with 10 µg/ml tetanus toxoid for 24 h.

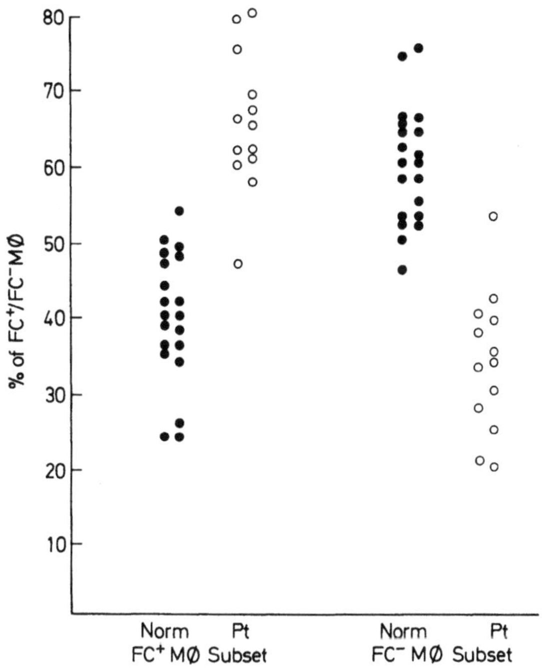

Fig. 1. Percentage ratio of FcRI-positive and -negative MØs in normals and patients. Monocytes were rosetted with anti-RH coated for O^+ human erythrocytes to separate out the MØ-subpopulation-enriched high-density FcRI ($FcRI^+$)-bearing cells. Nonrosetted MØs (those with low-density FcRI) were considered as the FcRI-negative subset

of their $FcRI^+$ to $FcRI^-$ MØ (Fig. 1). As we began to distinguish differences in functions of these two MØ subsets, we became more and more aware of the immune functional consequences that would befall patients who experienced a change in the proportion of their MØ subsets. In addition, we found that the $FcRI^-$ MØ population did not respond to bacterial stimulation with an elevation of its PGE_2 production sufficient to suppress MØ function, while the Fc^+ MØ subset did. We were also able to separate out the suppressor inducer contained in the $CD4^+$ T-helper-cell population by panning with the monoclonal antibody 2H4. After panning we had a population of $CD4^+$ T cells which could be evaluated for their helper activity without the presence of T_s. These preliminary experiments are allowing us to set up a test system for trauma patients' MØ antigen-presenting function which would actually examine the ability of patients' anti-presenting MØ to induce a tetanus toxoid proliferative response in their T-helper lymphocytes without the complicating presence of PGE_2-producing MØ or T-suppressor lymphocytes. Defective monokine production would still have to be examined before a dysfunction in MØ antigen presentation could be definitely delineated.

Although trauma-induced alterations in monokine production have been repeatedly reported, there are conflicting data in this area. Some investigators have reported post-trauma increases in Il-1 activity as measured in the thymocyte proliferation (LAF) assay [31]. Other investigators, using the murine D10, Il-1-dependent clone, have seen decreased Il-1 activity [32]. It is now understood that a wide family of monokines including Il-1, Il-6, and tumor necrosis factor (TNF) all have some proliferative effect in the LAF assay [33, 38]. It has even been suggested that Il-6 is the primary thymocyte stimulator and that the activities of Il-1 and TNF reflect their ability to induce Il-6 production by non-T cells contaminating the thymocyte preparations [20, 34, 35]. TNF, IL-1, and IL-6 share a number of similar biological activities. They are all pyrogenic, affect hepatocyte function, and can activate different types of T-cell proliferatioin [33, 36, 37, 39]. Consequently, data showing elevation in the ability of trauma patient's sera to stimulate thymocyte proliferation do not necessarily only indicate increased MØ Il-1 production. Aarden's group has reported elevated levels of Il-6 in the postburn patient sera using a specific Il-6 assay [33]. Whether these Il-6 elevations correlated to immunosuppression in these patients was not described. However, the elevations in Il-6 levels did correlate to appearance of the acute-phase response and metabolic derangement, and pyrogenic activity. Our laboratory has also seen elevated MØ leukocyte pyrogen activity after trauma in the face of an apparent Il-1 defect (Table 2). However, this pyrogenic activity has not been categorized to TNF, Il-1, or Il-6. Other data of ours and others indicate increased TNF levels in trauma patients [40]. Consequently the data showing depressed Il-1 production in an Il-1-specific D10 assay seem to provide evidence of altered post-trauma Il-1 functions. Nevertheless, recent examination of IL-1-mediated stimulation of the D10 clone in a cecal ligation and puncture model has implicated apparent increased IL-1 activity in the face of decreased MØ stimulation of the specific antigen response of the D10 clone [4]. Since the effect of TNF and/or Il-6 on the D10 clone is still undetermined, the definition of a post-trauma IL-1 MØ defect is still unresolved.

Evaluation of MØ Il-1 production after trauma is further complicated by the recent discovery that two genetically separate types of interleukin 1 are produced by monocytes [41, 42]. One of these monokines, Il-1α, is suggested as the membrane-bound form with two to ten times more T-cell-inducing activity than the second type, Il-1β [44]. Il-1α does not require as much processing and is active in its 30000-MW form while Il-1β appears more active in cytotoxity of pancreatic beta-cells [44]. Consequently there may be differences in the types of Il-1 produced by post-trauma MØ (i.e., more Il-1β than Il-1α) as well as in the quantity of Il-1 produced. Il-1α and Il-1β lack secretory sequences and the mechanism of their release from the MØ is still undefined. It has been suggested that plasmin-dependent plasminogen activator, or other MØ serine proteases, might be respon-

Table 2. Fc^+ – MØ subset contains the MØs which are producing leukocyte pyrogen (LP)

MØ population[a]	Patient		Normal	
	PGE_2	LP[b]	PGE_2	LP
Fc^+	12665	0.55	4058	0.25
Fc^-	1484	0	847	0

[a] Monocyte/macrophage populations (Pop) were selected for Fc receptor by rosetting with anti-RH-coated red cells.
[b] Leukocyte pyrogen was assayed as change in temperature (Δ temp) of mice injected with 0.3 ml MØ supernate.

sible for processing Il-1 into a biologically active form [46, 47]. Our laboratory has shown over a number of years that decreased MØ plasminogen activator (PA) production in trauma patients is correlated to decreased MØ immune functions, immunosuppression, and septic complications [48]. Such depressed MØ PA activity also correlates to depressed MØ-T interactions and could reflect decreased Il-1 processing.

Although the PA production of the total immunosuppressed patients' MØ population is reduced, our data indicate that when the PGE_2-producing $FcRI^+$ population is removed the remaining MØ subset can have normal PA activity. These data suggest that some of the MØ PA dysfunction is due to excessive MØ PGE_2 production. Our data do not preclude an additional trauma-induced defect in MØ Il-1 production or antigen processing.

Aberrant monokine function may represent an increase in production of certain monokines as well as a decrease in production of Il-1 [49]. Many of the metabolic derangements and pathological complications of septic shock are thought to be mediated by monokines [50, 51]. Tumor necrosis factor (TNF) is a monokine secreted only after intense and continuous stimulation of monocytes [52, 53]. TNF has both adverse metabolic effects and potential negative effects on immune function [50, 52]. TNF antagonizes the interferon-gamma (IFN-γ)-mediated induction of immune response antigen on macrophage surfaces [54]. This means that TNF can down-regulate MØ antigen-presenting function. TNF is a potent inducer of PGE_2 production in MØ fibroblast and endothelial cells [55]. Consequently, although increasing levels of MØ PGE_2 will eventually down-regulate MØ TNF synthesis, trauma-induced TNF can increase the levels of PGE_2 to immunosuppressive concentrations before it is itself down-regulated. In addition, TNF is an effective inducer of fibroblasts and endothelial cell production of Il-1 and more TNF [56]. These cell types are more resistant to PGE_2 down-regulation of their TNF while MØs are extremely sensitive. In a post-trauma microenvironment, elevated TNF levels could be maintained by activated fibroblast or endothelial cell types. As illustrated in Fig. 2, we have seen an increase in TNF production by immunosuppressed patients' monocytes, using suboptimal stimulation with 10 U/ml INF-γ and 20 µg/ml muramyl dipeptide (MDP), a synthetic analog

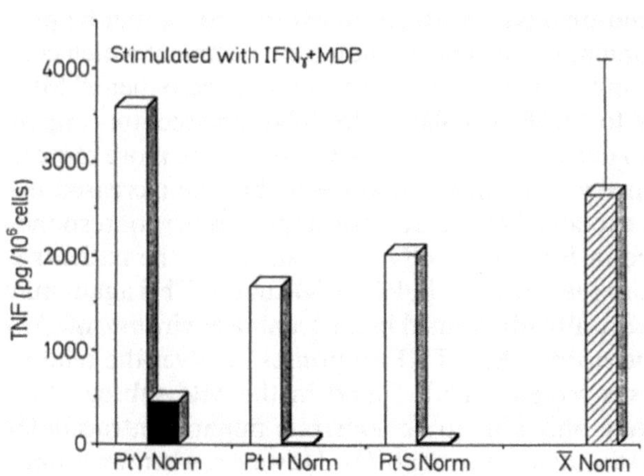

Fig. 2. Increased TNF production by the patients' monocytes after suboptimal stimulation. Monocytes from patients or normals were suboptimaly stimulated (10 U/10^6 cells IFN-γ + 20 µg/ml MDP). TNF was determined 20 h after stimulation in the serum-free L-M cell bioassay

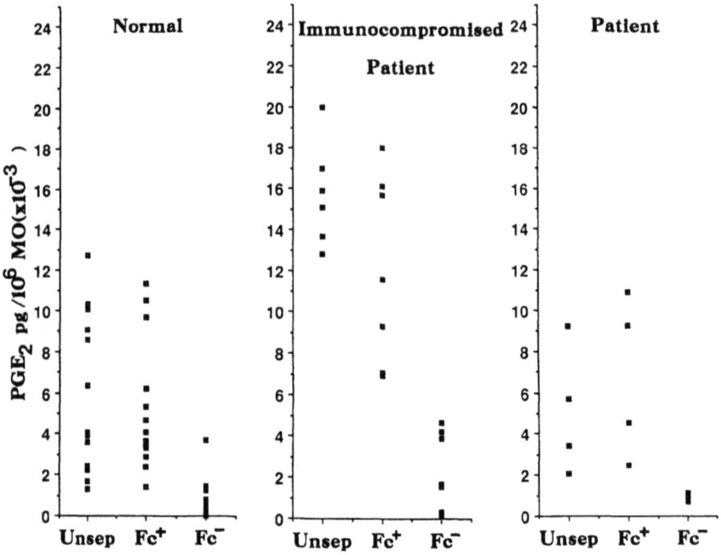

Fig. 3. The Fc^+ MØ subset of immunosuppressed patients produces the majority of their elevated PGE_2. PGE_2 produced by MØ subsets was determined in the cell-free MØ supernates with a sensitive ELISA method. MØ and MØ subsets were separated from immunocompromised and immunocompetent patients and from normals

of bacterial wall products. We interpret these data as implying that patient monocytes are already partially stimulated by lymphokines and bacterial products, whereas normal control MØs are not. We have identified a shift in the immunosuppressed patients' monocyte subset ratio which correlates to the onset of immunosuppression and appearance of elevated PGE_2 production (Fig. 3). The immunosuppressed patients' monocytes demonstrated increase in the proportion of their $FcRI^+$ MØ population. This $FcRI^+$ population is also primarily responsible for the TNF production in response to IFN-γ and MDP (Fig. 4). We interpret these data as implying that a shift toward an increase in the $FcRI^+$ MØ subset would have the following result on TNF production. More TNF would be produced by these altered MØ populations in a post-trauma environment which contains bacterial products and lymphokines. The immunosuppressed patients' MØs appear to be more responsive to MDP stimulation for TNF production (Fig. 5). Experiments are in progress to determine if patient MØ subsets are more responsive than controls. In preliminary experiments it appears that the increased patients' MØ TNF is not totally explained by an increase in the numbers of responding $FcRI^+$ MØ. As illustrated in Fig. 5 the $FcRI^+$ MØ subset of the patients is more responsive to stimuli than the normals' $FcRI^+$ MØ subset. This again may reflect that the patients' MØs are already primed in the trauma environment. Another difference in patient and normal MØ TNF responses involves the relative amounts of intracellular versus secreted TNF found in the MØ subsets. In a number of experiments we were only able to demonstrate minimal intracellular or membrane-bound TNF in stimulated normal MØs. However, when we looked

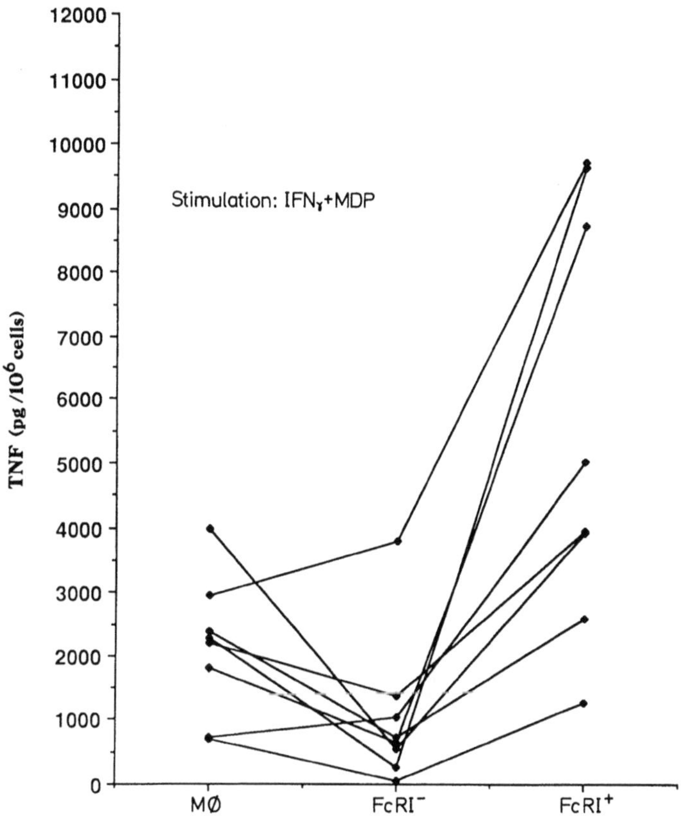

Fig. 4. Increased TNF secretion potential of stimulated FcRI-positive monocytes. Normal monocytes and MØ subsets were stimulated with 100 U IFN-γ and 20 µg/ml MDP for 20 h

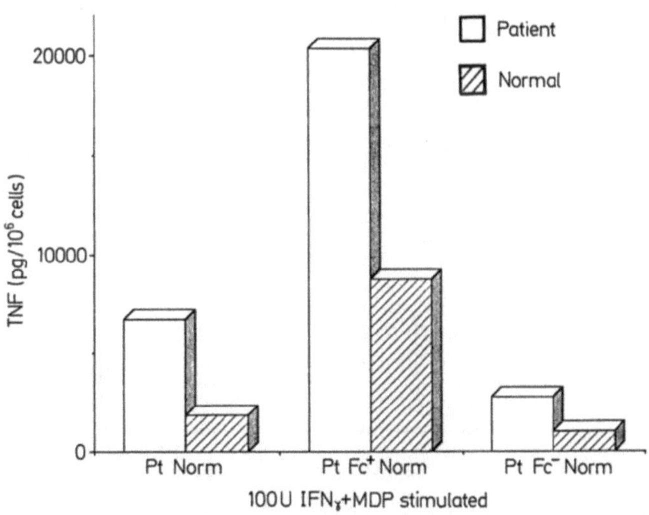

Fig. 5. Increased TNF production by the patients' FcRI$^+$ monocyte subset. Monocytes from normals and patients were separated into FcRI-positive and -negative subsets. Monocytes were stimulated with 100 U/10^6 IFN-γ plus 20 µg/ml MDP for 20 h. TNF was measured in the MØ supernates in the L-M cell bioassay

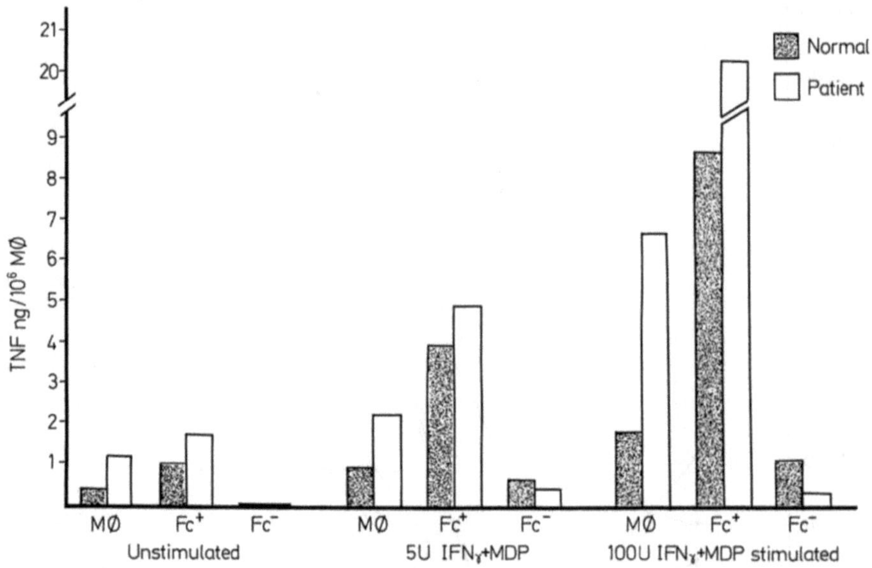

Fig. 6. Increased secreted TNF in immunocompromised patients. Monocytes and monocyte subsets from immunocompromised patients and normals were stimulated with 5 or 100 U IFN-γ/10^6 MØ plus 20 μg/ml MDP for 20 h. TNF was determined in the cell-free supernatant

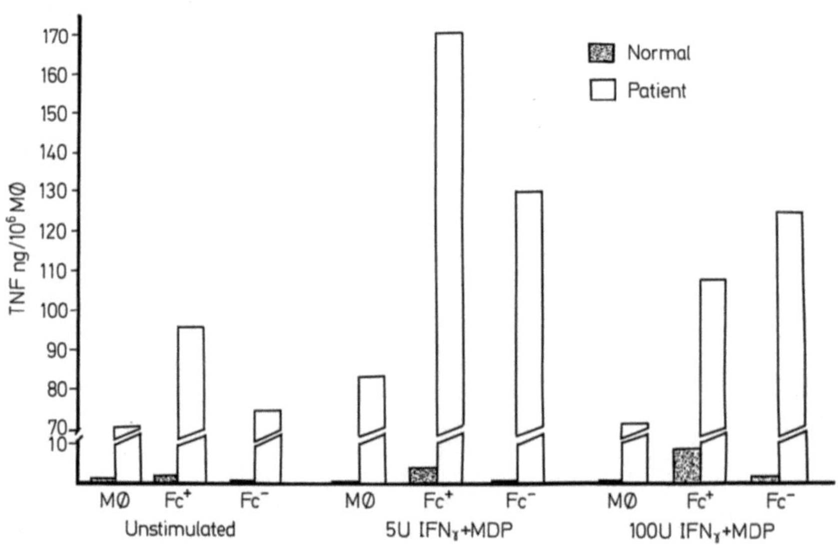

Fig. 7. Increased intracellular TNF in immunocompromised patients. Monocytes and monocyte subsets from immunocompromised patients and normals were stimulated with 5 or 100 U IFN-γ/10^6 MØ plus 20 μg/ml MDP for 20 h. Monocytes were freeze-thawed three times. Following sonification, TNF was measured in the membrane preparations

at immunosuppressed patients' MØs who showed increased secreted MØ TNF, these MØs also showed increased intracellular TNF. The FcRI$^+$ MØ subset produced the majority of both intracellular and secreted TNF (Figs. 6, 7). Consequently, patients with an increased FcRI$^+$ MØ ratio also have very different TNF production patterns.

A shift in the trauma patients' MØ ratio toward more FcRI$^+$ MØs would have a number of inimical consequences. As already demonstrated in Fig. 3, the FcRI$^+$ MØ subset is the primary producer of PGE_2 and is responsible for the elevated PGE_2 levels in post-trauma patients. The FcRI$^+$ MØ subset is also the primary producer of TNF (Fig. 4). Consequently TNF levels would be elevated in patients with increased numbers of FcRI$^+$ MØs. The FcRI$^+$ population is deficient in antigen-presenting cell function (Table 1). This deficiency is not totally reversed by addition of indomethacin and so may not be entirely due to elevated PGE_2 production. Consequently, patients with decreased FcRI$^-$ MØs would have decreased antigen-presenting activity in their total MØ population. The FcRI$^+$ population is not as active in the production of plasminogen activator (Fig. 8). Consequently, fibrinolysis and possibly IL-1 processing could be decreased in patients with decreased FcRI$^-$ MØ. Preliminary evidence indicates that both the FcRI$^+$ and FcRI$^-$ MØ. Preliminary evidence indicates that both the FcRI$^+$ and FcRI$^-$ MØ subsets produce IL-1 as measured in the D10 assay. However, we have no information on any difference in IL-1 type of these two MØ subsets.

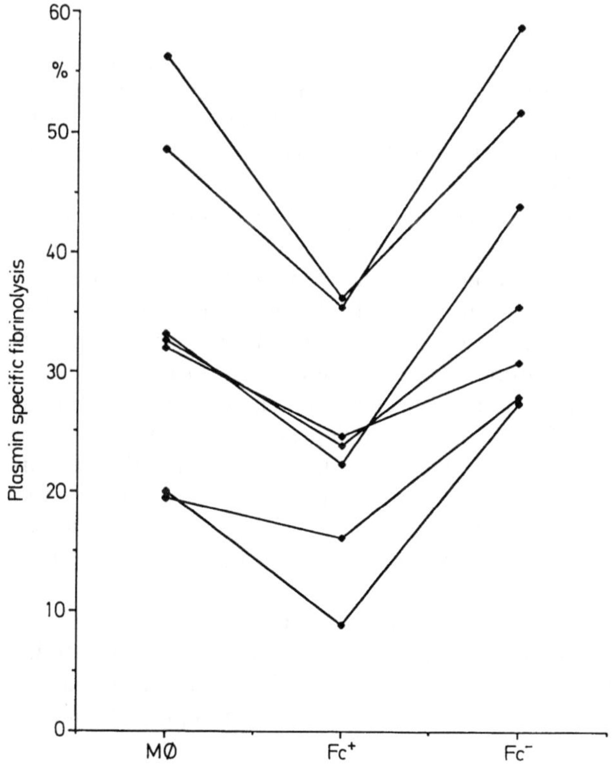

Fig. 8. Plasminogen activator production by monocyte subsets. Monocyte plasminogen activator capacity was measured as the percentage of plasmin-specific fibrinolysis

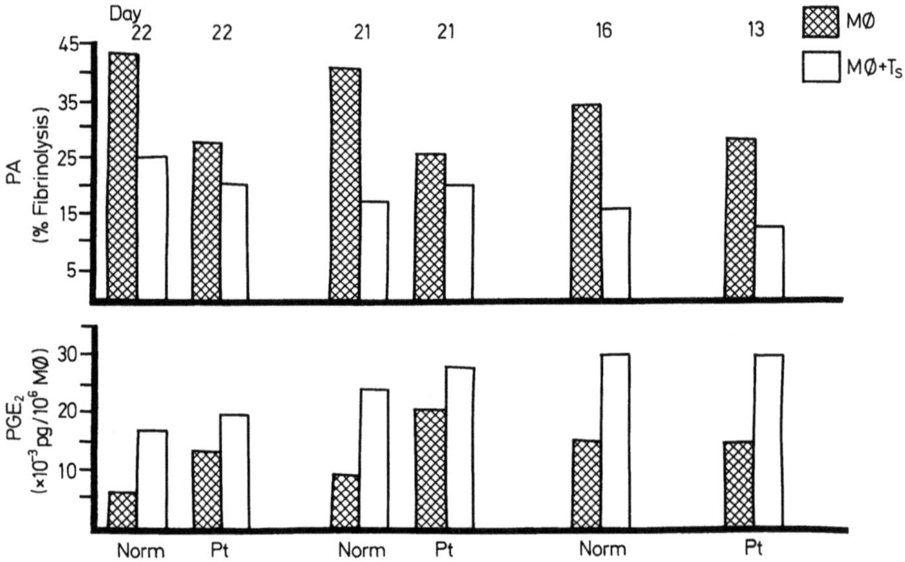

Fig. 9. Comparison of T_s activity of late T cells from immunosuppressed patients. Late T cells were collected 12 days after injury or later. T cells were recombined with monocyte that was collected 2–3 days earlier. T cells collected from patients with depressed monocyte PA activity were cocultured with equal numbers of allogenic monocytes from normal controls or monocytes from autologous patients. Monocyte PA and PGE_2 were measured after 48 h coculture

Monocyte/macrophage IL-1 is only one of the MØ functions that is down-regulated by elevation of PGE_2 levels. Expression of Ia on monocyte surfaces, expression of IL-2 receptors on T-lymphocyte surfaces, and expression of Ia on B-cell surfaces are all down-regulated by elevated PGE_2 levels [57]. In addition there is some evidence that elevated PGE_2 levels favor induction of T_s over induction of T_h [58, 59]. All of the data led us to postulate that a shift in MØ subsets toward a greater proportion of the $FcRI^+$, PGE_2-producing MØ subset could result in many of the post-trauma MØ aberrations described. One of the described effects of T_s developed in chronic infections is to induce PGE_2 production by MØs. Patient MØ populations containing a greater proportion of $FcRI^+$ MØs could respond to T_s with a greater production of PGE_2. As illustrated in Fig. 9 addition of immunosuppressed trauma patient T_s (collected from chronically infected patients) to either patient or normal MØs resulted in depressed MØ PA production and elevated PGE_2 production. We interpret these data as implying that immunosuppressed patients who develop septic complications may be maintained in their immunodepressed state by the action of late-appearing T_s. These late-appearing T_s increase the stimulation of PGE_2 production by the increased $FcRI^+$ MØ subset.

Considering the number of reports of increased immunosuppressive PGE_2 activity post-trauma, it would seem logical to treat patients' post-trauma by administration of cyclo-oxygenase inhibitors as immunomodulators. Clinical trials of ibuprophen have been initiated in some centers. As a prelude to patient trials of cyclo-oxygenase inhibitors, we have examined the in vitro effects of cyclo-oxygenase inhibitors on patient MØ monokine production. When we examined immunosuppressed trauma patients' MØ after in vitro treatment with indomethacin, we found that patients with increased intracellular MØ TNF secreted that TNF upon indomethacin treatment. These data imply that elevated PGE_2 levels, at least late in the patient's course, may be down-regulating some of the MØ TNF activity.

Our data imply that some of the immunologic dysfunctions seen in immunosuppressed trauma patients may be related to a shift in the MØ subset ratio with consequent MØ functional aberrations. Nevertheless, it is clear that a number of other dysfunctions also contribute to post-trauma immunosuppression. It is not clear what triggers the initial shift in MØ subsets. In addition, T_s arising early after trauma have been demonstrated by several investigators [59, 60]. We have shown that these T_s are of the CD4 type, and suppress monocyte PA function by some mechanism other than increasing PGE_2 production [61]. The immunosuppressed trauma patient syndrome is obviously complex. One of the more intriguing possibilities is that initial gut ischemia causes release of a cascade of mediators and endotoxin which initially affect the MØ subset ratio and consequently alter a number of subsequent immune functions. The data produced by a number of investigators seem to implicate MØ dysfunctions as pivotal in post-trauma immunosuppression.

Acknowledgements. The special cooperation of the Burn Unit at Worcester City Hospital and the nurses at the Trauma Intensive Are Unit of UMMC are gratefully acknowledged. The technical assistance of Karen Kodys, B. A., and Donna Catalano, B. S., is also gratefully acknowledged.

References

1. Stratta R, Warden G, Ninnemann J et al. (1986) Immunologic parameters in burned patients: effect of therapeutic interventions. J Trauma 26:7
2. Alexander J (1980) The role of host defense mechanisms in surgical infections. Surg Clin North Am 60:107
3. Hansbrough J, Zapata-Sirvent R, Peterson V (1987) Immunomodulation following burn injury. Surg Clin North Am 67:69
4. Baker C, Yamada A, Faist E et al. (1987) Interleukin-1 and T cell function following injury. JBCR 8:503
5. Faist E, Kupper T, Baker C et al. (1986) Depression of cellular immunity after major injury. Arch Surg 121:1000
6. Watters J, Bessey P, Dinarello C et al. (1986) Both inflammatory and endocrine mediators stimulate host responses to sepsis. Arch Surg 121:179
7. Deitch E, Bridges R, Dobke M et al. (1987) Burn wound sepsis may be promoted by a failure of local antibacterial host defenses. Ann Surg 206:340
8. Carrico J, Meakins J, Marshall J et al. (1986) Multiple-organ-failure syndrome. Arch Surg 121:196
9. Weinstein J, Taylor J (1987) Interleukin-1 and the acute-phase response: induction of mouse liver serum amyloid A mRNA by murine recombinant interleukin-1. J Trauma 27:1227
10. Warren R, Starnes F, Gabrilove J et al. (1987) The acute metabolic effects of tumor necrosis factor administration in humans. Arch Surg 122:1396

11. Moran K, Munster A (1987) Alterations of the host defense mechanism in burned patients. Surg Clin North Am 67:47
12. Hoyt D, Ozkan A, Ninnemann J (1987) Immunologic monitoring of infection risk in trauma patients: research questions and an approach to the problem. JBCR 8:549
13. Unanue E, Beller D, Lu C et al. (1984) Antigen presentation: comments on its regulation and mechanism. J Immunol 132:1
14. Ziegler H, Orlin C, Cluff C (1987) Differential requirements for the processing and presentation of soluble and particulate bacterial antigens by macrophages. Eur J Immunol 17:1287
15. Kaye J, Gillis S, Mizel S et al. (1984) Growth of a cloned helper T cell line induced by a monoclonal antibody specific for the antigen receptor: interleukin 1 is required for the expression of receptors for interleukin 2. J Immunol 133:1339
16. Kurt-Jones EA, Hamberge S, Ohara J et al. (1987) Heterogeneity of helper/inducer T lymphocytes. J Exp Med 166:1774
17. Kupper T, Horowitz M, Lee F (1987) Autocrine growth of T cells independent of IL-2: identification of interleukin 4 (IL-4, BSF-1) as an autocrine growth factor for a cloned antigen-specific helper T cell. J Immunol 138:4280
18. Killan L, MacDonald G, West J et al. (1987) Cloned, Ia-restricted T cells that do not produce interleukin 4 (IL-4) B cell stimulatory factor 1 (BSF-1) fail to keep antigen specific B cells. J Immunol 138:1674
19. Morimoto C, Letvin NL, Boyd AW et al. (1985) The isolation and characterization of the human helper inducer T cell subset. J Immunol 134:3762
20. Van Damme J, Opdenakker G, Simpson RJ et al. (1987) Identification of the human 26 kD protein, interferon β_2 (IFN-β_2), as a B cell hybridoma/plasmacytoma growth factor induced by interleukin 1 and tumor necrosis factor. J Exp Med 165:914
21. Taga T, Kawanishi Y, Hardy R et al. (1987) Receptors for B cell stimulatory factor 2. J Exp Med 166:967
22. Aarden LA, De Groot ER, Schaap OL et al. (1987) Production of hybridoma growth factor by human monocytes. Eur J Immunol 17:1411
23. Yasukawa K, Hirano T, Watanabe Y et al. (1987) Structure and expression of human B cell stimulatory factor-2 (BSF-2I, L-6) gene. EMBO 6:2939
24. Miller C, Claudy B (1979) Suppressor T cells induced by thermal injury. Cell Immunol 44:201
25. Kupper T, Baker C, Ferguson T et al. (1985) A burn induced Ly-2 suppressor T cell lowers resistance to bacterial infection. J Surg Res 38:606
26. Gibbons R, Martinez O, Horn J (1988) Early alterations in HLA class II antigen expression and response to tetanus toxoid by peripheral blood mononuclear cells from patients with severe injury or burns. Abstracts OR3. 1st International Congress on the Immune Consequences of Trauma, Shock and Sepsis. Mechanisms and therapeutic approaches. Munich, March 3–5, 1988
27. Zembala M, Uracz W, Ruggiero I et al. (1984) Isolation and functional characteristics of FcR^+ and FcR^- human monocyte subsets. J Immunol 133:1293
28. Ohkawa S, Martin L, Fukunishi Y et al. (1987) Regulatory role of FcR^+ and FcR^- monocyte subsets in *Mycobacterium leprae*-induced lymphoproliferative response in vitro. Clin Exp Immunol 67:43
29. Pryjma J, Flad H, Gruber M et al. (1986) Monocyte-T-cell interactions in the regulation of polyclonal B-cell response. Scand J Immunol 24:21
30. Looney R, Abraham G, Anderson C (1986) Human monocytes and U937 cells bear two distinct Fc receptors for IgG[1]. J Immunol 136:1641
31. Rodrick M, Wood J, Grbic J et al. (1986) Defective IL-2 production in patients with severe burns and sepsis. Lymphokine Res 5:S75
32. Faist E, Mewes A, Baker C et al. (1987) Prostaglandin E_2 (PGE_2)-dependent suppression of interleukin α (IL-2) production in patients with major trauma. J Trauma 27:837
33. Nijsten M, DeGroot E, TenDuis H et al. (1987) Serum levels of interleukin-6 and acute phase responses. Lancet II:921
34. Takai Y, Wong G, Clark S et al. (1988) B cell stimulatory factor-2 is involved in the differentiation of cytotoxic T lymphocytes. J Immunol 140:508

35. Zucali J, Elfenbein G, Barth K et al. (1987) Effects of human interleukin 1 and human tumor necrosis factor on human T lymphocyte colony formation. J Clin Invest 80:772
36. Helfgor D, May A, Sthoeger Z et al. (1987) Bacterial lipopolysaccharide (endotoxin) enhances expression and secretion of β_2 interferon by human fibroblasts. J Exp Med 166:1300
37. Garman R, Jacobs K, Clark S et al. (1987) B-cell-stimulatory factor 2 (β_2 interferon) functions as a second signal for interleukin 2 production by mature murine T cells. Proc Natl Acad Sci USA 84:7629
38. Le J, Vilcek J (1987) Tumor necrosis factor and interleukin 1: cytokines with multiple overlapping biological activities. Lab Invest 56:234
39. Dinarello C, Cannon J, Wolff S et al. (1986) Tumor necrosis factor (cachectin) is an endogenous pyrogen and induces production of interleukin 1. J Exp Med 163:1433
40. Damas P, Gysen P, Lopez M et al. (1988) Cachectin (TNFα) serum level in human during septic shock. 1st International Congress on the Immune Consequences of Trauma, Shock and Sepsis. Mechanisms and therapeutic approaches. Munich, March 3–5, 1988
41. March CJ, Mosley B, Larsen A et al. (1985) Cloning, sequence and expression of two distinct human interleukin-1 complimentary DNAs. Nature 315:641
42. Demuczuk S, Baumberger C, Mach B et al. (1987) Expression of human IL 1α and β messenger RNAs and IL 1 activity in human peripheral blood mononuclear cells. J Mol Cell Immunol 3:255
43. Kurt-Jones EA, Beller D, Mizel S et al. (1985) Identification of a membrane-associated interleukin 1 in macrophages. Proc Natl Acad Sci USA 82:1204
44. Conlon PJ, Grabstein KH, Alpert A et al. (1987) Localization of human mononuclear cell interleukin 1. J Immunol 139:98
45. Bendtzen K, Mandrup-Poulsen T, Nerup J (1986) Cytotoxicity of human pI7 interleukin-1 for pancreatic islets of Langerhans. Science 232:1545
46. Matsushima K, Taguchi M, Kovacs E et al. (1986) Intracellular localization of human monocyte associated interleukin 1 (IL1) activity and release of biologically active IL 1 from monocytes by trypsin and plasmin. J Immunol 136:2883
47. Auron P, Warner S, Webb A et al. (1987) Studies on the molecular nature of human interleukin 1. J Immunol 138:1447
48. Miller CL, Graziano CJ, Lim RC (1982) Human monocyte plasminogen activator production: correlation to altered MØ-T lymphocyte intersection
49. Cerami A, Beutler B (1988) The role of cachectin/TNF in endotoxic shock and cachexia. Immunol Today 9:28
50. Beutler B, Cerami A (1987) Cachectin: more than a tumor necrosis factor. N Engl J Med 316:379
51. Tracey K, Lowry S, Fahey T et al. (1987) Cachectin/tumor necrosis factor induces lethal shock and stress hormone responses in the dog. Surg Gynecol Obstet 164:415
52. Ruddle N (1987) Tumor necrosis factor and related cytotoxins. Immunol Today 8:129
53. Beutler B, Tbacenko V, Mibserk J et al. (1986) Effect of gamma interferon on cachectin expression by mononuclear phagocyte. J Exp Med 164:1791–1796
54. Hoffman M, Weinberg JB (1987) Tumor necrosis factor-α (TNF) stimulates peroxide production and expression of Fc receptors for IgG2b/Ia (FcR), but does not induce Ia expression on murine peritoneal macrophages (M.P.). J Leukocyte Biol 5:609
55. Dayer J, Beutler B, Cerami A (1985) Cachectin/tumor necrosis factor stimulates collagenase and prostaglandin E_2 production by human synovial cells and dermal fibroblasts. J Exp Med 162:2163
56. Le J, Weinstein D, Gubler U et al. (1987) Induction of membrane-associated interleukin 1 by tumor necrosis factor in human fibroblasts. J Immunol 138:2137
57. Tripp C, Wyche A, Unanue E et al. (1986) The functional significance of the regulation of macrophage Ia expression by endogenous arachidonate metabolites in vitro. J Immunol 137:3915

58. Wood J, Grbic J, Rodrick M et al. (1987) Suppression of interleukin 2 production in an animal model of thermal injury is related to prostaglandin synthesis. Arch Surg 122:179
59. Suzuki F, Pollard RB (1987) Suppressor cells generated in mice late after thermal injury. J Trauma 27:379
60. Green DR, Wang N, Zheng H (1987) A suppressor-inducer factor produced by burn trauma-associated T cells. JBCR 8:521
61. Miller-Graziano C, Fink M, Wu J et al. (1988) Mechanisms of altered monocyte prostaglandin E_2 production in severely injured patients. Arch Surg 123:293

Possible Use of the Monocyte/Macrophage Activation Marker Neopterin for Clinical Monitoring of Sepsis-Related Multiorgan Failure

H. Redl, W. Strohmaier, G. Schlag, R. Pacher, W. Woloszczuk, D. Inthorn, J. Troppmair, and C. Huber

Introduction

Multiorgan failure (MOF) is the result of the pathological sequence of a generalized inflammatory reaction with or without septic complications (Goris et al. 1985; Schlag and Redl 1987). The causal involvement of granulocytes in organ failure is reflected in the usefulness of measurements of the granulocyte-specific elastase alpha$_1$-antiprotease complex (Neumann et al. 1984) with respect to well-timed diagnosis of onset and severity of septicemia (Duswald et al. 1985), adult respiratory distress syndrome (ARDS), and MOF (Goris et al. 1987; Nuytinck et al. 1986). On the other hand, monocyte/macrophages may be stimulated as well in a generalized reaction by anaphylatoxins (Goodman et al. 1982), and especially by bacterial products (endotoxin) and lymphokines. When stimulated, macrophages release a broad spectrum of substances similar to granulocytes, and also important monokines [e.g., tumor necrosis factor (TNF)-cachectin]. In vitro evidence indicates that upon stimulation of macrophages with interferon-gamma, neopterin [D-erythro-neopterin (2-amino-4-oxo-6 (D-erythro-1,2,3-trihydroxypropyl)-dihydropteridine] – a metabolite derived from guanosine triphosphate (GTP) (Schödon et al. 1985) is secreted, which to date, is of unknown biological significance (Huber et al. 1984).

Since we have shown that neopterin might be of diagnostic value in septicemia (Strohmaier et al. 1987) and endotoxin is a central mediator, we evaluated both the effect of endotoxin on the release of neopterin from macrophages in vitro, as well as plasma levels of this activation marker in vivo, in patients prone to develop MOF.

Subjects and Methods

In Vitro Studies

A human macrophage cell line in long-term culture was treated with either recombinant interferon-gamma (Bender, Vienna) or endotoxin for 4–5 days.

Study I

Twenty-one postoperative or post-traumatic intensive care unit (ICU) patients with various underlying diseases, admitted to the Surgical Clinic, University Unit

Immune Consequences of
Trauma, Shock and Sepsis
Eds. Faist/Ninnemann/Green

Großhadern, Munich, FRG, were categorized by clinical evaluation and outcome. Seven patients had no complications (group Co), while 14 patients developed septic complications; of these five recovered (group SEP/SURV) and 9 died from septicemia (group SEP/NS).

Study II

Thirty-two patients (cardiac, orthopedic and tumor surgery, polytrauma, pneumonia) at the ICU of the Second Department of Internal Medicine, Vienna, with symptoms of nonviral septicemia (group SEP) were divided into non-survivors (group SEP/NS) and survivors (group SEP/SURV). Twenty-four postoperative patients (cardiac, orthopedic, and tumor surgery, polytrauma) without signs of septicemia served as the control group (group Co). Definition of septicemia was similar to that of Montgomery et al. (1985), except that if blood cultures were not positive three out of four additional hemodynamic criteria had to be fulfilled (Pacher et al. 1987). For classification of the clinical course we used the MOF score according to Goris et al. (1985). A total score of $\geqq 5$ was considered as the critical limit of outcome.

Blood samples were taken in EDTA tubes and were centrifuged within one hour after sampling. Plasma samples were stored frozen (−20 °C). Neopterin was determined using a radioimmunoassay distributed by Henning (FRG). The normal range in human plasma is 3–10 nmol/l. Granulocyte elastase alpha$_1$-protease inhibitor (E-alpha$_1$-PI) complex was measured by an enzyme immunoassay (Neumann et al. 1984) supplied in a kit by Merck (FRG), with a normal range of 60–110 µg/l.

Many other plasma parameters were analyzed and invasive hemodynamic measurements were made, but their results are beyond the scope of this paper. Statistical analysis between groups was performed with ANOVA and the Kruskal-Wallis test. The Spearman correlation coefficients were employed for the correlation matrix. To predict a clinical event the definitions of sensitivity, specificity, or accuracy were used.

Results

In vitro

Endotoxin stimulation of macrophages in long-term culture resulted in dose-dependent neopterin release (Fig. 1).

Study I

Values of group SEP/SURV were always higher than those of group Co; a significant difference was found on day 5 only (Table 1).

In group SEP/NS neopterin plasma concentrations were significantly elevated on each day during the observation period as compared with controls (Table 1).

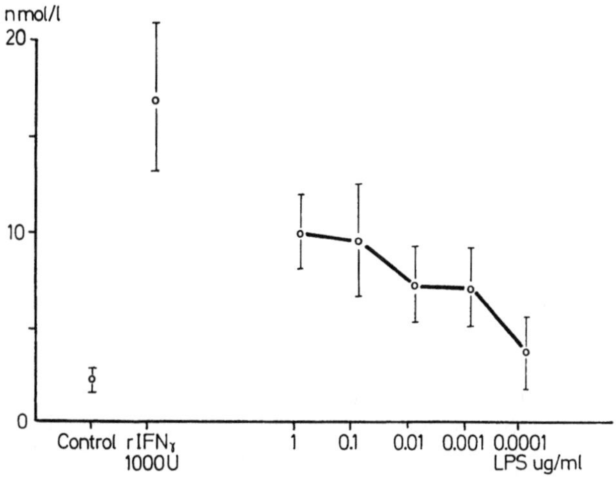

Fig. 1. Neopterin release from stimulated human macrophages into the supernatant fluid in long-term culture. Each data point is shown as mean ± SD of 3–9 individual experiments. *LPS*, Endotoxin; *gamma-IFN*, recombinant human interferon-gamma

Table 1. Plasma neopterin (nmol/l) in postoperative patients at the ICU without complications (Co) and with septic complications – survivors (SEP/SURV) and non-survivors (SEP/NS). Statistical analysis with ANOVA and linear contrasts according to Lindner (data are shown as mean ± SE)

	Days in the ICU								
	1 st		3 rd		5 th			Last	
Co $n=7$	7.30 ± 3.4		6.2 ± 8.6		9.7 ± 3.2	*		12.0 ± 2.6	***
		**		**			***		
SEP/SURV $n=5$	16.52 ± 1.6		28.6 ± 1.5		37.4 ± 1.5			30.4 ± 1.4 ***	
SEP/NS $n=9$	34.51 ± 2.1		59.8 ± 2.9		71.1 ± 2.9			193.2 ± 2.2	

* $P<0.05$; **$P<0.01$; *** $P<0.001$.

Study II

Significant differences in neopterin levels were revealed between septic patients and postoperative patients without complications ($P<0.001$) with normal neopterin levels (Fig. 2). Additionally, group SEP/NS vs. group Co and SEP/SURV vs. Co could be differentiated by neopterin levels on each day of the observation period (6 days). Groups SEP/NS and SEP/SURV revealed significant differences starting on the third day after admission to the ICU. Septic patients (groups SEP/SURV and SEP/NS) showed a significant correlation between neopterin and MOF score ($r=0.75$, $P<0.0001$, $n_{obs}=141$).

Similar results were found for the correlation between E-alpha$_1$-PI and MOF score ($r=0.67$, $P<0.001$, $n_{obs}=110$). Comparison of neopterin levels $\geqq 40$ nmol/l measured 1 day before evaluation of a MOF score $\geqq 5$ revealed a sensitivity of

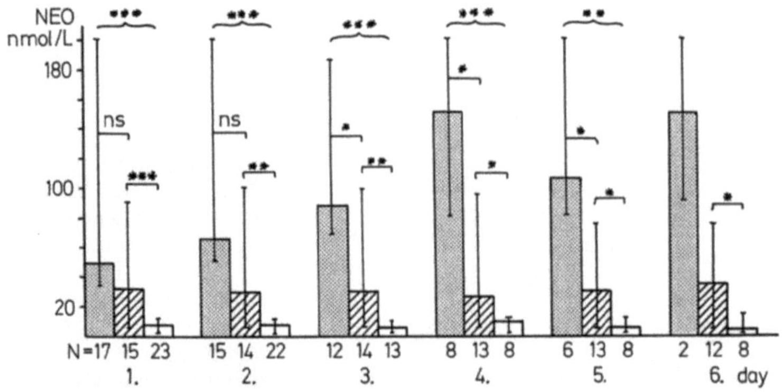

Fig. 2. Plasma levels of neopterin *(NEO)* in patients with sepsis [nonsurvivors, *spotted bars* (group SEP/NS), survivors (group SEP/SURV) *hatched bars*] and in postoperative patients without signs of septicemia (*open bars*, group Co). Significant differences: *** $P < 0.001$; ** *P*♀∊♀Γ′ * $P < 0.05$; median, 25th and 75th percentiles

96% and a specificity of 73% ($n_{obs} = 188$). The comparison of E-alpha$_1$-PI values $\geqq 400$ µg/l measured 1 day before evaluation of a MOF score $\geqq 5$ showed a sensitivity of 88% and had a specificity of 83% ($n_{obs} = 189$). A sensitivity of 91% and a specificity of 99% were achieved when patients fulfilled both criteria (neopterin $\geqq 40$ nmol/l and E alpha$_1$-PI $\geqq 400$ nmol/l; $n_{obs} = 151$). Furthermore, acute pulmonary insufficiency was predicted by elevated E-alpha$_1$ PI values (>400 µg/l) 1 day before mechanical ventilation had to be performed with a sensitivity of 81%, a specificity of 82% and an accuracy of 82%.

Discussion

Most systems to assess the severity of sepsis score the secondary effects of sepsis on various organ systems. We used the MOF score according to Goris et al. (1985), which evaluates organ failure on a three-point scale. Excellent correlations were established between mortality and the number of organ failures. Therefore it seems reasonable to use this score for comparison of biochemical parameters in MOF.

One of the mediators of organ failure, especially at a later stage, is endotoxin derived from endogenous (gut) and/or exogenous scources (Schlag et al. 1987).

Interestingly, endotoxin directly stimulates neopterin release in vitro. Whether high neopterin levels in vivo are the result of this direct action or are mediated via interferon-gamma cannot be decided. Parallel measurement of interferon-gamma with the highly sensitive test of Woloszczuk (1985) (data not shown) did not answer this question. Though the biological function of macrophage-derived neopterin is uncertain, it might serve as an excellent tool to monitor patients prone to develop sepsis and MOF. It is also much easier to perform and more reliable than the *Limulus* assay, and there are fewer pitfalls in blood sampling. A single test of neopterin might also be useful (because of the low variance from day to day and high reliability), while for endotoxin, serial plasma level measurements are strongly recommended (Grundman and Ingenhoff 1986).

The ability to demonstrate the activation of the T-lymphocyte/macrophage-axis in vivo in endotoxin related events is particularly important, because it was recently demonstrated that the TNF, which is recently demonstrated that the TNF, which is released from stimulated (e.g., by endotoxin) macrophages, is one of the major mediators of endotoxin shock (Tracey et al. 1986). The data presented demonstrate: (a) the possibility of direct neopterin release from macrophages in response to endotoxin; (b) that neopterin is released in vivo under conditions leading to organ failure, e.g., sepsis (generalized inflammation), which demonstrates the involvement of macrophages in MOF; (c) the involvement of granulocytes in MOF because of comparable results with elastase (data not shown); (d) that (besides E-alpha$_1$-PI) neopterin might become a helpful tool for evaluation of the clinical course in patients prone to develop sepsis and MOF, because of its correlation with the degree of organ failure.

References

Duswald KH, Jochum M, Schramm W et al. (1985) Released granulocytic elastase: an indicator of pathobiochemical alterations in septicemia after abdominal surgery. Surgery 98:892

Goodman MG, Chenoweth DE, Weigle WO (1982) Induction of interleukin 1 secretion and enhancement of humoral immunity by binding of human C5a to macrophage surface C5a receptor. J Exp Med 155:912

Goris RJA, Boekhorst TPA, Nuytinck JKS et al. (1985) Multi organ failure, generalized autodestructive inflammation? Arch Surg 120:1109

Goris RJA, Nuytinck HKS, Redl H (1987) Scoring systems and predictors of ARDS and MOF. In: Schlag G, Redl H (eds) Vienna shock forum, part B: monitoring and treatment of shock. Liss, New York, p 3 (Progress in clinical and biological research, vol 236-B)

Grundman R, Ingenhoff E (1986) Postoperative determination of plasma endotoxin levels. Dtsch Med Wochenschr 111:457

Huber C, Batchelor JR, Fuchs D et al. (1984) Immune-response associated production of Neopterin release from macrophages primarily under control of Interferon-gamma. J Exp Med 160:310

Montgomery AB, Stager MA, Carrico CJ et al. (1985) Causes of mortality in patients with the adult respiratory distress syndrome. Am Rev Respir Dis 132:485

Neumann S, Heinrich N, Gunzer G (1984) Enzyme linked immunoassay for human granulocyte elastase in complex with alpha1-proteinase inhibitor. In: Hörl WA, Heidland A (eds) Proteases: potential role in health and disease. Plenum, New York, p 379

Nuytinck JKS, Goris RJA, Redl H et al. (1986) Posttraumatic complications and inflammatory mediators. Arch Surg 121:886

Pacher R, Redl H, Woloszczuk W (1987) Neopterin and granulocyte elastase in septicemic patients prone to develop multi-organ failure. In: Blair JA, Pfleiderer H, Wachter H (eds) Biochemical and clinical aspects of pteridines, vol 5. Gruyter, Berlin, p 305

Schlag G, Redl H (1987) Mediators in sepsis. In: Vincent JL, Thijs LG (eds) Septic shock. Springer, Berlin Heidelberg New York, p 51 (Update in intensive care and emergency Medicine, vol 4)

Schödon G, Troppmair J, Huber C et al. (1985) Metabolism of pterins in human peripheral blood mononuclear cells. In: Curtius HC, Pfleiderer W, Wachter H (eds) Biochemical and clinical aspects of pteridines, vol 4. Gruyter, Berlin, p 369

Strohmaier W, Redl H, Schlag G et al. (1987) D-Erythro-neopterin plasma levels in intensive care patients with and without septic complications. Crit Care Med 15:757

Tracey KJ, Beutler B, Lowery SF et al. (1986) Shock and tissue injury induced by recombinant human cachectin. Science 234:470

Woloszczuk W (1985) A sensitive immunoradiometric assay for gamma interferon, suitable for its measurement in serum. Clin Chem 31:1090

Expression of Functional Interleukin 2 Receptors in Burn Patients May Be Regulated by Interleukin 3

J. A. Teodorczyk-Injeyan, G. B. Mills, B. G. Sparkes, and W. J. Peters

Introduction

In thermally injured patients the secretion of interleukin 2 (IL2) and acquisition of IL2-specific surface receptors (IL2R) by mitogen-activated T-lymphocytes is significantly suppressed (Wood et al. 1984; Teodorczyk-Injeyan et al. 1986). Exogenous recombinant IL2 (rIL2) can upregulate expression of its receptor (Tac antigen) in lymphocyte cultures from burn patients; however, the proliferative response of such cultures to rIL2 remains reduced (Teodorczyk-Injeyan et al. 1987). This may suggest that in the burn patient expression of functional (high-affinity) receptors is affected.

Recent reports demonstrated that another activated T-lymphocyte-derived growth factor, interleukin 3 (IL3) may be involved in regulation of IL2R expression (Birchenall Sparks et al. 1986). The present study examines the in vitro effect of IL3 on IL2-induced polyclonal proliferation of unstimulated peripheral blood mononuclear cells (PBMCs) from patients with severe burns. In addition the effect of IL2 and/or IL3 on expression of Tac antigen (IL2R) is reported, in parallel cultures of unstimulated and mitogen-activated PBMCs.

Materials and Methods

Six patients (five males and one female) ranging from 24 to 44 years of age were admitted to the burn center with injuries representing from 35% to over 50% total body surface area (TBSA). Five healthy volunteers aged 27–39 years were studied as controls. Burn patients' blood samples were collected at 8- to 12-day intervals after the injury.

Preparation of PBMCs for in vitro studies and for enumeration of Tac-positive cells by flow cytometry analysis was carried out as described elsewhere (Teodorczyk-Injeyan et al. 1986). Exogenous human rIL2 (Biogen Corp.) and purified IL2 (Electro-Nucleonics, Inc.) were used at concentrations of 20–40 U/ml and 10%–20% (V/V) respectively. WEHI-derived, purified IL3 (Ihle et al. 1983) was a gift from Dr. R. Cameron (University of Toronto) and was tested at concentrations ranging from 1% to 30%. The quadruplicate cultures of PBMCs (10^5/well) were incubated with or without IL2 and/or IL3 and the incorporation of [^{3}H]TdR (1 μCi/well, Amersham) was measured on day 6 after a 16-h pulse.

Immune Consequences of
Trauma, Shock and Sepsis
Eds. Faist/Ninnemann/Green

Results and Discussion

One of the six patients (31 years, TBSA 70%) died 30 days after the injury. The remaining patients had an average of four (range three to six) tests completed over the hospitalization period (Fig. 1). The mitogenic effect of rIL2 and of purified IL2 in cultures of unstimulated PBMCs from burn patients was optimal at a concentration of 20 U/ml and 20%, respectively. Figure 1 illustrates alternations in the magnitude of the proliferative response to IL2, expressed as a percentage of the (maximal) response observed at or close to discharge. The maximal response was comparable to that of the controls.

Interleukin 2-induced proliferation was significantly ($P<0.001$–0.05) suppressed (by 63% to over 90%, range 30%–98%) up to 12 days postburn and then increased in convalescent patients (Fig. 1). In concordance with our previous studies (Teodorczyk-Injeyan et al. 1987) PBMCs from nonsurviving patients did not proliferate in the presence of exogenous IL2 (not shown). Using PBMCs from the survivors, the addition of IL3 at the optimal concentrations (10%–20% v/v) to cultures with the reduced response to IL2 resulted in a significant augmentation of IL2-assisted proliferation (Fig. 1). The [^{3}H]TdR incorporation in such cultures represented 35% to over 100% of the optimal response to IL2 (Fig. 1). IL3 had no effect on IL2 – induced proliferation in PBMC cultures from the nonsurviving patient (not shown), from patients studied at 4 or more weeks after the

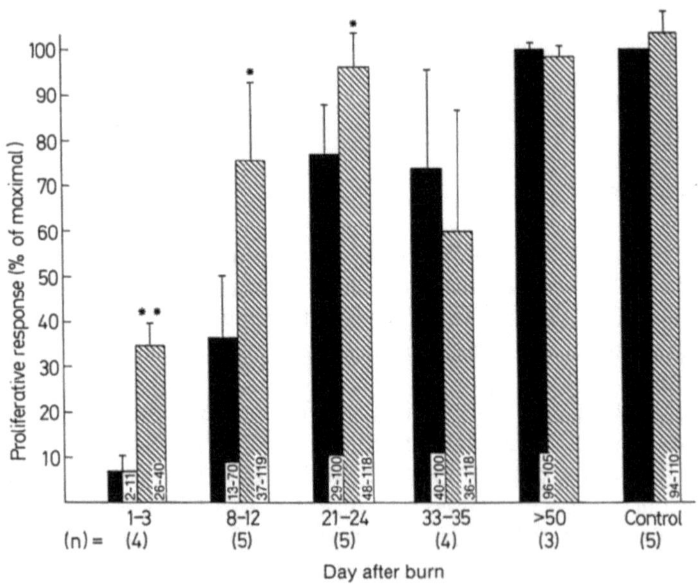

Fig. 1. Effect of IL3 (20% v/v) on IL2-induced proliferation of peripheral blood mononuclear cell cultures from burn patients. PBMC cultures were established at indicated time intervals after the burn and cultivated in the presence of IL2 alone (■) or IL2 with IL3 (▨). The cultures were pulsed with [^{3}H]TdR 16 h before harvesting on day 6. Results are expressed as a percentage of the maximal [^{3}H]TdR incorporation demonstrated by each patient during the postburn period. *$P<0.05$; **$P<0.001$

Table 1. Effect of IL2 and IL3 on Tac antigen (IL2R) expression by mitogen-stimulated and unstimulated PBMCs from burn patients (1–12 days postburn)

Culture conditions	% TC-positive cells at 72 h (range)	
	Patients	Controls
Con A (10 µg/ml)	19.9± 8.8 (9–37)	41.7± 6.9 (34–49)
Con A+IL2 (20 U/ml)	36.7±14.4 (14–62)	53.2±10.7 (42–67)
Con A+IL3 (20% v/v)	18.4±11.2 (11–34)	ND
Con A+IL2+IL3	32.9±12.1 (16–59)	ND
Tissue culture medium	4.7± 2.3 (4– 6)	ND
IL2	16.9±13.8 (6–29)	ND
IL3	9.6± 3.1 (5–11)	ND
IL2+IL3	31.3±24 (10–50)	ND

burn (convalescent) or from normal donors (Fig. 1). Moreover, IL3 was without effect on its own at all times tested.

To determine whether the effect of IL3 could result from an improved expression of IL2R, Con A-stimulated and unstimulated cultures of PBMCs were established from three burn patients at the time of the expected IL3-associated increase of IL2-induced proliferation (up to 2 weeks postburn). As reported previously (Teodorczyk-Injeyan et al. 1986) the numbers of Tac-positive cells in mitogen-activated cultures from burn patients had been found to be reduced compared with controls. This was confirmed for these patients and the addition of exogenous IL2-upregulated expression of Tac antigen to the control level (Table 1). In mitogen-stimulated cultures, IL3, used alone or combined with IL2, did not augment the percentage of IL2R-expressing cells over the number without it. In contrast, supplementation of PBMCs in mitogen-free medium with IL3 significantly ($P<0.05$) increased the number of Tac-positive cells (Table 1). Moreover, the combined treatment of such cultures with IL2 and IL3 appeared to have an additive effect on the percentage of Tac-expressing lymphocytes.

An increase in IL2-induced DNA synthesis (Fig. 1) and expression of IL2R (Table 1) may suggest acquisition of functional IL2 receptor densities in the presence of IL3. The efficacy of IL3 is potentially related to the thermal injury as it is apparent at the time of the reduced sensitivity of patients' PBMCs to exogenous IL2. The gradual improvement in response without IL3 could reflect a gradual reduction in the number of IL3-sensitive cells and/or a gradual restoration of such cells' ability to express functional IL2R, independently of exogenous IL3. Alternatively it may reflect the ability of cells to produce IL3 in response to IL2. Prior to the exposure to exogenous IL2, human PBMCs do not demonstrate sufficient amounts of high-affinity IL2R (Roosnek et al. 1986). Recent studies (Harel-Bellan et al. 1986) suggest that spontaneously IL2 proliferating cells may belong to the T-cell lineage.

The cellular target of IL3 activity in the burn patient is unclear. The lack of effect of this lymphokine on Con A-activated PBMCs may suggest an involvement of T-lymphocytes which do not normally express low-affinity IL2 receptors. The possibility that IL3 utilized in our studies contains another active cytokine cannot be entirely excluded. WEHI 3-derived IL3 was shown to have promoting activity on normal human cloned T cells (Palacios 1982) which could then secrete IL2 and/or IL3 (Palacios 1984). Both IL2 and IL3 are products of activated T-lymphocytes (Ihle et al. 1983; Palacios 1984) and their interactions with respective receptors initiate analogous intracellular events (Farrar and Anderson 1985; Farrar et al. 1985). IL3 increases IL2R gene expression in hematopoietic cell lines (Birchenall-Sparks et al. 1986). Conversely, IL2 regulates T-cell-mediated myelopoiesis (Burdach et al. 1987). Thermal-injury-induced disarray in the T-lymphocyte-mediated biological reponses may therefore reflect the disruption of homeostasis in the regulatory interactions of the lymphokine cascade within lymphoid and nonlymphoid compartments of the immune network.

Acknowledgments. The authors are grateful to Shelina Lalani for excellent technical assistance and to the nursing staff of The Ross Tilley Burn Centre for blood sample collection and for their unique commitment to burn care. The work was supported by the Defence & Civil Institute of Environmental Medicine (Contract #DSS W7711-6-9483/01-SE) and in part by the MRC of Canada grant #MA-8770, for flow cytometry.

References

Birchenall-Sparks MC, Farrar WL, Kilian PL, Ruscetti FW (1986) Regulation of expression of the interleukin-2 receptor on hematopoietic cells by interleukin-3. Science 233:455–458

Burdach S, Shatsky M, Wagenhorst B, Levitt L (1987) Receptor-specific regulation of myelopoiesis by recombinant DNA-derived interleukin 2. J Immunol 139:452–458

Farrar WL, Anderson WB (1985) Interleukin-2 stimulates association of protein kinase C with plasma membrane. Nature 315:233–235

Farrar WL, Thomas TP, Anderson WB (1985) Altered cytosol/membrane enzyme redistribution on interleukin-3 activation of protein kinase C. Nature 315:235–237

Harel-Bellan A, Bertoglio J, Quillet A, Marchiol C, Wakasugi H, Mishall Z, Fradelizi D (1986) Interleukin 2 (IL 2) upregulates its own receptor on a subset of human unprimed peripheral blood lymphocytes and triggers their proliferation. J Immunol 136:2463–2469

Ihle, Keller J, Oroszlan S, Henderson LE, Copeland TD, Fitch F, Prystowsky MB, Goldwasser E, Schrader JW, Palaszynski E, Dy M, Lebel B (1983) Biologic properties of homogeneous interleukin 3. I. Demonstration of WEHI-3 growth factor activity, colony-stimulating factor activity, and histamine-producing cell-stimulating factor activity. J Immunol 131:282–287

Palacios R (1982) Cloned lines of interleukin 2 producer human T lymphocytes. J Immunol 129:2586–2593

Palacios R (1984) Production of lymphokines by circulating human T lymphocytes that express or lack receptors for interleukin 2. J Immunol 132:1833–1836

Roosnek EE, Brouwer MC, Kipp JB, Aarden LA (1986) Monocyte-dependent induction of proliferation of human peripheral T cells by recombinant interleukin 2. Eur J Immunol 16:35–40

Teodorczyk-Injeyan JA, Sparkes BG, Mills GB, Peters WJ, Falk RE (1986) Impairment of T cell activation in burn patients: a possible mechanism of thermal injury-induced immunosuppression. Clin Exp Immunol 65:570–581

Teodorczyk-Injeyan JA, Sparkes BG, Mills GB, Falk RE, Peters WJ (1987) Impaired expression of interleukin-2 receptor (IL2R) in the immunosuppressed burned patient: reversal by exogenous IL2. J Trauma 27:180–187

Wood JJ, Rodrick ML, O'Mahony JB, Palder SB, Saporoschetz I, D'Eon P, Mannick JA (1984) Inadequate interleukin 2 production. A fundamental immunological deficiency in patients with major burns. Ann Surg 200:311–320

Role of Monocyte HLA-DR Expression Following Trauma in Predicting Clinical Outcome

W. G. Cheadle, M. J. Hershman, S. R. Wellhausen, and H. C. Polk, Jr.

Introduction

The majority of late deaths following trauma are due to infection, mostly of pulmonary and abdominal origin (Goris and Draaisma 1982). There is no trauma score that incorporates the host defense capability of the victim or is predictive of infection or septic death. We have (Polk et al. 1986) examined various parameters thought to be markers of host response capability, and found that both reduced monocyte DR antigen expression (Mo2-DR) and serum-opsonizing capacity were highly correlated with major sepsis and death from infection. We report the results of both initial and serial measurements of monocyte DR expression in the construction of an outcome predictive score (OPS) of patients following major trauma.

Patients and Methods

This study consisted of 60 patients who sustained major trauma or burns, which resulted in an injury severity score (ISS) of at least 20, and were admitted consecutively to University Hospital in Louisville, Kentucky. They were divided into three groups: (1) a good outcome group of patients who did not develop major sepsis ($n=17$), (2) a major sepsis group ($n=28$), and (3) a group of patients who died ($n=5$). Thirteen of the 15 patients in the third group died of multiple organ failure resulting from infection. Major sepsis included all cases with bacteremia, pneumonia, major wound or soft tissue infection, or intraabdominal abscess. The components of the OPS are percentage LD_{50} of the ISS (%LD_{50}), degree of bacterial contamination, and monocyte DR antigen expression (Mo2-DR). Venous blood for Mo2-DR measurements was obtained from each patient within 24 h of admission and then serially measured throughout their hospital course.

The %LD_{50} for each patient was calculated by the following formula: %LD_{50} = (ISS/LD_{50} for age) $\times$ 100. The LD_{50} for age values used were 40 for the 15- to 44-year-old age group, 29 for the 45- to 65-year-old age group, and 20 for those 65 years of age or older (Bull 1975). Contamination at the time of admission or surgery was graded massive soft-tissue contamination or large bowel spillage (2+), minor soft-tissue, intrathoracic or abdominal contamination (1+), or no contamination (0).

The Mo2-DR value is the percentage of monocytes that expresses the class II human leukocyte antigen DR (HLA-DR) on the surface. This value was deter-

Immune Consequences of
Trauma, Shock and Sepsis
Eds. Faist/Ninnemann/Green

mined using fluorochrome-labeled monoclonal antibodies and flow cytometry as previously described (Polk et al. 1986). The normal range for Mo2-DR is 70% –100%, based on studies of healthy individuals. Monocytes were also incubated with lipopolysaccharide (10 μg/ml) for 2 h and DR expression compared with appropriate controls.

The OPS for each patient was calculated by multiplying the %LD_{50} by scaling factors of 1, 1.5, or 3 according to the degrees of contamination, 0, 1+, and 2+, respectively. These values were then multiplied by the scaling factors:

Mo_2DR	<40	41–50	51–60	61–70	>71
Factor	1.5	1.25	1.0	0.80	0.67

The result obtained was termed the OPS. Student's *t*-tests, Fischer's exact tests, and linear regression analyses were used to compare components of the OPS. Results are expressed as the mean ± standard error of the mean.

Results

The overall mean ISS for the study group was 34.9±1.4 and the overall mean Mo2-DR was 46.5±3.0. The mean %LD_{50} was 99.9±5.1 and the mean OPS was 214±19. The mean ISS, %LD_{50}, Mo2-DR, and OPS of each outcome group are shown in Table 1. There were no statistical differences in ISS between any of these outcome groups. The mean %LD_{50} of the good outcome group was 91.0±6.5, which was significantly less than 134±12.7, the mean of the dead group ($P<0.005$). The mean %LD_{50} of the septic group was 85.0±4.5, which was similar to the good outcome group but significantly less than that of the dead group ($P<0.001$). Therefore, neither ISS nor %LD_{50} could distinguish between all three outcome groups. The mean Mo2-DR value of the good outcome group was 57.4±6.2, significantly greater than the mean of the major sepsis group (41.7±3.9), but just failing to reach significance above the mean (40.3±6.9) of the dead group ($P=0.079$). Although monocyte DR expression in the surviving patients was stimulated to within the normal range following 2-h incubation with LPS throughout their hospital course, those destined to die had a progressive deterioration and never reached normal.

Table 1. Relationship between patient outcome and injury severity score, %LD_{50}, Mo2-DR, and outcome predictive score

	ISS	%LD_{50}	Mo2-DR	OPS
No species	33.9±2.3	91.0+ 6.8	57.4±6.2	110±10.1***
Major infection	32.0±2.3	85.0± 6.1	41.7±3.9*	215±19.4
Dead	39.9±3.5	135.0±12.7**	40.3±6.9	363±51.0**

*** Significantly different from both major infection and dead groups ($P<0.001$).
** Significantly different from both major infection and dead groups ($P<0.01$).
* Significantly different from both major infection and dead groups ($P<0.05$).

The mean OPS of the good outcome group was 110 ± 10.1, which was significantly less than 215 ± 19.4, the mean OPS of the septic group ($P<0.0002$) and 363 ± 51.0, the mean OPS of the dead group ($P<0.00001$). There was also a significant difference between the major infection group and those who died ($P<0.002$). Only 1 of 17 patients in the good outcome group had OPS values greater than 149, significantly less than the 24 of 28 in the septic group ($P<0.00002$) and the 14 of 15 in the dead group ($P<0.00002$) with OPS values greater than 149. Eleven of 15 patients in the dead group had OPS values above 299, which was significantly more than the 4 of 24 in the septic group ($P<0.005$) and the 0 of 17 in the good outcome group ($P<0.0002$) who had OPS values above 300.

Discussion

In an ongoing study of host defense mechanisms in severely injured patients, we have identified several important factors that are highly correlated with outcome (Polk et al. 1986). These include $\%LD_{50}$, degree of contamination, monocyte HLA-DR antigen expression, and the ability of patient serum to support phagocytosis. The level of contamination was especially important in the determination of outcome, as virtually all patients with heavy contamination became infected or died. Although each of the factors was generally associated with overall outcome, they were unable by themselves to predict particular outcome groups. However, the OPS was able clearly to distinguish between the three clinical outcome groups within 24 h of admission to the hospital.

Incorporation of monocyte DR antigen expression in the OPS enables an important aspect of host defense to be assessed. Class II histocompatability antigens are present on the monocyte cell surface and the HLA class II antigen DR appears to be of major importance (Lehner and Jones 1984). Foreign antigen presentation on the monocyte is necessary for interaction with both B and T cells, and DR antigen expression may be a measure of such antigen-presenting capacity of the monocyte (Unanue et al. 1984). Only those cells that express the HLA-DR antigen are capable of presenting foreign antigen to specific helper T cells and are therefore generalized markers of immune capability of the host (Tsakalos et al. 1984). Identification of patients at particular risk of infection or death because of reduced immune capability and prompt institution of appropriate therapy during this time may reduce the additional risk of infection in these patients.

References

Bull JP (1975) Measures of severity of injury. Injury 9:184

Committee on Medical Aspects of Automotive Safety (1971) Rating the severity of tissue damage. I. The Abbreviated Scale. JAMA 215:277

Goris RJA, Draaisma J (1982) Causes of death after blunt trauma. J Trauma 22:141

Lehner T, Jones T (1984) The role of MHC class II antigenic determinants in the function of human antigen binding T8+ cells, monocytes and helper and suppressor factors. Clin Exp Immunol 56:683

Polk HC Jr, George CD, Wellhausen SR et al. (1986) A systematic study of host defense processes in badly injured patients. Ann Surg 204:282
Tsakalos ND, Lachman LB, Newhouse YG et al. (1984) Lipopolysaccharide (LPS) modulation of human monocyte accessory cell function in promoting T-cell colonies: inability of LPS and IL-1 to abrogate the need for monocytes with high HLA-DR expression. Cell Immunol 83:229
Unanue ER, Beller DR, Christopher YL et al. (1984) Antigen presentation: comments on its regulation and mechanism. J Immunol 132:1

Early Alterations in HLA Class II Expression and Response to Tetanus Toxoid by Peripheral Blood Monocytes from Patients with Injury from Burns or Trauma *

R. A. S. Gibbons, O. M. Martinez, V. Lim, R. Lim, J. Horn, and M. R. Garovoy

Introduction

Sepsis is a major complication of injuries from burn and trauma [1]. CD4+ lymphocytes, which play a prominent role in the elimination of microbes from the host, require human class II antigen (HLA)-bearing accessory cells for activation and proliferation [2]. Monocytes that are HLA class II+ can serve as accessory cells by internalizing and processing antigen [2]. The antigen is then transported to the membrane of the monocyte, where it is found in association with monocyte HLA class II antigens [2]. CD4+ lymphocytes recognize the antigen/HLA complex and proliferate [2]. The efficiency of antigen processing and presentation is dependent on the percentage of cells that bear HLA class II molecules and the density of HLA class II molecules on the surfaces of cells [3]. We were interested, therefore, in determining whether monocytes from individuals injured by burns or trauma had altered expression of class II which affected accessory function. We measured the expression of HLA class II molecules on monocytes within 24 h of injury and correlated the results with proliferation of lymphocytes to a soluble antigen, tetanus toxoid, in a monocyte-dependent response.

Materials and Methods

Expression of HLA-DR, DO, and DP by Leu-M3+ Monocytes

Peripheral blood mononuclear cells (PBMNCs) were isolated by Ficoll-Paque density centrifugation. The percentage of monocytes bearing HLA class II molecules HLA-DR, DQ, and DP and the density of HLA class II molecules on cells was determined by double-staining PBMNCs with fluorescent monoclonal antibodies (mabs). The first mab was against Leu-M3, which stains 78%–90% of peripheral blood monocytes [4], and the second mabs were against HLA-DR, DQ, or DP [5]. Anti-Leu-M3 mabs were conjugated to phycoerythrin (PE) and antibodies to HLA class II molecules were conjugated to fluorescein (FITC). All monoclonal antibodies were obtained from Becton-Dickinson and the results analyzed with a Becton-Dickinson FACS Analyzer or FACSCAN.

---

* R.A.S.G. was supported by Grant #GM07032-05 from the National Institute of Health.

Immune Consequences of
Trauma, Shock and Sepsis
Eds. Faist/Ninnemann/Green

Response of Cells to Tetanus Toxoid

One hundred thousand PBMNCs were incubated with 0.27 LF/ml tetanus toxoid for 7 days and the rate of proliferation of lymphocytes determined by labeling the cultures with tritiated thymidine for the last 21 h. Results were obtained by harvesting the cells and counting in a liquid scintillation counter and were expressed as a stimulation index (SI) = CPM cultures with tetanus toxoid/CPM cultures without tetanus toxoid.

Results

Early Changes in Class II Expression Postburn

Six patients were evaluated during the first 24 h after admission to hospital. Table 1 shows that the percentage of peripheral blood Leu-M3+ cells bearing DR was reduced in the burn patients as early as 24 h postburn. The percentage of cells bearing DQ and DP were also significantly reduced. These results suggested that changes in class II antigen expression occur very soon after thermal injury or trauma. The percentage of cells expressing Leu-M3 postburn, however, was not significantly different from the controls (control = 75% ± 2%, patient = 78% ± 4%.

Relative Density of HLA-Class II Antigen Expression by Monocytes

The amount of fluorescence detected by flow cytometry can give a relative estimate of the quantity of antibody bound to the surface of the cell. Figure 1 shows dual-parameter histograms that compare control and patient PBMNCs which have been stained with anti-Leu-M3-PE (y-axis) and anti-HLA-DR-,DQ-, or DP-FITC (x-axis). The data are presented on a log scale. By using appropriate control antibodies it was established that cells (Fig. 1A) in the monocyte gate with fluorescence intensity above channel 84 on the x-axis were considered DR+ and those falling above channel 88 on the y-axis were Leu-M3+.

For patients samples, cells falling above channel 88 on the x-axis and channel 92 on the y-axis were designated HLA-DR+ and Leu-M3+ populations, respectively. By similar criteria it was determined that 76% of the control sample cells

Table 1. Reduction in HLA-DR, HLA-DQ, and HLA-DP expression by Leu-M3^{+} monocytes 24 h postinjury

Group	%HLA-DR	%HLA-DQ	%HLA-DP
Controls ($n=6$)	94±2	20±2	19±3
Burns ($n=6$)	4±8	7±3	7±2
P-value	< 0.001	< 0.01	< 0.01
Trauma ($n=3$)	34±3	5±2	4±2
P-value	< 0.001	< 0.01	< 0.01

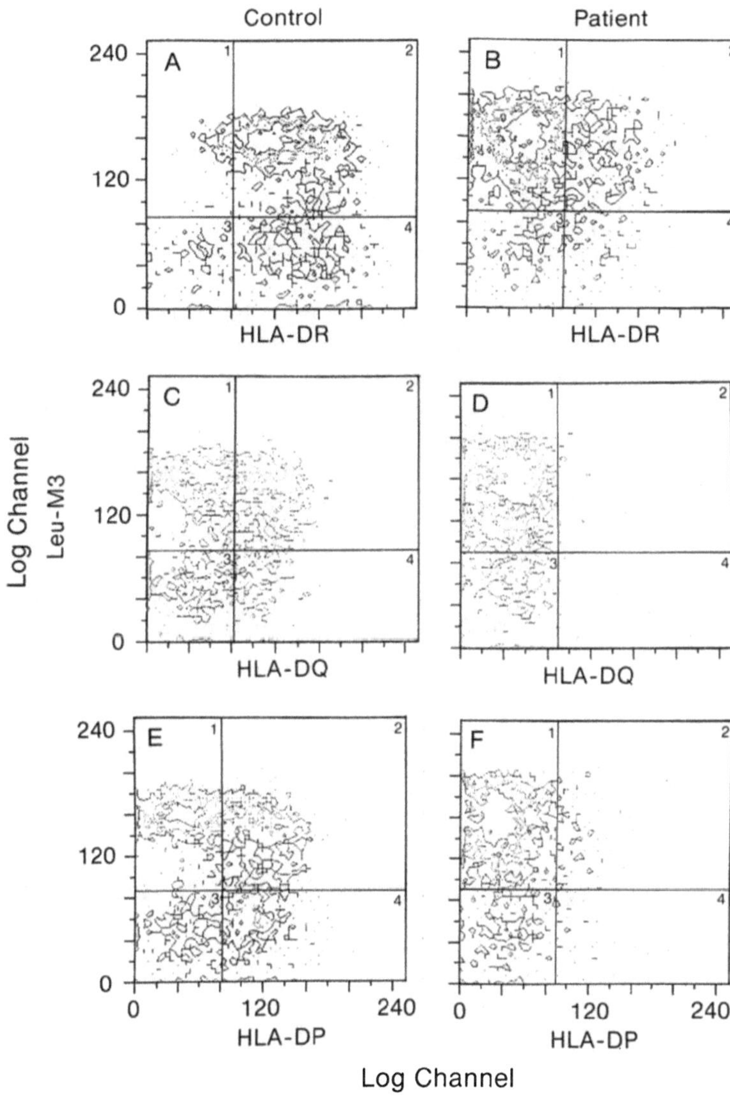

Fig. 1. Dual-parameter histogram of monocytes from controls and patients. 1 × 10 000 000 PBMNCs from one control and one patient were stained with anti-Leu-M3-PE and anti-HLA-DR-FITC, anti-HLA-DQ-FITC, or anti-HLA-DP-FITC mabs. Cells in the monocyte gate were analyzed by flow cytometry. Values shown on the *x*- and *y*-axis are logarithmic channels

were Leu-M3+ (Fig. 1A, quadrant 1 and 2) while 92% of the patient sample cells were Leu-M3+ (Fig. 1B, quadrant 1 and 2). Quadrant 1 represents those cells which were M3+DR- (control = 6%, patient = 77%). Unstained cells and debris appeared in quadrant 3.

By utilizing Consort 30 software it was possible to calculate the mean channel fluorescence (MCF) for each of these populations (Table 2). Monocytes from the

Table 2. Cell surface phenotype of Leu-M3-positive monocytes: percentage of positive cells and mean channel fluorescence (MCF)

Leu M3+	DR−		DR+		DQ−		DQ+		DP−		DP+	
	%	MCF	%	MCF	%	MCF	%	MCF	%	MCF	%	MCF
Control	7	68	93	132	65	44	35	112	64	40	36	116
Patient	77	48	14	124	99	40	1	40	99	28	0.3	116

patient staining with anti-Leu-M3 mabs and anti-DR mabs had a lower MCF for DR compared with the controls. The reduction in MCF was more marked for monocytes from the patient stained with anti-HLA-DQ as compared with controls. The percentage of cells from the patient staining with anti-Leu-M3 mab and anti-HLA-DP mab were too low to evaluate.

By calibration of the analyzer, which determined that a difference of 25 channels on the log scale corresponded to a doubling in fluorescence, it was possible to calculate the relative antigen density between two populations based on the differences in MCF. Consequently, while 93% of the control cells stained brightly for DR only, 14% of the patient cells did. When comparing the MCF for the major populations of control samples (MCF = 132) and patient samples (MCF = 48), we found that the brightly stained DR+ control cells had an antigen density tenfold greater than the dimly stained 77% DR-cells of the patient. It was observed that 35% of the control Leu-M3+ cells stained positively for DQ while only 1% of the patient cells did. Control Leu-M3+ cells expressing DQ (35%, MCF = 112) were sevenfold greater in antigen density than the major subpopulation of patient cells (89%, MCF = 40).

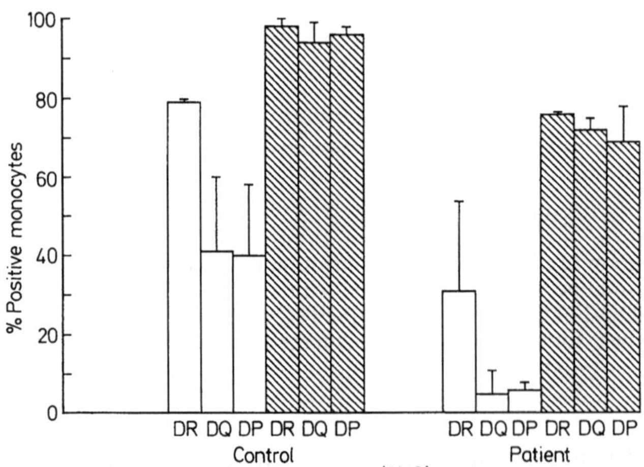

Fig. 2. The effect of IFN-gamma on HLA class II expression by Leu- M3+ cells from burn patients. 1 × 10000000 PBMNCs/ml were incubated with or without 1000 U/ml IFN-gamma for 72 h. 1 × 10000000 cells were double-stained with anti-Leu-M3-PE mab and anti-HLA-DR-FITC, anti-HLA-DQ-FITC, or anti-HLA-DP-FITC mabs and analyzed by flow cytometry. □, no IFN-gamma; ▨, 1000 U/ml IFN gamma

Effect of Interferon-Gamma on Percentage Leu-M3+ Cells Bearing HLA-Class II Antigens

Figure 2 shows the effect of incubating class II deficient PBMNCs from two burn patients and two controls with 1000 U/ml interferon (IFN)-gamma for 72 h. The percentage of Leu-M3+ cells staining with anti-HLA-DR, DQ, and DP mabs increased in both the patients and controls, with the most dramatic change being in the percentage of HLA-DQ- and DP-bearing cells.

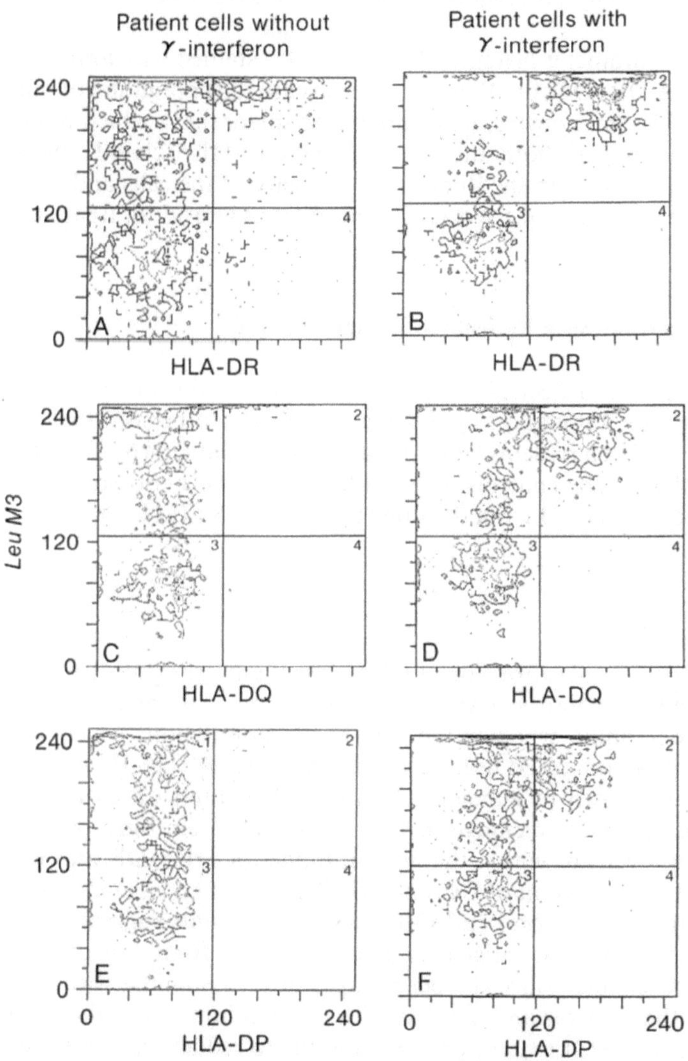

Fig. 3. Dual-parameter histogram of patient monocytes with or without treatment with 1000 U/ml IFN-gamma for 72 h. 1 × 10 000 000 PBMNCs were stained with anti-Leu-M3-PE and anti-HLA-DR-FITC, anti-HLA-DQ-FITC, or anti-HLA-DP-FITC mabs and cells in the monocyte gate analyzed by flow cytometry. Values shown on the *x*- and *y*-axis are on a logarithmic scale

Table 3. In vitro response of peripheral blood mononuclear cells to stimulation by tetanus toxoid postinjury

	Stimulation index
Control ($n=6$)	66 ± 20
Burn patients ($n=6$)	5 ± 2
Trauma patients ($n=3$)	6 ± 3

Density of HLA Class II Molecules Induced with Interferon-Gamma

Figure 3 shows a dual-parameter histogram of monocytes stained with anti-Leu-M3 mab and anti-HLA DR, DQ, or DP mabs. In each case the population of cells in quadrant 1 (Leu-M3+ monocytes) was shifted into quadrant 2, which represents cells double-staining with both anti-Leu-M3 and anti-HLA class II mabs. These changes reflect increases in the fluorescent intensity of the cells and, consequently, an increase in density of the class II molecules as a result of treatment with IFN-gamma.

Response of PBMNCs from Burn Patients to Tetanus Toxoid

Table 3 shows the response of PBMNCs isolated from burn and trauma patients within 24 h postinjury to stimulation by tetanus toxoid. It can be seen that the mean SI response of the burn patients was 5 ± 2 and trauma patients 6 ± 3, which was far lower than that of the controls 66 ± 20 ($P = 0.001$). This correlates with the reduced expression of class II from the same patient's cells (Table 1).

Discussion

In the present study, decreased expression of HLA class II antigens (DR, DQ, and DP) by Leu-M3+ cells was observed within 24 h of trauma or thermal injury. It was of interest to determine whether the Leu-M3+ population, which was deficient in class II molecules, could be induced to express HLA class II antigens. IFN-gamma, which is known to augment HLA class II expression by normal monocytes [6], increased the percentage of Leu-M3+ cells from burn patients bearing the class II antigens to within the normal range for HLA-DR and well above the basal level of expression of DQ and DP. The treatment also increased the density of class II molecules on Leu-M3+ cells. These results suggested that the decreased expression of these antigens on Leu-M3+ cells from patients with thermal injury was reversible. Since the percentages of cells staining with anti-Leu-M3 mabs from the controls and patients with thermal injury was about the same, changes in HLA class II expression were not due to reductions in the percentages of circulating monocytes. HLA class II expression remained very low throughout the duration of the patient's illness. When clinical symptoms abated and septic episodes resolved the level of HLA class II expression became normal (data not shown).

The response to soluble antigens requires the expression of HLA class II molecules [2]. The expression on all HLA class II-D region gene products is reduced within 24 h of injury and HLA-DQ and DP virtually disappear a few days postinjury (data not shown). It was not surprising to find, therefore, a decreased response to tetanus toxoid by peripheral blood cells from burn and trauma patients soon after injury.

Many other immune functions that are altered in burn and trauma patients require class II+ monocytes. For example, stimulation by some mitogens [7] and responses to alloantigens require class II+ cells [8]. Alterations in class II expression by monocytes from patients with injuries from burns or trauma, therefore, could have profound implications on the immune status of the individual.

References

1. Munster AM (1984) Immunologic response of trauma and burns. Am J Med:142–145
2. Unanue ER, Allen PM (1987) The basis for the immunoregulatory role of macrophages and other accessory cells. Science 236:552–557
3. Janeway CA, Bottomly K, Jones B, Katz M, Kaye J, Su G, Tite J (1985) Quantitative variation in Ia and non-Ia B cell surface molecules regulates T-cell: B-cell interactions. In: Pernis B, Vogel HJ (eds) Cell biology of the major histocompatibility complex. Academic, London, pp 259–271
4. Dimitriu-Bona A, Burmester GR, Waters SJ, Winchester RJ (1983) Human mononuclear phagocyte differentiation antigens. I. Patterns of antigenic expression on the surface of human monocytes and macrophages defined by monoclonal antibodies. J Immunol 130:145
5. Haas JG, Riethmuller G, Ziegler-Heitbrock HWL (1987) Monocyte phenotype and function in patients with the acquired immune deficiency syndrome (AIDS) and aids-related disorders. Scand J Immunol 26:371–379
6. Gonwa TA, Frost JP, Karr RW (1986) All human monocytes have the capability of expressing HLA-DQ, and HLA-DP molecules upon stimulation with interferon-gamma. J Immunol 137:519–524
7. Kohno K, Kakiuchi T, Takeuchi M, Taira S, Noriuchi H (1987) Cell Immunol 106:250–259
8. Owens T, Czitrom AA, Gascoigne NRJ, Crispe IN, Ratcliffe MJH, Lai PK, Mitchison NA (1984) The presentation of cell surface alloantigens to T-cells. Immunobiology 168:189–201

Lymphocyte Surface Antigen Expression Following Lectin Stimulation: An Index of Early T-Cell Dysfunction After Controlled Murine Injury

M.A. Gadd, C.S. Soderberg, A.N. Ozkan, and J.F. Hansbrough

Introduction

The depression in cell-mediated immunity following severe injury contributes to increased sepsis and mortality. The possible mechanisms behind the development of immune dysfunction include the generation of suppressor T-cell subpopulations [1], decreased helper T-cell function [2], the appearance of immunosuppressive factors [3], depressed interleukin-2 production and receptor expression [2, 4], and enhanced activation of prostaglandin pathways [4, 5]. The maintenance of normal T-cell activities and proliferation is obviously disrupted prior to and following these changes in the immune system. Recent studies have shown that after thermal injury T-cell clonal expansion is depressed because of reduced production of and response to interleukin-2 [6].

A commonly used assay of T-cell proliferation measures the incorporation of radioactive thymidine into DNA following mitogen stimulation or mixed lymphocyte reactions. The results from these tests are markedly variable and provide no information about the cell types undergoing proliferation. There is also evidence to suggest that DNA synthesis may not parallel blast transformation [7].

We therefore utilized a potentially more useful type of lymphocyte stimulation test to study immunity in injured mice. In addition to measuring isotope incorporation into DNA, we followed the expression of lymphocyte surface antigens during the culture period using monoclonal antibodies and two-color flow cytometry.

Stimulation and proliferation of small, resting T-lymphocytes has been shown to be accompanied by the appearance of new surface antigens, which are now termed T-cell activation antigens. The earliest antigens to appear prior to DNA synthesis include the transferrin receptor [8], the insulin receptor [9] and "Tac" or IL-2 receptor [10]. Ia or HLA-DR [11] is expressed after DNA synthesis has begun. In addition, cell surface coexpression of both "helper" and "suppressor" MHC antigens has been shown to be an early step in T-cell blastogenesis [12]. We describe in this report the lectin-induced expression of surface markers on murine splenic lymphocytes following controlled injury. The results indicate that characterization of lymphocyte surface antigen expression after culture and stimulation may be a useful indicator of postinjury T-cell dysfunction, and that the block in T-cell blastogenesic potential following severe injury occurs early in the activation process.

Immune Consequences of
Trauma, Shock and Sepsis
Eds. Faist/Ninnemann/Green

Materials and Methods

Female, CF-1 mice underwent either musculoskeletal trauma by crushing and amputating the distal hindlimb or burn injury producing a full-thickness steam burn of approximately 25% total body surface area. Spleens were harvested 10 days after injury. Mitogen-stimulated cultures were established with 2.5 μg/ml purified phytohemagglutinin (PHA) (Wellcome, Beckenham, England) for 48 h. On the 2nd day cultures were pulsed with 1 μCi [^{3}H]thymidine. Following mitogen stimulation, the splenocytes were harvested from the wells and labeled with the following monoclonal antibodies (Moabs): anti-L3T4 and anti-Lyt-2 (rat anti-mouse, direct phycoerythrin or fluorescein conjugates, Becton Dickinson Co., Sunnyvale CA; in some experiments biotinylated Lyt-2 was used), anti-Ia (rat anti-mouse, unconjugated, Hybritech, La Jolla, CA), and anti-IL-2 receptor (IL-2R) (rat anti-mouse, unconjugated, Boehringer-Mannheim, FRG). Fluorescein-labeled goat anti-rat IgG (Becton Dickinson) was used as the second antibody for the indirect assays. All experiments included controls using goat anti-rat IgG-fluorescein. Cell population percentages in control and test animals are expressed as mean ± SEM, and values were compared utilizing Student's *t*-test. Statistical significance was assumed at $P < 0.05$.

Results

L3T4 Surface Antigen Expression. L3T4 surface antigen expression increased in control cells after 48 h of PHA stimulation (37.4% ± 2.3% to 52.9% ± 2.5%, $P > 0.05$). Marked suppression of L3T4 was seen at the initiation and throughout the culture period, as shown in Fig. 1 A, using cells from burned animals. Minimal changes in L3T4 expression were seen in traumatized animals.

Lyt-2 Surface Antigen Expression. Lyt-2 surface expression increased on cells from noninjured animals during PHA stimulation culture (from 13.6% ± 0.8% to 49.9% ± 2.4% of cells, $P < 0.05$). The percentage of Lyt-2 expression was markedly depressed in cells from burn-injured animals (Fig. 1 B) but increased compared with normal animals after skeletal trauma.

Ia Antigen Expression. In cultures from control mice, Ia expression by T_h and T_s subpopulations markedly increased after stimulation. Burn injury resulted in marked depression in percentages of L3T4$^+$/Ia$^+$ and Lyt-2$^+$/Ia$^+$ lymphocytes following PHA stimulation (Fig. 1 C, D). Skeletal trauma produced minimal alterations in Ia expression by T_h but markedly increased in T_s subpopulations (Fig. 1).

IL-2 Receptor (IL-2R) Expression. A small percentage (approximately 4%) of splenic T-lymphocytes bound IL-2 at time 0 (initiation of culture). Following culture and PHA stimulation, the overall percentage of IL-2R$^+$ cells increased to approximately 73%. Both T_h (L3T4$^+$) and T_s (Lyt-2$^+$) cells from noninjured animals demonstrated increased percentage expression of IL-2R (Fig. 1 E–F). Burn injury resulted in a marked defect in the ability of both L3T4$^+$ and Lyt-2$^+$ cells to express IL-2R. Musculoskeletal trauma produced minimal T_h changes compared with normal animals but increase in T_s IL-2R expression.

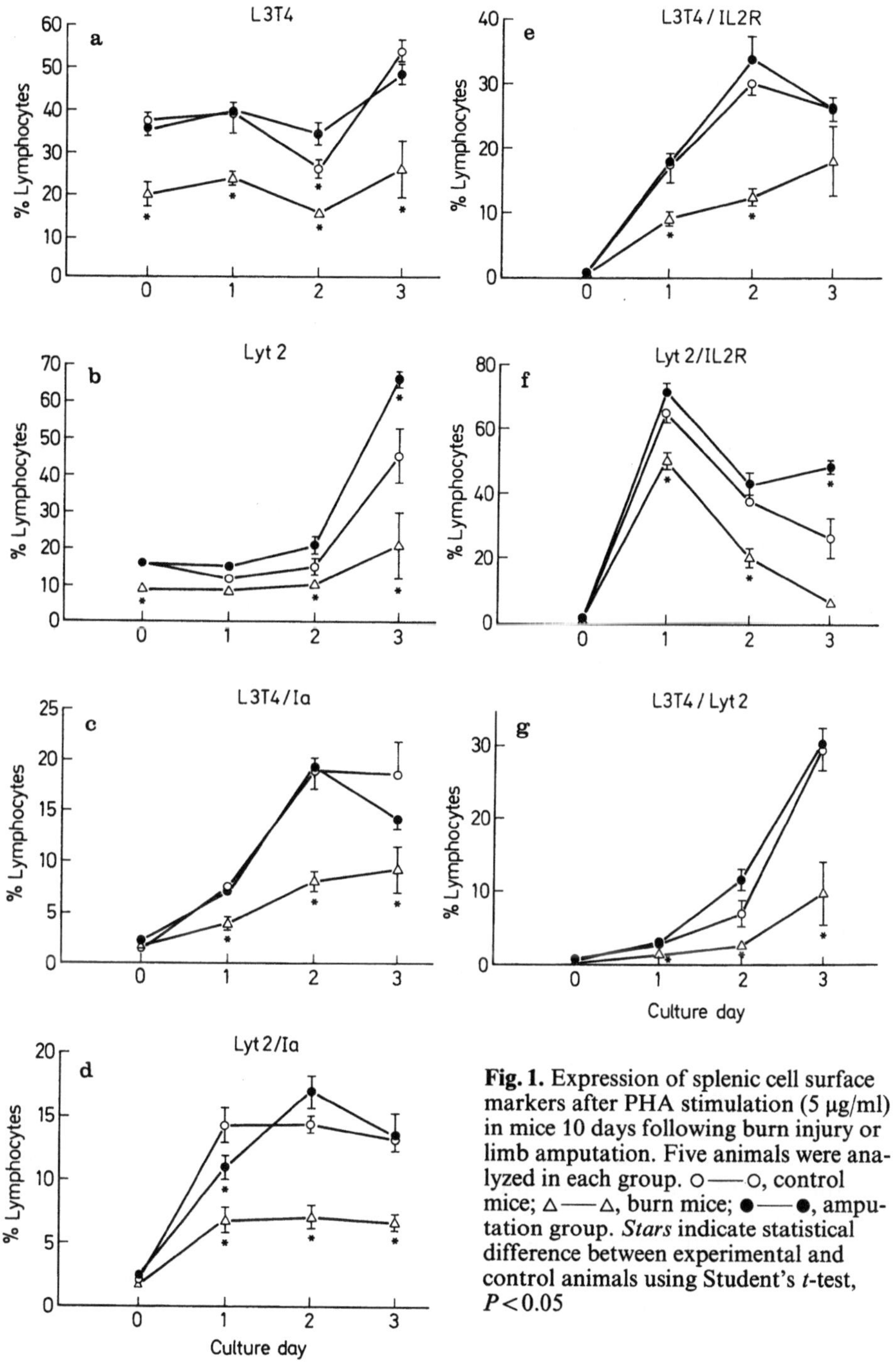

Fig. 1. Expression of splenic cell surface markers after PHA stimulation (5 μg/ml) in mice 10 days following burn injury or limb amputation. Five animals were analyzed in each group. ○—○, control mice; △—△, burn mice; ●—●, amputation group. *Stars* indicate statistical difference between experimental and control animals using Student's *t*-test, $P<0.05$

L3T4/Lyt-2 Coexpression. Coexpression of these surface antigens has been shown to occur during mitogen-induced lymphocyte blastogenesis [12]. We noted striking increases in $L3T4^+/Lyt\text{-}2^+$ cell percentages in cultures from control mice. L3T4/Lyt-2 coexpression was markedly depressed following burn injury, but coexpression was minimally altered following skeletal trauma (Fig. 1 G).

[^{3}H]Thymidine Incorporation. Thymidine incorporation after 72 culture hours was 37400 ± 7740 CPM in controls compared with 10570 ± 2881 CPM in burned mice.

Discussion

Studies now indicate that T-cell proliferation, whether initiated by antigen or lectin, is mediated by the lymphocytotrophic hormone interleukin-2, and IL-2-T cell interaction is effected via specific receptor molecules which increase their expression following cell stimulation. T-cell activation is highly complex, and a diversity of biochemical responses are correlated with different steps in the cascade of T-cell activation leading to proliferation. IL-2 receptors are expressed early following lymphocyte stimulation, prior to DNA synthesis [13]; IL-2R expression may be transient, and receptor appearance and disappearance is mirrored by the proliferative rate of the cells [14]. We noted a marked depression in IL-2R surface expression in cultured lymphocytes from burn-injured mice.

In studies of lectin-stimulated human lymphocytes [15] it has been shown that the transferrin receptor and IL-2R are early antigens, appearing prior to DNA synthesis, and both are expressed on all proliferating cells. HLA-DR (Ia) is expressed later (after the proliferation stage is entered), and does not appear on all proliferating cells. Further evidence in support of this sequence comes from experiments which show that antibodies to HLA-DR fail to inhibit mitogen-dependent T-cell proliferation [16], whereas antibodies to early activation markers reproducibly (but partially) block proliferation [8]. Although we have shown that L3T4/Ia and Lyt-2/Ia antigen coexpression is markedly depressed in burn-derived cells following lectin stimulation, the studies reported here were not able to discern clear differences in the temporal expression of IL-2R and Ia antigens after stimulation. However, from the previously cited work it appears that the block in lymphocyte activation following murine burn injury occurs early in the blastogenic response, as evidenced by the inhibition of IL-2R appearance, and before DNA synthesis and Ia expression.

The expression of T_h and T_s surface glycoproteins appears to be linked closely to maturation of T cells since both L3T4 and Lyt-2 antigens play critical roles in MHC antigen recognition or differentiation. Our studies found that L3T4 expression was greatly decreased in postburn spleen cells at the time of initiation of cultures; the percentage of $L3T4^+$ cells rose slightly during culture of cells from normal animals, while L3T4 expression remained depressed in burn-derived cells. T3T4 expression increased after stimulation in the traumatized animals but was depressed compared with controls. In contrast, the percentage of cells expressing Lyt-2 greatly increased after culture of splenocytes from normal animals; this increase was almost completely blocked in burn-derived cells, while the percentage of Lyt-2^+ cells from animals after skeletal trauma actually increased during culture.

Our studies confirm those of others using human cells [12] which demonstrate the appearance of lymphocytes which coexpress "helper" and "suppressor" antigens following lectin stimulation. Although the functional roles of these cells which coexpress "helper" and "suppressor" markers remain to be defined, they have been shown to highly express activation antigens such as IL-2R and have been suggested as potentially important immunoregulatory cells [12]. Our data indicate that the overall percentage of L3T4^+ cells did not increase after lectin stimulation, while the percentage of cells expressing Lyt-2 increased markedly very early in the culture period. Therefore, it appears likely that many cells which are originally L3T4^+/Lyt-2^- subsequently coexpress Lyt-2 antigen before cell division, as opposed to the appearance of both antigens occurring only on newly divided cells. We found that a profound decrease in the percentage of L3T4^+/Lyt-2^+ cells was a very reproducible alteration following lectin stimulation of cells from burn-injured mice.

In conclusion, these studies demonstrate that burn-derived splenic lymphocytes are markedly deficient in their ability to express surface activation markers (IL-2R, Ia, T_h/T_s antigen coexpression) following lectin stimulation. However, in trauma-derived cells, surface antigen expression is minimally affected. Thus, murine burn injury results in marked defects in mitogen-induced lymphocyte maturation as reflected by surface membrane antigen expression. This assay should prove useful for further study of the complex immunoregulatory events and immune dysregulation which occur following severe injury.

References

1. Wang BS, Heacock EH, Wu AVO, Mannick JA (1980) Generation of suppressor cells in mice after surgical trauma. J Clin Invest 66:200
2. Antonacci AC, Calvano SE, Reaves LE, Prajapati A, Bockman R, Welte K, Mertelsmann R, Gupta S, Good RA, Shires GT (1984) Autologous and allogeneic mixed-lymphocyte responses following thermal injury in man: the immunomodulatory effects of interleukin 1, interleukin 2, and a prostaglandin inhibitor, WY-18251. Clin Immunol Immunopathol 30:304
3. Ozkan NA, Ninnemann JL (1985) Circulating mediators in thermal injuries: isolation and characterization of a burn injury-induced immunosuppressive serum component. J Burn Care Rehabil 6:147
4. Faist E, Mewes A, Baker CC, Strasser T, Alkan SS, Rieber P, Heberer G (1987) Prostaglandin E_2 (PGE_2)-dependent suppression of IL-2 production in patients with major trauma. J Trauma 27:837
5. Ninnemann JL (1982) Immunologic defenses against infection: alterations following thermal injuries. J Burn Care Rehabil 3:355
6. Teodorczyk-Injeyan JA, Sparkes BG, Mills GB, Peters WJ, Falk RE (1986) Impairment of T cell activation in burn patients: a possible mechanism of thermal injury-induced immunosuppression. Clin Exp Immunol 65:570
7. Rogers JC, Boldt D, Kornfeld A, Skinner A, Valeri CR (1972) Excretion of deoxyribonucleic acid by lymphocytes stimulated with phytohemagglutinin or antigen. Proc Natl Acad Sci USA 69:1685
8. Trowbridge IS, Omary MB (1981) Human cell surface glycoprotein related to cell proliferation is the receptor for transferrin. Proc Natl Acad Sci USA 78:3039

9. Helderman JH, Strom TB (1979) Role of protein and RNA synthesis in the development of insulin binding sites on activated thymus-derived lymphocytes. J Biol Chem 254:7203
10. Uchiyama T, Broder S, Waldman TA (1981) A monoclonal antibody (anti-Tac) reactive with activated and functionally mature human T cells. J Immunol 126:1393
11. Evans RL, Faldetta J, Humphreys RE, Pratt DM, Yunis EJ, Schlossman SF (1978) Peripheral human T cells sensitized in mixed leukocyte culture synthesize and express Ia-like antigens. J Exp Med 148:1440
12. Blue M-L, Daley JF, Levine H, Schlossman SF (1985) Coexpression of T4 and T8 on peripheral blood T cells demonstrated by two-color fluorescence flow cytometry. J Immunol 134:2281
13. Braylan RC, Benson NA, Nourse V, Kruth HS (1982) Correlated analysis of cellular DNA, membrane antigens and light scatter of human lymphoid cells. Cytometry 2:337
14. Cantrell DA, Smith KA (1983) Transient expression of interleukin 2 receptors. Consequences for T cell growth. J Exp Med 158:1895
15. Cotner T, Williams JM, Christenson L, Shapiro HM, Strom TB, Strominger J (1983) Simultaneous flow cytometric analysis of human T cell activation. Antigen expression and DNA content. J Exp Med 157:461
16. Palacios R (1982) Concanavalin A triggers T lymphocytes by directly interacting with their receptors for activation. J Immunol 128:337

Role of T-Cell Lymphocyte Populations and Their Products as Mediators of Immune Depression in Thermal Burns

J. Demarinis and S. E. Briggs

Helper T cells and suppressor T cells represent critical immunologicalsubsets involved in resistance to bacteria in thermally injured patients [1–4]. Activated T cells secrete soluble mediators of immune reactions called lymphokines [5, 6]. Two lymphokines, interleukin 1 and interleukin 2, have been demonstrated to be of particular importance to host defense mechanisms against microbial invasion [7–10].

Much of the early research on the effect of thermal injury on T-lymphocytes focussed on measurements of total T-cell activity. Bauer demonstrated that the number of T cells is depressed during the first 24–48 h after trauma or operation [11]. The degree of depression was related to the severity of injury. Ishizawa et al. reported decreased T-cell function in burned patients [12]. Menon and associates documented significant depression of T-cell function in burns involving more than 25% total body surface area (TBSA). This depression of T-cell function as measured by the leukocyte migration inhibition test (LMT) started after the 7th postburn day and continued until the 60th postburn day [13].

Such studies were important in documenting the role of thermal injury in adversely modifying host defense mechanisms. They failed, however, to delineate the cellular mechanisms and interactions in the generation of human T-cell depression following thermal injury. Several notable advances have made possible the elucidation of the major T-lymphocyte subsets in man and their unique functional characteristics. The development of in vitro methods for characterization and identification of human T-lymphocyte subsets by cell surface markers and the development of new techniques for the isolation of highly purified subclasses of human T-lymphocytes depending on cell surface markers significantly influenced the direction of research on the effect of thermal injury on T-lymphocyte activity. Wood related burn-induced immunosuppression to a decrease in the number of circulating T cells [14] rather than to any dysfunction at the level of the individual T cell. Antonacci and associates enumerated T-cell subsets as defined by receptors for immunoglobulin isotypes at 24–48 h postburn. T cells possessing surface receptors for the Fc fragment of IgM represented a population of cells with helper activity, while T cells possessing surface receptors for the Fc fragment of IgG represented a population of cells with suppressor-cytotoxic function [15]. A decrease in total T cells was accompanied by a decrease in IgM-Fc-binding lymphocytes in all burns greater than 20% TBSA. An increase in IgG-Fc-binding lymphocytes was seen in patients with greater than 60% TBSA burn or greater than 25% third-degree burn.

Immune Consequences of
Trauma, Shock and Sepsis
Eds. Faist/Ninnemann/Green

These changes correlated linearly with the amount of full-thickness injury, and the ratio of helper: suppressor T cells was significant in their study at 24–48 h postburn in predicting the risk of septic death. Ninnemann reported evidence for the occurrence of an immunosuppressive serum component following thermal injury [16, 17]. A direct correlation was found between serum suppressor activity in vitro and prolonged survival of skin allografts applied for burn therapy and the increased frequency of opportunistic infection of the burn wound [18, 19].

Munster postulated that post-traumatic immunosuppression is due to activation of suppressor T cells. [20] McIrvine and associates in a study of 22 patients with thermal burns greater than 30% TBSA, used monoclonal antibodies to identify T-lymphocyte subsets known to have suppressor/cytotoxic (OKT8) and helper/inducer (OKT4) function [18]. They documented an inversion of the normal ratio between suppressor/cytotoxic (OKT8) and helper/inducer (OKT4) subsets which occurred soon after the burn injury reached a peak in 5–7 days, and then returned to normal levels by 14 days. Later in the postburn course, systemic sepsis in 8 patients was associated with a return of increased suppressor to helper cell ratios. Calvano and associates utilized fluorescence flow cytometry to assess the effect of thermal injury on rat lymphoid organ lymphocyte subpopulations and noted that thermal injury induces significant changes in lymphocyte trafficking pattens including a relative increase in T-helper cells in the bone marrow [19].

Researchers [7–9, 21, 22] have suggested that immunosuppression of thermally injured patients is brought on by an increase in the suppressor population and a deficit in the production and/or release of IL-2, which is dramatically reduced as compared with normal controls. This depression is mediated via an elaborate reorganization of the cell-mediated immune network. In patients who have recovered from nonfatal septic episodes, it was found that their helper/suppressor ratio and the amount of IL-2 being produced gradually decreased 24–48 h postburn, with a mean depression occurring 5–7 days postburn. Following this depression a gradual increase to preburn levels takes place 10–29 days postburn. Those patients who succumbed to fatal septicemia were found to follow the course of the nonfatal episodes in every fashion except that their levels of IL-2 remained depressed.

Animal data generated from our laboratory support the findings of other researchers working along the same lines utilizing different methods. A standardized rat burn model was utilized to investigate levels of helper T cells and suppressor T cells in the rat following thermal injury. Virus-free Sprague-Dawley rats weighing (200–300) normal total T-cell count (W3/13), helper T cells (W3/25), suppressor T cells (OX8) and monocyte (OX4) activity prior to thermal injury. A model was developed for cannulation of the jugular vein according to a procedure described by Axelson. Use of a cannula instead of the conventional heart puncture or tail bleed in the rat model allows blood to be drawn on a daily basis without further traumatizing or anesthetizing the animal, procedures which may in themselves stimulate immune depression. One milliliter of blood was drawn daily and subsequent analysis was performed with monoclonal technology and fluorescence flow cytometry for measurement of T-cell subpopulations. Following the establishment of normal values in the rat, a standardized burn model was developed using a modification of the technique of Walker. The rat model was chosen because of the similarity of the rat immune system, especially proliferative lymphocytes, to that of the human and the feasibility of inducing a significant (50%) thermal burn without significant mortality. After burn injury, it was found that the helper/suppressor ratio became depressed and the total amount of T cells circulating in the body was also depressed. The depression of this ratio was demonstrated to be an increased suppressor population rather than a decrease of the helper populations. Peak depression for these populations occurred between 5 and 7 days postburn and returned to normal or near normal levels around the 10th day following injury (Figs. 1–4).

A major objective of immunological monitoring of patients with inhalation injury is the development of practical, predictive assays of host defense which both accurately reflect the complex totality of host defense and allow identification of patients at greater risk for septic complications following inhalation in-

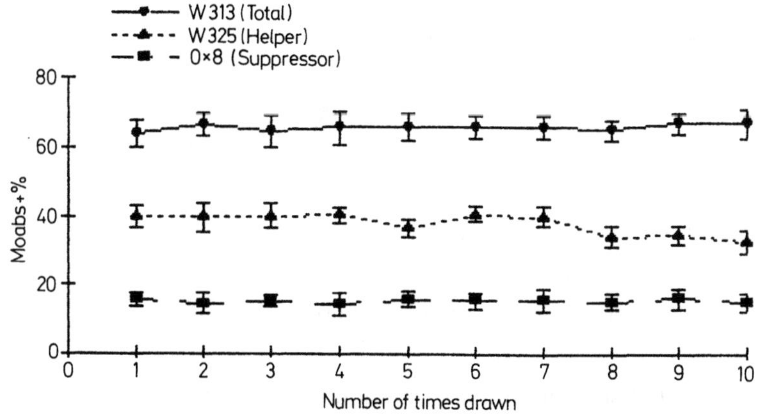

Fig. 1. Mean value for each antibody prior to burn

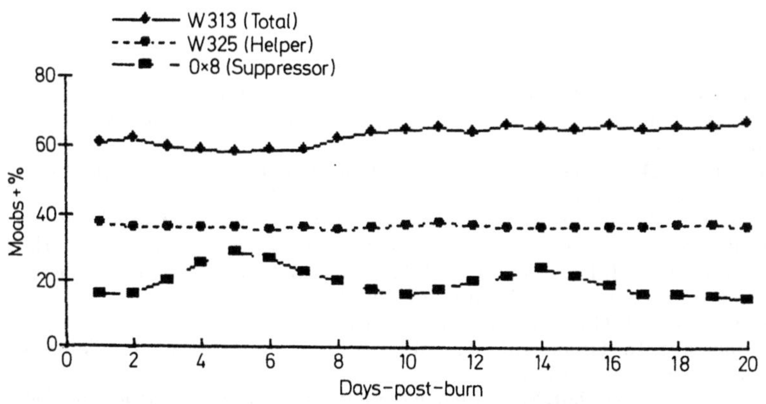

Fig. 2. Means for each antibody for all animals postburn

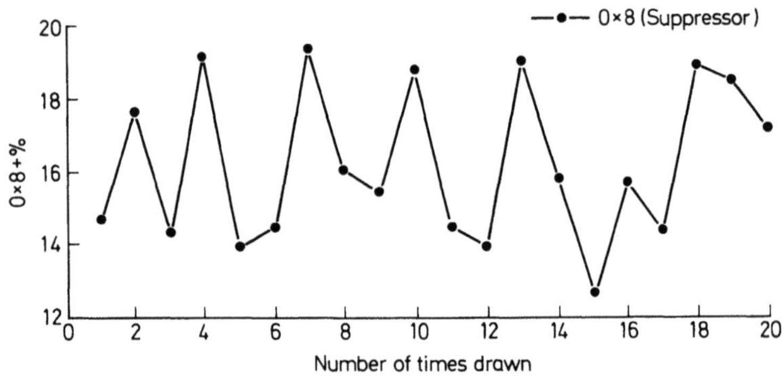

Fig. 3. Specific values for suppressor T cells (OXB) preburn for one animal

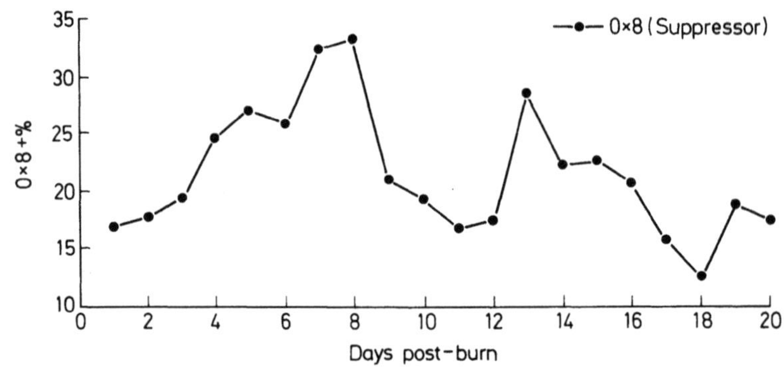

Fig. 4. Specific values for suppressor T cells (OXB) postburn for one animal

jury. The ultimate goal of such immunological monitoring is the development of prophylactic and therapeutic modalities which alter an individual's susceptibility to infection.

References

1. Loor F, Roelants GE (1977) B and T cells in immune recognition. Wiley, London
2. Miller CL (1981) Secondary immunodeficiency in burns and after surgical trauma. Clin Immunol Allergy 1 (3):641
3. Waldman TA (1978) Disorders of suppressor immunoregulatory cells in the pathogenesis of immunodeficiency and autoimmunity. Ann Intern Med 88:226
4. Cantor H, Boyse E (1977) Regulation of immune response by T cell subclasses. In: Stutman O (ed) Contemporary topics in immunobiology, vol 7. Plenum, New York
5. Gebel HM, Radaj PA, Holmes D et al. (1981) Functional characteristics of Tg and Tnong cells in a three party MLR. J Immunol 126:118
6. Gerson RK, Naidorf KF (1980) Information transfer between T cell sets: the macrophage is the message. In: Unane ER, Rosenthal AS (eds) Macrophage regulation of immunity. Academic, New York, p 431
7. Unane ER, Rosenthal AS (1980) Macrophage regulation of immunity. Academic, New York

8. Reinherz EL, Moretta L, Roper M et al. (1980) Human T lymphocyte subpopulations defined by Fc receptors and monoclonal antibodies. J Exp Med 151:969
9. Miller SE, Miller CL, Trunkey DD (1982) The immune consequences of trauma. Surg Clin North Am 62 (no 1)
10. Miller CL, Trunkey DD (1977) Thermal injury: defects in immune response induction. J Surg Res 22:621
11. Bauer AR, McNeil C, Trentelman E et al. (1978) The depression of T lymphocytes after trauma. Am J Surg 136:674
12. Ishizawa S, Sakai H, Sarles HE et al. (1984) Effect of thymosin on T lymphocyte functions in patients with acute thermal burns. J Trauma 24:220
13. Menon T, Sundararaj T, Subramanian S et al. (1984) Kinetics of peripheral blood T cell numbers and functions in patients with burns. J Trauma 24:220
14. Wood GW, Volenec FJ, Mani MM, Humphrey LJ (1978) Dynamics of T lymphocyte subpopulations and T lymphocyte function following thermal injury. Clin Exp Immunol 31:291
15. Antonacci AC, Good RA, Gupta S (1982) T cell subpopulations following thermal injury. Surg Gynecol Obstet 155:1
16. Ninneman JL, Fisher JC, Wachtel TL (1979) Thermal injury associated immunosuppression: occurrence and in vitro blocking effect of post recovery serum. J Immunol 122:1736
17. Ninneman JL, Fisher JC, Frank HA (1978) Prolonged survival of human skin allografts following thermal injury. Transplantation 25:69
18. McIrvine AJ, O'Mahoney JB, Saporoschetz I, Mannick JA (1982) Depressed immune response in burn patients. Ann Surg 196:297
19. Calvano Se, Chiao J, Antonacci AC, Shires GT (1984) Changes in rat lymphoid organ lymphocyte subpopulations following thermal injury. Surg Forum
20. Munster AM (1977) Post-traumatic immunosuppression is due to activation of suppressor T cells. Lancet I:1329
21. Miller CL (1979) Burns and the immune network. J Trauma 19:880
22. Miller CL (1981) Alteration in macrophage function following thermal injury. In: Ninneman JL (ed) The immune consequences of thermal injury. Williams and Wilkins, Baltimore, p 49
23. Thompson S, Bowen K, Burton RC (1986) Sequential monitoring of peripheral blood lymphocytes subsets in rats. Cytometry 7:184–193

2.2 Trauma and B-Cell Function

The Influence of Mechanical Trauma on the B-Cell System: Phenotypes, Terminal B-Cell Maturation, Immunoglobulin Synthesis and Influence of Lymphokines

W. Ertel and E. Faist

Introduction

While many investigators agree that the trauma-induced breakdown of the lymphokine cascade (interleukins 1 and 2; IL-1, IL-2) is responsible for the lack of T-lymphocyte activation and proliferation following injury [7–9], its potential effect on B-cell responses has not been investigated extensively so far. While there have been some studies on specific and unspecific humoral immune responses in burned individuals [25, 30], there have been only a very limited number of observations made of humoral immune responses following major trauma. It is known that in patients who develop severe sepsis, the antibody-forming cell responses are profoundly depressed compared to those of patients who did not develop sepsis and who had normal amounts of antibody-forming cells [4]. Nohr et al. [20, 21] studied humoral immunity in surgical patients in vivo and in vitro. They found a deficiency of in vitro B-cell responses to tetanus toxoid compared to those of controls, who showed a population of B-cells that spontaneously secreted tetanus toxoid in vitro following immunization. In vitro antibody production in their study reflected the in vivo antibody responses. Nohr et al. concluded from their results that the failure of specific antibody production might be caused by a failure of the antigen recognition and/or lymphocyte activation in unresponsive surgical patients.

To gain further insight into the pathogenesis of the immune dysorders acquired after trauma in terms of altered B-cell function, a number of studies were undertaken in our laboratory. The capacity of B-cells for immunoglobulin synthesis following mitogenic activation was used as a functional B-cell assay. The pokeweed mitogen (PWM)-induced polyclonal immunoglobulin production of B-cells is highly reproducible and the response has been shown to depend on T-cells [12, 15].

In addition, the capacity for terminal B-cell maturation, i.e., differentiation into plasma cells, was evaluated by staining B-lymphocytes for intracellular immunoglobulin by direct immunofluorescence in fixed smears of cultured cells [13]. Together with the phenotyping of mononuclear leukocytes, the two assays appeared to be a reliable in vitro measure for terminal B-cell maturation and B-cell function.

We wanted to investigate the time course and extent of trauma-induced alterations of in vitro terminal B-cell maturation and immunoglobulin (Ig) synthesis. We also wanted to determine whether major trauma has different effects on synthesis of the three Ig subclasses A, G, and M.

Immune Consequences of
Trauma, Shock and Sepsis
Eds. Faist/Ninnemann/Green

In a recent study, we investigated B-cell proliferation and Ig synthesis in purified B-cell cultures where negative regulatory macrophages were excluded. The influence of recombinant lymphokines like IL-2 and IL-4 on these B-cell functions was studied.

Material and Methods

Patients and Controls. Studies were initiated in 30 multiply injured patients (20 male, 10 female, mean age 32.1 ± 2.4 years, range 16–59 years). All patients had major trauma that was considered on initial assessment to be life-threatening. The injury severity scores (ISS) [11] ranged from 25 to 57 points (mean 39.1 ± 1.9 points). Twenty-five healthy volunteers aged from 20 to 36 years (mean age 27.8) were studied as controls.

Preparation of Peripheral Blood Mononuclear Cells. Serial blood samples of the patients were obtained on days 1, 3, 5, 7, 10, 14, and 21 posttrauma. Peripheral blood mononuclear cells (PBMCs) were separated by density gradient centrifugation using Ficoll Hypaque (Sp.G. 1.077).

PBMC phenotyping was performed using the indirect immunofluorescence technique. OKT4 (Ortho) was used to detect peripheral CD4+ T-helper/inducer cells, B1 (Coulter) for B-lymphocytes and LeuM3 (Becton Dickinson) for peripheral monocytes. The number of cells that were restained with antibodies labeling individual subpopulations was assayed using fluorescence microscopy.

PBMC Culture Conditions. PBMC cultures were incubated over 7 days at 37 °C in a humid atmosphere with 6% CO_2, with and without pokeweed mitogen at 1.6 µg/ml (PWM; Seromed). At the end of the incubation time, PBMCs were centrifuged and the supernatants collected and frozen until tested for Ig contents.

Assessment of Ig Levels in PBMC Cultures. The amount of IgM, IgG, and IgA produced in the PBMC cultures was quantified using a double sandwich enzyme-linked immunosorbent assay (ELISA) technique modified from the method of Engvall and Perlman [6]. Enzymatic cleavage was measured spectrophotometrically at 405 nm with a Titertek Multiscan Plate Reader. The sample Ig concentrations were calculated from the standard curve.

Staining of Cytoplasmic Ig. Cells from PBMC cultures with and without PWM were harvested, pooled, counted, and deposited on slides with a cytocentrifuge. Cytoplasmic Ig (CIg) was labeled with a rabbit antihuman Ig(M+G+A)-FITC conjugated antibody (Behring). The percentage of CIg+ cells was calculated on counts of at least 300 cells.

B-Cell Preparations. Mononuclear lymphocytes were obtained from peripheral blood by Ficoll Hypaque density gradient centrifugation. Adherent cells were removed by incubating PBMCs on plastic dishes for 1–2 h at 37 °C. The B-cells were separated from the T-cell population by the rosetting technique with 2-aminoethylisothiouronium bromide treated sheep red blood cells. In the B-cell fraction we found less than 2% of CD3+ T-lymphocytes and less than 3% of LeuM3+ monocytes.

B-Cell Growth Factor Assay. The purified B-cell preparation (1×10^5 B-cells/0.2 ml well) was stimulated with *Staphylococcus aureus* Cowan I (SAC; 1:13500,

Sigma) for 72 h in the presence or absence of the lymphokines IL-2 (250 U/ml) or IL-4 (250 U/ml). The proliferative response was measured by pulsing the B-cell cultures with [^{3}H]thymidine (1 μCi/ml) during the final 18 h. Cells were harvested with an automatic cell harvester.

B-Cell Differentiation Factor Assay. The purified B-cell cultures (3.74×10^5 B-cells/0.5 ml) were stimulated with SAC (1:13500) for 7 days in the presence or absence of IL-2 (185 U/ml) or IL-4 (370 U/ml). At the end of the incubation time, cell cultures were centrifuged. IgM and IgG contents in supernatants were measured using an ELISA technique [6].

Statistics. Student's *t*-test, paired or unpaired, was used to test for statistical significance. Statistical significance was defined as a *P* value of less than 0.05.

Results

PBMC Phenotyping

The posttraumatic course of the patients studied was characterized by a distinct monocytosis and a highly significant reduction of the CD4+ helper/inducer T-cell population (Fig. 1). At the same time, the B-cell population showed no essential shift from the normal range during the whole observation period. The phenotype profile of circulating B-cells was quite stable compared to the norm of 15±2% positive cells (Fig. 1). The reduction of B-cells was never significant, the

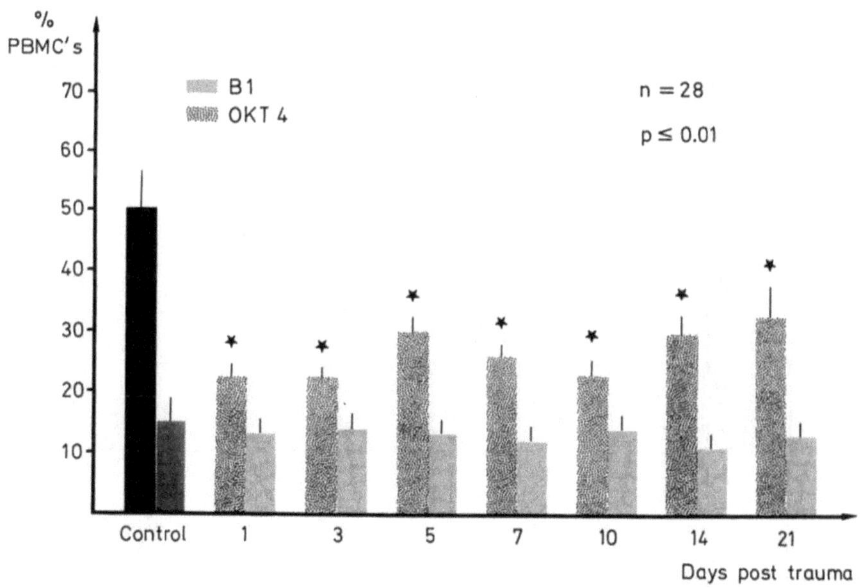

Fig. 1. Changes in T-cell (OKT4) and B-cell (B1) phenotypes compared to controls following trauma (means ± SEM). *$p<0.01$, difference in percentage of phenotypically positive PBMCs from control

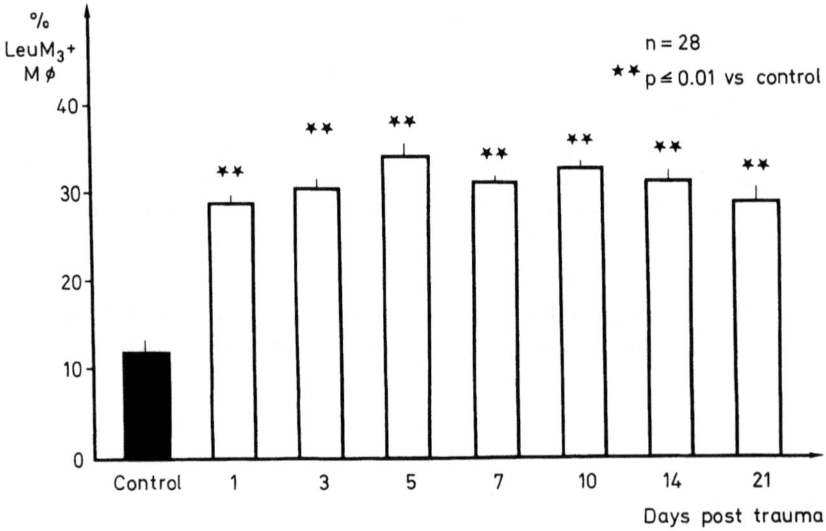

Fig. 2. Changes in the monocyte (LeuM3) phenotypes compared to controls following trauma (means ±SEM). ** $P<0.01$, difference in percentage of phenotypically positive PBMCs from control

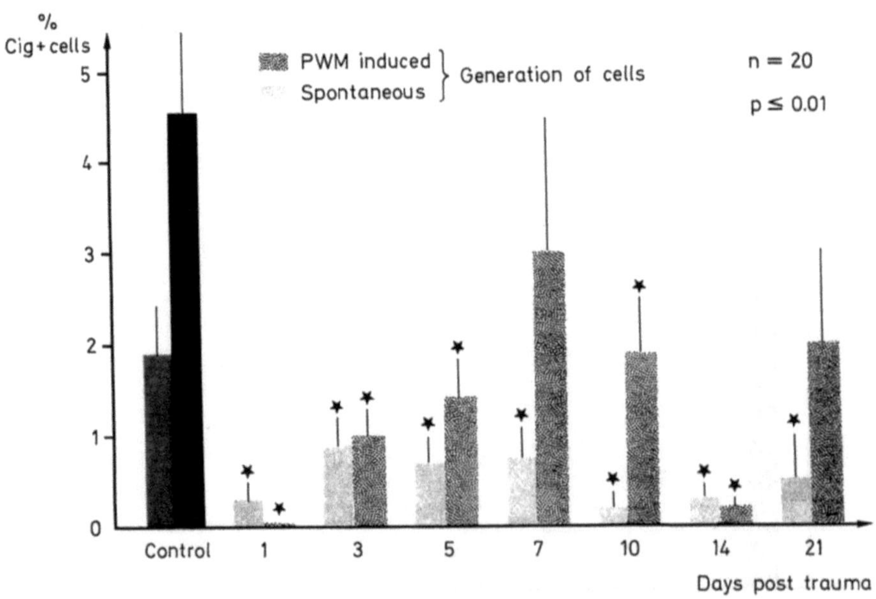

Fig. 3. The percentage of CIg+ PBMCs that represent plasma cells. Spontaneous and PWM-induced differentiation of B-cells to plasma cells (CIg+ cells) on various days that were generated spontaneously or induced with PWM through differentiation from B-cells following major trauma. * $P \leq 0.01$, difference in percentage of phenotypically positive PBMCs from control

numbers being in the range 12%–15%. In contrast to the B-cell population, a significant reduction of the CD4+ population was evident over 21 days post-trauma, with reductions of more than 50% compared to controls. The phenotyping of the monocyte subpopulation (Fig. 2) with the LeuM3 antibody showed a significant elevation of LeuM3+ cells from day 1 through day 21, with a peak value of 34%.

Terminal B-Cell Maturation

The number of PBMCs showing terminal B-cell maturation after PWM stimulation was significantly reduced in patients with major injuries compared to controls (Fig. 3). CIg+ B-cells were suppressed during the whole post-trauma course. Controls had 5% ± 1% CIg+ cells after PWM stimulation; by comparison, there were no CIg+ cells on day 1, 1.0% CIg+ cells on day 3, and only 1.3% CIg+ cells on day 5 post-trauma. The average rate of spontaneous B-cell maturation showed a similar profile of suppression throughout the post-trauma course.

In Vitro Ig Synthesis

Spontaneous Ig synthesis of the subclasses IgG and IgM was significantly suppressed until day 3 post-trauma, while IgA output was low only on day 1. On day 5, IgA and IgG synthesis returned to normal, while IgM synthesis, after recovering initially, decreased again and remained low for the remainder of the observation period (Fig. 4).

PWM-induced synthesis of IgM, IgG, and IgA was significantly supressed until day 3 post-trauma compared to control values (Fig. 5). On day 5, synthesis of

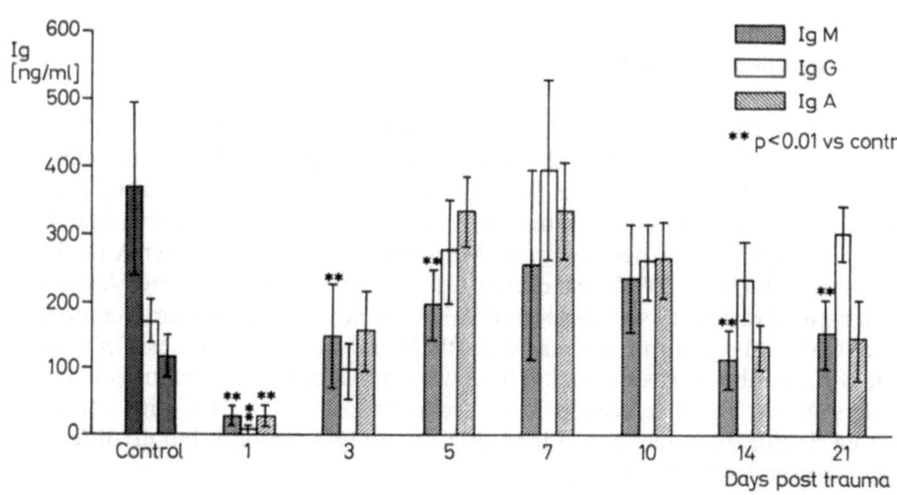

Fig. 4. The changes in spontaneous Ig (subclasses M, G, A) production (ng/ml) of PBMC cultures (1×10^6 cells/ml) after 7 days incubation. ** $p \leqq 0.01$, difference in Ig synthesis from control

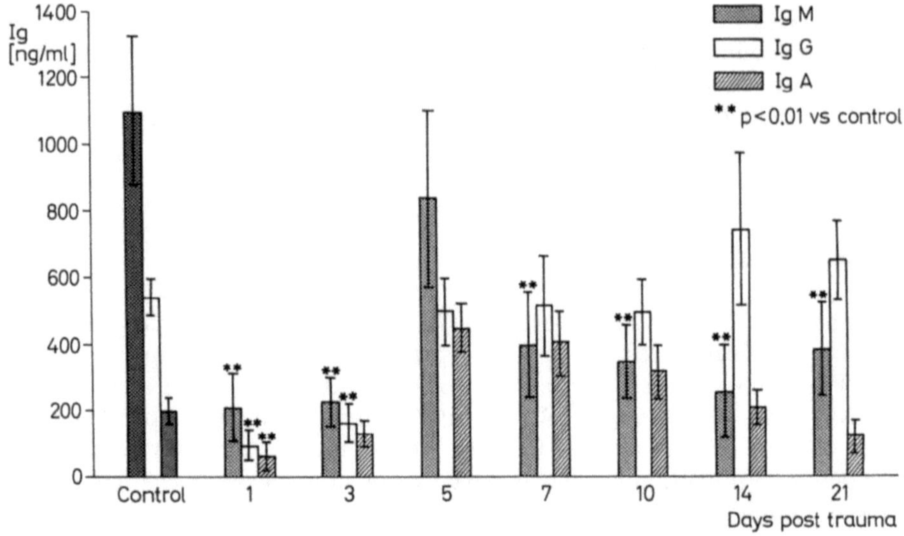

Fig. 5. Changes in PWM-induced Ig (subclasses M, G, A) synthesis of PBMC cultures (1×10^6 cells/ml) after 7 days incubation (means ±SEM). ** $p \leqq 0.01$, difference in Ig synthesis from control

all Ig subclasses was normal. Subsequently, while IgG and IgA synthesis remained normal, IgM synthesis dropped back to subnormal values and remained significantly suppressed, never reaching more than 40% of the control value. While 65% of the patients showed a normal or increased amount of IgG and IgA synthesis, at least on day 7 and later, only 10% of patients had normal rates of mitogen-induced IgM synthesis.

PBMC Monocytes and in Vitro Ig Synthesis

The potential role of monocytes (Mø) in the regulation of Ig synthesis following trauma was studied by relating the quantity of IgA, IgG and IgM to the number of Mø present in PBMC cultures. Analyses of 30 control samples and 101 patient samples at various times post-trauma are depicted in Table 1. The patient samples were subdivided by the percentage of Mø present as follows: cluster A (<30%, Mø), cluster B (30%–60%), and cluster C (>60%). Samples in cluster A showed significant elevations of spontaneous and PWM-induced IgA synthesis compared to controls and significant decreases in PWM-induced IgM synthesis ($p \leqq 0.05$), while IgG synthesis was normal. There were no significant differences between clusters A and B, while comparison of cluster C (>60% Mø) with cluster A showed significant reductions in IgM (Fig. 6) and IgG synthesis but no difference in IgA synthesis (Table 1).

Table 1. Spontaneous and PWM-induced Ig synthesis in relation to the percentage of Mø in the the PBMC cultures (means ± SEM)

	Ig synthesis (ng/ml)			
	Control ≈22% Mø	Cluster A ≦30% Mø	Cluster B >30% Mø	Cluster C ≧60% Mø
IgM	366 ± 121	245 ± 78	204 ± 68	100 ± 37*
IgM + PWM	1086 ± 231	589 ± 143*	353 ± 82*	277 ± 80*
IgG	165 ± 31	288 ± 65	294 ± 59	178 ± 34*
IgG + PWM	537 ± 78	596 ± 112	504 ± 106	274 ± 44*
IgA	118 ± 33	240 ± 42*	261 ± 58*	214 ± 41
IgA + PWM	194 ± 33	334 ± 53*	298 ± 57	273 ± 47
No. of samples	30	38	26	37

* $p \leqq 0.05$ vs control.

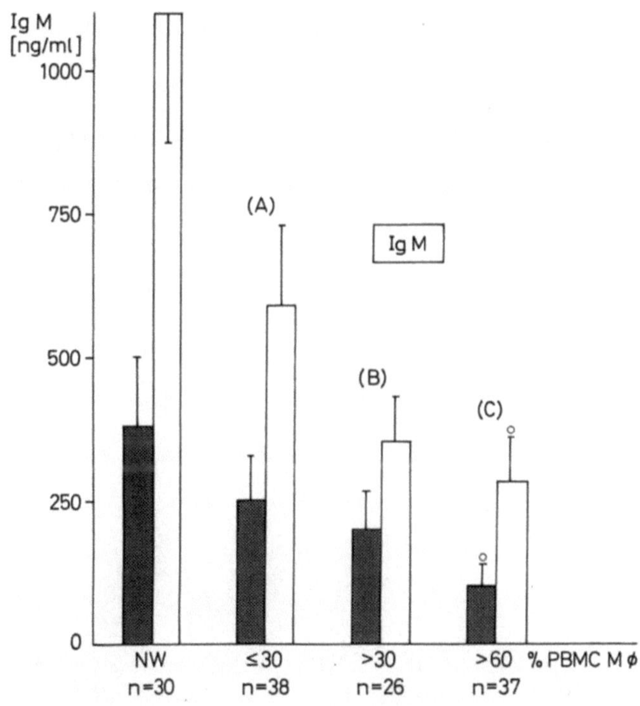

Fig. 6. Changes of spontaneous and PWM-induced IgM synthesis in relation to the percentage of Mø in corresponding PBMC cultures (means ± SEM). ° $P \leqq 0.05$ vs cluster A; *NW*, control value

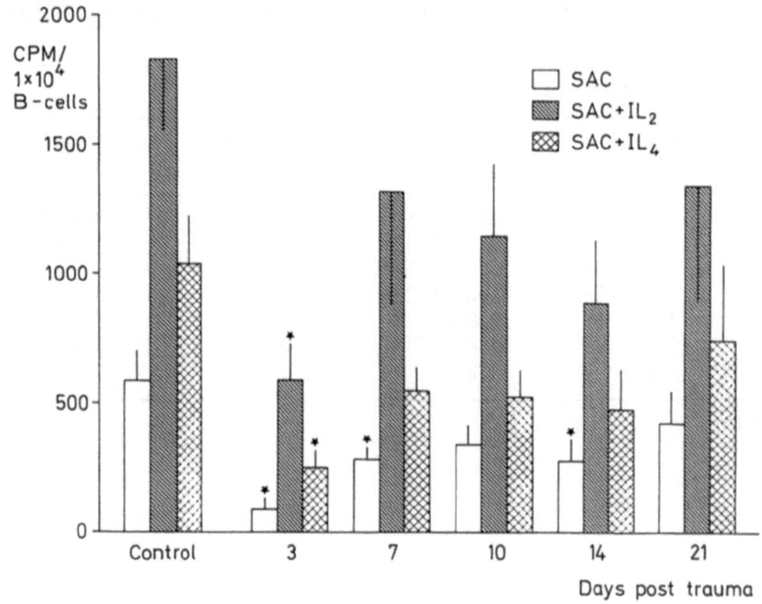

Fig. 7. Effect of IL-2 (250 U/ml) and IL-4 (250 U/ml) on proliferation in SAC-stimulated B-cell cultures (1×10^5 B-cells/0.2 ml/well). Cells of multiply traumatized patients ($n=5$) were prepared on days 3, 7, 10, 14, and 21 post-trauma and compared to controls ($n=14$). Means ±SEM, * $P \leqq 0.05$ vs control

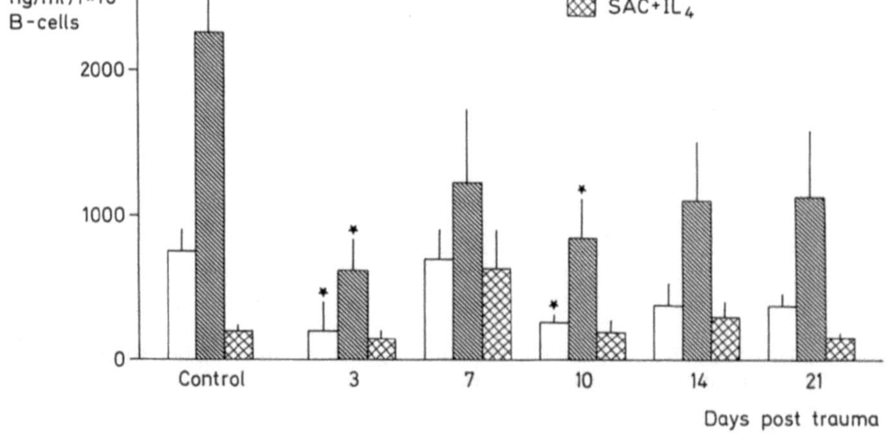

Fig. 8. Impact of IL-2 (185 U/ml) and IL-4 (370 U/ml) on IgM synthesis in SAC-stimulated B-cell cultures (3.64×10^5 B-cells/0.05 ml). After 7 days' incubation cells of multiply traumatized patients ($n=5$) were prepared on days 3, 7, 10, 14, and 21 post-trauma and compared to controls ($n=14$). Means ±SEM, * $P \leqq 0.05$ vs controls

Effect of IL-2/IL-4 on Proliferation in SAC-Stimulated B-Cell Cultures

Addition of IL-2 and IL-4 caused significant increases ($P \leqq 0.05$) in B-cell proliferation in the control group (Fig. 7) with an elevation of 213% for IL-2 and of 76% for IL-4. B-cell proliferation in the patient group was significantly lower than in controls on day 3 post-trauma after stimulation with SAC alone as well as with IL-2 or IL-4 ($P \leqq 0.05$). There was a tendency towards normalization until day 21 post-trauma, but the absolute amounts of the control group could not be reached. The capacity of IL-2 or IL-4 to augment SAC-induced B-cell proliferation was not depressed in the patient group. The stimulation index for IL-2 (B-cells + SAC + IL-2)/(B-cells + SAC) in the patient group was 4.16 (controls 3.13) and the stimulation index for IL-4 (B-cells + SAC + IL-4)/(B-cells + SAC) was 1.98 (controls 1.76).

Effect of IL-2/IL-4 on IgM Synthesis in SAC-Stimulated B-Cell Cultures

IL-2 induced a significant increase of IgM synthesis in the control group, with a stimulation index of 3.0, while IL-4 did not show any positive influence on IgM synthesis (Fig. 8). In parallel to the B-cell proliferation absolute levels of patients' IgM synthesis were depressed on all days post-trauma. The stimulation index of IL-2 for IgM synthesis was similar in the two groups (patients 2.8; controls 3.0).

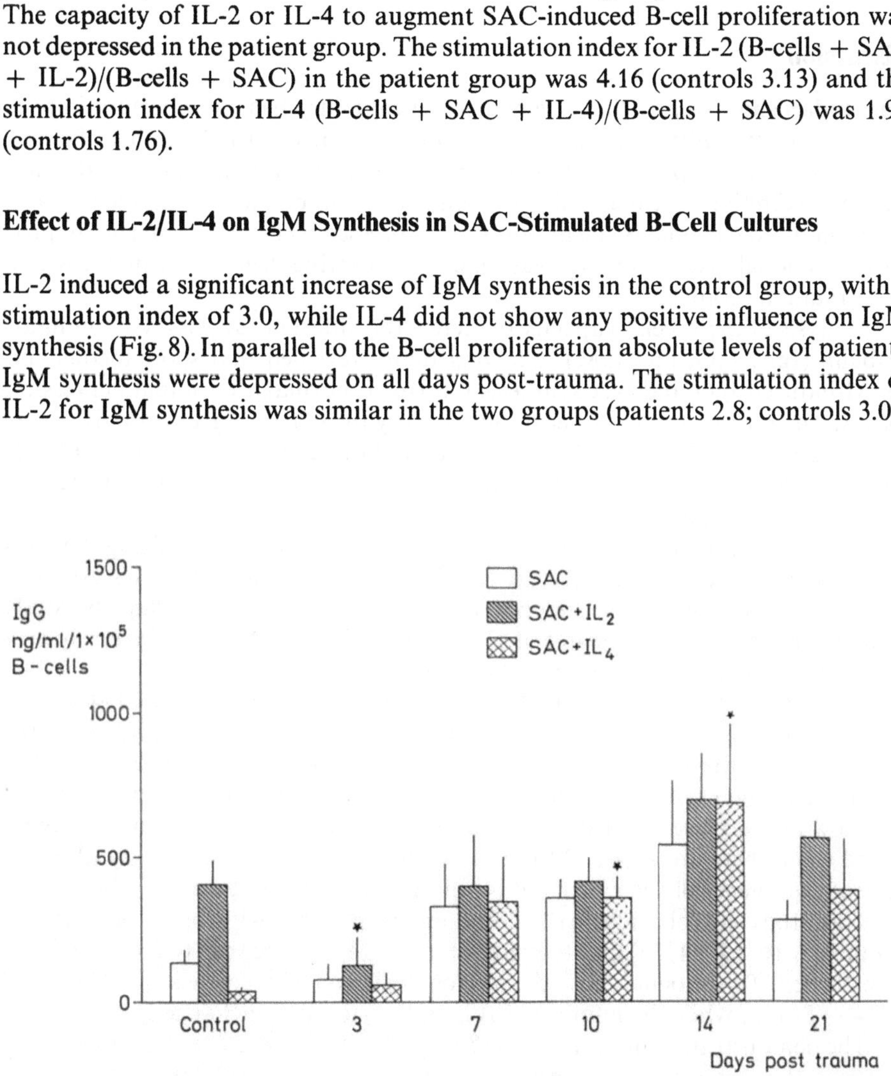

Fig. 9. Impact of IL-2 (185 U/ml) and IL-4 (370 U/ml) on IgG synthesis in SAC-stimulated B-cell cultures (3.64×10^5 B-cells/0.05 ml) after 7 days' incubation. Cells of multiply traumatized patients ($n = 5$) were prepared on days 3, 7, 10, 14, and 21 post-trauma and compared to controls ($n = 14$). Means $\pm$SEM, *$p \leqq 0.05$ vs controls

Impact of IL-2/IL-4 on IgG-Synthesis in SAC-stimulated B-Cell Cultures

In parallel to IgM synthesis, IL-4 was not found to have any influence on IgG production, while IL-2 significantly induced IgG synthesis ($P \leqq 0.05$) (Fig. 9). We found a depression of IgG synthesis on day 3. On day 7 post-trauma and later, the IgG levels of the patient group were elevated up to 300% (day 14). In contrast to IgM synthesis, the capacity of IL-2 to induce IgG synthesis was reduced in patients (1.46) compared to controls (3.01).

Discussion

Our studies show clearly that severe mechanical injury has an important impact on humoral immunity. Although there is an apparently normal number of circulating B-cells, the capacity of those lymphocytes to mature into functional intact antibody-secreting plasma cells is significantly impaired. Spontaneous and PWM-induced terminal B-cell maturation, expressed by the cells' capacity to produce polyclonal cytoplasmic Ig, was reduced to varying degrees during the whole post-traumatic course.

Analysis of the B-cells' capacity to secrete the different subclasses of immunoglobulin (IgA, IgG, and IgM) following injury revealed that spontaneous and PWM-induced IgG and IgA synthesis returns to normal after initial depression (day 3). In contrast to the rather rapid recovery of IgG and IgA synthesis, a persisting deficiency of IgM synthesis was found. After an initial recovery of PWM-induced IgM synthesis by day 5, IgM synthesis remains insufficient throughout the post-trauma course.

One reason for the differences between cells in terms of synthesizing the individual Ig subclasses is apparently the Mø/T-cell ratio within the PBMCs. Analysis of all Ig-containing PBMC supernatants that were collected during the study showed strikingly that the degree of suppression of IgM synthesis is inversely proportional to the percentage of peripheral Mø.

An excess of Mø is accompanied by a decrease in T-cells, mainly CD4+ cells. As the percentage of CD8+ T-cells and B-cells does not vary significantly, the sensitivities of the various Ig subclasses to this phenomenon appear to differ. Spontaneous IgG synthesis, independent of the Mø/T-cell ratio, is not suppressed to below normal levels and PWM-induced IgG synthesis is only significantly reduced when there are $\geqq 60\%$ Mø in the PBMC cell suspension. IgA synthesis in patients was generally elevated and is not influenced by an excess of Mø.

This study corroborates earlier findings in patients with burn and surgical trauma [2, 16, 23, 24, 26] that the quantitative Mø/T helper cell (CD4+) balance is disturbed. The patients showed a monocytosis and a severe lack of CD3+ and CD4+ T-cells, while the number of B-lymphocytes was unchanged.

The demonstration of normal numbers of B-cells has been used in recent years to argue that the trauma-induced disturbances of humoral immunity would be minor compared to the disturbances that develop within the cell-mediated immune system. On the other hand, a number of studies dealing with the formation of antibody to bacterial antigens [20, 30] have demonstrated that there is serious impairment of the response to tetanus toxoid, for example.

In contrast, several authors have reported that burned patients exhibited enhancement of spontaneous and PWM-stimulated polyclonal Ig secretion in vitro. Because of these differences in antibody response following specific and polyclonal stimulation, it has been suggested that there is no intrinsic B-cell abnormality, but that T-cell regulation of B-cell function is abnormal. Further support for this notion comes from the findings of Miller and Chaudry [18], who showed that normal antibody synthesis was restored when the B-cells of burned mice received adequate T-cell support from T-cells of healthy animals. Our studies give information about intrinsic B-cell function and on the Mø/T cell interaction-dependent functional capacity.

Spontaneous terminal B-cell maturation was severely suppressed on all days post-trauma compared with spontaneous B-cell activity in controls. Quantitative and qualitative tests of putative CD8+ T suppressor function which were carried out in this laboratory along with other functional studies revealed that the regulatory role of T suppressor cells in trauma patients does not differ importantly from that in controls. Therefore, we might assume that the discrepancy between the apparently normal numbers of B-cells and the deficiency of spontaneously generating CIg+ cells is due to the fact that, after trauma, we see B-cells that may not be differentiated far enough to synthesize CIg, and/or that they may have been blocked through the contact with possible inhibitory serum factors [19].

Theodorczyk-Injeyan et al. [26] studied PWM-induced monoclonal Ig production in vitro in burned patients and found an elevation of both IgG and IgM secretion during the first 14–21 days after burn injury. This was then followed by a period of relative depression lasting several weeks. This study, however, provides a possible explanation, in that suppression and augmentation of the PWM-stimulated Ig synthesis were well correlated with alterations in T-cell reactivity measured in mixed lymphocyte reaction (MLR). It may be that burned patients have depressed production of Ig secondary to T suppressor cell activity [17] or due to the failure of T helper cell activity [29]. In other studies in our laboratory major changes in T suppressor cell numbers (CD8+) have not been demonstrated. These facts may explain some of the above-mentioned differences in Ig synthesis between trauma and burn patients [26].

When Wood and coworkers studied the in vitro response of tetanus toxoid (TT)-specific antibodies in burned patients, the impaired antibody response correlated with severely suppressed T lymphocyte IL-2 production [30]. They concluded that inadequate IL-2 production was followed by reduced T-cell help, which then ultimately might have been responsible for the lack of a persistent antibody response in burned patients. In addition, they found that the TT-specific antibody produced was primarily of the IgG subclass. The authors' interpretation of this finding was that, because of the IL-2 deficiency, adequate IgM secretion in activated B-cells was not possible, as IL-2 directly and selectively induces IgM synthesis and secretion in long-term tissue cultures [5]. In patients with multiple trauma, there is a severe persistent IL-2 deficiency, as described by us and others [1, 9]. Thus, a lack of lymphokine output could very well be one factor responsible for the pronounced deficiency of IgM synthesis.

Further work done by us showed that the defective Mø/T-cell interaction following major trauma is due to the generation of an excessive amount of negative regulatory Mø, which have an effect via prostaglandin E_2 (PGE_2) mainly on IL-2-synthesizing T-helper cells [7, 8, 29]. Knapp and Baumgartner [14] found that the addition of high numbers of normal human Mø to PBMC-stimulated cultures suppresses various immune responses. These responses include T- and B-lymphoproliferation, terminal B-cell differentiation, suppression of Ig synthesis, and the switching from IgM to IgG production. They showed that cocultivation of strongly adherent Mø with partially adherent-cell depleted PBMCs led to a significant suppression of plasma cell differentiation. Partial depletion of adherent cells not only led to an increase in differentiation and proliferation of human B-cells, but also to a shift in the Ig class distribution of CIg+ cells from IgM to IgG. The clinical correlate of their observation was found in myeloma patients with an excess of adherent Mø and suppressed B-cell capacity for PWM-induced differentiation to CIg+ plasma cells. Depletion of Mø led to a significantly increased B-cell differentiation in normal subjects and patients. This is accord with our present observations of the predominantly downregulatory role of Mø. A correlation between the quantity and quality of Ig synthesis and the percentage of Mø in the PBMC population was found. IgM synthesis was particularly severely depressed in patients with a high proportion of Mø. Independent of the excess of Mø, IgA synthesis was elevated in patients, and IgG synthesis was depressed in patients with a Mø share of $\geqq 60\%$.

It is our hypothesis that the excess of Mø and the lack of CD4+ cells act together to impair IgM synthesis. The suppression of IL-1 synthesis following trauma might be responsible for further suppression of Ig synthesis, as an effect of IL-1 on B-cell differentiation and Ig synthesis is well accepted. Parallel to its downregulating effect on IL-2 synthesis, PGE_2 can also act as a suppressor of Ig production or B-cell differentiation. Goodwin et al. [10] were successful in enhancing humoral responses with the cyclooxygenase inhibitor indomethacin. Addition of indomethacin to PWM-driven cultures in our laboratory did not show a persistent enhancement of Ig synthesis. Furthermore, another monokine, leukotriene B_4, has been found to have a potent negative regulatory effect on Ig synthesis [3] and might thus also impair humoral immunity of trauma patients with high numbers of Mø.

Similarly to the deficiency of IL-2 synthesis following trauma or burn injury, it seems evident that a lack of other lymphokines like interferon-γ or IL-4 might also downregulate T-cell-induced B-cell activation.

Besides the influence of negative regulatory macrophages, other possible causes of the downregulation of B-cell function and the possible shift from IgM to IgG synthesis had to be investigated. These included depression of receptor expression on B-cells for lymphokines like IL-2 or IL-4 as well as a functional defect of the B-lymphocyte itself. While our original studies were carried out in PBMC cultures, we could not examine the alterations of B-lymphocyte function post-trauma. By using purified B-cell cultures, further investigations on B-cell function became possible.

We found a reduction of the absolute amounts of B-cell proliferation after stimulation with SAC on all days post-trauma compared to controls. IL-2 and IL-4 could induce a certain increase in the proliferation rate, but this never reached control levels. The capacity of lymphokines to increase the rate of B-cell proliferation was identical in patients and controls. Profiles of IgM synthesis after trauma showed rather similar results. IL-4 did not stimulate Ig synthesis. These findings confirm results of previous studies [22] showing that IL-4 can induce an increase in B-cell proliferation but is not involved in Ig synthesis.

Finally, in these recent studies we showed that the downregulation of the B-cell system following severe mechanical trauma is not exclusively caused by negative regulatory Mø. The considerable reduction of proliferative capacity and IgM synthesis seems to be also a consequence of intracellular defects. The fact that IgM synthesis was massively depressed while IgG production was elevated from day 7 to day 21 may indicate altered intracellular behaviour. The shift from IgG to IgM had already been shown in earlier studies by Nohr et al. [20]. Molecular biological investigations will be necessary to get better information about this phenomenon. A further explanation for the depression of B-cell function following trauma might be altered receptor expression on B-cells for certain lymphokines. However, we found that the capacity of IL-2 and IL-4 to increase B-cell proliferation was identical in patients and controls.

The PWM, B-cell growth factor, and B-cell differentiation factor assays which were used in this study for the in vitro analysis of B-cell function in patients after major mechanical trauma appear to be very attractive, in spite of their complexity. They might be of great value, combined with other test systems, in delineating further mechanisms of immune dysfunction and in obtaining more information about intracellular mechanisms.

References

1. Abraham E, Lee RJ, Chang Y (1986) The role of interleukin-2 in hemorrhage induced abnormalities of Lymphocyte proliferation. Circ Shock 18:205
2. Antonacci AC, Reaves LE, Calvano SE, Amand R, DeRiesthal HF, Shires GT (1984) Flow cytometric analysis of lymphocyte subpopulations after thermal injury in human beings. Surg Gynecol Obstet 159:1
3. Atluru D, Goodwin JS (1984) Control of polyclonal immunoglobulin production from human lymphocytes by leukotrienes, leukotriene B4 inducts an OKT8+, radiosensitive suppressor cell from resting, human OKT8− T-cells. J Clin Invest 74:1444
4. Baker CC (1986) Immune mechanisms and host resistance in the trauma patient. Yale J Biol Med 59:387
5. Brooks K, Yuan D, Uhr JW et al. (1983) Lymphokine-induced IgM secretion by clones of neoplastic B-cells. Nature 302:825
6. Engval E, Perlman P (1971) Enzyme-linked immunosorbent assay (ELISA): quantitative assay for immunoglobulin G. Immuno Chem 8:871
7. Faist E, Kupper TS, Baker CC, Chaudry IH, Dwyer J, Baue AE (1986) Depression of cellular immunity after major injury. Arch Surg 121:1000
8. Faist E, Mewes A, Baker CC, Strasser Th, Alkan SS, Rieber P, Heberer G (1987) Prostaglandin E_2 (PGE_2) dependent suppression of interleukin (IL-2) production in patients with major trauma. J Trauma 27:837
9. Faist E, Mewes A, Strasser Th, Walz A, Alkan S, Baker CC, Ertel W, Heberer G (1988) Alteration of monocyte function following major injury. Arch Surg 123:287
10. Goodwin JS, Selinger DS, Messner RP, Reed WP (1978) Effect of indomethacin in vivo on humoral and cellular immunity in humans. Infect Immun 19:430
11. Greenspan L, McLellan B, Greg RW (1985) Abbreviated injury scale and injury: a scoring chart. J Trauma 25:60

12. Hirano T, Kuritani T, Kishimoto T, Yamamura Y (1977) In vitro immune response of human peripheral lymphocytes. J Immunol 119:1236
13. Keightley RG, Cooper MD, Lawton AR (1976) The T-cell dependence of B-cell differentiation induced by pokeweed mitogen. J Immunol 117:1538
14. Knapp W, Baumgartner G (1978) Monocyte-mediated suppression of human B-lymphocyte differentiation in vitro. J Immunol 121:1177
15. Kondo N, Orii T, Uetake H (1983) Competence of B-cells for T-cell help in pokeweed mitogen-induced immunoglobulin production. Clin Immunol Immunopathol 26:192–200
16. Lennard TWJ, Shenton BK, Borzotta A, Donnely PK, White M, Gerrie LM, Proud G, Taylor RMR (1985) The influence of surgical operations on components of the human immune system. Br J Surg 72:771
17. Miller CL, Baker CC (1976) Changes in lymphocyte activity after thermal injury: the role of suppressor cells. J Clin Invest 63:202–210
18. Miller CL, Chaudry BJ (1979) Suppressor T-cell activity induced as a result of thermal injury. Cell Immunol 44:201
19. Ninnemann JL (1982) Immunologic defenses against infection: alterations following thermal injuries. J of Burn Care Rehabil 3,6:355–398
20. Nohr CW, Christou NV, Rode H, Gordon J, Meakins JL (1984) In vivo and in vitro humoral immunity in surgical patients. Ann Surg 200:373
21. Nohr CW, Christou NV, Broadhead M, Meakins JL (1986) Failure of humoral immunity in surgical patients. Surg Forum 34:127–129
22. Nossal GJ (1988) Triumphs and trials of immunology in the 1980s. Immunol Today 9,10:286
23. Polk HC, George CD, Wellhausen SR, Cost K, Davidson PR, Regan MP, Borzotta AP (1986) A systematic study of host defense processes in badly injured patients. Ann Surg 204:282
24. Rodrick ML, Wood JJ, Grbic JT, O'Mahony JB, Davis CF, Moss NM, Blazat BA, Demling RH, Mannick JA (1986) Defective IL-2 production in patients with severe burns and sepsis. Lymphokine Res 5:75
25. Shorr RM, Ershler WB, Gamelli RL (1984) Immunoglobulin production in burned patients. J Trauma 24,4:319
26. Theodorzyk-Injeyan JA, Sparkes BG, Falk RE, Peters WJ (1986) Polyclonal immunoglobulin production in burned patients – kinetics and correlations with T-cell activity. J Trauma 26:834
27. Twomey JJ (1982) Excessive immunosuppression. In: the pathophysiology of human immunologic disorders. UL Schwarzenberg 8:125
28. Winkelstein A (1984) What are the immunological alterations induced by burn injury? J Trauma 24,9:72
29. Wood JJ, Grbic JT, Rodrick ML, Jordan A, Mannick JA (1987) Suppression of interleukin-2 production in an animal model of thermal injury is related to prostaglandin synthesis. Arch Surg 122:179
30. Wood JJ, O'Mahony JB, Rodrick ML, Eaton R, Demling RH, Mannick JA (1986) Abnormalities of antibody production after thermal injury. Arch Surg 121:108

Activation of B Cells Spontaneously Secreting Ig After Surgery

F. Di Padova and M. Dürig

Introduction

Following surgery a state of immunosuppression or immunodeficiency, in which cellular immune responses are more heavily depressed, has been described (Antonacci 1986). On the other hand the appearance in the circulation of lymphoblastoid B cells spontaneously secreting IgG and IgA shows that B cells are activated (Di Padova et al. 1986). Analogous B-cell subsets are observed after in vivo immunization and represent a sensitive marker of antigenic exposure (Di Padova et al. 1983). Lymphoblastoid B cells are actively synthesizing low titers of antibodies against bacterial antigens like tetanus toxoid, pneumococcal capsular polysaccharides, and the lipopolysaccharides of several enteropathogenic *Escherichia coli* (Di Padova et al. 1988). Now the relationship between spontaneous Ig secretion and DNA synthesis in recently operated subjects has been analyzed.

Methods

Patients

Ten women aged 18–75 years (50.3 ± 5.8 years) and two men aged 49 and 68 years entered this study (eight cholecystectomies, two thyroidectomies, one abdominal incisional hernia, one lymphedema). The patients received similar premedication, anesthetic agents, and postoperative analgesia. Antibiotic prophylaxis with cephalosporins was used. Pre- and postoperative complications were not observed. No subject had evidence of anemia, jaundice, infection, autoimmune disease, or malignancy. No patient was receiving drugs known to have immunological effects, nor did any receive blood transfusions. Informed consent was obtained from each patient.

Spontaneous Ig Secretion and [^{3}H]Thymidine Incorporation

Blood samples were obtained in the morning at specified times after surgery. Peripheral blood mononuclear cells (PBMCs) were separated and cultured as previously described (1 or 2×10^6 cells/ml) (Di Padova et al. 1986). No mitogen was added. After 4 days of culture the supernatants were carefully collected for the determination of spontaneous Ig secretion. To measure proliferation 1 µCi [^{3}H]thymidine was added 20 h before the end of the culture period. Cells were

Immune Consequences of
Trauma, Shock and Sepsis
Eds. Faist/Ninnemann/Green

harvested with a Titertek cell harvester (Flow Laboratories) and thymidine incorporation was measured using a liquid scintillation counter (Packard Tricarb 4640).

Cytoplasmic Ig (cIg) and BrdU Detection by Immunofluorescence

Peripheral blood mononuclear cells were centrifuged onto slides with a Shandon cytofuge (5×10^4 cells/slide). The slides were fixed and stained with 50 µl TRITC-conjugated goat anti-human Ig (Cappel; 1/100 dilution). Positive cells were detected with a fluorescence microscope (Leitz). For the determination of labeling indices 2000 cells were counted by two independent investigators.

Measurement of Specific Antibodies and of Total Ig

An enzyme-linked immunosorbent assay (ELISA) was used to measure total IgG, IgA, and IgM (Di Padova et al. 1986).

Statistical Analysis

All values are reported as means and standard errors (SE).

Results

Spontaneous Ig Secretion by PBMCs

Spontaneous Ig secretion was very low before and 1 and 3 days following surgery, became evident at day 5, reached its maximum on day 7, and decreased at day 11 (Fig. 1). Mainly IgG and IgA antibodies were found; a modest and earlier IgM peak was also observed. Individual variations in the magnitude of the response were seen.

Spontaneous Incorporation of [^{3}H]Thymidine

DNA synthesis was studied by [^{3}H]thymidine incorporation before and at the specified times after surgery (Fig. 2). Proliferative activity increased after surgery and reached its maximum on days 5 and 7. Eleven days after the intervention DNA synthesis was still sustained, indicating the persisting presence of actively proliferating cells.

Cytoplasmic Ig-Positive (cIg+) Cells

The kinetics of cIg+ cells in the peripheral blood paralleled spontaneous Ig secretion in culture supernatants (Fig. 3). A significant rise was observed on day 5; the highest level was documented on day 7. At day 11 cIg+ B cells had returned to basal values.

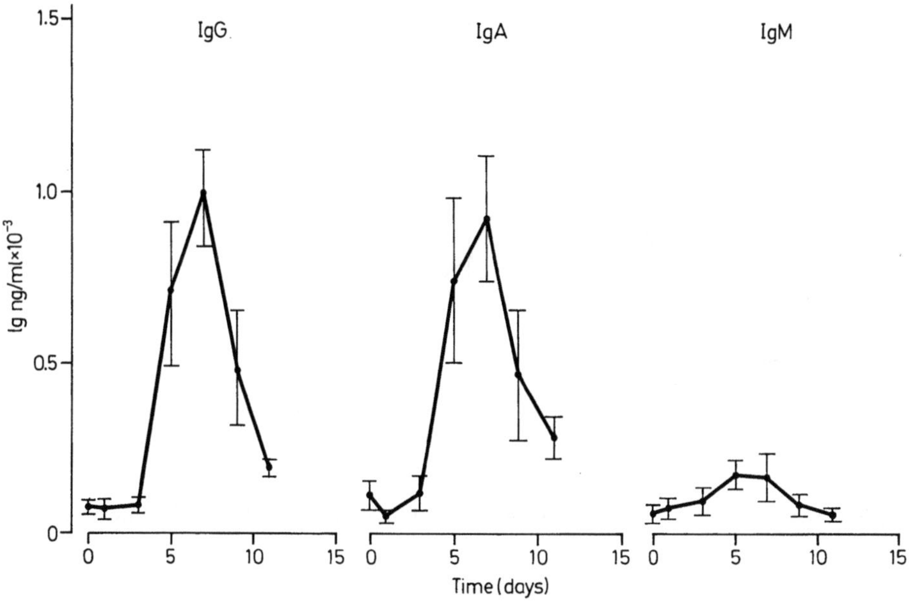

Fig. 1. Spontaneous Ig secretion by PBMCs after surgery. PBMCs (1×10^6 cells/ml) were collected at the indicated times and cultured for 4 days

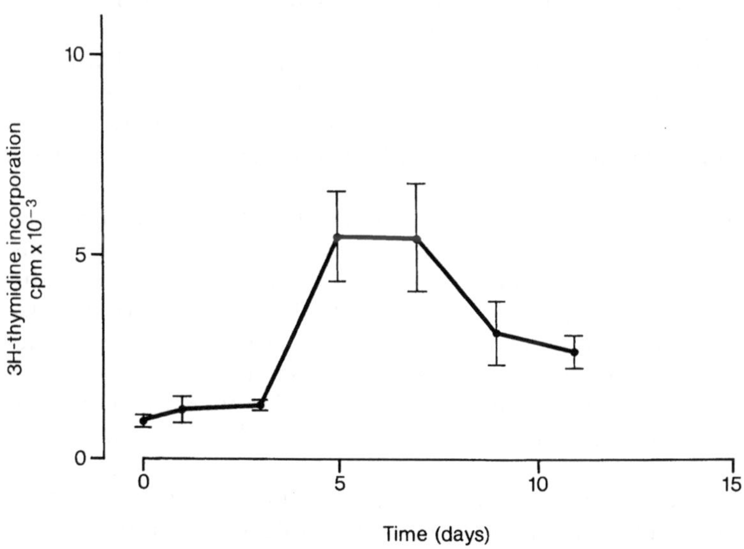

Fig. 2. Kinetics of spontaneous incorporation of [^{3}H]thymidine. PBMCs (2×10^6 cells/ml), collected at the specified times, were cultured for 24 h

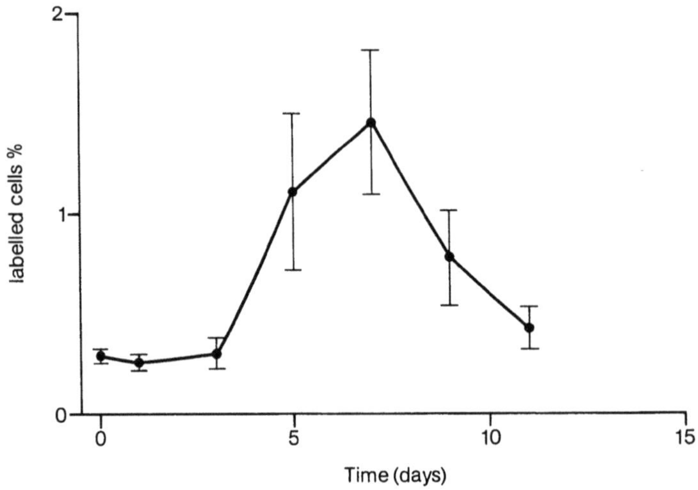

Fig. 3. Percentage of cIg+ cells in the peripheral blood before and after the intervention

Discussion

This study demonstrates that in surgical patients the immune system is activated as evident from the appearance in the peripheral blood of B cells spontaneously secreting Ig and by an increase in DNA synthesis.

This study shows a correlation between the appearance of lymphoblastoid B cells and the increase in DNA synthesis. The sensitivity of lymphoblastoid B cells to radiation and to BrdU strongly suggests that these cells require DNA synthesis before Ig secretion (Brieva and Stevens 1984; Di Padova et al. 1986; De La Sen et al. 1987).

Even if the origin, destination, and regulation of lymphoblastoid B cells remain obscure, they are considered the progeny of recently activated memory cells. These B cells are not only involved in the antibody response but also in the dissemination of the immune response (Thiele et al. 1981). In bone marrow transplant recipients, transfer of lymphoblastoid B cells provides for specific immunologic memory in addition to an active adoptive antibody response (Saxon et al. 1986; Wimperis et al. 1986). The appearance of lymphoblastoid B cells after a surgical intervention might have an important role in the defense against infections.

In conclusion, after elective surgery several changes in circulating cell populations are detectable. In contrast with the present prevalent opinion that defines a condition of immunodeficiency or immunosuppression in surgical patients (Antonacci 1986), our data indicate that the immune system is actively synthesizing Ig.

Summary

Immunosuppression or immunodeficiency have been described following surgery. However, the appearance of lymphoblastoid B cells spontaneously secreting IgG and IgA in surgical patients proves B-cell activation. In this study the kinetics of appearance of lymphoblastoid B cells and the relationship between spontaneous Ig secretion and DNA synthesis have been analyzed. Peaks of spontaneous IgG and IgA secretion and of [^{3}H]thymidine incorporation become evident 5 and 7 days after surgery.

Acknowledgments. We thank Dr. M. H. Schreier, Preclinical Research, Sandoz, Basel, for advice and criticism and M. J. Tondre for excellent technical assistance.

References

Antonacci AC (1986) Immune dysfunction and immunomodulation following trauma. In: Gallin JI, Fauci AS (eds) Advances in host defense mechanisms, vol 6. Raven, New York, pp 81–109

Brieva JA, Stevens RH (1984) Human in vivo antigen induced lymphoblastoid B cells are capable of cyclical antibody production in vitro. J Immunol 133:147–153

De La Sen M, Garcia-Alonso A, Brieva JA (1987) Human B lymphocytes capable of spontaneous Ig production in short term cultures. II. Relationship with the spontaneous DNA-synthesizing B cells. Cell Immunol 104:281–289

Di Padova F, Di Padova C, Rovagnati P, Tritapepe R (1986) Appearance of spontaneously Ig secreting B cells in human peripheral blood after surgery. Clin Exp Immunol 65:582–588

Di Padova F, Dürig M, Di Padova C, Pozzoli M, Tritapepe R (1988) Spontaneous and polyclonal Ig secretion by circulating B cells after surgery. Surgery 103:547–552

Di Padova F, Dürig M, Wadstrom J, Harder F (1983) Role of spleen in immune response to polyvalent pneumococcal vaccine. Br Med J 287:1829–1832

Saxon A, Mitsuyasu R, Stevens R, Champlin RE, Kimata H, Gale RP (1986) Designed transfer of specific immune responses with bone marrow transplantation. J Clin Invest 78:959–967

Thiele CJ, Morrow CD, Stevens RH (1981) Multiple subsets of anti-tetanus toxoid antibody producing cells in human peripheral blood differ by size, expression of membrane receptors, and mitogen reactivity. J Immunol 126:1146–1153

Wimperis JZ, Brenner MK, Prentice HG, Reittie JE, Karayannis P, Griffiths PD, Hoffbrand AV (1986) Transfer of a functioning humoral immune system in transplantation of T-lymphocyte-depleted bone marrow. Lancet I:339–343

Section 3

Trauma and Non-Specific Immune Mechanisms

Pathobiochemical Mechanisms in Inflammation

M. Jochum and H. Fritz

Introduction

The primary response of the organism to an inflammatory stimulus (tissue destruction after multiple trauma, invasive microbae, endotoxins of exogenous and endogenous origin, immune complexes etc.) is directed physiologically towards inactivating and eliminating the agent and to initiating the process of healing and repair. The activation of the complex interacting humoral and cellular defence mechanisms necessary for this purpose carries with it, however, the risk of damaging healthy tissue and thus perpetuating the inflammatory process. The relation of stimuli, mediators, effectors, and inhibitors to each other finally determines the effectiveness or failure of the inflammatory response [1].

Out of the multitude of factors investigated hitherto, proteolytic enzymes, both of the plasma cascade systems (clotting, fibrinolysis, complement, kallikrein/kinin system) and also of lysosomal origin [from polymorphonuclear (PMN) granulocytes, monocytes, macrophages, mast cells], have proved to be potent mediators of inflammation [2].

Mediators of the Humoral and Cellular Systems

The contact between proenzymes of the cascade systems and damaged vascular endothelium together with the activators liberated from those cells results in the formation of system-specific proteases, whose activity is largely responsible for hemostasis and closure of the wound. Some of these proteolytic enzymes (plasma kallikrein, thrombin, plasmin, complement esterases), however, also produce additional mediators of inflammation such as the vasoactive kinins, the hemostatic and edema-forming fibrin monomers and fibrin peptides, or the anaphylactic complement factors (C3a, C4a and C5a) (Fig. 1). System-specific proteases themselves, together with a series of polypeptides formed as a result of their proteolytic activity, act as potent chemotaxins and bring about the sequestration and activation of inflammatory cells (particularly PMN granulocytes) in the area of the wound [2, 3].

The primary task of these cells is to remove the inflammatory stimulus by phagocytosis and thus to limit the inflammatory process to a significant extent [2–4]. Even during the binding and ingestion of "foreign" material in the infective focus, however, the phagocytic cells also liberate numerous aggressive substances (oxygen radicals, hydrolytic and proteolytic enzymes, etc.) into the surrounding

Immune Consequences of
Trauma, Shock and Sepsis
Eds. Faist/Ninnemann/Green

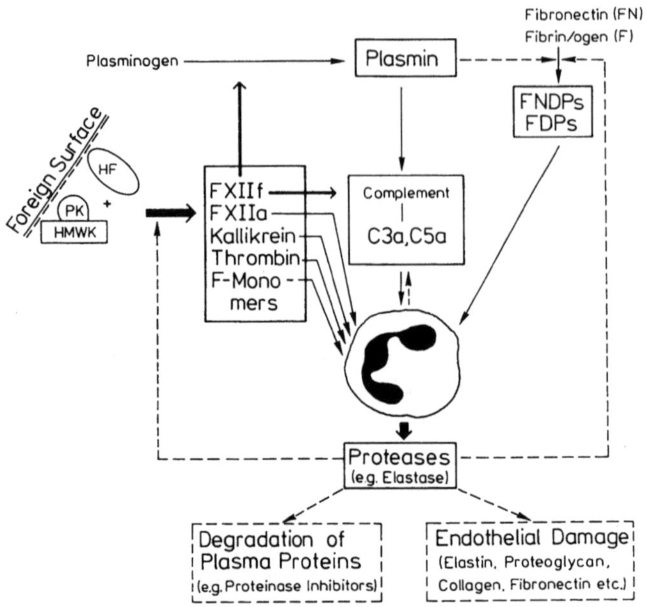

Fig. 1. The interaction between humoral system (clotting, fibrinolysis, complement, kallikrein/kinin system) and the polymorphonuclear (PMN) granulocytes; FNDP = Fibronectin degradation product; FDP = Fibrin/ogen degradation product; FXIIf = Factor XIIf; FXIIa = Factor XIIa; HF = Hageman factor; HMWK = high molecular weight kininogen; PK = Prokallikrein

environment. Once there, these substances are able to cause lasting damage to structural elements (basement membranes, elastin, collagen, fibronectin etc.) and to humoral factors (particularly proteins of the cascade systems). In this way they augment the inflammatory process to a significant degree [5, 6].

When there is restricted activity of an inflammatory stimulus, activation of the proteolytic mediators of inflammation remains confined mainly to the local event by potent protease inhibitors [7]. If the primary defense mechanisms of the organism are not, however, in a position to counteract a massive stimulus (e.g., invasive micro-organisms in severe infection) in time, the increased formation of system-specific proteases and the liberation of proteolytic enzymes and oxidizing substances from inflammatory cells eventually leads to the exhaustion of the functional capacity of the inhibitory regulators. As a consequence, the destructive processes caused by proteases and the systemic manifestations of a local inflammatory process can no longer be prevented adequately or at all [5].

With regard to the pathological mechanisms involved in severe inflammation, the neutral proteases, elastase and cathepsin G, from the azurophilic granules of the PMN granulocytes, stand out as being significant among the lysosomal enzymes currently recognized. They are not only numerically predominant, but also have practically no substrate specificity [8]. After extracellular liberation, these proteases inactivate a series of plasma proteins, such as the protease inhibitors antithrombin III, α_2-plasmin inhibitor, and C1 inactivator [9, 10] only by a very few proteolytic cleavages if they are not inhibited immediately by their natural antagonists, α_1-protease inhibitor, α_1-antichymotrypsin and α_2-macroglobulin,

Myeloperoxidase, another enzyme localized in the azurophilic granules, catalyzes the reaction of hydrogen peroxide (H_2O_2) with chloride ions (Cl^-) in the phagolysosomes. Thus it produces highly bactericidal oxidizing substances which also have extracellular activity and destroy humoral and structurally-bound proteins [11].

The antibacterial activity of lactoferrin, a protein formed mainly in the specific granules of granulocytes, but which is also produced by cells such as those of the glandular epithelium, is also well documented. It depends, in part, upon the catalytic function of the protein in the formation of highly reactive hydroxyl radicals [12]. Patients with lactoferrin deficiency suffer recurrent infections. Lactoferrin has been described as having a large number of other activities in addition, but many of these effects have not been confirmed by other investigators. The functional role of lactoferrin in inflammation can, therefore, be regarded as still being largely unclarified [12].

Studies in Patients and Experimental Animals

Methodology

Fundamental information relating to the extent to which proteases participate in an inflammatory process is obtained from thc following studies:

1. Quantitative demonstration of the liberation of lysosomal proteins and activation of system-specific proteolytic enzymes.
2. Simultaneous demonstration of the consumption of protease inhibitors and plasma factors susceptible to proteolytic degradation.
3. Use of specific exogenous protease inhibitors and antioxidants in therapeutic studies in experimental animals.

Measurement of the lysosomal PMN granulocyte proteins elastase [13], myeloperoxidase [14], and lactoferrin [15] was carried out by means of highly specific sandwich enzyme immuno assays (ELISA). The normal concentrations of these proteins in the cells and plasma are shown in Fig. 2. With regard to elastase, it should be noted that the protease released extracellularly into the circulation can no longer be demonstrated as the active enzyme, but only as an inactive complex with α_1-protease inhibitor (α_1 PI). The levels mentioned in the following discussion relate, however, only to the elastase moiety and not to the whole complex.

Protease inhibitors and plasma factors susceptible to proteolytic degradation were quantified in accordance with the methods outlined in [5].

The methods used in the therapeutic studies are extensively described in [16] and [17].

Clinical Studies

Abdominal Surgery and Sepsis

In order to measure exactly the rapid liberation and elimination of elastase during the acute stages of inflammation, blood samples were taken at frequent intervals (6–12 hourly) from patients undergoing abdominal surgery in a prospective clini-

	Elastase	Myeloperoxidase	Lactoferrin
Localisation		PMN Granula	
	azurophilic	azurophilic	specific Body Secretions Glandular Epithelial Cells
M_r	30 000	145 000	70 000
Concentration			
$\mu g/10^6$ PMNs	4- 7	2- 3	4- 7
ng/ml Plasma	60-120	20-60	100-300
Method		Enzyme Immunoassay (ELISA)	
	E-α_1PI	MPO	LF

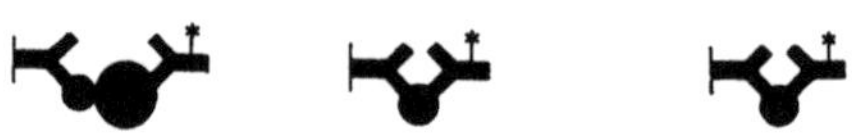

Fig. 2. Localization, method of determination, and normal concentrations of the lysosomal proteins elastase (complexed with α_1-protease inhibitor; *E-α_1 PI*), myeloperoxidase (*MPO*), and lactoferrin (*LF*)

cal study (Director: Professor Duswald, City Surgical Clinic, University of Munich) and the amount of complexed elastase in the plasma was measured [18]. Patients with no postoperative infection (group A) had only a moderate increase (up to three times) after operation in comparison with the preoperative levels (60–120 ng/ml), while in patients with sepsis, markedly increased concentrations were repeatedly determined in the course of the sepsis. At the time of diagnosis of sepsis, concentrations of complexed elastase were measured and these showed a mean six fold increase in group B (postoperative sepsis which was eventually overcome) or tenfold increase in group C (postoperative sepsis with a fatal outcome). Individual peak levels up to 2500 ng/ml occurred in both groups. In patients with persisting sepsis (group C) the E-α_1 PI level remained significantly elevated, as a mean, until death, while the recovery phase in group B was accompanied by an obvious return to normal levels. At the same time as complexed elastase increased in the plasma, a significant reduction in the inhibitory activity of antithrombin III and α_2-macroglobulin together with the fibrin-stabilizing activity of factor XIII was detected in the patients with sepsis. The reduced activity of the factors named above at the onset of sepsis was restored to normal again in patients who overcame infection (group B), while a further decrease occured in those who perished (group C).

Multiple Trauma

In patients with multiple trauma, the concentration of the complexed elastase in plasma correlated with the degree of severity of the injury [19]. The group of patients under investigation (Director of the study: Dr. Dittmer, Surgical Clinic Munich-Großhadern, University of Munich) with widely differing injuries showed very high increases in the mean levels of elastase (up to ten times normal) up to about 12 h after the accident, followed by a well-defined return to normal. Independent of each other, the whole group could be divided into three individual identical groups on the basis of clinical criteria, aided by a scale of severity as well as in accordance with the peak amount of elastase liberated. With these patients, it was not possible to establish a correlation between the concentration of the elastase and the consumption of circulating plasma factors because of the large volumes of blood transfused, particularly in the early days following multiple injury.

Sequential studies of the bronchoalveolar lavage fluid of eight patients with multiple trauma (the samples were collected for us by Dr. Joka, Surgical Clinic, University of Essen) revealed a possible pathogenetic relationship between a permeability injury in the lung and the release of lysosomal proteins together with the oxygen products formed during the "respiratory burst" [20]. Even before the increase in extracellular fluid in the lung (as a measure of pulmonary edema), extremely high concentrations of complexed elastase, together with myeloperoxidase and lactoferrin, could be measured in the lavage fluid in some patients. Since the latter two proteins mentioned are involved in secondary oxidative processes which, among other things, inactivate α_1-protease inhibitor [7], the demonstration of enzymatically active elastase, in addition to E-α_1 PI-complex, in a number of these samples is entirely comprehensible (Fig. 3).

General Surgical Patients and Bacterial Infections

In an extensive clinical study (Director of the study: Dr. Inthorn, Surgical Clinic Munich-Großhadern, University of Munich), the effect of operative trauma and bacterial infection of varying degrees of severity upon the release of granulocyte contents and upon humoral mediators of the inflammatory process was investigated [21]. Elastase and lactoferrin were measured in almost identical amounts in plasma in individual cases. The time course of the release of both proteins showed a pattern of behavior that was often to a large degree identical; myeloperoxidase was generally detected in substantially smaller amounts than the other two lysosomal factors. On general review, of the measurements, however, the amount of elastase showed a continual rise corresponding to the extent of the inflammation, while mild and moderate inflammation could not be differentiated on the basis of lactoferrin and myeloperoxidase; the extracellular levels of these two proteins only reflected the degree of severity of the infection when sepsis was present (Fig. 4). The activation of humoral cascade systems in accordance with the severity of the inflammation was clearly documented by the increases in the anaphylatoxin C3a in plasma and by the consumption of plasma prokallikrein, prothrombin, antithrombin III, and fibronectin.

Therapeutic Studies in Experimental Animals

The results shown in the clinical studies described above may be seen as a clear demonstration of the release of lysosomal enzymes from granulocytes and the ensuing extracellular proteolysis or oxidation of vital structural and humoral proteins in the course of a severe inflammatory process. As a means of avoiding a deleterious endogenous imbalance of proteases and protease inhibitors, it appeared to us that the early administration of effective exogenous inhibitors and antioxidants in animal experiments was promising.

In a preliminary study of sepsis in young pigs (Director of the study: Dr. Welter, City Surgical Clinic, University of Munich), we were able to show that

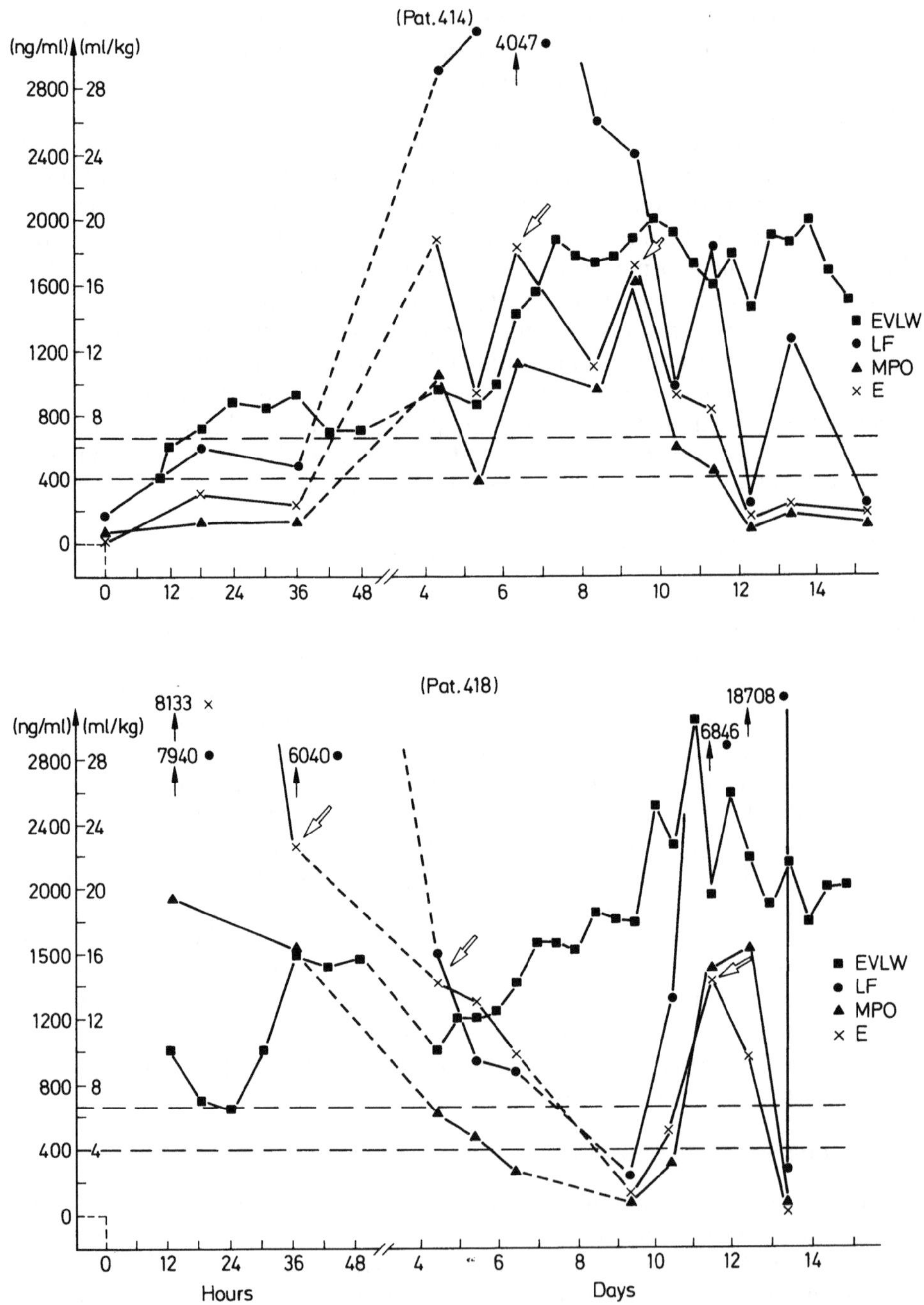

Fig. 3. Granulocyte elastase (*crosses*) in complex with α_1-protease inhibitor and in proteolytically active form (*arrows*) together with myeloperoxidase (*triangles*) and lactoferrin (*circles*) in sequential bronchoalveolar lavage samples from two patients with multiple trauma. The change in extravascular lung water is added (*squares*) as a measure of pulmonary edema

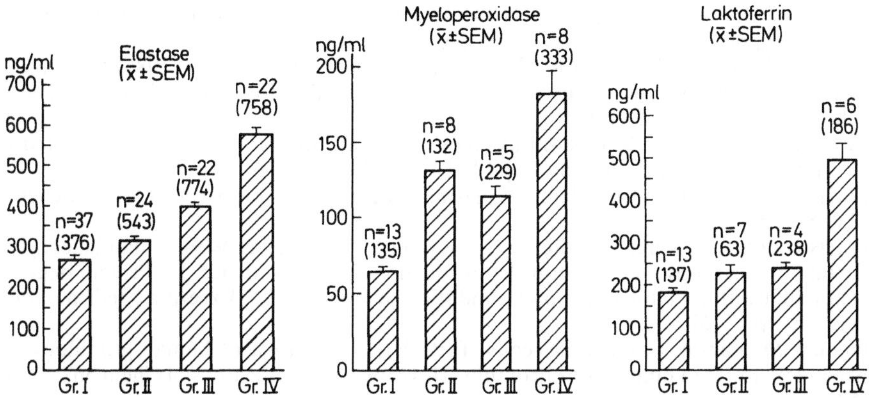

Fig. 4. Increasing concentrations of granulocytic proteins in the plasma of patients following operative trauma with varying degrees of severity of postoperative inflammation. The number of patients (*n*) and the actual number of samples (in brackets) tested in each severity group are shown. *Gr. I,* uncomplicated course; *Gr. II,* a wound infection, locally confined peritonitis, basal pneumonia; *Gr. III,* extensive soft tissue inflammation, peritonitis >1 quadrant, severe bronchial pneumonia; *Gr. IV,* clinically diagnosed sepsis

the relatively specific recombinant elastase cathepsin G inhibitor Eglin (isolated initially from the leech) significantly reduced consumption of protease inhibitors (antithrombin III, α_2-macroglobulin) and other plasma proteins (e.g., factor XIII) and also the formation of interstitial pulmonary edema [16]. Meanwhile, we found in a more sophisticated model of sepsis (Director of the study: Dr. Siebeck, City Surgical Clinic, University of Munich), that Eglin in suitable doses clearly prevented edema in general in the organism and thus is active in counteracting sepsis-related hypotension and multiple organ failure [22].

We achieved similar, though less obviously therapeutic effects by the administration of C1 inactivator, of an inhibitor of system-specific proteases (complement esterases, plasma kallikrein, plasmin), and of the antioxidant superoxide dismutase [17]. A further improvement in inflammatory symptoms may therefore be achievable in future by the combined administration of protease inhibitors and antioxidants.

Acknowledgements. We owe thanks to the named participating clinical colleagues for their intensive collaborations and also to Dr. S. Neumann and Dr. H. Lang, Biochemical Research Department, E. Merck, Darmstadt, for their generous provision of test kits.

References

1. Kalden JR (1983) Klinische Befunde und klinisch-experimentelle Untersuchungen zur Pathogenese entzündlicher Erkrankungen. In: Lang H, Greiling H (eds) Pathobiochemie der Entzündung. Springer, Berlin, pp 9–19
2. Neuhof H (1987) Humorale Veränderungen im Schock: Die pathogenetische Bedeutung der Mediatoren. In: Kilian J, Meßmer K, Ahnefeld FW (eds) Schock. Springer, Berlin pp 37–52
3. Gustafson EJ, Colman RW (1987) Interaction of polymorphonuclear cells with contact activation factors. Semin Thromb Hemostasis 13:95–105

4. Klebanoff SJ, Clark RA (eds) (1987) The Neutrophil. Function and clinical disorders. North Holland, Amsterdam New York Oxford
5. Jochum M, Witte J, Duswald K-H, Inthorn D, Welter HF, Fritz H (1986) Pathobiochemistry of sepsis: role of proteinases, proteinase inhibitors and oxidizing agents. Behring Inst Mitt 79:121–130
6. Havemann K, Gramse M (1984) Physiology and pathophysiology of neutral proteinase of human granulocytes. Adv Exp Med 167:1–20
7. Travis J, Salvesen GS (1983) Human plasma proteinase inhibitors. Ann Rev Biochem 52:655–709
8. Travis J, Giles PJ, Porcelli L, Reilly CF, Baugh R, Powers J (1980) Human leucocyte elastase and cathepsin G: structural and functional characteristics. In: Protein degradation in health and disease. Ciba Foundation Symposium 75. Excerpta Medica, Amsterdam, pp 51–68
9. Jochum M, Lander S, Heimburger N, Fritz H (1981) Effect of human granulocytic elastase on isolated human antithrombin III. Hoppe Seyler's Z Physiol Chem 362:103–112
10. Brower MS, Harpel PC (1982) Proteolytic cleavage and inactivation of α_2-plasmin inhibitor and C1-inactivator by human polymorphonuclear leucocyte elastase. J Biol Chem 257:9849–9854
11. Clark RA (1983) Extracellular effects of the myeloperoxidase-hydrogen peroxide-halide system. In: Weismann G (ed) Advances in inflammation research, vol 5. Raven Press, New York, pp 107–146
12. Birgens HS (1984) The biological significance of lactoferrin in haematology. Scand J Haematol 33:225–230
13. Neumann S, Jochum M (1984) Elastase-α_1-proteinase inhibitor complex. In: Bergmeyer HU, Bergmeyer J, Graßl M (eds) Methods of enzymatic analysis, 3rd edn, vol 5. Verlag Chemie, Weinheim, pp 184–195
14. Neumann S, Gunzer G, Lang H, Jochum M, Fritz H (1986) Quantitation of myeloperoxidase from human granulocytes as an inflammation marker by enzyme-linked immunosorbent assay. Fresenius Z Anal Chem 324:365
15. Rautenberg W, Neumann S, Gunzer G, Lang H, Jochum M, Fritz H (1986) Quantitation of human lactoferrin as an inflammation marker by an enzyme-linked immunosorbent assay (ELISA). Fresenius Z Anal Chem 324:364
16. Jochum M, Welter HF, Siebeck M, Fritz H (1987) Proteinase inhibitor therapy of severe inflammation in pigs. First results with eglin, a potent inhibitor of granulocyte elastase and cathepsin G. In: Taylor JC, Mittmann C (eds) Pulmonary emphysema and proteolysis: 1986. Academic Press, Orlando, pp 85–90
17. Welter HF, Thetter D, Siebeck M, Wiesinger H, Elster U, Fritz H (1985) Versuche zur Therapie der Schocklunge mittels Superoxiddismutase (SOD) und C1-Inaktivator (C1-INA). Langenbecks Arch [Suppl], Chir Forum '85, pp 63–67
18. Duswald K-H, Jochum M, Schramm W, Fritz H (1985) Released granulocytic elastase: an indicator of pathobiochemical alterations in septicemia after abdominal surgery. Surgery 98:892–898
19. Dittmer H, Jochum M, Fritz H (1986) Freisetzung von granulozytärer Elastase und Plasmaproteinveränderungen nach traumatisch-hämorrhagischem Schock. Unfallchirurg 89:160–169
20. Joka Th, Obertacke U, Schönfeld W, Oberste-Beulmann S, Pison U, Kreutzfelder E, Jochum M, Zilow G (1987) Reaction pattern of alveolar cells in posttraumatic lung failure. In: Schlag G, Redl H (eds) Progress in clinical and biological research. (Subseries): Vienna Shock Forum. Part A. Pathophysiological role of mediators and mediator inhibitors. Liss, New York, pp 509–515
21. Inthorn D (1986) Untersuchungen zum Einfluß des operativen Traumas und bakterieller Infektionen auf neutrophile Leukozyten und humorale Entzündungsparameter. Habilitationsschrift der Med. Fakultät der Ludwig-Maximilians-Universität München
22. Siebeck M, Hoffmann H, Jochum M, Welter H, Fritz H (1987) Therapeutische Effekte der Inhibition lysosomaler Proteasen im Schock. Langenbecks Arch [Suppl] Chir Forum '87, pp 325–328

Cytokines and Oxygen Radical Responses

P. A. Ward, J. S. Warren, K. J. Johnson, and J. Varani

Introduction

There is much current interest in the biological role of cytokines and their ability to modify the outcome of biological reactions. Cytokines are soluble peptides/proteins which are released by macrophages or lymphocytes and have effects on similar or different cells. Cytokines may have direct or indirect effects, as will be pointed out below. The two cytokines that are the subject of our studies are interleukin 1 (IL-1) and tumor necrosis factor (TNF), each of which has a multitude of biological activities [1]. There is evidence that these cytokines can function in a synergistic manner and under conditions in which the effect of either cytokine is minimal. For example, IL-1 and TNF in combination can protect rats from death caused by hyperoxia, whereas either cytokine alone has little if any protective effect [2]. In the studies to be presented we will deal only with the effects of individual cytokines, not their combination. The examples given below serve to demonstrate fundamental mechanisms of cytokine action in biological systems.

As shown in Table 1, the effects of the cytokines IL-1 and TNF can be broadly classified into *direct* and *indirect* effects. Examples of direct effects include stimulation of phagocytic cells with resultant enhanced oxygen radical production and enzyme secretion [3–7]. Other direct effects of the cytokines include complex pathophysiological changes such as hypotension, diminished cardiac output and bradycardia [8–11], the result of which can be tissue or organ ischemia. Indirect effects of the cytokines include alterations in effector cells (phagocytes) and changes in target cells. The recognition of these diverse and complex effects may lead to a better understanding of the complex biological effects of cytokines.

Table 1. Biological effects of cytokines

1. Direct effects
   a) Direct stimulation of phagocytic cells
   b) Pathophysiological changes
2. Indirect effects
   a) "Priming" of phagocytic cells for enhanced oxygen radical responses
   b) Alteration of target cells

Immune Consequences of
Trauma, Shock and Sepsis
Eds. Faist/Ninnemann/Green

Direct Effects of Cytokines

TNF and IL-1 appear to have important direct roles in the activation of neutrophils. Purified IL-1 has been shown to be chemotactic for neutrophils in vitro and to activate their respiratory burst, as demonstrated by increased oxygen consumption and enhanced reduction of nitroblue tetrazolium [4, 5]. Similarly, TNF can directly stimulate the neutrophil respiratory burst and bring about degranulation [6, 7]. Both IL-1 and TNF have been shown to induce 1.5–2-fold increases in the expression of the surface glycoprotein CDw18 (which is required for optimal neutrophil adherence) and enhanced expression of the complement (CR3) receptor [12, 13]. The former, which functions as a neutrophil adhesion molecule, is regulated through a mechanism that is quite different from a companion ability of IL-1 or TNF to enhance neutrophil adherence through modification of endothelial cells.

There is considerable evidence that cytokines, notably TNF, trigger many of the fundamental pathophysiological manifestations of the endotoxemic shock syndrome. In 1980, Rouzer and Cerami [14] noted that rabbits infected with *Trypanosoma brucei* became cachectic and markedly lipemic. It was subsequently shown that "cachectin" (later identified as being identical to TNF) is responsible for suppression of lipoprotein lipase activity in endotoxin-sensitive animals [15]. Cachectin (TNF) appears to be the primary mediator of gram-negative (endotoxin induced) shock. Injections of TNF mimic endotoxemic shock and trigger pathophysiologic changes such as neutropenia followed by neutrophilia [9, 10, 16]. Immunization of animals against TNF protects animals from the lethal effects of endotoxin [9, 10].

It has been relatively recently that the identity of IL-1 and endogenous pyrogen has been established [17–19]. IL-1 (and TNF) triggers many of the metabolic changes associated with the acute-phase response [20–22]. Both IL-1 and TNF have been shown to possess a wide variety of biological activities relating to T-cell activation, cytotoxicity for tumor cells, regulation of hematopoiesis and effects on bone and cartilage metabolism [1]. These examples serve to illustrate the pleiotypic nature of these cytokines.

Indirect Effects of Cytokines

Like a variety of other agonists that at very low concentrations can interact with phagocytic cells (e.g., neutrophils and macrophages) causing a "priming" effect on these cells, IL-1 and TNF can modify macrophages for enhanced oxygen radical responses to other agonists. Examples of this phenomenon are shown in Table 2 in which we have employed rat alveolar macrophages and recombinant human IL-1 or TNF, or supernatant fluids from alveolar macrophages that have been incubated with opsonized zymosan particles.

In these experiments rat alveolar macrophages and peritoneal neutrophils were employed as the responder cells and incubated in the presence or absence of IgG immune complexes. In data plotted as percent increase in oxygen radical responses, recombinant human interleukin 1 (hu IL-1r) in a dose-dependent manner caused enhancement of oxygen radical responses in immune complex stimulated alveolar macrophages with a 48% increase in the presence of 0.5 units IL-1. However, in the absence of immune complexes the cytokine did not by itself cause an oxygen radical response (data not shown). In the case of recombinant human TNF (hu TNFr), similar data were obtained, although the magnitude of the enhanced oxygen radical response was less impressive. Finally, supernatant fluids from rat alveolar macrophages that had been activated by contact with opsonized zymosan particles were also able to cause enhanced oxygen radical responses in immune complex stimulated alveolar macrophages.

Interestingly, in none of the conditions described above were we able to demonstrate that the cytokines can affect oxygen radical responses of rat peritoneal neutrophils (Table 2), although, as described above, there is abundant evidence that cytokines can directly stimulate neutrophils. This may represent a species specificity, at least for recombinant cytokines, or the data may imply that macrophages are intrinsically more responsive to influences of cytokines. The data indicate that the cytokines IL-1 and TNF can interact synergistically with macrophages stimulated with agonists such as immune complexes to bring about enhanced oxygen radical responses.

A second example of indirect effects of cytokines occurs when they come into contact with endothelial cells. It has recently been reported that TNF and IL-1

Table 2. Indirect effects of cytokines on phagocytic cells

Cytokine employed	Dose	Immune complex[a]	Percent increase in oxygen-radical generation[b]	
			Alveolar macrophages	Neutrophils
hu ILlr	0.1 unit	+	19	<5
	0.3 unit	+	33	<5
	0.5 unit	+	48	<5
hu TNFr	0.03 n*M*	+	11	<5
	0.3 n*M*	+	16	<5
	3.0 n*M*	+	19	<5
	30 n*M*	+	19	<5
Supernatant fluid from nonactivated alveolar macrophages	100 µl	+	12	<5
Supernatant fluid from from activated alveolar macrophages	100 µl	+	43	<5
	200 µl	+	58	<5
	200 µl	–	–	–

Rat alveolar macrophages (5×10^5) or rat peritoneal neutrophils (2×10^6) were incubated with immune complexes in the presence of increasing doses of recombinant human IL1 (hu Il1r) or TNF, or with supernatant fluids from alveolar macrophages that had been incubated with opsonized zymosan particles. The agonist employed was immune complexes consisting of rabbit polyclonal IgG antibody to bovine serum albumin.

[a] Immune complexes containing 10 µg IgG rabbit antibody to bovine serum albumin.

[b] Percent increases in oxygen radical generation are relative to cells activated with immune complexes alone.

can modify endothelial cells in a manner that increases adherence interactions with neutrophils [12, 13]. This phenomenon is dependent on protein synthesis within endothelial cells, is time dependent (requiring several hours for expression), and is thought to be associated with elaboration on endothelial cells of an adhesive factor(s) interactive with the adhesive-promoting glycoproteins on the surface of the neutrophil (see above).

In order to explore these interactions, we have treated arterial endothelial cells with human recombinant TNF or IL-1 for 18 h, followed by washing, and have found increased adherence interactions with human neutrophils. Adherence increases from 21% to 57% (data not shown). Using a similar protocol, the effects of pretreatment of endothelial cells with TNF and IL-1 under a variety of conditions have been assessed for endothelial cell killing by phorbol myristate acetate (PMA) activated human neutrophils. The data are shown in Fig. 1. In this experiment the amount of specific ^{51}Cr release (with spontaneous release value being subtracted) was 21.4%. Pretreatment of the endothelial cells with 3×10^{-12} *M* TNF for 5 and 18 h resulted in 37.3% and 47.1% cytotoxicity, respectively. If TNF was first heat-inactivated (100 °C, 30 min) or its activity blocked by the addition of antibody, the cytotoxicity value fell to the reference positive control values. When endothelial cells were pretreated with three separate doses (0.5, 1.0, and 2.0 units) of IL-1 for 18 h, then washed, followed by addition of neutrophils and phorbol ester, there was a similar enhancement in neutrophil-mediated cytotoxicity (Fig. 1). Thus, TNF and IL-1 are potent modifiers of endothelial cells, making them more susceptible to killing by activated neutrophils. Whether increased adherence interactions between neutrophils and altered endothelial cells account for this phenomenon or the enhanced susceptibility of endothelial cells

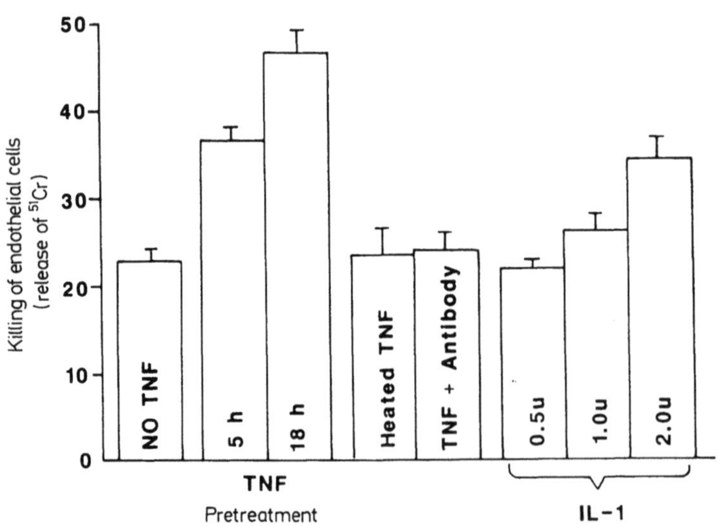

Fig. 1. Enhanced neutrophil killing of endothelial cells by TNF and IL-1. Composite results of preexposure of bovine pulmonary-artery endothelial cells to TNF or IL-1 and subsequent sensitivity to cytotoxic effects (measured by ^{51}Cr release) of phorbol ester activated neutrophils

to neutrophil-mediated killing is ascribable to some other modification of endothelial cells is currently unknown.

These findings have implications for the increasing body of evidence that cytokines may place the microvasculature at risk, as suggested by the evidence that TNF is a principle mediator in the pathogenesis of the shock syndrome triggered by infusion of bacterial endotoxin or gram-negative bacteria into animals [9]. In other studies it has been demonstrated that early microvascular injury which follows the infusion of recombinant human TNF into mice or rats involves the small-intestinal mucosa with resultant sloughing of the villous tips of the small bowel [10]. There is also evidence in these animals of intrapulmonary hemorrhage, indicating that damage of the lung interstitial capillaries has also occurred. Since TNF can also cause activation of neutrophils with resultant oxygen radical production [6, 7], it is likely that TNF can alter both effector cells (neutrophils) and target (endothelial) cells, as documented above. It can be speculated that cytokines alter the microvasculature in vivo such that it is highly susceptible to neutrophil mediated injury.

Cytokines can, therefore, interact with phagocytic cells or with target cells (such as endothelial cells), or in combination, to cause greatly accentuated injury of cells and of organs. An altogether separate consideration is synergy that may occur as the result of the presence of multiple types of cytokines, a situation that would be expected to be present in vivo. An understanding of how the cytokines can enter into pathophysiological pathways to affect the outcome of an inflammatory reaction is central to an understanding of how cytokines can amplify oxygen radical mediated damage of cells, tissues and organs.

References

1. Le J, Vilcek J (1987) Tumor necrosis factor and interleukin 1: cytokines with multiple overlapping biological activities. Lab Invest 56:234–248
2. White CW, Ghezzi P, Dinarella CA, Caldwell SA, McMurtry IF, Repine JE (1987) Recombinant tumor necrosis factor/cachectin and interleukin 1 pretreatment decreases lung oxidized glutathione accumulation, lung injury, and mortality in rats exposed to hyperoxia. J Clin Invest 79:1868–1873
3. Klempner MS, Dinarello CA, Gallin JI (1978) Human leukocytic pyrogen induces release of specific granule contents from human neutrophils. J Clin Invest 61:1330
4. Luger TA, Charon JA, Colot M, Micksche M, Oppenheim JJ (1983) Chemotactic properties of partially purified human epidermal cell-derived thymocyte-activating factor (ETAF) for polymorphonuclear and mononuclear cells. J Immunol 131:816
5. Sauder DN, Mounessa NL, Katz SI, Dinarello CA, Gallin JI (1984) Chemotactic cytokines: the role of leukocytic pyrogen and epidermal cell thymocyte-activating factor in neutrophil chemotaxis. J Immunol 132:828
6. Klebanoff SJ, Vadas MA, Harlan JM, Sparks LH, Gamble JR, Agosti JM, Waltersdorph AM (1986) Stimulation of neutrophils by tumor necrosis factor. J Immunol 136:4220
7. Tsujimoto M, Yokota S, Vilcek J, Weissman G (1986) Tumor necrosis factor provokes superoxide anion generation from neutrophils. Biochem Biophys Res Commun 137:1094
8. Tracey KJ, Lowry SF, Fahey TJ, Albert JD, Fong Y, Hesse D, Beutler B, Manogue KR, Calvano S, Wei H et al. (1987) Cachectin/tumor necrosis factor induces lethal shock and stress hormone responses in the dog. Surg Gynecol Obstet 164:415–422

9. Tracey KJ, Beutler B, Lowry SF, Merryweather J, Wolpe S, Milsark IW, Hariri RJ, Fahey TJ, Zentella A, Albert JD et al. (1986) Shock and tissue injury induced by recombinant human cachectin. Science 234:470–474
10. Remick DG, Kunkel RG, Larrick JW, Kunkel SL (1987) Acute in vivo effects of human recombinant tumor necrosis factor. Lab Invest 56:583–590
11. Bauss F, Droge W, Mannel DN (1987) Tumor necrosis factor mediates endotoxic effects in mice. Infect Immun 55:1622–1625
12. Gamble JR, Harlan JM, Klebanoff SJ, Vadas MA (1985) Stimulation of the adherence of neutrophils to umbilical vein endothelium by human recombinant tumor necrosis factor. Proc Natl Acad Sci USA 82:8667
13. Pohlman TH, Stanness KA, Beatty PG, Ochs HD, Harlan JM (1986) An endothelial cell surface factor(s) induced in vitro by lipopolysaccharide, interleukin 1, and tumor necrosis factor-alpha increases neutrophil adherence by a CDw18-dependent mechanism. J Immunol 136:4548
14. Rouzer CA, Cerami A (1980) Hypertriglyceridemia associated with trypanosoma brucei infection in rabbits: role of defective triglyceride removal. Mol Biochem Parasitol 2:31–38
15. Kawakami M, Cerami A (1981) Studies of endotoxin-induced decrease in lipoprotein lipase activity. J Exp Med 154:631–639
16. Remick DG, Larrick J, Kunkel SL (1986) Tumor necrosis factor-induced alterations in circulating leukocyte populations. Biochem Biophys Res Commun 141:818–824
17. Sztein MB, Vogel SN, Sipe JD, Murphy PA, Mizel SB, Oppenheim JJ, Rosenstreich DL (1981) The role of macrophages in the acute-phase response: SAA inducer is closely related to lymphocyte activating factor and endogenous pyrogen. Cell Immunol 63:164
18. Kampschmidt RF, Upchurch HF, Worthington ML (1983) Further comparisons of endogenous pyrogens and leukocytic endogenous mediators. Infect Immun 41:6
19. Dinarello CA (1984) Interleukin-1. Rev Infect Dis 6:51
20. Darlington GJ, Wilson DR, Lachman LB (1986) Monocyte-conditioned medium, interleukin-1, and tumor necrosis factor stimulate the acute phase response in human hepatoma cells in vitro. J Cell Biol 103:787–793
21. Evans E, Courtois GM, Kilian PL, Fuller GM, Crabtree GR (1987) Induction of fibrinogen and a subset of acute phase response genes involves a novel monokine which is mimicked by phorbol esters. J Biol Chem 262:10850–10854
22. Koj A, Kurdowska A, Magielska-Zero D, Rokita H, Sipe JD, Dayer JM, Demczuk S, Gauldie J (1987) Limited effects of recombinant human and murine interleukin 1 and tumor necrosis factor on production of acute phase proteins by cultured rat hepatocytes. Biochem Int 14:553–560
23. Beutler B, Cerami A (1986) Cachectin/tumor necrosis factor: an endogenous mediator of shock and inflammation. Immunol Res 5:281–293

Structure and Properties of a Novel Neutrophil-Activating Factor (NAF) Produced by Human Monocytes

A. Walz, P. Peveri, H. Aschauer, B. Dewald, and M. Baggiolini

Neutrophils are the main cellular elements of antimicrobial defense and acute inflammation. Their activity depends largely on the release of cytotoxic, tissue-damaging, and cell-activating products. A variety of stimulatory molecules of different origin are known to condition neutrophil activity in inflamed tissues. Among the best-characterized ones are *N*-formyl-methionyl peptides (e.g., fMLP) related to bacterial products (Showell et al. 1976), C5a formed upon complement activation (Fernandez et al. 1978), and two lipids, platelet-activating factor (PAF) and leukotriene B_4 (LTB_4) (Dewald and Baggiolini 1986), which are released by stimulated phagocytes (Baggiolini et al. 1988). At sites of chronic inflammation, neutrophils are exposed to the products of activated mononuclear phagocytes which are prominent in such lesions. We have studied the production of neutrophil-activating factors by human monocytes stimulated in different ways, and describe here one of these factors, termed NAF, which binds to human neutrophils via a selective surface receptor and acts like the chemotactic agonists C5a and fMLP.

Neutrophil-activating factor production by blood mononuclear cells was dependent on stimulation by LPS, ConA, or phytohemagglutinin (PHA). Figure 1 shows the time course of NAF release into the culture medium and its dependence on the concentration of LPS. Experiments with mononuclear phagocytes purified by adherence or elutriation indicated that NAF is produced by the monocytes and that lymphocytes have little influence on this process. NAF production was sensitive to cycloheximide, suggesting that de novo protein synthesis is required. The peptide does not appear to be stored since virtually no cell-associated activity could be found.

Amino acid sequencing of a pure preparation indicated that NAF is a novel peptide (Walz et al. 1987). Edman degradation analysis showed that the first 32 amino-terminal residues of NAF correspond to those of a peptide, termed MDNCF for monocyte-derived neutrophil chemotactic factor, described by Yoshimura et al. (1987), and to part of a cDNA-deduced sequence (starting with Ser 28) recently reported by Schmid and Weissmann (1987). On SDS-PAGE electrophoresis, pure NAF showed an apparent MW of 6000. We recently found, however, that the peptide extends to amino acid 99 of the above cDNA, its MW being 8386.

The activity of NAF on human neutrophils was studied in comparison to that of fMLP, C5a, PAF, and LTB_4 (Peveri et al. 1988). NAF was found to induce a rapid and transient increase in cytosolic-free calcium as revealed by intracellular indicators like quin-2 or fura-2. The time course of calcium-associated fluorescence changes was virtually identical to that of the known receptor agonists, and

Immune Consequences of
Trauma, Shock and Sepsis
Eds. Faist/Ninnemann/Green

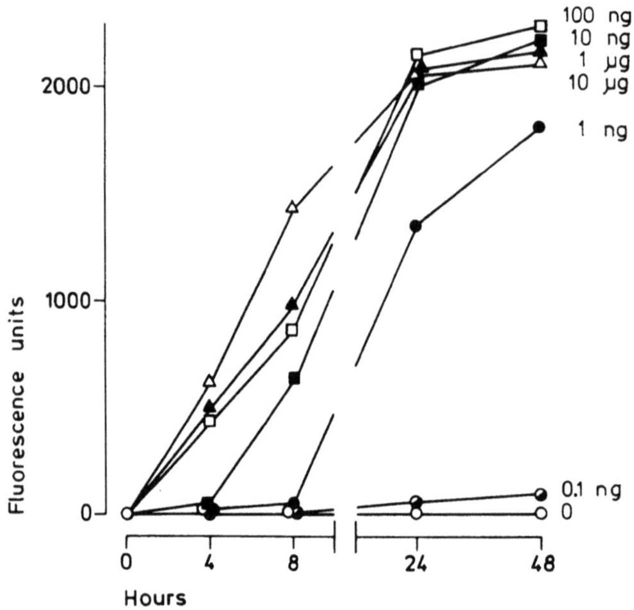

Fig. 1. Stimulus-dependent NAF production. Mononuclear cells were seeded in 24-well culture plates (5×10^6 cells in 1 ml) and were stimulated with LPS (0.1 ng to 10 µg/ml as indicated). At given times, the media were collected, cleared by centrifugation, and NAF activity was determined (see Peveri et al. 1988 for details)

showed the characteristic concentration-dependent initial lag described by von Tscharner et al. (1986). The effects of NAF on the two main release functions of neutrophils, exocytosis of granule contents and formation of superoxide, were also examined. NAF induced exocytosis of specific granules only (release of vitamin B_{12}-binding protein), unless the neutrophils were pretreated with cytochalasin B, in which case release from the azurophil granules (β-glucuronidase or elastase) was observed as well. In terms of potency, NAF compared well with the peptide agonists. On a molecular basis, it was somewhat less potent than C5a and more potent than fMLP as shown in Fig. 2.

A detailed analysis of the mechanism of neutrophil activation by NAF was done on the basis of the respiratory burst response, which can be monitored more accurately than exocytosis. NAF induced a progressive, concentration-dependent increase in the rate of superoxide generation up to a maximum, which corresponded closely to that obtained with optimum concentrations of other peptide agonists. Recordings of the time-dependent changes of the rate of H_2O_2 formation as measured by chemiluminescence (Fig. 3) showed that the respiratory burst induced by NAF, C5a, or fMLP is similar in time course, extent, and duration. In particular, the onset time of the responses was identical, i.e., approximately 2 s, a value previously observed upon stimulation of human neutrophils with fMLP, C5a, PAF, or LTB_4 (Wymann et al. 1987). The remarkable similarity of the respiratory burst responses described suggested that NAF, like the chemotactic pep-

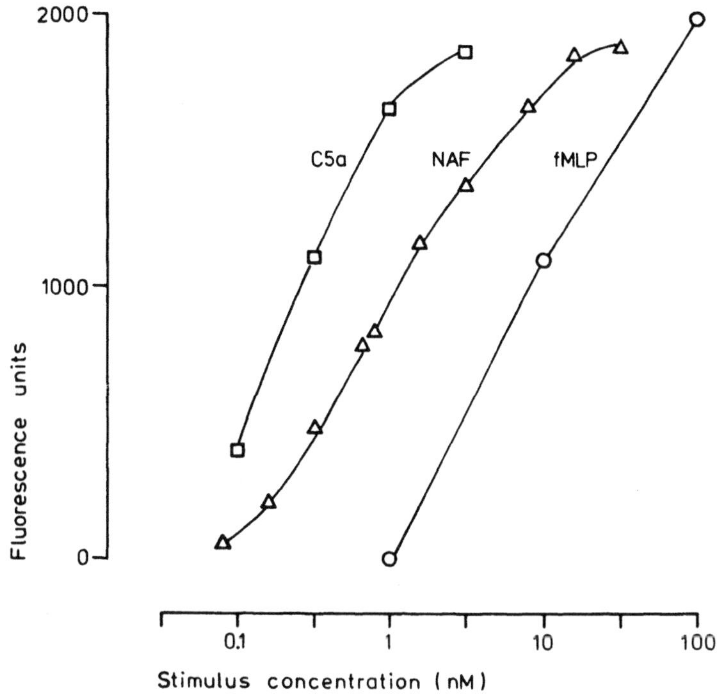

Fig. 2. Exocytosis of elastase induced by NAF, C5a, and fMLP in cytochalasin B-treated human neutrophils

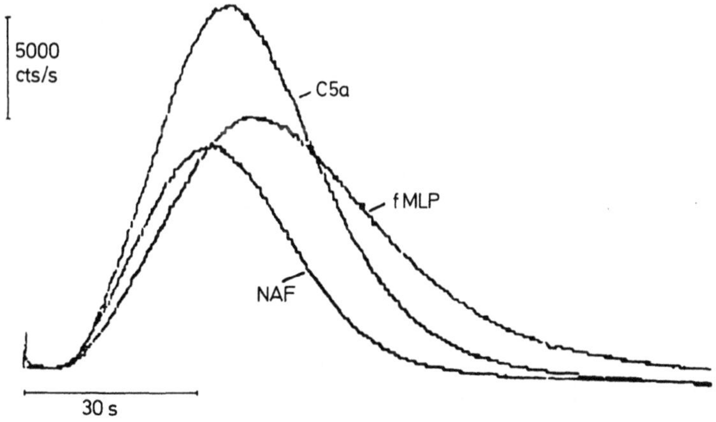

Fig. 3. Respiratory burst. H_2O_2-dependent chemiluminescence by human neutrophils stimulated with NAF and approximately equally active concentrations of C5a or fMLP

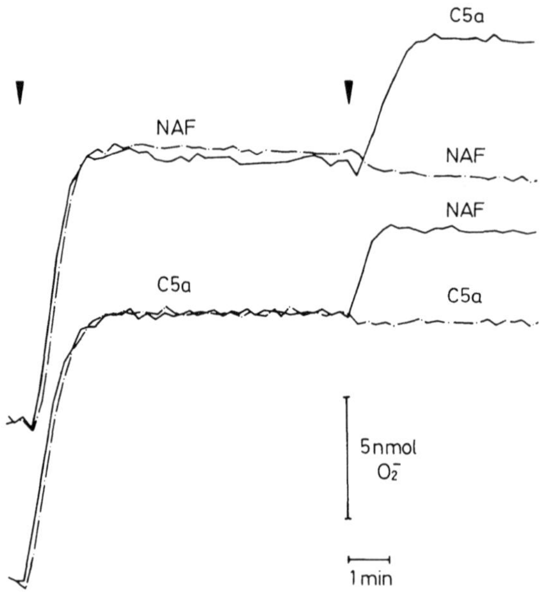

Fig. 4. Superoxide production by human neutrophils stimulated with NAF and C5a. The cells were first stimulated with NAF or C5a and then either with the same or the alternate stimulus as indicated. Recordings of cytochrome *c* reduction are shown

tides, acts through a surface receptor. Since neutrophils show marked desensitization upon repeated agonist challenge, the characteristics of the NAF receptor were studied with different agonist combinations. A typical experiment is shown in Fig. 4. When the cells were first stimulated with NAF and then with C5a or vice versa, two independent respiratory burst responses were obtained. However, when the same stimulus was applied a second time, the cells failed to respond again. This experiment showed complete desensitization to either NAF and C5a, but no cross-desensitization. Similarly, no cross-desensitization was observed between NAF and fMLP, PAF, or LTB_4 (data not shown). These results support the notion that NAF acts via a receptor and indicate that the NAF receptor is unrelated to those of known agonists.

NAF-like factors were reported some years ago as products of alveolar macrophages (Kazmierowski et al. 1977; Merrill et al. 1980; Hunninghake et al. 1980; Pennington et al. 1983). They were shown to exert chemotactic activity and to enhance bacterial killing by neutrophils (Pennington et al. 1985), Granulocyte-activating mediators (GRAM) produced by LPS-stimulated human monocytes were described more recently (Kapp et al. 1986), and a mononuclear cell-derived chemotaxin (MOC) was reported by Kownatzki et al. (1986). Most recently, Schroeder et al. (1987) described a monocyte-derived, weight similar to NAF. Due to the lack of structural information, it is impossible to compare the various NAF-like factors. It is conceivable, however, that several of them may turn out to be identical.

In functional terms, NAF may be regarded as homologous to fMLP and C5a. NAF differs, however, in some important aspects from either chemotactic peptide. It is of host origin, like C5a, but is generated by inflammatory cells (the mononuclear phagocytes) rather than by the activation of a humoral cascade.

Most importantly, unlike C5a, NAF is not inactivated by peptidases in plasma or exudate and could therefore accumulate in inflamed tissues. While C5a and *N*-formyl-methionyl peptides are early mediators of neutrophil activation upon infection, NAF is likely to act as a second-wave mediator, generated at later stages, when a lesion is postulated by mononuclear phagocytes.

References

Baggiolini M, Dewald B, Thelen M (1988) Effects of PAF on neutrophils and mononuclear phagocytes. Prog Biochem Pharmacol 22:90

Dewald B, Baggiolini M (1986) Platelet-activating factor as a stimulus of exocytosis in human neutrophils. Biochim Biophys Acta 888:42

Fernandez HN, Henson PM, Otani A, Hugli TE (1978) Chemotactic response to human C3a and C5a anaphylatoxins. J Immunol 120:109

Hunninghake GW, Gadek JE, Fale HM, Crystal RG (1980) Human alveolar macrophage-derived chemotactic factor for neutrophils. J Clin Invest 66:473

Kapp A, Luger TA, Maly FA, Schoepf F (1986) Granulocyte-activating mediators (GRAM): I. Generation by lipopolysaccharide-stimulated mononuclear cells. J Invest Dermatol 86:523

Kazmierowski JA, Gallin JI, Reynolds HY (1977) Mechanism for the inflammatory response in primate lungs. J Clin Invest 59:273

Kownatzki E, Kapp A, Uhrich S (1986) Novel neutrophil chemotactic factor derived from human peripheral blood mononuclear leukocytes. Clin Exp Immunol 64:214

Merrill WW, Naegel GP, Matthay RA, Reynolds HY (1980) Alveolar macrophage-derived chemotactic factor. J Clin Invest 65:268

Pennington JE, Rossing TH, Boerth LW (1983) The effect of human alveolar macrophages on the bactericidal capacity of neutrophils. J Infect Dis 148:101

Pennington JE, Rossing TH, Boerth LW, Lee TH (1985) Isolation and partial characterization of a human alveolar macrophage-derived neutrophil-activating factor. J Clin Invest 75:1230

Peveri P, Walz A, Dewald B, Baggiolini M (1988) A novel neutrophil-activating factor produced by human mononuclear phagocytes. J Exp Med 167:1547

Schmid J, Weissmann C (1987) Induction of mRNA for a serine protease and a beta-thromboglobulin-like protein in mitogen-stimulated human leukocytes. J Immunol 139:250

Schroeder JM, Mrowietz U, Morita E, Christophers E (1987) Purification and partial biochemical characterization of a human monocyte-derived, neutrophil-activating peptide that lacks interleukin 1 activity. J Immunol 139:3474

Showell HJ, Freer RJ, Zigmond SH, Schiffmann E, Aswanikumar S, Corcoran B, Becker EL (1976) The structure-activity relations of synthetic peptides as chemotactic factors and inducers of lysosomal enzyme secretion for neutrophils. J Exp Med 143:1154

von Tscharner V, Prod'hom B, Baggiolini M, Reuter H (1986) Ion channels in human neutrophils activated by a rise in free cytosolic calcium concentration. Nature 324:369

Walz A, Peveri P, Aschauer H, Baggiolini M (1987) Purification and amino acid sequencing of NAF, a novel neutrophil-activating factor produced by monocytes. Biochem Biophys Res Commun 149:755

Wymann MP, von Tscharner V, Deranleau DA, Baggiolini M (1987) The onset of the respiratory burst in human neutrophils. J Biol Chem 262:12048

Yoshimura T, Matsushima K, Tanaka S, Robinson EA, Appella E, Oppenheim JJ, Leonard EJ (1987) Purification of a human monocyte-derived chemotactic factor that shares sequence homology with other host defense cytokines. Proc Natl Acad Sci USA 84:9233

The Effect of Injury on Murine Neutrophil Oxidative Metabolism

M. A. Gadd and J. F. Hansbrough

Introduction

The ability of the inflammatory or nonspecific immune system to respond to antigenic stimuli is extremely important. Neutrophils (PMNs) are the leukocytes most responsive and capable, in the normal host, of controlling bacterial invasion. However, neutrophil dysfunction occurs after injury, including defects in chemotaxis [1], phagocytosis, and microbial killing [2]. In addition, depressed serum opsonic capacity and the presence of inhibitory substances further compromise neutrophil function in the burn victim [3].

The microbicidal and cytotoxic activity of neutrophils begins with reduction of NADPH to superoxide, which rapidly converts to H_2O_2. The peroxidase enzyme system then acts on H_2O_2 to produce hydroxyl radicals. Hydroxyl radicals and H_2O_2 have been implicated as primary mediators of bacterial killing, and are toxic toward normal tissues [4, 5].

Assays commonly used to measure neutrophil oxidative metabolism include chemiluminescence, which is the production of chemical light during the excitation of the cell, and redox reactions using tetrazolium dye [6]. These assays provide an overall measure of the ability of cell populations to respond to stimuli. The precise defect in oxidative metabolism must be identified with a more specific test.

In the present study we used dichlorodihydrofluoroscein diacetate (DCFH-DA) and flow cytometry in an assay described previously by Keston and Brandt [7] to measure the ability of neutrophils from thermally injured mice to produce H_2O_2 after stimulation with phorbol 12-myristate 13-acetate (PMA). DCFH-DA, a stable nonfluorescent compound, diffuses through the cell membrane and is hydrolyzed to DCFH. In the presence of H_2O_2, DCFH is oxidized to fluorescent DCF. To determine whether there was a serum inhibitory component of neutrophil H_2O_2 production after burn injury, the assay was performed in the presence of control or postburn serum on days 1, 5, and 10 following injury.

Methods

Thermal Injury

Female mice were anesthetized with brief exposure (3–5 min) to methoxyfluorane vapor (Penthrane, Abbott Laboratories, North Chicago, IL). A demarcated area

Immune Consequences of
Trauma, Shock and Sepsis
Eds. Faist/Ninnemann/Green

of the shaved dorsal skin was burned by a 6 s exposure to steam, similar to previously described methods [8]. This produced a full-thickness burn of 25% total body surface area (TBSA). Animals received fluid resuscitation with 3.0 ml 0.9% NaCl injected intraperitoneally (i.p.) and one i.p. injection of morphine (15 ml/kg) for analgesia. Control animals received similar anesthesia, morphine, and i.p. saline, and were evaluated on each test day. Peritoneal cells and serum were obtained from individual groups of mice on days 1, 5, and 10 postinjury.

Measurement of H_2O_2 Production

Control or burn PMNs, 10^6/ml, were preincubated in Dulbecco's phosphate-buffered saline with 5 mM glucose and 0.1% gelatin (PBSg) and with 10% control or burn serum for 15 min at 37 °C. The cells were washed once then 20 μM DCFH-DA in PBSg was added to the PMN suspension and incubated for 15 min at 37 °C with shaking (150 rev/min). Fluorescence of the cells was measured following the second incubation by flow cytometry (FACStar, Becton Dickinson),

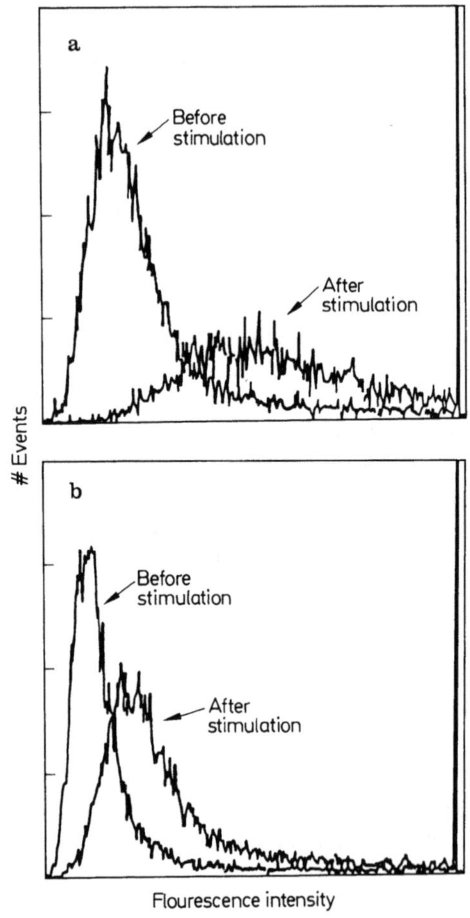

Fig. 1 a, b. Fluorescence distribution of neutrophils obtained from control **a** or burn **b** mice in the presence of control serum at *To* and 15 min after stimulation 5 days postburn. The left most peak represents fluorescence at *To*. A graded response is apparent after 15 min, with the fluorescence histogram shifted further to the right (i.e., toward higher intensity) in the control group compared with the burn group and designated as zero time, *To*. The suspension was then stimulated with 100 ng/ml PMA for 15 min at 37 °C, shaking, and reanalyzed by the cytometer to detect the percentage change in fluorescence at 15 and 60 min (Fig. 1).

Results

The ability of burn neutrophils to produce H_2O_2 on day 1 postinjury was equal to control (Fig. 2). Burn neutrophils demonstrated a significant defect in their ability to produce H_2O_2 compared with control neutrophils on postburn day 5 (Fig. 2). Similarly, the addition of postburn day 5 serum to control neutrophils significantly reduced control neutrophils' production of H_2O_2. Burn serum in the presence of burn neutrophils did not appear to have an additional inhibitory effect on burn neutrophil H_2O_2 production. On postburn day 10, burn neutrophil H_2O_2 production remained significantly depressed compared with controls (Fig. 2). The presence of burn serum in the assays with control or burn neutrophils slightly enhanced H_2O_2 production compared with the same assay in control serum. A relatively high fluorescent intensity region lies between channels 180 and 250 on the FACstar linear fluorescence scale. The percentage of positive fluorescence at time zero and 15 and 60 min in the high-intensity region was calculated for each experimental group. Control PMNs with control serum exhibited significantly higher fluorescence intensities at 15 and 60 min compared with groups with burn PMNs or burn serum (Fig. 3).

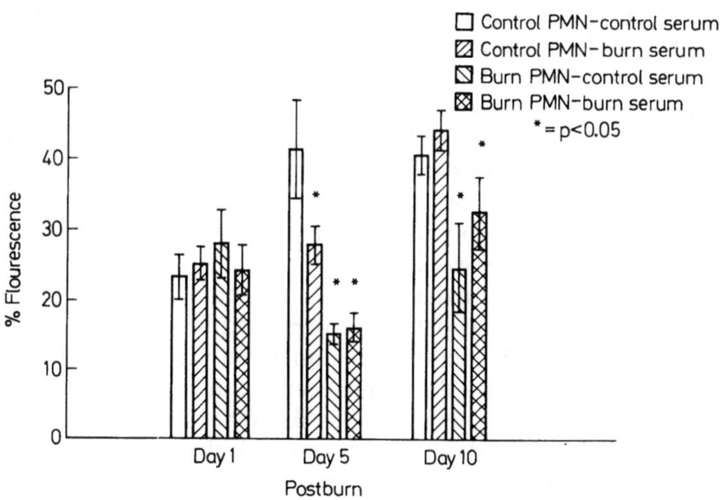

Fig. 2. The change in percentage fluorescence between *To* and 15 min after stimulation as a reflection of H_2O_2 production by murine neutrophils (*$P<0.05$ compared with control). On days 5 and 10 postburn, the burn neutrophils' response was depressed. On day 5, the addition of burn serum to control neutrophils depressed H_2O_2 production

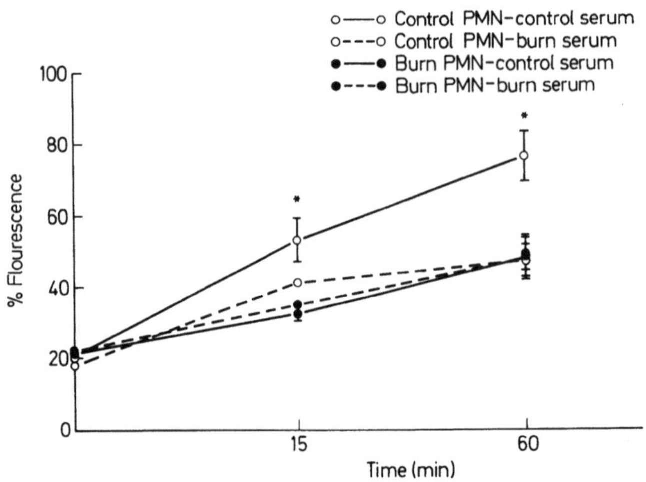

Fig. 3. Percentage of positive fluorescence at time 0, 15, and 60 min in the high-intensity channels on postburn day 5. Control PMNs with control serum exhibit significantly higher fluorescence intensities than the other three groups at 15 and 60 min following stimulation

Discussion

These experiments clearly identify a defect in neutrophil oxidative metabolism on days 5 and 10 after uncomplicated thermal injury in the mouse. The significance of this finding relates to its temporal association with the increasing frequency of clinical infections at 1–2 weeks after injury in burned humans and the concurrent appearance of a number of additional immune defects. Studies have shown that between days 5 and 10 suppressor lymphocytes appear [3, 9]; conversely helper and Ia-positive lymphocytes are depressed [10], IgG levels are depressed [11] a serum immunosuppressive factor is present [3], and neutrophils exhibit impaired bactericidal activity against particular organisms [2]. Previous studies from this laboratory have shown that the burned mouse is increasingly susceptible to infectious challenge after the first postburn week [12].

In addition to a neutrophil defect on days 5 and 10 postburn, a serum inhibitory effect was noted on day 5. Similar data were presented by Duque et al. in rats after a 20% TBSA burn [13]. The fact that a serum defect was no longer seen by day 10 and that there was actually a slight enhancement in H_2O_2 production in the presence of burn serum is interesting. It is possible that there is a factor in the serum which is relatively dilute by day 10 and therefore lacks inhibitory properties at the concentrations used in the assay. A second explanation is that the subset of originally responsive neutrophils were depleted or inactivated and unable to react to the inhibitor. A heterogeneous population of neutrophils is likely to exist especially in an injury model [14, 15].

The role of H_2O_2 in microbial killing, local tissue destruction, and the development of adult respiratory disease in being actively investigated. It is clear that there is probably a defect in production, metabolism, and clearance of hydrogen compounds in particular instances after injury. Further studies will help better to define neutrophil activity after severe burns and possibly prevent the occurrence of these defects.

References

1. Van Dijk WC, Verbrugh HA, Van Rijswijk REN, Vos A, Verhoe J (1982) Neutrophil function, serum opsonic activity, and delayed hypersensitivity in surgical patients. Surgery 92:21–29
2. Bjornson AB, Bjornson HS, Altemeier WA (1981) Serum-mediated inhibition of polymorphonuclear leukocyte function following burn injury. Ann Surg 94:568–575
3. Wolfe JHN, Saporoschetz I, Young AE, O'Connor NE, Mannick JA (1981) Suppressive serum, suppressor lymphocytes, and death from burns. Ann Surg 193:513–520
4. Babior BM (1983) The respiratory burst of phagocytes. J Clin Invest 73:599–601
5. Klebanoff SJ (1980) Oxygen metabolism and the toxic properties of phagocytes. Ann Intern Med 93:480–489
6. Van Dyke K (1987) Helpful hints for chemiluminescence assay. In: Van Dyke K, Castranova V (eds) Cellular chemiluminescence. CRC Press, Florida, pp 39–45
7. Keston AS, Brandt R (1965) The fluorometric analysis of ultramicro-quantities of H_2O_2. Anal Biochem 11:1–5
8. Zapata-Sirvent RL, Hansbrough JF (1985) Postburn immunosuppression in an animal model: III. Maintenance of normal helper and suppressor lymphocyte subpopulations by immunomodulating drugs. Surgery 97:721–727
9. Kupper TS, Baker CC, Ferguson TA, Green DR (1985) A burn induced Ly-2 suppressor T cell lowers resistance to bacterial infection. J Surg Res 38:606–612
10. Hansbrough JF, Soderberg C, Gadd MA Temporal analysis of murine lymphocyte subpopulations by monoclonal antibodies and dual-color flow cytometry following injury. J Surg Res (in press)
11. Munster AM, Hoagland HC, Pruitt BA (1970) The effect of thermal injury on serum immunoglobulins. Ann Surg 172:965–969
12. Zapata-Sirvent RL, Hansbrough JF, Bender EM, Bartle EJ, Mansour MA (1986) Postburn immunosuppression in an animal model. IV. Improved resistance to septic challenge with immunomodulating drugs. Surg 99:53–58
13. Duque RE, Phan SH, Hudson JL, Till GO, Ward PA (1985) Functional defects in phagocytic cells following thermal injury. Am J Pathol 118:116–127
14. Bass DA, Obrantz P, Szejda P, Seeds MC, McCall CE (1986) Subpopulations of neutrophils with increased oxidative product formation in blood of patients with infection. J Immunol 136:860–866
15. Klempner MS, Gallin JI (1978) Separation and functional characterization of human neutrophil subpopulations. Blood 51:659–669

Opsonophagocytosis in Patients Undergoing Abdominal Surgery

C. G. Gemmell, J. Gardner, Y. Wilson, and H. G. Burns

Introduction

It has been estimated that 7.5% of all surgical wounds become infected (Altemeir et al. 1971) and such infections, as well as those occurring within the respiratory and urinary tracts, can result in disability, delayed healing morbidity and even mortality. Anaesthesia, trauma and cardiopulmonary bypass affect many components of the immune system such as neutrophil chemotaxis and bacterial opsonophagocytosis (Mayer et al. 1976; Van Velzen-Blad et al. 1985). In other studies (Alexander et al. 1979) abnormal neutrophil function was associated with an increased incidence of bacteraemia. Bactericidal activity towards *Staphylococcus aureus* was impaired but that towards *Escherichia coli* was not altered. However, changes in phagocytic ingestion rates of potential bacterial pathogens have not been measured hitherto in relation to the incidence of postoperative infection.

In this study an assessment has been made of preoperative phagocytic efficiency as an index of high or low risk of subsequent infection. Similar measurements were made for up to 7 days postoperatively.

Patients and Methods

Blood samples were taken from each of the patients 24 h before and 24 h and 7 days after the operation. In each case a modification of the method of Boyum (1968) was used to separate polymorphonuclear leucocytes (PMNs) by dextran sedimentation and centrifugation (1200 g/30 min) on lymphocyte separation medium. The purified PMNs were standardised to a concentration of 2×10^6/ml.

Suspensions of *Staphylococcus aureus* and *Proteus mirabilis* (1×10^7/ml) were opsonised with either pooled normal human serum (heterologous) or patient's own serum (homologous). For bacterial opsonisation the serum was used at 10% (v/v). Thereafter the bacteria were centrifuged (3000 g/15 min) and resuspended to 1×10^7/ml in gel-Hank's solution. Phagocytic ingestion of either opsonised bacterium was followed by measuring the uptake of the radiolabelled cells over a 15-min incubation period (method of Peterson et al. 1977) and results for each organism and serum were expressed as percentages of the bacteria added to the PMNs actually ingested by the PMNs.

Immune Consequences of
Trauma, Shock and Sepsis
Eds. Faist/Ninnemann/Green

Results

Twenty-eight patients undergoing several forms of abdominal surgery (see Table 1) have been included in this study. Details of patient age, sex, weight, clinical diagnosis, and operation were taken in each case. Serum albumin levels were taken before and after the operation. Subsequently the incidence or otherwise of postoperative infection was noted.

Hitherto nutritional status has been used to determine those patients at risk of postoperational infection and in such patients albumin levels have been followed. In the present study only two patients had levels of albumin of 28 mg/litre and in neither was there any postoperative infection. However, in four other patients some sign of infection was detected (Table 2). The infections involved the upper respiratory tract (2), the urinary tract (1) and bacteraemia (1).

Measurement of PMN phagocytic efficiency amongst the patients included in this study showed considerable variation both *inter allos* and in different blood donations from the same patient. The overall pattern was similar whether or not the bacteria were opsonised in homologous or heterologous serum. Lowered levels of phagocytic ingestion were apparent when *Proteus mirabilis* was used as target compared with *Staphylococcus aureus*. However, the majority of preparations of PMNs displayed some depression of phagocytic efficiency compared with the normal range for PMNs from control subjects (age-matched) not undergoing any surgical procedure. These results are illustrated in Figs. 1 and 2.

Table 1. Patients in the study

Patient groups	No. with carcinoma	Mean age (range)	Sex ratio (M:F)
Upper GI tract surgery (4)	2	52 (38–71)	2:2
Laparotomy (4)	4	58 (31–77)	3:1
Cholecystectomy (8)	0	56 (40–68)	3:5
Colorectal surgery (11)	11	65 (51–75)	4:7

Table 2. Albumin levels pre- and postoperatively in patients undergoing abdominal surgery

Patient group	Low albumun levels pre-operarively	(28 mg/litre) post-operatively	Incidence of postoperative infection
Upper GI tract surgery (4)	0/4	0/4	0/4
Laparotomy (4)	0/4	0/4	2/4
Cholecystectomy (8)	0/8	0/8	0/8
Colorectal surgery (11)	2/11	2/11	2/11 [a]

[a] Neither patient had low albumin levels.

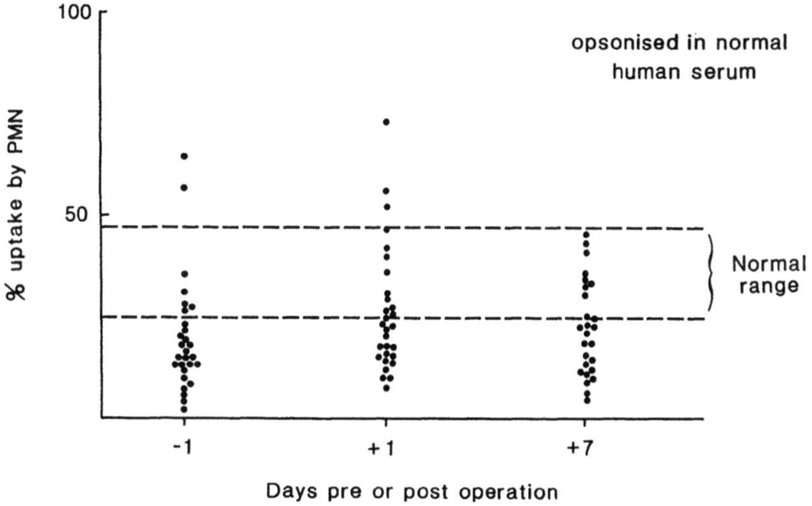

Fig. 1. Opsonophagocytosis of *Proteus mirabilis* by PMNs from patients undergoing abdominal surgery

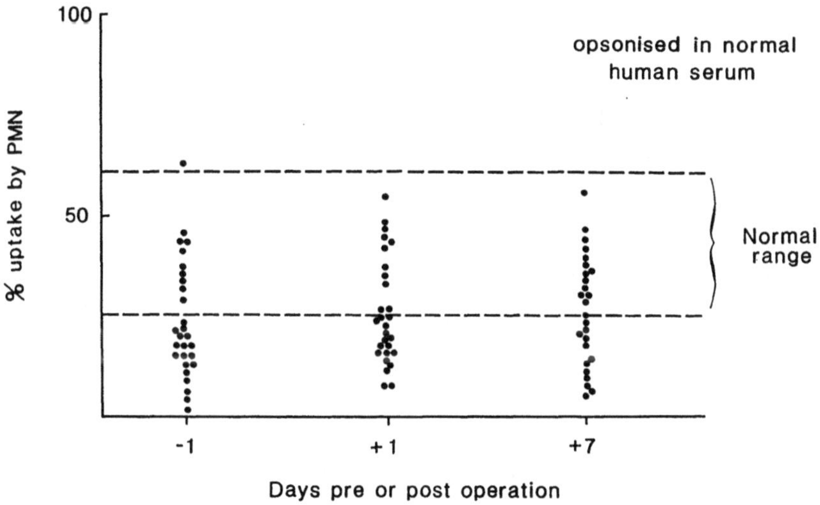

Fig. 2. Opsonophagocytosis of *Staphylococcus aureus* by PMNs from patients undergoing abdominal surgery

Discussion

Of the four patients with a history of postoperative infection sequential measurement of phagocytic cell function showed that there was a low preoperative level of phagocytosis in three out of four which did not improve postoperatively (Table 3). Throughout, levels of phagocytic function in these patients remained below normal.

Table 3. Sequential measurement of phagocytic cell function

Patient	% phagocytosis of target bacterium after			
	Staphylococcus aureus		*Proteus mirabilis*	
	−1 day	+7 days	−1 day	+7 days
B. S.	39.5	32.4	22.5	25.1
A. M.	12.6	19.3	8.5	16.2
H. B.	5.4	4.4	4.1	5.7
H. C.	11.5	22.6	16.7	25.1

Our results have shown that individual patients undergoing abdominal surgery display unique phagocytic ingestion efficiencies. In some there was marked postoperative depression of ingestion probably due to anaesthesia which did or did not recover over the next 6 days. However, in the four patients with evidence of postoperative infection three showed poor phagocytic activity. Albumin levels as a measure of nutritional status did not correlate with phagocytic function or susceptibility to infection in this study.

References

Alexander JW, Stinnett JD, Ogle CK, Ogle JD, Morris MJ (1979) A comparison of immunologic profiles and their influence on bacteraemia in surgical patients with a high risk of infection. Surgery 86:94–103

Altemeir WA, Culbertson WR, Fullen WD (1971) Sepsis and gastrointestinal bleeding. Ann Surg 175:759–770

Boyum A (1968) Isolation of mononuclear cells and granulocytes from human blood. Isolation of mononuclear cells by one centrifugation, and of granulocytes by combining centrifugation and sedimentation at 1 g. Scand J Clin Lab Invest 21 [Suppl 97]:77–89

Mayer JE, McCullough J, Wieblen BJ, Kaplan EL, Lindsay WG, Nicoloff DM (1976) Effects of cardiopulmonary bypass on neutrophil chemotaxis. Surg Forum 27:285–287

Peterson PK, Verhoef J, Schmeling D, Quie PG (1977) Kinetics of phagocytosis and bacterial killing by human polymorphonuclear leukocytes and monocytes. J Infect Dis 136:502–509

Van Velzen-Blad H, Dijkstra YJ, Schurink GA, Verbrugh HA, Verhoef J, Zegers BJM et al. (1985) Cardiopulmonary bypass and host defense functions in human beings: I serum levels and role of immunoglobulins and complement in phagocytosis. Ann Thorac Surg 39:207–211

Effects of Pyocyanine, Liberated by *Pseudomonas aeruginosa*, on the Oxidative Burst of Phagocytes

P. K. Müller and P. F. Mühlradt

Pseudomonas aeruginosa is known sometimes to cause severe and persistent infections, particularly in immunocompromised patients or those suffering from burns. *P. aeruginosa* infections are difficult to control as these bacteria carry antibiotic resistance genes. They may also produce a number of exoenzymes such as elastase, collagenase, and phospholipase C, and an exotoxin A. In addition, 95% of clinical isolates of these bacteria produce a blue phenazine dye, pyocyanine (Pyo), a compound to which no major role for the infection process has yet been ascribed. In vitro measurements of T-lymphocyte response in the presence of Pyo had shown Pyo to be inhibitory (Sorensen et al. 1983), and detailed analysis with mouse T cells revealed that it acts by preventing the expression of the interleukin 2 receptor while not inhibiting interleukin 2 release (Mühlradt et al. 1986). Data obtained with human lymphocytes differed somewhat in that interleukin 2 formation was also inhibited (Nutman et al. 1987).

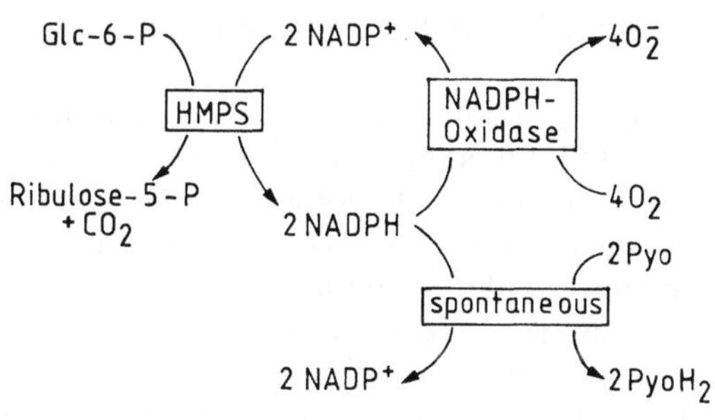

Since phagocytes may play a decisive primary role in the defense against *Ps. aeruginosa,* we now studied the possible influence of Pyo on polymorphonuclear cell (PMN) functions such as phagocytosis, and bacterial killing dependent on the oxidative burst. This biochemical event generates superoxide anions which then give rise to bacteriocidal products such as hydroxyl radical and hypochlorite anion (reviewed by Babior 1984). Molecular oxygen is reduced by NADPH oxidase at the cost of NADPH. Pyo was shown spontaneously to react with reduced pyridine nucleotides (Hassan and Fridovich 1980) and could thus interfere with O_2-production as shown above. Our experiments presented here were aimed at determining the extent to which this might occur and the possible consequences for the capacity of PMN to kill bacteria.

Immune Consequences of
Trauma, Shock and Sepsis
Eds. Faist/Ninnemann/Green

Results and Discussion

Superoxide anion is usually determined by the ferricytochrome c or nitroblue tetrazolium reduction test. In the presence of Pyo these assays are problematic, however, since, contrary to a recent report (Miller et al. 1987), Pyo interferes with both tests. Pyo is reduced by living cells to the colorless leukopyocyanine ($PyoH_2$) (our unpublished data) which can only be observed under anaerobic conditions, because it is spontaneously reoxidized by molecular oxygen. In the presence of cyt. c_{red}, however, $PyoH_2$ reacts faster with this substrate than with O_2, giving false-positive values for superoxide. This is shown in Fig. 1 for unstimulated PMN, along with data from 12-$^{\theta}$-tetradecanoyl-phorbol-13-acetate (TPA)-stimulated PMN. Only in the latter case was cytochrome c reduction inhibitable by superoxide dismutase (SOD), proving that O_2- had indeed been produced by the stimulated cells, but not by the Pyo-treated ones. Addition of Pyo to TPA-stimulated cells led to a considerable SOD noninhibitable fraction of cyt. c_{red}, indicating inhibition of O_2-production (Fig. 1).

When O_2-production was calculated from the SOD-inhibitable fraction of cyt. c_{red}, it became evident that superoxide production was to some extent suppressed by Pyo. Percentagewise this effect was more pronounced in PMN stimulated with zymosan, a less unphysiologic stimulant than TPA (Fig. 2). Phagocytes, newly arriving at the site of a *Pseudomonas* infection, are likely to be exposed to Pyo some time before the oxidative burst is triggered by contact with the bacteria. We tested, therefore, whether the inhibitory action of Pyo would be more pronounced after a preincubation of up to 2 h. This was not the case (data not shown).

The oxidative burst is accompanied by a stimulation of the hexose monophosphate shunt (HMPS) replenishing NADPH used up by the NADPH oxidase (see review by Babior 1984). If Pyo, as delineated in our hypothesis above, acts by oxidizing NADPH, thus depleting the substrate for the O_2-generating enzyme system, one would expect a Pyo-dependent stimulation of the HMPS through the appearance of $NADP^+$ in otherwise unstimulated cells. The HMPS was monitored by determination of $^{14}CO_2$ liberated from (1-^{14}C)-labeled glucose. The data shown in Fig. 3 indicate a moderate stimulation of the HMPS by Pyo alone, which is considerably increased in zymosan-stimulated cells. The partial inhibition of zymosan-stimulated O_2-release may thus be due to partial oxidation of NADPH by Pyo.

We next tested killing of opsonized *Staphylococcus aureus* by PMN in the presence of 50 μM Pyo. When assayed with fluorescent yeast particles (data not shown) Pyo did not inhibit phagocytosis at even tenfold higher concentration. As shown in Fig. 4, Pyo had no influence on bacterial killing in our experimental system.

We are well aware of the great uncertainties which arise from extrapolating data from well-defined cell cultures to conditions prevailing in living and inflamed tissue. No data as to actual Pyo concentrations in infected tissue are available, nor do we know at this stage of our investigations how critical the glucose concentration might be for an effective oxidative burst, and what concentration of glucose can be expected in infected tissue. Our data suggest, however, that Pyo

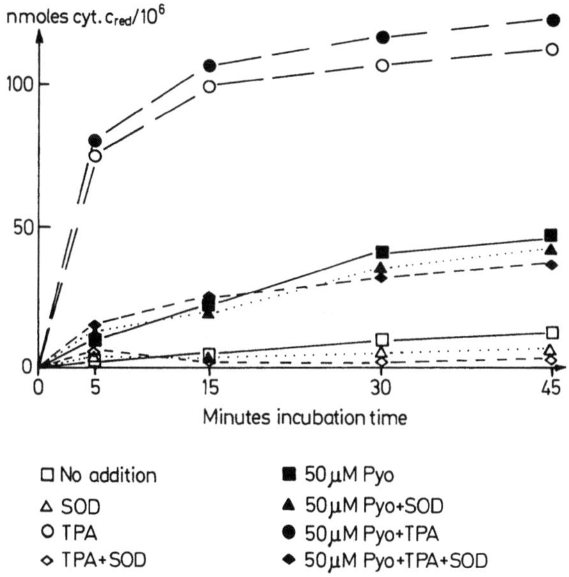

Fig. 1. Cytochrome c reduction by human PMNs. Conditions of incubations were similar to those described by Rajkovic and Williams (1985). Cell concentrations were 10^6/ml PMNs. Where indicated, 50 μM Pyo was present, TPA was added at 0.4 μM concentration, and SOD was used at 300 u/mol. OD_{546} was followed in an ELISA reader

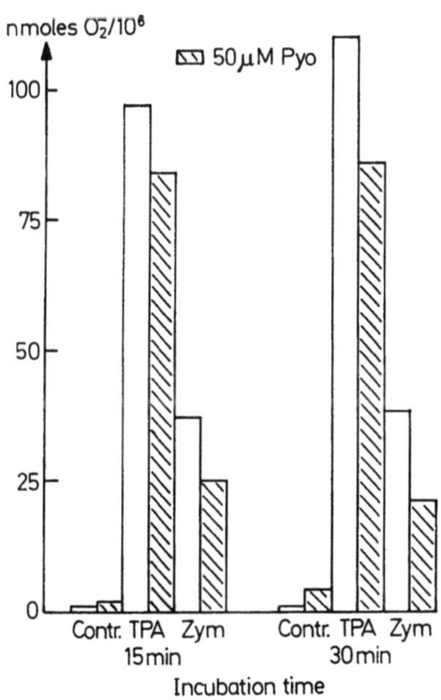

Fig. 2. Superoxide anion production by human PMNs. Incubations were as in Fig. 1. Superoxide was calculated from the SOD inhibitable fraction of reduced cytochrome c. Where indicated, 1 mg/ml opsonized zymosan was added

under conditions prevailing in infectious tissue may not only inhibit lymphocyte proliferation but also interfere with the most effective, oxygen-dependent microbicidal mechanism of the phagocytes, thus contributing to the ability of *P. aeruginosa* to persist at the site of infection.

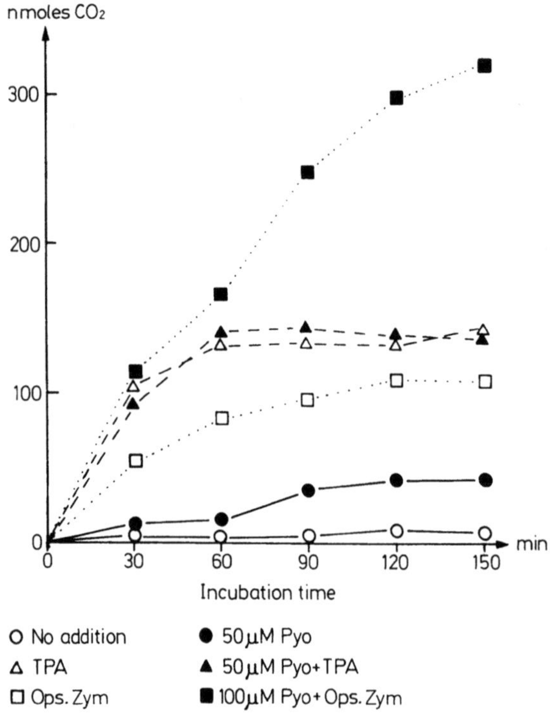

Fig. 3. Measurement of the hexose monophosphate shunt. Determination of CO_2 release from 1-^{14}C-labeled glucose was done as described by Metcalf et al. (1986). Concentration of PMNs was 3.25×10^6/ml, glucose concentration 5.5 m*M*. TPA and opsonized zymosan were added at 0.1 µg/ml and 70 µg/ml, respectively; the Pyo concentration was 50 µ*M* and 100 µ*M* as indicated. The cells for each pair of curves were from different batches

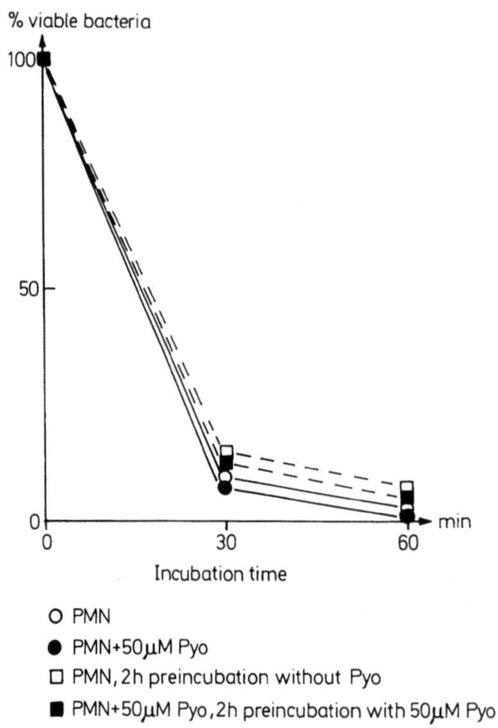

Fig. 4. Killing of *Staphylococcus aureus* by human PMNs. Intracellular killing in vitro after phagocytosis in vitro was done according to Leijh et al. (1986). Briefly, 10^7/ml PMNs and 10^7/ml preopsonized *S. aureus* were mixed and incubated at 37 °C for 5 min. Phagocytes were spun down, washed thoroughly, and allowed to kill the internalized bacteria for the indicated times. Internalized viable bacteria were determined as colonies after lysis of the phagocytes in distilled water. Where indicated, PMNs were preincubated with 50 µ*M* Pyo, and phagocytosis and killing was done in the presence of 50 µ*M* Pyo

References

Babior BM (1984) Oxidants from phagocytes: agents of defense and destruction. Blood 64:959–966

Hassan HM, Fridovich I (1980) Mechanism of the antibiotic action of pyocyanine. J Bacteriol 141:156–163

Leijh PCJ, van Furth R, van Zwet RL (1986) In vitro determination of phagocytosis and intracellular killing by polymorphonuclear and mononuclear phagocytes. In: Weir DM (ed) Handbook of experimental immunology, vol 2. Blackwell, Oxford, pp 46.1–46.21

Metcalf JA, Gallin JI, Nauseef WM, Root RK (1986) Laboratory manual of neutrophil function. Raven, New York, pp 105–106

Miller KM, Dearborn DG, Sorensen RU (1987) In vitro effect of synthetic pyocyanine on neutrophil superoxide production. Infect Immun 55:559–563

Mühlradt PF, Tsai H, Conradt P (1986) Effects of pyocyanine, a blue pigment from *Pseudomonas aeruginosa,* on separate steps of T cell activation: interleukin 2 (IL2) production, IL2 receptor formation, proliferation and induction of cytolytic activity. Eur J Immunol 16:434–440

Nutman J, Berger M, Chase PA, Dearborn DG, Miller KM, Waller RL, Sorensen RU (1987) Studies on the mechanism of T cell inhibition by the *Pseudomonas aeruginosa* phenazine pigment pyocyanine. J Immunol 138:3481–3487

Rajkovic IA, Williams R (1985) Rapid microassays of phagocytosis, bacterial killing, superoxide and hydrogen peroxide production by human neutrophils in vitro. J Immunol Methods 78:35–47

Sorensen RU, Klinger JD, Cash HA, Chase PA, Dearborn DG (1983) In vitro inhibition of lymphocyte proliferation by *Pseudomonas aeruginosa* phenazine pigments. Infect Immun 41:321–330

Polymorphonuclear Leukocyte Function Following Burn and Mechanical Injury: Regulation and Kinetics *

R. D. Nelson, S. R. Hasslen, D. H. Ahrenholz, and L. D. Solem

Microbicidal functions of the circulating neutrophil are well known to be temporally compromised following thermal or blunt traumatic injury. One function of the neutrophil grossly affected by injury is chemotaxis, or the ability to exit the vasculature and migrate directionally in response to one or more chemical signals generated at a site of inflammation. Defective patient neutrophil chemotactic function ex vivo has been reported by multiple laboratories using a variety of techniques [1–3] and has been reproduced in an animal model [4]. A decrease in the chemotactic response of neutrophils in vivo has also been documented for patients and animals with severe burns [5–7]. A defect in chemotactic function limits emigration of neutrophils from the circulation and likely contributes to the increased susceptibility to infection associated with thermal and traumatic injuries.

Precisely how much the loss of neutrophil chemotactic function contributes to infection susceptibility following thermal and traumatic injury remains unknown. For some clinicians, the absence of this information is viewed as compromising the utility of continuing efforts to identify mechanisms of injury-associated neutrophil chemotactic dysfunction. Thus it becomes frustrating to recognize that the answer to this question is not readily available. For these patient populations the contribution of defective neutrophil chemotaxis to postinjury infectious complications cannot be directly assessed because neutrophil chemotaxis is not the only leukocyte function affected – other functions of the neutrophil as well as other components of host defense are also compromised by these injuries. Ironically, the answer must depend upon the availability of a therapy which corrects the injury-associated neutrophil chemotactic dysfunction and accumulation of clinical evidence which proves that application of the therapy results in fewer and less morbid infectious complications following thermal and traumatic injuries.

Therapies which prevent or restore the temporal loss of neutrophil chemotactic function acquired in response to thermal or traumatic injury have yet to be identified. Their development has not progressed because of a lack of knowledge about the mechanism(s) involved, only clues to these mechanisms are currently available. Some of the clues available derive from our research efforts at the St. Paul-Ramsey Burn Center and the University of Minnesota to discover the mechanisms involved in the neutrophil chemotactic dysfunction that follows thermal

* Supported in part by grants from the St. Paul-Ramsey Foundation, St. Paul-Ramsey Medical Center, St. Paul, Minnesota, by grant AI 22374 from the National Institutes of Health, DHHS, and by a grant from the International Fire Fighters Union.

Immune Consequences of
Trauma, Shock and Sepsis
Eds. Faist/Ninnemann/Green

injury. Our presentation will emphasize the results of research carried out in these laboratories.

We will not review the literature describing the phenomenon of acquired neutrophil chemotactic dysfunction associated with thermal and traumatic injury. That literature is well known, as is the fact that temporal loss of chemotactic function occurs and that this change is maximum during the second week after injury, coincident with a period of gross bacterial challenge [8]. Rather, we propose to describe evidence that there are specific and nonspecific components of chemotactic function loss that alterations of both cell surface and cytoplasmic components are involved, and will proceed to identify two of the possible mediators involved.

Specificity of Chemotactic Dysfunction

Among the numerous reports that describe patient neutrophil chemotactic dysfunction, there are no studies which thoroughly characterize the specificity or selectivity of loss of chemotactic sensitivities. Considering the number of chemotactic factors identified to date, this would become a major task if thoroughly evaluated. Knowledge of the specificity is important, however, because it would direct experimental approaches to identification of the mechanism(s) involved as well as provide an important clue to the clinical significance of patient neutrophil chemotactic dysfunction ex vivo. For example, limited specificity would suggest a receptor-dependent mechanism, possibly involving desensitization of cells through downregulation or inactivation of selected receptor populations; an absence of specificity would suggest a receptor-independent mechanism, possibly involving loss of motility. Limited specificity would also suggest that patient neutrophil chemotactic dysfunction ex vivo has limited significance in vivo because preserved sensitivities would ensure effective delivery of circulating neutrophils; an absence of specificity would more likely limit the protective role of the neutrophil in vivo.

To begin to test the selectivity of loss of neutrophil chemotactic function following thermal injury, we evaluated temporal changes in chemotactic responses of patient neutrophils under agarose to two chemoattractants: C5a, as zymosan-activated serum, and the synthetic tripeptide, *N*-formyl-methionyl-leucyl-phenylalanine (FMLP) [3]. The data derived from neutrophils isolated from patients with major degrees of thermal injury (third-degree injury involving $\geqq 40\%$ of body surface area) demonstrate that patient neutrophils become deficient in chemotaxis to both of these attractants (Fig. 1). Considering Arturson's observation [8] that neutrophil chemotaxis in response to casein is also compromised following thermal injury, it becomes tempting to believe that there may be either no or limited selectivity for chemotactic dysfunction following thermal injury – that chemotactic dysfunction is a "global" phenomenon related at least in part to a receptor-independent mechanism.

The possibility that a receptor-independent mechanism may explain reduced chemotactic responses to unrelated attractants is further supported by results of assays for the expression of surface receptors for C5a and FMLP on patient neu-

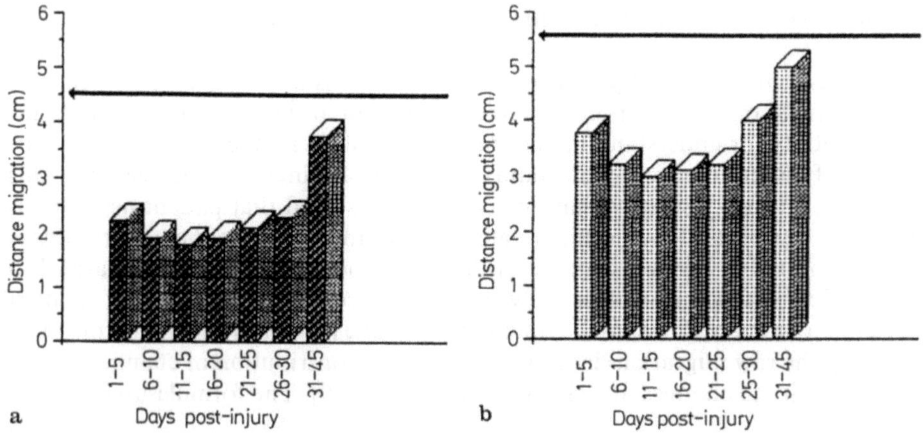

Fig. 1 a, b. Temporal changes in neutrophil chemotaxis ex vivo following major thermal injury. Chemotaxis was measured under agarose in terms of projected (40 ×) distance of migration. *Black arrow,* control. **a** Chemotaxis in response to C5a as zymosan-activated serum. **b** Chemotaxis in response to the synthetic tripeptide FMLP. Figure adapted from published data [3]

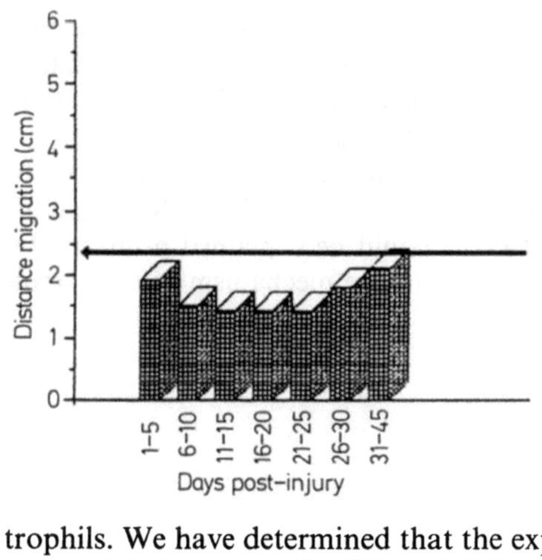

Fig. 2. Temporal changes in neutrophil random motility ex vivo following major thermal injury. Random migratory function was measured under agarose in terms of projected (40 ×) distance of migration. *Black arrow,* control. Figure adapted from published data [3]

trophils. We have determined that the expression of surface receptors on patient neutrophils is reduced for C5a only (Fig. 2) [3]. Thus, reduced receptor expression cannot account for reduced chemotaxis to both attractants in our studies. We therefore attempted to identify a receptor-independent mechanism to account for the observations described.

Loss of random motility provides one receptor-independent mechanism which could affect responses to multiple chemoattractants. Alteration of the cell membrane and cytoplasmic components providing for cell movement would render the neutrophil unable to respond to any chemotactic factor, independent of the availability of functional receptors for these factors. Put in human terms, your ability to walk will determine your ability to run any race: being unable to walk or to walk with a limp will limit your pace, no matter how well you perceive the course and the finish line.

Contribution of Reduced Motility to Chemotactic Dysfunction

The measurement of leukocyte chemotactic functions under agarose also enables measurement of random motility. Given the potential significance of altered random motility for understanding the mechanisms of chemotactic dysfunction, our assays of patient neutrophil chemotaxis have always included the testing of this function. In such testing we have consistently observed that patient neutrophils exhibit a loss of random motility related in time and degree to the pattern of loss of chemotaxis to FMLP. Data describing this phenomenon are summarized in Fig. 3. To evaluate more objectively the possible contribution of loss of random motility to reduced chemotactic functions, we have proposed a formula for transforming the raw migration data to factor out the contribution of changes in random motility to changes in a chemotactic function [9]. The formula used is:

$$\text{CI} = (\text{distance chemotaxis} - \text{distance random}) \div \text{distance random}.$$

It provides a chemotactic index (CI) which we interpret in the following way: a constant CI over time indicates that reduced chemotaxis in reponse to an attractant is related primarily to reduced random motility; a changing CI would suggest that reduced chemotaxis is related secondarily to reduced random motility and primarily to some other phenomenon. On transformation of the data presented in Fig. 1, we discovered that the CIs for chemotaxis toward FMLP were constant and that the CIs for chemotaxis toward C5a varied over time (Fig. 4). We interpret these patterns of CIs to mean that loss of chemotaxis to the tripeptide is attributable primarily to reduced random motility and that loss of chemotaxis to C5a is only secondarily attributable to reduced random motility. This apparent selective loss of chemotactic sensitivity to C5a could be explained primarily by loss of C5a receptor expression or function. Thus, the mechanism of neutrophil

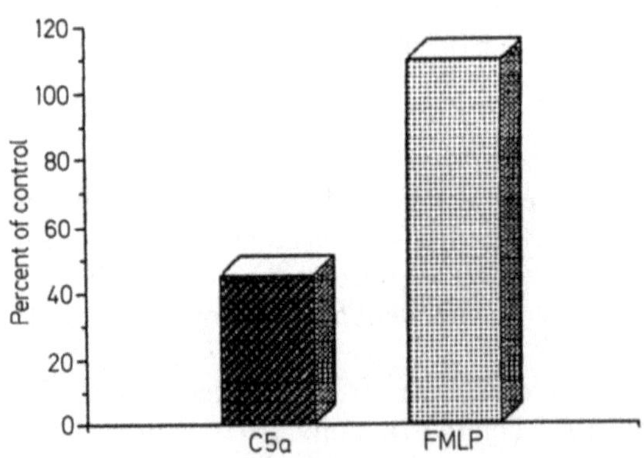

Fig. 3. Influence of major thermal injury on expression of receptors for chemotaxins on patient neutrophils. Neutrophils were isolated from patients at a time when migratory functions were known to be near maximally depressed. Receptors for C5a were measured using ^{125}I-C5a and receptors for FMLP were measured using ^{3}H-FMLP. Control levels of binding each of the radiolabeled ligands were established using neutrophils isolated from healthy control donors. Figure adapted from published data [3]

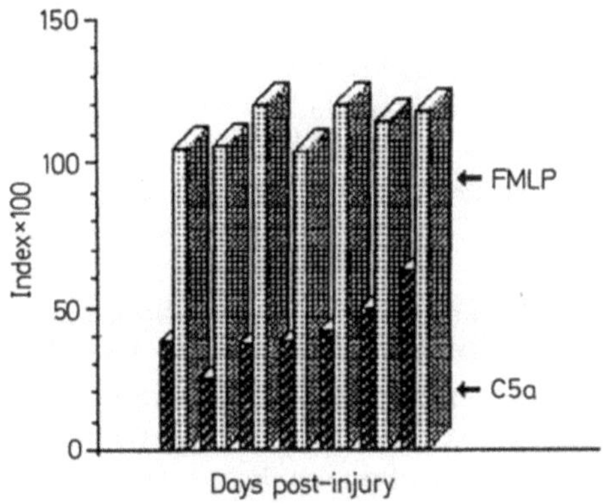

Fig. 4. Chemotactic indices (× 100) describing patient neutrophil chemotactic responses to C5a and FMLP. Indices were generated by transformation of the raw data summarized in Figs. 1 a, b using the formula, CI = (distance chemotaxis − distance random motility) ÷ distance random motility. The purpose of the CI is to factor out the contribution of reduced random motility to reduced chemotactic responses and so determine if reduced random motility contributes primarily or secondarily to chemotactic dysfunction. Figure adapted from published data [9]

chemotactic dysfunction following thermal injury is complex and involves both nonspecific and specific components. Understanding the mechanism will require evaluation of patient cells in terms of the expression and function of receptors for multiple chemoattractants and function of external and cytoplasmic elements which mediate adherence and motility.

Neutrophil C5a Receptor Expression Following Thermal Injury

We have reported that the ability of patient neutrophils to bind ^{125}I-labeled C5a is reduced during a time when chemotactic sensitivity to C5a is minimal or absent [3]. More recently we have applied fluorescein-labeled C5a (Fl-C5a) and flow cytometry to evaluate C5a receptor expression on patient neutrophils. Results deriving from application of this alternative technique for monitoring C5a receptor expression confirm our earlier findings and provide several additional pieces of information. When patient neutrophils were followed over time after injury in terms of staining with Fl-C5a at 25 °C, we found that a relatively small number (<25%) of receptor negative cells accumulate and that the greater number of receptor-positive cells lose no more than 50% of their ability to bind the ligand. Gross accumulation of receptor negative cells does not therefore account fully for loss of patient neutrophil chemotactic sensitivity to C5a.

Human neutrophils normally express approximately 200 000 C5a receptors per cell [10] and approximately 20 000 FMLP receptors per cell [1]. Given that an order of magnitude fewer FMLP receptors are sufficient to mediate chemotactic sensitivity to the tripeptide and that fewer still are required if chemotaxis is mediated by a high-affinity subpopulation of receptors [12], it would seem untenable that loss of patient neutrophil chemotactic sensitivity to C5a could occur with 100 000 residual C5a receptors available. An explanation would require that binding of the ligand and signal transduction are or become dissociated for these residual C5a receptors. Whether or not such uncoupling of binding and response is acquired or represents a preexisting subpopulation of C5a receptors then becomes the question. It has been reported that C5a receptors share a common affinity for C5a, unlike the peptide and LTB_4 receptors for their respective ligands

[12, 13], so subpopulations of C5a receptors would have to be based upon some other receptor quality. Support for the existence of C5a receptor subpopulations and a clue to a quality which distinguishes them are provided by results deriving from more recent experiments in our laboratory.

We have determined that binding of Fl-C5a by control neutrophils can be reduced by 50% by staining the cells at 4° vs 25 °C (Fig. 5). This observation reproduces results previously reported by Bender et al. [14] and Huey and Hugli [15]. We offer that this phenomenon identifies two C5a receptor subpopulations of approximately equal number, one temperature dependent and the other temperature independent in terms of ligand binding function. We therefore considered that the maximum 50% decrease in binding of Fl-C5a observed for patient neutrophils might reflect the selective loss or inactivation of one of these receptor subpopulations.

Identification of the C5a receptor subpopulation altered in response to thermal injury can be easily accomplished by comparing staining of patient cells incubated with Fl-C5a at 25° and 4 °C. Data summarized in Fig. 5 illustrate the utility of this protocol. For neutrophils from the patient studied, staining with Fl-C5a at the lower temperature did not further reduce binding of Fl-C5a. This result demonstrates that the temperature-dependent C5a receptor subpopulation has been selectively inactivated or lost. Our current working hypothesis is, therefore, that C5a receptors exist in two subpopulations of approximately equal number: a temperature-sensitive subpopulation, mediating chemotaxis, and a temperature-insensitive subpopulation, either nonfunctional or mediating other responses to C5a/C5adesArg. We have yet to identify the mechanism involved in the effect of low temperature on the expression and functional state of half of the human neutrophil C5a receptors, though preliminary evidence on hand suggests that the cytoskeleton plays a role.

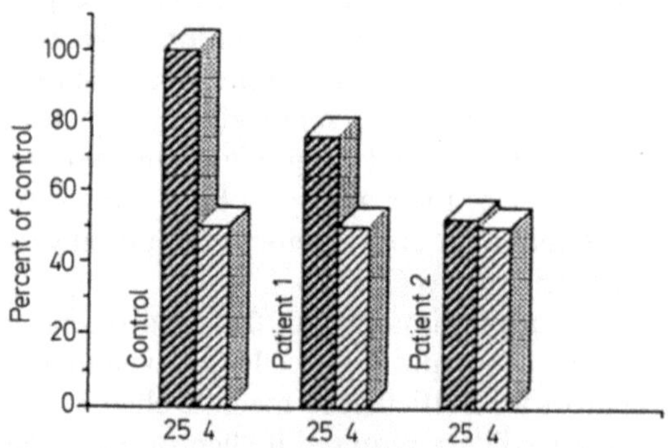

Fig. 5. Influence of temperature on expression/function of receptors for C5a on control and patient neutrophils. Receptors were monitored by flow cytometric analysis of cells stained with fluorescein-conjugated C5a (Fl-C5a). Relative fluorescence was recorded in terms of mean channel fluorescence on a linear scale. Cells were incubated with Fl-C5a using time and ligand concentration conditions providing for saturation of functional receptors. The temperature for the staining reaction was either 25° or 4 °C. Control values were obtained using neutrophils isolated from healthy donors; two patients with major degrees of thermal injury were studied during the second week postinjury

Mediators of Loss of C5a Receptor Function

Given the numerous examples of desensitization of cells to an agonist as a result of receptor downregulation by the agonist itself, it is reasonable to expect that the same mechanism must explain loss of neutrophil C5a receptor expression following thermal injury. This would require activation of complement on a systemic scale in response to injury to provide sufficient ligand to saturate all available C5a receptors. To determine if C5a accumulates systemically in response to thermal injury, we assayed patient plasma specimens for C5a/C5adesArg using a radioimmunoassay kit available at that time from Upjohn Diagnostics (now available from Amersham, Arlington Heights, Illinois) [3]. C5adesArg is the primary product of C5 activation measured in this assay because C5a not binding to cells expressing C5a receptors will be quickly converted to its anaphylatoxin-inactive analog, C5adesArg. This conversion involves enzymatic removal of the carboxy-terminal arginine residue by a plasma carboxypeptidase, known alternatively as anaphylatoxin inactivator [16]. Although impotent as a spasmogen, C5adesArg retains a portion of the activity of C5a as a neutrophil chemoattractant [17].

Results summarized in Fig. 6 demonstrate that C5a is present in patient plasma following major thermal injury, that its concentration begins to rise during the second week after injury, and that its maximum concentration can reach more than six times the normal level of 20 ng/ml. Although these results demonstrate generation of C5a in response to thermal injury, they may not accurately characterize either the time at which C5a generation begins or the true level at which activation occurs. Such underestimation of C5a activation occurs because C5adesArg, having residual biological activity, will not accumulate in patient plasma until C5a receptors on neutrophils and other cells approach saturation [18].

To circumvent the difficulties associated with using C5adesArg as a marker for time and level of C5 activation, measurements of C3adesArg and iC3b were added. Measurement of C3adesArg was done using a radioimmunoassay kit also manufactured by Upjohn Diganostics; measurement of iC3b was accomplished in collaboration with Dr. William Kolb at Cytotech, Inc., San Diego, California,

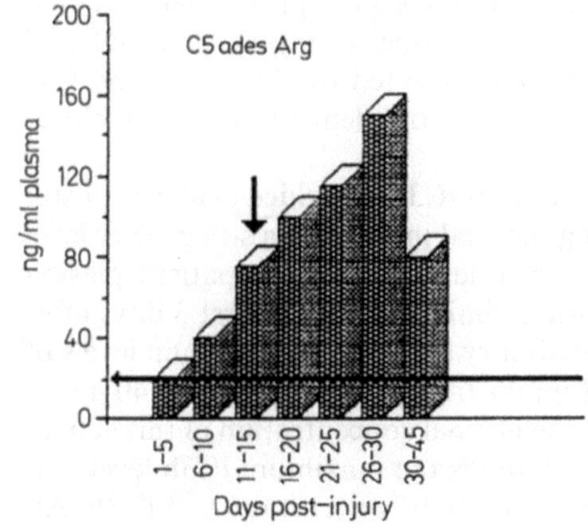

Fig. 6. Influence of major thermal injury on complement activation: C5a. C5a present in control and patient plasma (EDTA) specimens as C5adesArg was assayed by radioimmunoassay using a kit available from Upjohn Diagnostics. The *vertical arrow* denotes the time postinjury at which patient plasma C5adesArg levels were considered to first exceed the control level (*horizontal arrow*). Figure adapted from published data [3]

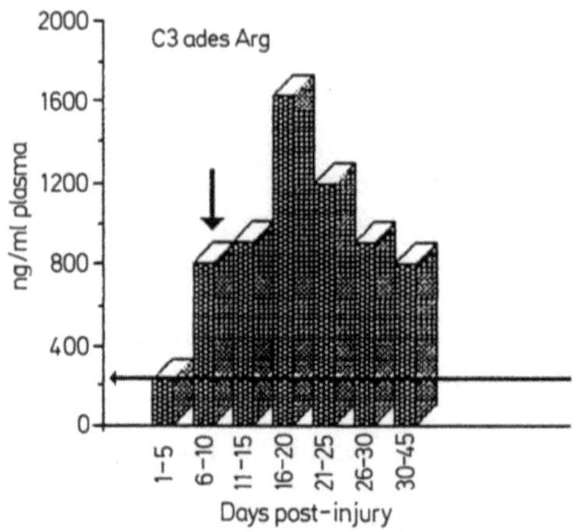

Fig. 7. Influence of major thermal injury on complement activation: C3a. C3a present in control and patient plasma (EDTA) specimens as C3adesArg was assayed by radioimmunoassay using a kit available from Upjohn Diagnostics. The *vertical arrow* denotes the time postinjury at which patient plasma C3adesArg levels were considered to first exceed the control level (*horizontal arrow*). Figure adapted from published data [3]

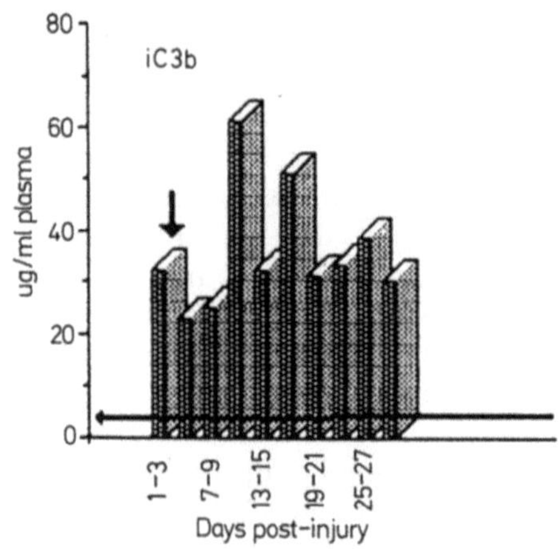

Fig. 8. Influence of major thermal injury on complement activation: iC3b. iC3b present in control and patient plasma (EDTA) specimens was assayed by enzyme-linked immunoassay, using reagents now available in kit form from Cytotech, Inc., San Diego, California. The *vertical arrow* denotes the time postinjury at which patient plasma iC3b levels were considered to first exceed the control level (*horizontal arrow*)

using an enzyme-linked immunoassay now available commercially. Because these C3 derivatives have grossly reduced biological activity, we expected that the temporal patterns of their accumulation would more closely approximate the real time and level of complement activation induced by thermal injury. Data in Fig. 7 illustrate that plasma C3adesArg levels become elevated by the end of the first week after injury. These results move the time of complement activation closer to the time of injury by 3–5 days.

Data in Fig. 8, deriving from measurements of iC3b, provided evidence of still earlier activation of complement following thermal injury and a still greater level of injury-induced complement activation. The level of iC3b in patient plasma specimens was observed to rise above normal limits during the first 3 days after injury and was elevated in several 24-h postinjury specimens. Maximum levels of iC3b in plasma specimens from 11 of 18 major injury patients were ≧40 μg/ml iC3b, representing a tenfold increase over the normal concentration of this activation product (4 μg/ml). For 5 of these 11 patients the maximum iC3b levels exceeded 100 μg/ml, or more than 20 times the normal concentration of iC3b. Al-

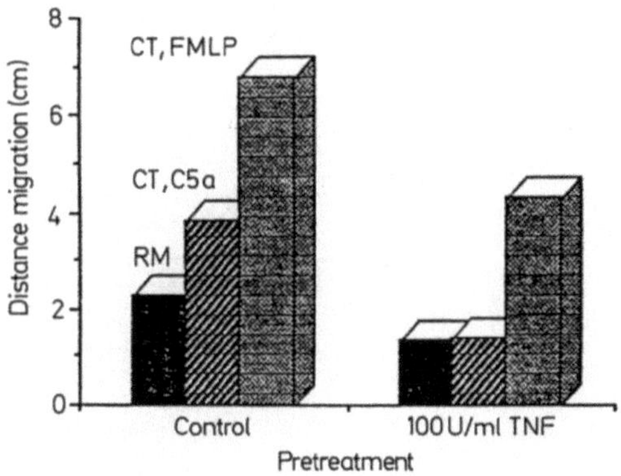

Fig. 9. Influence of preexposure to tumor necrosis factor (TNF) on chemotaxis of control neutrophils under agarose to two chemoattractants, C5a as zymosan-activated serum and the synthetic tripeptide, FMLP. Ten million neutrophils isolated from healthy donors were preincubated for 30 min at 37 °C with 100 U/ml TNF (0.5 ml total volume), washed, and tested for chemotactic function. Control neutrophils were incubated under the same conditions in the absence of TNF

though knowledge of the rate of clearance of iC3b in vivo is required to fully evaluate the significance of these plasma iC3b values, we suggest that these results demonstrate that complement activation following major thermal injury occurs earlier and at levels not appreciated by data deriving from assays for either C3adesArg or C5adesArg. In addition, the 4-week duration over which iC3b remains elevated after major injury may indicate that complement activation in this situation is a chronic rather than an acute phenomenon. Finally, we suggest that these results support the long-term availability of C5a/C5adesArg in the systemic circulation to influence neutrophil C5a receptor expression.

Until recently we were content to believe that C5a activation products were the exclusive mediators of loss of patient neutrophil chemotactic sensitivity to C5a. Within the past year we have discovered, however, that a cytokine, tumor necrosis factor (TNF), may also influence C5a receptor expression. This activity of TNF is illustrated in Fig. 9 by the differentially greater inhibitory influence of rhTNF on chemotaxis of control neutrophils toward C5a as zymosan-activated serum than toward an unrelated attractant, FMLP [19]. This conclusion was based upon the comparable distance of migration values of the TNF-treated cells for random motility and chemotaxis toward C5a and their contrasting positive response to the tripeptide. Because TNF and C5a share no structural homology, this phenomenon is likely not the result of TNF binding directly to the C5a receptor, but we have yet to discover the mechanism involved. We consider it a reasonable possibility that TNF is not a unique cytokine in this respect and that other agonists to which the neutrophil is sensitive may also negatively influence C5a receptor expression. Bender et al. [14] provided support for this possibility with the observation that preexposure of human neutrophils to phorbol myristate acetate also decreases the ligand-binding function of C5a receptors.

Auto-oxidative Loss of Random Motility

Some years ago we described experimental results which suggested that excessive stimulation of neutrophil respiratory function by chemotactic factors can cause auto-oxidative injury to the cells, resulting in depression of random motility [20].

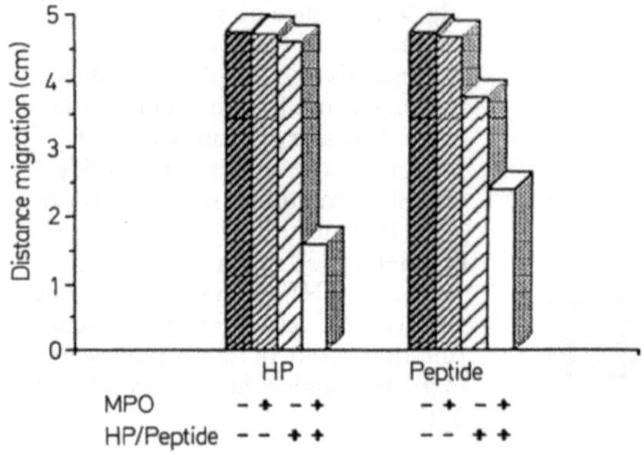

Fig. 10. Influence of myeloperoxidase (*MPO*) on loss of random motility induced by preincubation of control neutrophils with hydrogen peroxide (*HP*) or *N*-formyl-norleucyl-leucyl-phenylalanyl-norleucyl-tyrosyl-lysine (*peptide*). Concentrations of HP and peptide are cited in the text. Human neutrophil MPO was isolated by chromatography and used without estimation of activity. A contribution of MPO to loss of random motility was noted only when added 5–10 min prior to addition of HP or peptide

One experiment involved pretreatment of neutrophils from healthy control donors and from patients with chronic granulomatous disease (CGD) to chemotactic factors, followed by measurement of random migratory function. We observed that random motility of the CGD neutrophils was unaffected by such treatment and attributed this result to the well-known inability of CGD neutrophils to generate reactive oxygen species.

We have since found no major reason to change our conclusion that auto-oxidation resulting from excessive stimulation of the neutrophil respiratory burst can contribute to loss of random motility and, in fact, have accumulated several additional observations which further support this proposal [21]. These observations are summarized in Table 1. Though the protective influence of catalase would suggest that hydrogen peroxide is involved, another observation, which is not listed in the table, would appear not to support this conclusion. This observation is that exposure of neutrophils to exogenous hydrogen peroxide at concentrations less than 10 m*M* does not negatively influence their random motility. Still another observation, however, further supports a role for hydrogen peroxide and provides a clue to how it is involved. The latter observation was the product of a preliminary experiment to consider a role for myeloperoxidase in auto-oxidation, based in part upon the proposal by Gallin et al. [22] that secreted lysosomal enzymes contribute to loss of neutrophil chemotactic function. Our experimental data presented in Fig. 10 illustrate that when neutrophils were preincubated with exogenous human myeloperoxidase and subsequently exposed to 100 μ*M* hydrogen peroxide or 10^{-4} *M* FMLP, random motility of the treated cells was considerably less than that resulting from exposure of the cells to hydrogen peroxide or tripeptide alone. These results support a contribution of hydrogen peroxide through hypochlorous acid to oxidative injury and suggest that a cell membrane component to which myeloperoxidase can bind may be one target of injury. Ad-

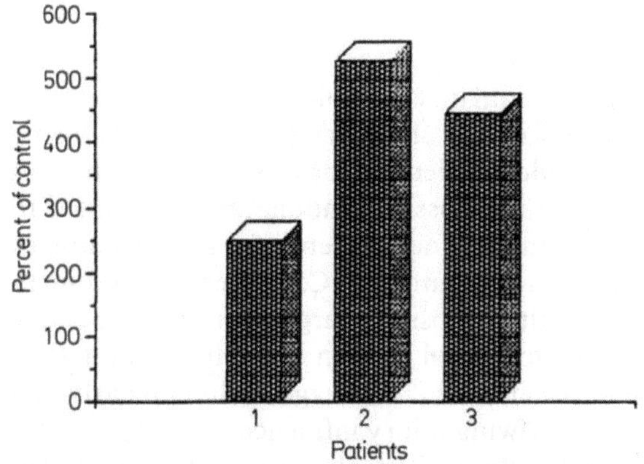

Fig. 11. Polymerization of actin in neutrophils from patients with major thermal injury. Actin polymerization was quantified using NBD-phallacidin in association with flow cytometry. NBD-phallacidin binds selectively to polymerized (filamentous, F) actin; therefore, increased staining denotes polymerization. The data shown derive from three patients with major thermal injury studied during the second week after injury. Control levels of staining were established using neutrophils isolated from healthy control volunteers. No increase in staining was observed for patient lymphocytes

ditional work is required to evaluate the contributions of other oxygen reduction products to this phenomenon and to identify the specific target substrate(s) involved.

A recent report by Hinshaw et al. [23] stating that exposure of cell-line fibroblasts to hydrogen peroxide results in significant polymerization of cytoplasmic actin suggests one target substrate of the neutrophil which can be modified by oxidation. Because of the known role of actin gelation and solvation in cell motility, we have more recently begun to evaluate the polymerized state of actin in patient neutrophils. This is possible using flow cytometry in conjunction with NBD-phallacidin, a fluorescent reagent which binds specifically to actin in the polymerized/filamentous form [24]. Our preliminary results, summarized in Fig. 11, demonstrate that patient neutrophils bind up to five times the NBD-phallacidin of control cells, demonstrating that actin becomes highly polymerized in circulating neutrophils following major thermal injury. We have also observed that exposure of patient cells to 4 °C does not reduce binding of NBD-phallacidin, suggesting further that the polymerized state of actin is not reversible in the patient neutrophil. This conclusion is consistent with the observation by Hinshaw et al. that polymerization of actin associated with oxidant injury of the cell line cells appears to be essentially irreversible [23]. We therefore speculate that an accumulation of filamentous actin must certainly account for some of the loss of patient neutrophil motility functions.

Summary

I have reviewed and updated our experimental observations and thoughts relating to mechanisms of acquired loss of neutrophil chemotactic function following thermal injury. Older observations provided evidence of desensitization of patient neutrophils to C5a as a chemoattractant and loss of random motility related to auto-oxidative injury. Newer information provides evidence for selective loss of a previously unrecognized subpopulation of neutrophil C5a receptors and identifies cell membrane and cytoplasmic actin as possible targets for auto-oxidative "injury" to affect random motility. The temporal pattern of complement activation we observed in assays of patient plasma for iC3b suggests that an early and continuing activation of complement following injury influences vascular permeability as well as leukocyte migratory functions. The observation that TNF can influence neutrophil chemotactic sensitivity to C5a suggests that one or more cytokines may additionally contribute to neutrophil chemotactic dysfunction in response to injury. Although our research has concentrated on the thermal injury patient, I offer that the same phenomena likely occur to some degree in patients with blunt traumatic injury or chronic infection, and, although we have emphasized chemotactic function of the neutrophil, I offer that loss of chemotactic function of the monocyte would compromise the accumulation of this cell at sites of injury, limiting the availability of monocyte-derived growth factors to initiate the healing response. Studies of acquired neutrophil chemotactic dysfunction therefore have broad implications and the identification of therapies to control this injury-associated phenomenon has considerable potential.

References

1. Warden GD, Mason AD Jr, Pruitt BA Jr (1974) Evaluation of leukocyte chemotaxis in vitro in thermally injured patients. J Clin Invest 54:1001–1004
2. Davis JM, Dineen P, Gallin JI (1980) Neutrophil degranulation and abnormal chemotaxis after thermal injury. J Immunol 124:1467–1471
3. Solomkin JS, Nelson RD, Chenoweth DE, Solem LD, Simmons RL (1984) Regulation of neutrophil migratory function in burn injury by complement activation products. Ann Surg 200:742–746
4. Davis JM, Gallin JI (1988) Abnormal rabbit heterophil chemotaxis following thermal injury. Arch Surg 123:752–755
5. Yurt RW, Pruitt BA Jr (1985) Decreased wound neutrophils and indiscrete margination in the pathogenesis of wound infection. Surgery 98:191–197
6. Balch HH (1963) Resistance to infection in burn patients. Ann Surg 157:1–19
7. McCabe WP, Rebuck JW, Kelly AP, Ditmore DM (1973) Leukocyte response as a monitor of immunodepression in burn patients. Arch Surg 106:155–159
8. Arturson G (1985) Neutrophil granulocyte functions in severely burned patients. Burns 11:309–319
9. Nelson RD, Hasslen SR, Ahrenholz DH, Solem LD (1987) Mechanisms of loss of human neutrophil chemotaxis following thermal injury. J Burn Care Rehabil 8:496–502
10. Chenoweth DE, Hugli TE (1978) Demonstration of specific C5a receptor on intact human polymorphonuclear leukocytes. Proc Natl Acad Sci USA 75:3943–3947
11. Fletcher MP, Gallin JI (1980) Degranulating stimuli increase the availability of receptors on human neutrophils for the chemoattractant f-Met-Leu-Phe. J Immunol 124:1585–1588

12. Yuli I, Tomonaga A, Snyderman R (1982) Chemoattractant receptor functions in human polymorphonuclear leukocytes are divergently altered by membrane fluidizers. Proc Natl Acad Sci USA 79:5906–5910
13. Goldman DW, Goetzl EJ (1984) Heterogeneity of human polymorphonuclear leukocyte receptors for leukotriene B_4. J Exp Med 159:1027–1041
14. Bender JG, Van Epps DE, Chenoweth DE (1987) Independent regulation of human neutrophil chemotactic receptors after activation. J Immunol 139:3028–3033
15. Huey J, Hugli TE (1985) Characterization of a C5a receptor on human polymorphonuclear leukocytes. J Immunol 135:2063–2068
16. Bokisch VA, Muller-Eberhard HJ (1970) Anaphylatoxin inactivator of human plasma: its isolation and characterization as a carboxypeptidase. J Clin Invest 49:2427–2436
17. Perez HD, Goldstein IM, Webster RO, Henson PM (1981) Enhancement of the chemotactic activity of human C5adesArg by an anionic polypeptide ("cochemotaxin") in normal serum and plasma. J Immunol 126:800–804
18. Chenoweth DE, Cooper SW, Hugli TE, Stewart RW, Blackstone EH, Kirklin JW (1981) Complement activation during cardiopulmonary bypass. Evidence for generation of C3a and C5a anaphylotoxins. N Engl J Med 304:497–503
19. Fast DJ, Schlievert PM, Nelson RD (1988) Non-purulent response to toxic shock syndrome toxin-1 producing *Staphylococcus aureus:* relationship to toxin-stimulated production of tumor necrosis factor. J Immunol 140:949–953
20. Nelson RD, McCormack RT, Fiegel VD, Herron MJ, Simmons RL, Quie PG (1979) Chemotactic deactivation of human neutrophils: possible relationship to stimulation of oxidative metabolism. Infect Immun 23:282–286
21. Nelson RD, Fiegel VD, Herron MJ, Gracyk JM, Bauman MP, McCormack RT, Simmons RL (1980) Chemotactic deactivation of human neutrophils: role of stimulation of hexose monophosphate shunt activity in nonspecific deactivation. Acta Physiol Scand [Suppl] 492:31–41
22. Gallin JI, Wright DC, Schiffmann E (1979) Role of secretory events in modulating humane neutrophil chemotaxis. J Clin Invest 62:1364–1374
23. Hinshaw DB, Sklar LA, Bohl B, Schraufstatter IU, Hyslop PA, Rossi MW, Spragg RG, Cochrane CG (1986) Cytoskeletal and morphologic impact of cellular oxidant injury. Am J Pathol 123:454–464
24. Wulf E, Deboren A, Bantz FA, Faulstich H, Wieland T (1979) Fluorescent phallotoxin, a tool for the visualization of cellular actin. Proc Natl Acad Sci USA 76:4498–4502

The Role of Complement in Injury

M. Heideman

Complement is of importance for restricting microorganisms to their normal sites such as skin and gut as well as for clearing the blood stream of these invaders. During evolution organisms had complement for host defence before they were provided with antibodies (Muller-Eberhard 1975). This cascade system can be activated by an antibody fixed to an antigen but also in a more nonspecific way without antibodies. Chemotaxis, opsonization, and lysis of bacteria or injured or foreign cells are influenced by products formed when complement is activated, a process modulated by inhibitors. Hereditary defects leading to reduced amounts of complement from the alternative pathway are associated with repeated and sometimes life-threatening infections (Muller-Eberhard 1978). The same effect can be observed after extensive injuries leading to consumption of complement or after starvation or by prolonged medication with corticosteroids (Alexander et al. 1979; Alexander 1980; Atkinson et al. 1973).

Under normal circumstances the complement system will guide leukocyte migration to the area of injury or infection. A dose-related accumulation of radiolabelled leukocytes to endotoxin has been found in healthy animals. However, when hypoperfusion, peritonitis, or pretreatment with methylprednisolone has preceded the deposition of endotoxin this does not occur (Bengtson et al. 1987 a). Similar findings have been observed following extensive trauma or burns, ischemia of intestine or limbs, and in patients with multiple abscesses. One explanation for impaired leukocyte function in this situation is altered availability of complement leading to impaired chemotaxis. Another is generation of large quantities of C3a which may produce an immunosuppressive response with impaired B-cell function. Large quantities of C5a or C5a des-Arg will also impair the chemotactic response (Chenoweth et al. 1980).

Damaged cells and foreign invaders are eliminated by components of the immune and inflammatory systems (Hansson et al. 1984). A local activation of complement in tissues changed by injury can be seen following burns, acute vascular occlusions and in association with abscesses. Products of the complement system can then be traced to the area of injury, e.g., the burn bullae or in the abscess fluid (Bengtson et al. 1987 b). When complement is activated in the area of injury stimulation to remove altered autologous cells and foreign invaders will occur. However, when widespread appearance of activated products exists in the bloodstream a generalized reaction can be observed. This can be seen in patients with widespread deep burns, multiple soft-tissue injuries, bacteremia or extensive areas with impaired tissue perfusion (Bengtson et al. 1986, 1987 c; Heideman et al. 1984). When altered foreign tissue or microorganisms are reached by blood com-

Immune Consequences of
Trauma, Shock and Sepsis
Eds. Faist/Ninnemann/Green

ponents involved in chemotaxis and opsonization, they will be removed. However, these mechanisms will be dangerous when they occur in a more generalized fashion. Then impaired microvascular flow, increased permeability with edema, e.g., in the lung, or lysis of bystanding cells can be life-threatening for the individual in whom this occurs (Weigelt et al. 1987; Weinberg et al. 1984). This might be one of the reasons for the high incidence of multisystem organ failure in patients with extensive tissue injury or infections for a longer period. However, only temporary effects on arterial oxygenation and blood pressure can be seen when toxic material reaches the bloodstream for only a short period in association with fixation of hip prostheses with methylmethacrylate (Bengtson et al. 1987d), or when extensive abscesses or limbs without arterial perfusion are promptly drained or resected.

Activating factors can replace and enhance each other. One example of this situation is the initially noninfected burn which later is complicated by burn-wound sepsis. Then, further appearance of activated complement components can be seen in the bloodstream due to the additive effect of bacteremia to burn injury (McPhaden et al. 1985).

In patients with extensive tissue injury or bacteremia a cytolytic effect by the complement cascade will occur, leading to lysis of damaged cells or foreign invaders. Lysis of cells primarily not involved in triggering the complement cascade will also occur. This might be one of the reasons for hemolysis and anemia in patients with this kind of injury (Heideman et al. 1988). Cells other than erythrocytes such as leukocytes and platelets might also be injured by this mechanism, leading to release of products which will enhance the inflammatory reaction, e.g., release of prostaglandins, superoxides and platelet-activating factors.

The initial complement reaction serves to recognize injured tissue and foreign microorganisms. This will recruit and coordinate multiple-effector systems involved in inflammation. Such systems are plasma proteins, e.g., the Hageman factor and components from the fibrin, kinin and prostaglandin systems, resident mastcells and macrophages, supraoxides and leukotrienes and, ultimately, circulating cellular elements including platelets, neutrophils, and monocytes. The cellular effectors are the major destructive elements of the inflammatory response. The intensity of the initial noncellular response is central in determining whether infection will progress and to what extent tissue will be destroyed (Solomkin et al. 1983).

The humoral and cellular systems involved in the inflammatory reaction have many activators and inactivators in common (Goldstein et al. 1973; Ninnemann 1987; Solomkin and Simmons 1983). This is the reason why *E. coli* affect coagulation and fibrinolysis, the kinin systems, and the complement systems but also release the platelet-activating factors and leukotrienes. Examples of common inactivators for prostaglandin and complement systems are cortisone and methylprednisolone. Proteolytic effects have also been observed when macrophages have been triggered to release their content following complement activation (George et al. 1983; Goldstein et al. 1973).

The activation process of complement is dependent on the amount of triggering factors as well as the amount of bacteria, soft-tissue injury or introduced foreign and toxic material. The biological effects are also dependent on the time span allowed for these factors to work which can be limited by the treatment. Pharmacological treatment by cortisone but also lidocain (Bengtson et al. 1987c; Heideman et al. 1985) and calcium blockers has been shown to reduce release of biologically active complement components. Plasmapheresis is one way of removing products such as anaphylatoxins from the blood (Warden et al. 1983).

In the future, prompt identification and elimination of the activating process and more selective methods of modulating the defence mechanisms will be of value for patients with extensive injuries.

References

Alexander JW (1980) Symposium on surgical infections. Surg Clin North Am 60:107–116

Alexander JW, Stinnett JD, Ogle CK et al. (1979) A comparison of immunologic profiles and their influence on bacteremia in surgical patients with a high risk of infections. Surgery 86:94–101

Atkinson JP, Frank MM (1973) Effect of cortisone therapy on serum complement components. J Immunol 111:1061–1066

Bengtson A, Heideman M (1986) Altered anaphylatoxin activity during hypoperfusion in acute and elective abdominal aortic surgery. J Trauma 26:631–637

Bengtson A, Heideman M (1987b) Anaphylatoxin formation in plasma and burn bullae fluid in the thermally injured patient. Burns Incl Therm Inj 13:185–189

Bengtson A, Hansson GK, Heideman M (1987a) In vivo determination of modulated migration of radiolabelled leukocytes. Arch Surg 122:909–912

Bengtson A, Lannsjö W, Heideman M (1987c) Complement and anaphylatoxin responses to cross-clamping of the aorta. Studies during general anaesthesia with or without extradural blockade. Br J Anaesth 59:1093–1097

Bengtson A, Larsson M, Gammer W, Heideman M (1987d) Anaphylatoxin release in association with methylmethacrylate fixation of hip prostheses. J Bone Joint Surg 69:46–49 [Am]

Chenoweth DE, Hugli TE (1980) Human C5a and C5a analogs as probes of the neutrophil C5a receptor. Mol Immunol 17:152–161

George BC, Clowes GHA Jr, Saravis C, Heideman M, Lane B (1983) Plasmaproteolysis inducing factor produced by human macrophages. Fed Proc 42:1039–1045

Goldstein IM, Brai M, Osler AG, Weissman G (1973) Lysosomal enzyme release from human leukocytes: mediation by the alternative pathway of complement activation. J Immunol 111:33–37

Hansson GK, Starkebaum GA, Benditt EP, Schwartz SM (1984) Fc-mediated binding of IgG to vimentin-type intermediate filament in vascular endothelial cells. Proc Natl Acad Sci USA 81:3103–3107

Heideman M, Bengtson A (1985) Immunological interference of high dose corticosteroids. Acta Chir Scand [Suppl] 526:48–55

Heideman M, Bengtson A (1988) Terminal complement complexes and anaphylatoxins in septic and ischemic patients. Arch Surg 123:188–192

Heideman M, Hugli TE (1984) Anaphylatoxin generation in multisystem organ failure. J Trauma 24:1038–1043

McPhaden AR, Whaley K (1985) The complement system in sepsis and trauma. Br Med Bull 41:281–286

Muller-Eberhard HJ (1975) Complement. Annu Rev Biochem 44:697–724

Muller-Eberhard HJ (1978) Complement abnormalities in human disease. Hosp Pract [Off] 13:65–76

Ninnemann JL (1987) Trauma, sepsis, and the immune response. JBCR 8:462–468

Solomkin JS, Simmons RL (1983) Cellular and subcellular mediators of acute inflammation. Surg Clin North Am 63:225–243

Warden GD, Stratta RJ, Saffle JR et al. (1983) Plasma exchange therapy in patients failing to resuscitate from burn shock. J Trauma 23:945–951

Weigelt JA, Borman KR (1987) Complement and severity of pulmonary insufficiency. J Trauma 27:834

Weinberg PF, Matthay MA, Webster RO, Roskos KV, Golstein IM, Murray JF (1984) Biologically active products of complement and acute lung injury in patients with the sepsis syndrome. Am Rev Respir Dis 130:791–796

Control of Acute-Phase Protein Production *

G. E. Brown and M. E. Lanser

Injury induces characteristic alterations in the circulating levels of specific plasma proteins, referred to as the acute-phase proteins. Their major known functions are to serve as antiproteases, transport proteins, and opsonins. The acute-phase proteins, synthesized primarily in the liver, have been the focus of considerable study, since their altered levels presumably contribute to an improved ability of the host to survive injury. When interpreting the significance of the acute-phase response, it should not be forgotten that these proteins may represent only a few of the proteins synthesized in the liver whose synthesis changes following injury. The acute-phase protein profile may thus give an incomplete picture of the adaptive processes that occur (consider intracellular "stress proteins" and extracellular non-plasma proteins). However, the classic acute-phase proteins do give an indication of the extent of the body's response to injury, and they have the clinical advantage of being easy to sample and assay.

The acute-phase proteins fall into several categories: those whose levels are greatly increased, moderately increased, and decreased following injury. Table 1 lists the better-known acute-phase proteins in man, indicates into which category each falls, and indicates the functions of each. Note that this categorization may be misleading because the changes in circulating levels often underestimate the increased rate of synthesis due to enhanced utilization of many of these proteins. Thus, decreased circulating levels do not necessarily imply a decrease in synthesis.

Table 1. Acute-phase proteins in man

Protein	Response	Function
Albumin	Decrease	Transport
Alpha-1-antitrypsin	Increase	Antiprotease
Alpha-2-macroglobulin	Increase	Antiprotease
Ceruloplasmin	Increase	Transport; oxidase
Complement C3	Increase	Opsonization, lysis
C-reactive protein	Increase	Opsonization?
Factor B	Increase	Complement activation
Fibrinogen	Increase	Hemostasis
Fibronectin	Decrease/increase	Opsonization
Serum amyloid A	Increase	?
Transferrin	Decrease	Transport

* Supported in part by NIH grants GM36258 and GM00511

Immune Consequences of
Trauma, Shock and Sepsis
Eds. Faist/Ninnemann/Green

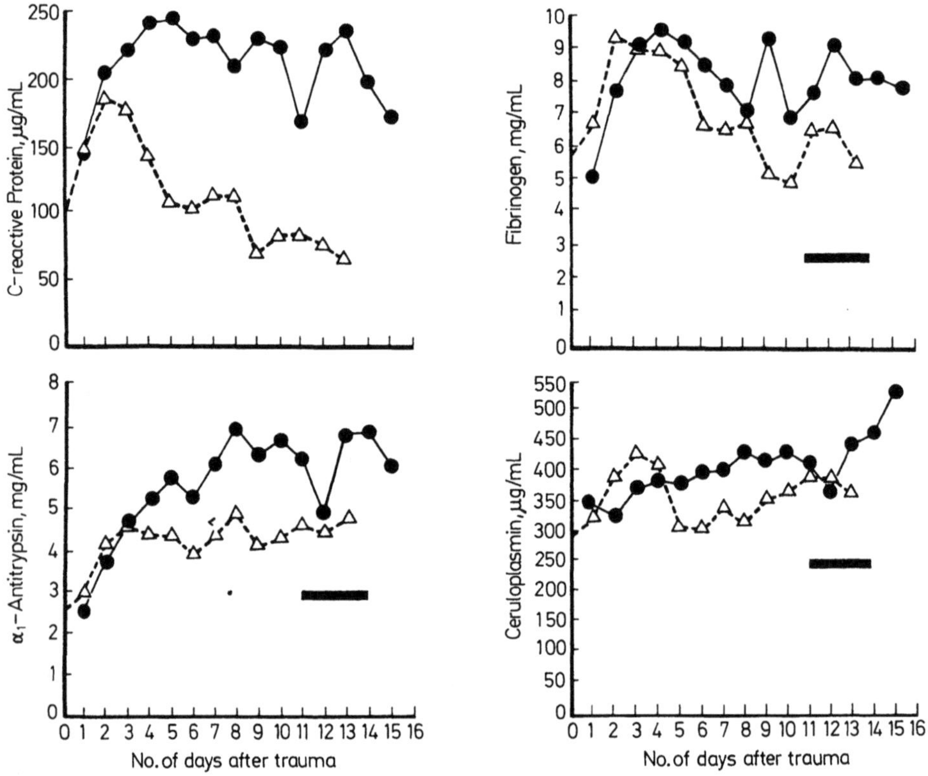

Fig. 1. Time course of positive acute-phase protein levels in septic and nonseptic trauma patients. (From Sganga et al. 1985)

The time course and the changes in levels of some of the acute-phase proteins following severe blunt trauma are given in Figs. 1–3. In Fig. 1 the levels of four proteins that increase (positive acute-phase proteins) are shown for two groups of trauma patients: those who eventually became septic and those who remained free of sepsis. Levels of all four proteins increased within a day or so in both groups of patients. The most dramatic changes occurred with C-reactive protein, which went from <1 µg/ml in control noninjured subjects to several hundred micrograms per milliliter in both groups of trauma patients. The increase in C-reactive protein was much more prolonged in patients who eventually became septic.

Figure 2 contains data on three plasma proteins that decrease following trauma. These proteins (negative acute-phase proteins) exhibited prolonged suppression that was similar in both groups of patients. Presumably, decreased levels of these proteins also contribute to the survival of the host. Lower levels of transferrin, for example, result in decreased amounts of iron being available for bacterial growth.

In man, fibronectin is a unique acute-phase protein (Fig. 3). Severe burn injury results in a transient decrease in plasma fibronectin, followed by elevated levels

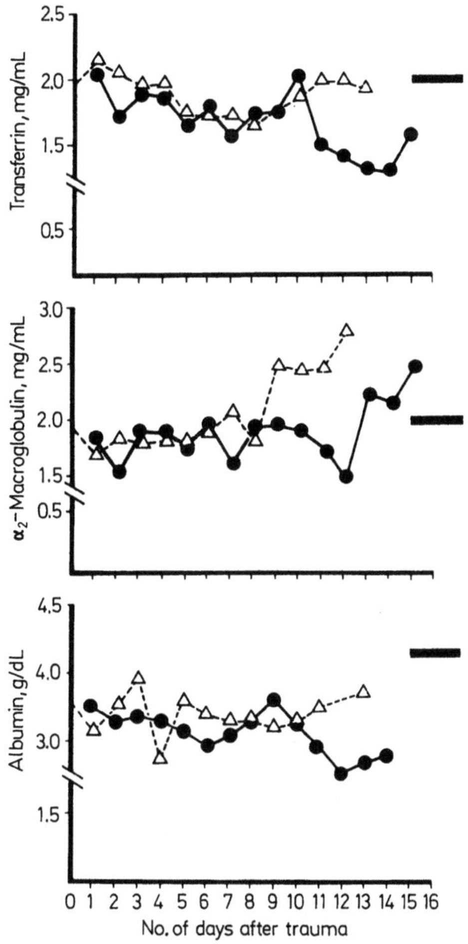

Fig. 2. Time course of negative acute-phase protein levels in septic and non-septic trauma patients. (From Sganga et al. 1985)

after about 2 days. In animals, this initial decrease is not seen (Pick-Korber et al. 1986). The initial decrease in man is probably due to increased peripheral binding of circulating fibronectin to injured tissue.

The acute-phase protein response is quite complicated in that acute-phase proteins differ in the extent to which their levels are altered and in the time course of these alterations. Furthermore, proteins that are acute-phase reactants in one species are sometimes not acute-phase proteins or are modulated to different extents in other species. For example, C-reactive protein is a very strong acute-phase protein in man in that its levels can increase a thousandfold within 24 h (Kushner et al. 1981) while its levels change only slightly in rats. Alpha-2-macroglobulin increases a fewfold in man, but a hundredfold in rats. Fibronectin levels increase severalfold almost immediately in rats, while in man fibronectin initially decreases then doubles after 2 days. The extreme diversity of changes in acute-phase protein levels raises the important question as to whether such disparate changes in production of these proteins (with such disparate biological functions) are controlled by the same mechanisms.

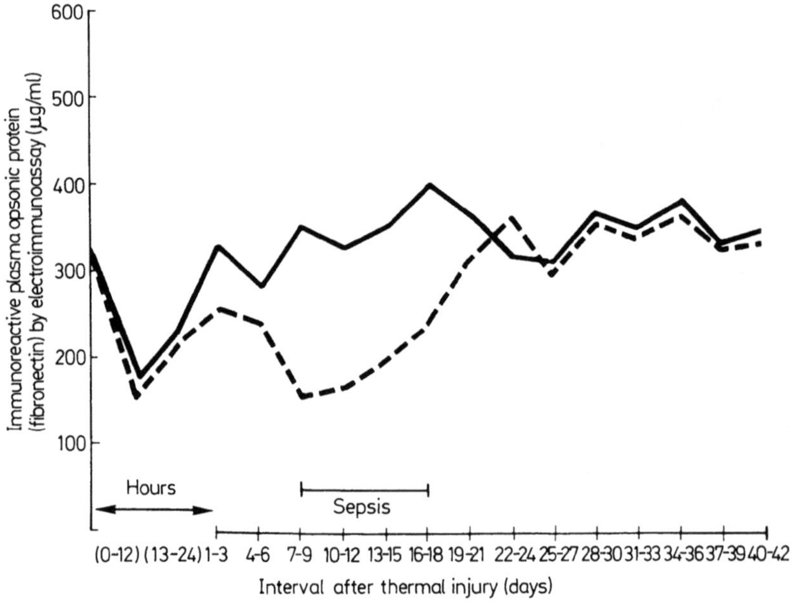

Fig. 3. Effect of burn on plasma fibronectin levels in both septic and nonseptic patients. (From Lanser et al. 1980)

A number of agents influence the acute-phase response in vivo. Substances secreted by stimulated monocytes are powerful modulators of acute-phase protein production when injected into experimental animals (Ramadori et al. 1985; Woloski et al. 1985). However, these in vivo studies must be interpreted with great care because they leave open the question as to whether the agent is acting directly on the hepatocytes or through an intermediary messenger.

Crude monokine preparations also affect the synthesis of acute-phase proteins by cultured hepatocytes and hepatoma cells, as shown in Table 2, which lists the effects of monocyte culture supernatants upon the synthesis of various acute-phase proteins by cultured rat hepatocytes, mouse hepatocytes, and human hepatoma cells. It is clear from these data that monocyte supernatants can induce almost all of the reported changes in acute-phase protein synthesis. The most notable exception is the inability of human hepatoma cells to be stimulated to produce large amounts of C-reactive protein. However, it is possible that monocyte supernatants could induce normal human hepatocytes to produce this protein.

Three specific proteins have been isolated from monocyte culture supernatants that affect the production of acute-phase proteins: interleukin 1 (IL-1), interleukin 6 (IL-6), and tumor necrosis factor (TNF). IL-1 was the first of these proteins to be implicated as the biological regulator of the acute-phase protein response. Table 3 lists the effect of purified IL-1 upon the synthesis of acute-phase proteins by cultured rat and mouse hepatocytes and by human hepatoma cells.

Several precautions need to be emphasized in interpreting these data. First, hepatocyte cultures are always contaminated by unknown amounts of nonparenchymal cells, such as Kupffer's cells. Since both Kupffer's cells and endothelial

Table 2. Monokine and cytokine modulation of acute-phase protein production by murine hepatocytes and human hepatoma cells

Inducing agent	Proteins affected	Assay cell	Ref.
Monocyte supernatants	Alpha-2-macroglobulin, Fibrinogen, Serum amyloid A	Hepatocytes	Bauer et al. (1986) Fuller et al. (1985) Selinger et al. (1980)
	Albumin, C3, Alpha-1-acid glycoprotein, Alpha-1-acute-phase protein, Alpha-1-antichymotrypsin, Alpha-1-fetoprotein, Fibrinogen, Haptoglobin, Transferrin	Hepatoma	Baumann et al. (1984) Darlington et al. (1986)
Colo-16 supernatants	Albumin, Alpha-1-acid glycoprotein, Alpha-1-acute-phase protein, Alpha-1-antichymotrypsin, Alpha-1-acute-phase protein, Alpha-1-cysteine proteinase inhibitor, Alpha-2-macroglobulin, Fibrinogen, Hemopexin, Haptoglobin	Hepatocytes	Baumann et al. (1984, 1986)
	Alpha-1-antichymotrypsin	Hepatoma	Baumann et al. (1985, 1986)
Keratinocyte supernatants	Alpha-1-cysteine proteinase inhibitior, Alpha-1-acid glycoprotein, Alpha-1-macroglobulin, Alpha-2-macroblobulin, Fibrinogen, Haptoglobin, Hemopexin, Serum amyloid A	Hepatocytes	Baumann et al. (1986) Sztein et al. (1982)
	Alpha-1-antichymotrypsin	Hepatoma	Baumann et al. (1984)
MCA-3 supernatants	Alpha-1-macroglobulin	Hepatocytes	Baumann et al. (1986)

Table 3. Modulation of acute-phase protein production by purified and recombinant

Inducing agent	Proteins affected	Assay cell	Ref.
Purified IL-1	Albumin, Factor B, Serum amyloid A, Serum amyloid P	Hepatocytes	Le and Mortensen (1984) Ramadori et al. (1985)
	Albumin, C3, Factor B	Hepatoma	Darlington et al. (1986) Perlmutter et al. (1986)
Recombinant IL-1	Albumin, Alpha-2-macroglobulin, Factor B, Serum amyloid A	Hepatocytes	Bauer et al. (1985) Ramadori et al. (1985)
	Albumin, C3	Hepatoma	Darlington et al. (1986)

cells can be induced to produce factors that affect synthesis of acute-phase proteins, the IL-1 preparation might not, in some cases, be affecting hepatocyte protein synthesis directly, but via its action on contaminating cells. Data obtained using hepatoma cell cultures avoid this difficulty. Second, monokines are notoriously difficult to purify away from contaminating bioactive proteins. Since monokines are often effective at sub-nanogram per milliliter concentrations, even very minor impurities could be responsible for the reported activities. For example, commercial IL-1 preparations have often been contaminated with significant amounts of IL-6. Preferably, recombinant IL-1 should be used in conjunction with neutralizing antibody specific for IL-1 (and for other monokines such as IL-6 and TNF) for such experiments. The effects of recombinant IL-1 upon the synthesis of acute-phase proteins are also listed in Table 3. Fortunately, data obtained with recombinant IL-1 largely confirm those obtained with purified IL-1.

Tumor necrosis factor has been reported to stimulate production of certain acute-phase proteins (Table 4). Once again care must be taken in interpreting these data since TNF can induce IL-1 production (Dinarello et al. 1986), which may be responsible for some of the reported effects of TNF. Nevertheless, TNF does appear to induce synthesis of some of the acute-phase proteins which are also induced by IL-1.

A third monokine, hepatocyte-stimulating factor (HSF), appears to be very important in the control of acute-phase protein production. HSF (also known as IL-6, B-cell-stimulating factor 2, and interferon-B_2) has a variety of biological actions, including stimulation of IgG synthesis by B cells, pyrogenic activity, and antiviral activity, in addition to its effects on hepatocyte protein synthesis. This factor, isolated by Fuller et al. (1987), was initially characterized by its ability to stimulate the production of fibrinogen. The production of many acute-phase proteins is probably modulated by IL-6.

We have been studying the ability of crude monokine preparations and of recombinant IL-6 to control hepatocyte production of fibronectin. This protein appears to be critical for opsonization of certain types of foreign particles and for activation of the phagocytic capacity of neutrophils and macrophages. Furthermore, control of production of this protein may be unusual because of its two-phase response to injury in man. Plasma fibronectin is produced primarily by hepatocytes (Tamkun and Hynes 1983). Crude monokine preparations stimulate fibronectin synthesis by cultured hepatocytes (Table 5). Furthermore, monokine preparations derived from lipopolysaccharide (LPS)-stimulated monocyte cultures are more potent than preparations derived from control or from polymyxin B-treated cultures. Recombinant IL-6 strongly stimulates fibronectin synthesis,

Table 4. Modulation of acute-phase protein production in human hepatoma cells by TNF

Inducer	Proteins affected	Ref.
Purified TNF	Albumin, C3	Darlington et al. (1986)
Recombinant TNF	Albumin, Alpha-1-antichymotrypsin, C3, Factor B, Transferrin	Perlmutter et al. (1986)

Table 5. Regulation of fibronectin synthesis by a crude monokine preparation

Inducer	Fibronectin (μg/ml)	Fold stimulation
None[a]	1.22±0.16 (n=8)	1.00
Supernatant	1.50±0.23 (n=7)	1.26±0.19
Polymyxin B supernatant	1.38±0.32 (n=3)	1.16±0.17
Lipopolysaccharide supernatant	2.45±0.40 (n=7)	2.08±0.52

[a] Fifty microliters of either control media or monocyte culture supernatant was added to hepatocyte cultures fed with 300 μl complete medium. Monocytes were cultured for 24 h at 37° C in RPMI 1640 (Gibco), 5% fetal bovine serum, 100 μ/ml penicillin, 100 μg/ml streptomycin, and plus or minus 20 μg/ml polymyxin B sulfate or 5 μg/ml lipopolysaccharide (LPS, Re595).

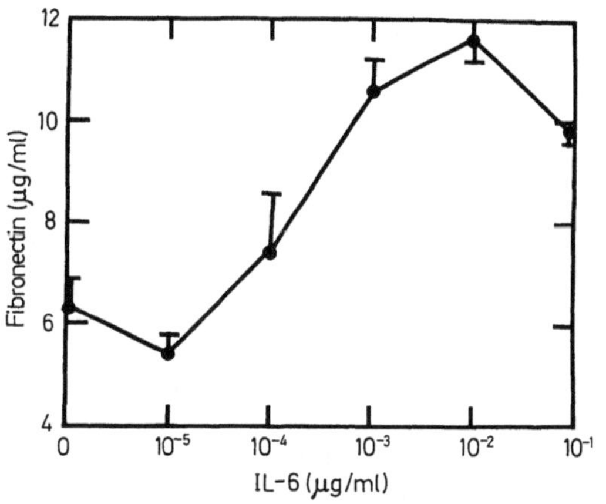

Fig. 4. Effect of recombinant IL-6 on fibronectin production by rat hepatocytes in vitro

even at doses as low as 100 pg/ml (Fig. 4). Stimulating activity peaks at 10 ng/ml, followed by lesser stimulation at higher doses. This suggests that hyperinduction of IL-6 might actually suppress synthesis of some of the acute-phase proteins.

Are there other factors that modulate the production of acute-phase proteins? While IL-1, TNF, and IL-6 appear to be capable of directly controlling synthesis of acute-phase proteins, many other factors both induce the synthesis of these three monokines and modulate their function. For example, interferon-gamma augments production of TNF-alpha induced by IL-2 (Nedwin et al. 1985). Furthermore, in a wide variety of systems, interferons modify the effectiveness of TNF (Williamson et al. 1983). The possibility that individual monokines modulate the haptocyte-stimulating activity of other monokines has yet to be carefully investigated.

Steroids may regulate the acute-phase response. Steroids inhibit the response to IL-1 in vivo. Since IL-1 injection increases glucocorticoid levels (Besedovsky et al. 1986), glucocorticoids might function in a negative feedback manner to limit the acute-phase response. Newer data, obtained in vitro, indicate that suppression of acute-phase protein production by steroids is due to inhibition of the production of monokines that modulate hepatocyte protein synthesis (Beutler et al.

1986). Steroids (dexamethasone) can also directly stimulate production of some acute-phase proteins [e.g., alpha-1-acid glycoprotein (Baumann and Held 1981), fibrinogen (Otto et al. 1987), fibronectin (Nimmer et al. 1987)] and can make hepatocytes more responsive to hepatocyte-stimulating factors (Bauer et al. 1986; Otto et al. 1987). Thus, steroids can simultaneously have both suppressive and stimulatory effects on acute-phase protein production. Certainly, in vivo, the effect of natural steroids is undoubtedly very complicated and might serve to help fine-tune the production of the acute-phase proteins.

Do cells other than monocytes and macrophages make factors that control production of acute-phase proteins and, if so, how important is their contribution to this control? Endothelial cells can be stimulated by TNF to produce IL-1 (Nawroth et al. 1986). In addition, keratinocytes make factors that stimulate production of several acute-phase proteins (Bauer et al. 1986; Sztein et al. 1982). Keratinocytes may make several such factors (Baumann et al. 1986). However, whether these factors are identical to IL-1, IL-6, TNF, or other known monokines has not been determined. Since these cells appear to produce these factors constitutively, the possibility exists that these cytokines are produced as an artifact of tissue culture. Nonetheless, it is clear that cells other than monocytes and macrophages do have the capacity of producing factors with potent hepatocyte-stimulating activity.

What agents induce the production of these hepatocyte-stimulating monokines? Two categories of agents have been reported. Tissue products, i.e., fibrinogen fragments D and E (Ritchie and Fuller 1983), appear to be sufficient to induce IL-6. Other tissue products induced by injury can also induce production of these monokines. Products from gram-negative bacteria, i.e., LPS, are also powerful inducers of monokine production. The ability of other bacterial products, e.g., formylated peptides, to induce hepatocyte-stimulating factors has not been systematically investigated. Thus, both tissue-derived and infectious agent-derived products can induce monocytes and macrophages to produce hepatocyte-stimulating factors.

By what mechanisms do hepatocyte-stimulating factors enhance production of acute-phase proteins? Messenger RNA levels have been investigated for several proteins following induction of the acute-phase response. In vivo, the acute-phase response is associated with increased mRNA levels (Glibetic and Baumann 1986). In cultured hepatocytes, treatment with monocyte supernatants also results in increased levels of specific mRNAs (Baumann et al. 1986; Fuller et al. 1985; Hayashida et al. 1985; Northemann et al. 1985; Otto et al. 1987; Perlmutter et al. 1986; Ramadori et al. 1985). Furthermore, experiments with isolated nuclei have shown that injury results in increased mRNA transcription (Northemann et al. 1985). Thus, hepatocyte-stimulating activities appear to control the transcription of mRNA for the acute-phase proteins.

The obvious conclusion to be drawn from these data is that there is considerable redundancy in the control of acute-phase protein production. That is, although the production of some proteins appears to be stimulated by only one monokine, the production of others is stimulated by all three monokines and sometimes by other cytokines. In addition, agents that stimulate monokine production commonly induce many monokines. But what is the biological significance of this redundancy? This redundancy probably evolved in order to ensure this response following injury even in the absence of one or more of these monokines. Additionally, by virtue of the tissues affected and the nature of the injury, production of variable amounts of different hepatocyte-stimulating factors may be induced. Since these factors alter the production of overlapping but nonidentical groups of proteins, different types of injury may induce different acute-phase protein responses. We hypothesize that the evolution of this ability to induce different responses results in a "tailored" response to ensure survival from a variety of insults.

References

Bauer J, Weber W, Tran-Thi T-A, Northoff G-H, Decker K, Gerok W, Heinrich PC (1985) Murine interleukin 1 stimulates alpha-2-macroglobulin synthesis in rat hepatocyte primary cultures. FEBS 190:271–274

Bauer J, Tran-Thi T-A, Northoff H, Hirsch F, Schlayer H-J, Gerok W, Heinrich PC (1986) The acute-phase induction of alpha-2-macroglobulin in rat hepatocyte primary cultures: action of a hepatocyte-stimulating factor, triiodothyronine and dexamethasone. Eur J Cell Biol 40:86–93

Baumann H, Held WA (1981) Biosynthesis and hormone-regulated expression of secretory glycoproteins in rat liver and hepatoma cells. J Biol Chem 256:10145–10155

Baumann H, Jahreis GP, Sauder DN, Koj A (1984) Human keratinocytes and monocytes release factors which regulate the synthesis of major acute phase plasma proteins in hepatic cell from man, rat, and mouse. J Biol Chem 259:7331–7342

Baumann H, Hill RE, Sauder DN, Jahreis GP (1986) Regulation of major acute-phase plasma proteins by hepatocyte-stimulating factors of human squamous carcinoma cell. J Cell Biol 102:370–383

Besedovsky H, del Rey A, Sorkin E, Dinarello CA (1986) Immunoregulatory feedback between interleukin-1 and glucocorticoid hormones. Science 233:652–654

Beutler B, Krochin N, Milsark IW, Luedke C, Cerami A (1986) Control of cachectin (tumor necrosis factor) synthesis: mechanisms of endotoxin resistance. Science 232:977–980

Darlington GJ, Wilson DR, Lachman LB (1986) Monocyte-conditioned medium, interleukin-1, and tumor necrosis factor stimulate the acute phase response in human hepatoma cells in vitro. J Cell Biol 103:787–793

Dinarello CA, Cannon JG, Wolff SM, Bernheim HA, Beutler B, Cerami A, Figari IS, Palladino MA Jr, O'Connor JV (1986) Tumor necrosis factor (cachectin) is an endogenous pyrogen and induces production of interleukin 1. J Exp Med 163:1433–1450

Fuller GM, Otto JM, Woloski BM, McGary CT, Adams MA (1985) The effects of hepatocyte stimulating factor on fibrinogen biosynthesis in hepatocyte monolayers. J Cell Biol 101:1481–1486

Fuller GM, Bunzel RJ, Woloski BM, Nham S-U (1987) Isolation of hepatocyte stimulating factor from human monocytes. Biochem Biophys Res Commun 144:1003–1009

Glibetic MD, Baumann H (1986) Influence of chronic inflammation on the level of mRNA for acute-phase reactants in the mouse liver. J Immunol 137:1616–1622

Hayashida K, Okubo H, Noguchi M, Yoshida H, Kangawa K, Matsuo H, Sakaki Y (1985) Molecular cloning of DNA complementary to rat alpha-2-macroglobulin mRNA. J Biol Chem 260:14224–14229

Kushner I, Gewurz H, Benson MD (1981) C-reactive protein and the acute-phase response. J Lab Clin Med 97:739–749

Lanser ME, Saba TM, Scovill WA (1980) Opsonic glycoprotein (plasma fibronectin) levels after thermal injury. Ann Surg 188:521–529

Le PT, Mortensen RF (1984) Mouse hepatocyte synthesis and induction of the acute phase reactant: serum amyloid P-component. In Vitro Cell Devel Biol 20:505–511

Mortensen RF, Sarlo K, Le PT (1984) Monokine-induced hepatocyte synthesis of acute-phase reactants in mice. Lymphokine Res 3:17–22

Nawroth PP, Bank I, Handley D, Cassimeris J, Chess L, Stern D (1986) Tumor necrosis factor/cachectin interacts with endothelial cell receptors to induce release of interleukin 1. J Exp Med 163:1363–1375

Nedwin GE, Svedersky LP, Bringman TS, Palladino MA Jr, Goeddel DV (1985) Effect of interleukin 2, interferon-gamma, and mitogens on the production of tumor necrosis factors alpha and beta. J Immunol 135:2492–2497

Nimmer D, Bergtrom G, Hirano H, Amrani DL (1987) Regulation of plasma fibronectin biosynthesis by glucocorticoids in chick hepatocyte cultures. J Biol Chem 262:10369–10375

Northemann W, Heisig M, Kunz D, Heinrich PC (1985) Molecular cloning of cDNA sequences for rat alpha-2-macroglobulin and measurement of its transcription during experimental inflammation. J Biol Chem 260:6200–6205

Otto JM, Grenett HE, Fuller GM (1987) The coordinated regulation of fibrinogen gene transcription by hepatocyte-stimulating factor and dexamethasone. J Cell Biol 105:1067–1072

Perlmutter DH, Dinarello CA, Punsal PI, Colten HR (1986) Cachectin/tumor necrosis factor regulates hepatic acute-phase gene expression. J Clin Invest 78:1349–1354

Perlmutter DH, Goldberger G, Dinarello CA, Mizel SB, Colten HR (1986) Regulation of class III major histocompatability complex gene products by interleukin-1. Science 232:850–852

Pick-Kober KH, Munker D, Gressner AM (1986) Fibronectin is synthesized as an acute phase reactant in rat hepatocytes. J Clin Chem Clin Biochem 24:521–528

Ramadori G, Sipe JD, Dinarello CA, Mizel SB, Colten HR (1985) Pretranslational modulation of acute phase hepatic protein synthesis by murine recombinant interleukin 1 (IL-1) and purified human IL-1. J Exp Med 162:930–942

Ritchie DG, Fuller GM (1983) Hepatocyte-stimulating factor: a monocyte-derived acute-phase regulatory protein. Ann NY Acad Sci 408:490–499

Selinger MJ, McAdam KPWJ, Kaplan MM, Sipe JD, Vogel SN, Rosenstreich DL (1980) Monokine-induced synthesis of serum amyloid A protein by hepatocytes. Nature 285:498–500

Sganga G, Siegel JH, Brown G, Coleman WP, Wiles CI III, Belzberg H, Wedel S, Placko R (1985) Reprioritization of hepatic plasma protein release in trauma and sepsis. Arch Surg 120:187–199

Sztein MB, Luger TA, Oppenheim JJ (1982) An epidermal cell-derived cytokine triggers the in vivo synthesis of serum amyloid a by hepatocytes. J Immunol 129:87–90

Tamkun JW, Hynes RO (1983) Plasma fibronectin is synthesized and secreted by hepatocytes. J Biol Chem 258:4641–4647

Williamson BD, Carswell EA, Rubin BY, Prendergast JS, Old LJ (1983) Human tumor necrosis factor produced by human b-cell lines: synergistic cyktotoxic interaction with human interferon. Proc Natl Acad Sci USA 80:5397–5401

Woloski BMRNJ, Gospodarek E, Jamieson JC (1985) Studies on monokines as mediators of the acute phase response: effects on sialytransferase, albumin, alpha-1-acid glycoprotein and beta-*N*-acetylhexosaminidase. Biochem Biophys Res Commun 130:30–36

Elastase from Polymorphonuclear Leukocytes, Complement, and C-Reactive Protein in Multiple Trauma Patients

K. H. Muhrer, P. Quoika, M. Schütterle, and P. Martin

Introduction

The severity of injury in multiple trauma is classified as a rule according to anatomical injury patterns and pathological alterations of vital functions (Oestern et al. 1985). The immunological reactions to a severe mechanical trauma with extensive tissue and organ lesions have been inadequately investigated up to now. The objective of this study was to investigate the effects of mechanical trauma on defense mechanisms of the body in relation to the severity of injury. Nonspecific humoral and cellular defense mechanisms are more prominent compared with the specific immune response delay in time. Leukocyte immigration and phagocytosis, release of lysosomal enzymes, and mobilization of acute-phase proteins constitute so to speak the "first line of defense."

Methods

Measurement of Nonspecific Defense Mechanisms (Fig. 1)

Elastase from Polymorphonuclear Leukocytes (PMN Elastase)

PMN elastase has a biological function in the breakdown of phagocytosed material within the cell (Havemann and Janoff 1978). In the degranulation of leukocytes, this enzyme is released from the cells into the surrounding medium. In massive enzyme secretion, the inhibitor concentration of this enzyme is exceeded locally, so that it is flushed into the bloodstream. Here, the PMN elastase is bound to inhibitors as a complex. The concentration of this PMN-elastase inhibitor complex in the serum serves as a measure for the PMN elastase released. It is determined by means of an enzmye immunoassay (Merck, Darmstadt).

Complement Factors C_3 and C_4

By quantitative determination of the complement factors C_3 and C_4, the involvement of the complement system in mechanical trauma is to be investigated. The complement protein C_4 reacts immediately after C_1 (recognition unit) and elicits the "classical reaction pathway." C_3 belongs to the activation unit in the cascade chain and takes a central place in the "alternative pathway." C_3 and C_4 were determined quantitatively by radial immunodiffusion (Behringwerke Ltd., Marburg/Lahn).

Immune Consequences of
Trauma, Shock and Sepsis
Eds. Faist/Ninnemann/Green

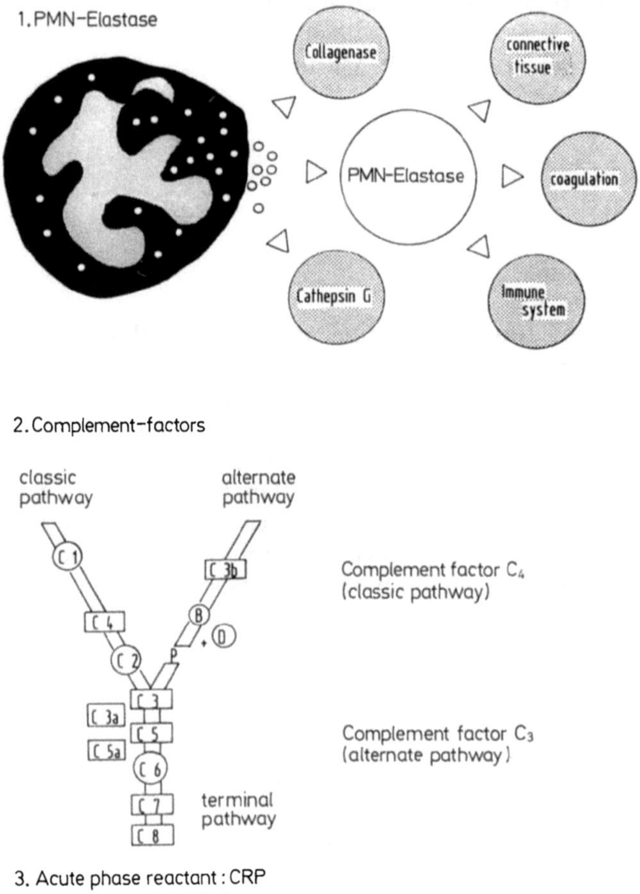

Fig. 1. Methods: laboratory parameters

C-Reactive Protein

C-Reactive protein (CRP) is regarded as a classical acute-phase protein. The acute-phase reaction is based on an intensified synthesis and release of a heterogeneous group of plasma proteins by the liver within 24 h. The quantitative detection was also carried out by radial immunodiffusion (Behringwerke Ltd., Marburg/Lahn).

Antithrombin III (AT III)

Antithrombin III inactivates thrombin and factor Xa and is the most important natural inhibitor of blood clotting. AT III is inter alia the substrate of free PMN elastase. An intensified degradation of AT III can given rise to disseminating intravascular coagulation. The determination of AT III was carried out by radial immunodiffusion (Behringwerke Ltd., Marburg/Lahn).

Patients

The investigations were carried out in 31 patients (21 men, 10 women, average age 30 years) who displayed a different severity of injury. In accordance with the Hannover classification of the degree of severity (Oestern 1985), 10 patients each were assigned to the severity grades I and II, 5 patients to the severity grade III, and 6 patients to the severity grade IV. Twenty-two patients survived, and nine patients died of their injuries.

Results

1. The PMN elastase was raised in all injured persons a few hours after the accident event and in the further course. In surviving patients, a tendency to fall was noticeable within 6 days. Lethal courses showed values which were highly raised initially without a tendency to normalization (Fig. 2). Severe multiple trauma cases (groups III and IV) displayed higher elastase values than patients with a lower injury severity (groups I and II) (Fig. 2).
2. The complement factor C_3 was always in the normal range in the multiple-trauma phase, and there was no difference between survivors and lethal courses. A dependence on the degree of severity of multiple trauma could not be demonstrated. In nonseptic course, the values did not fall below the normal range (Fig. 2).

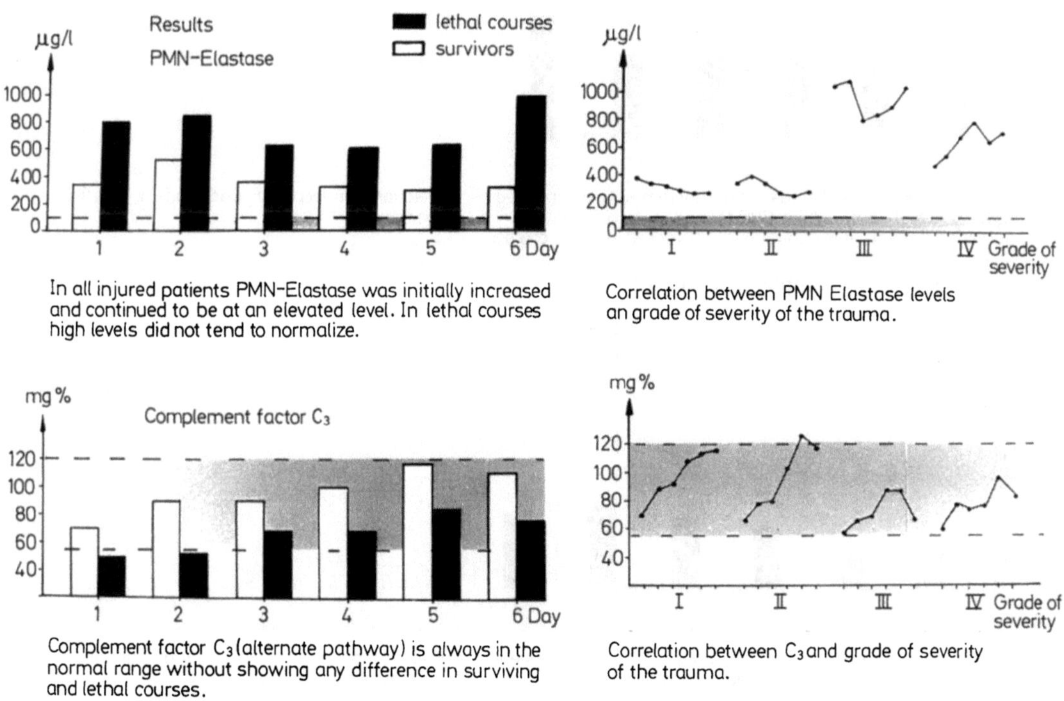

Fig. 2. Results: PMN elastase and complement factor C_3

3. The complement factor C_4 (classical reaction pathway) was within the normal range after the accident and in the post-traumatic phase. Lethal courses did not differ significantly from surviving patients. A dependence on the degree of severity of multiple trauma was not apparent (Fig. 3).
4. The acute-phase protein CRP was initially raised in all injured persons and was several times higher than normal in the further course. Whereas a tendency to fall could be discerned in the survivors within 6 days, the values rose con-

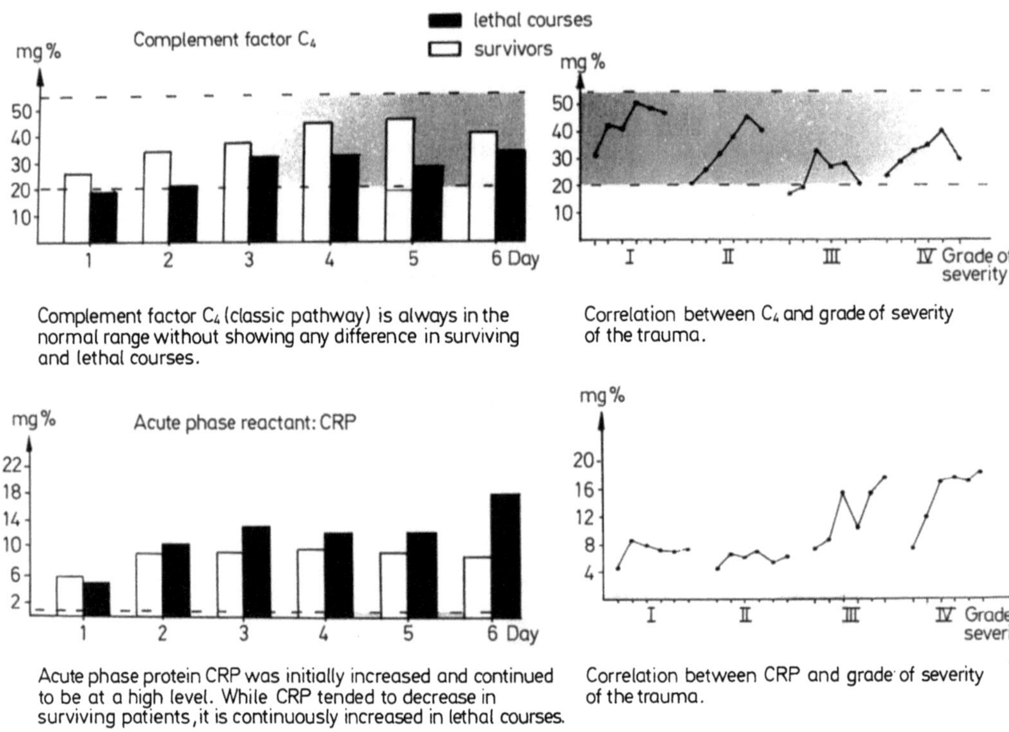

Fig. 3. Results: complement factor C_4

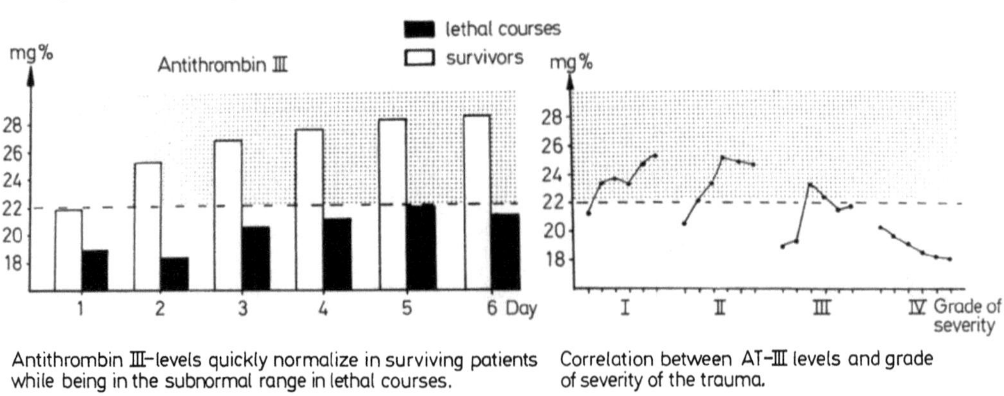

Fig. 4. Results: antithrombin III

tinuously in patients with a lethal course (Fig. 3). Severely injured patients showed higher CRP values than patients with less-pronounced injuries (Fig. 3).
5. The antithrombin III values of surviving patients normalized within 3 days, whereas the values of lethal courses were always in the subnormal range (Fig. 4). A dependence of the AT III level on the degree of severity of multiple trauma could be demonstrated (Fig. 4).

Discussion

The humoral and cellular mechanisms of nonspecific resistance to tissue traumatization are complex. The results of this study show that proteinases are released like elastase from polymorphonuclear leukocytes after severe trauma. The extent of their release correlates with the degree of severity of multiple trauma.

Besides elastin, biological substrates of PMN elastase are also immunoglobulins, the clotting factors AT III, factor XIII, and complement factors. Although natural inhibitors such as the alpha 1 proteinase inhibitor and alpha 2 macroglobulin neutralize the PMN elastase, in massive release of PMN elastase disturbances of the clotting system by degradation of antithrombin III can result. The complement system can be defined as cytotoxic activity which leads to cell lysis after activation. According to the present investigations, the complement system does not appear to be activated primarily in the early phase after a mechanical trauma. This applies in particular to the classical reaction pathway (C_4), for which a specific antigen-antibody reaction (immune complex) is a prerequisite "trigger." The "alternative pathway" is antibody independent, bypasses the early reaction, and leads directly to activation (cleavage) of C_3 by certain autologous or bacterial components such as endotoxin. A consumption of the complement factor C_3 could not be demonstrated in the first post-traumatic phase. Serum endotoxin determinations performed in parallel did not reveal any indications of endotoxinemia.

The acute-phase reaction is regarded as a general, nonspecific response to tissue damage of the most diverse kind. After acute tissue lesion, there is a distinct, measurable rise in the C-reactive protein within 24 h. The duration and level of the CRP rise proved to depend on the extent of tissue damage. This is known to be true for inflammatory lesions. CRP is also mobilized at a very early stage after trauma. The serum levels correlated with the degree of severity of the trauma.

Summary and Conclusion

In patients afflicted with multiple trauma, elastase from PMNs is set free shortly after the accident. The quantity of liberated elastase is correlated with the grade of severity of the trauma. Lethal courses initially show extremely high levels without a tendency to normalize.

Early after injuries the acute-phase protein CRP is mobilized. Its level correlates to the grade of severity of the injuries.

In the early phase after trauma the complement system does not yet seem to be activated.

Decreased AT-III levels in patients with third- or fourth-grade traumas have to be interpreted as latent DIC.

References

Havemann K, Janoff A (eds) (1978) Neutral proteases of human polymorphonuclear leukocytes. Urban and Schwarzenberg, Baltimore

Oestern H-J, Tscherne H, Sturm J, Nerlich M (1985) Klassifizierung der Verletzungsschwere. Unfallchirurg 88:465–472

Flow Cytometric Analysis of Phagocytosis, Respiratory Burst, Intracellular pH, and Cytosolic Free Calcium of Granulocytes of Post-traumatic and Septic Patients *

G. Rothe, W. Kellermann, and G. Valet

Sepsis and trauma-related organ failure is intimately related to granulocyte functions. Granulocytes protect the organism against bacterial invasion but may also cause endothelial damage due to the release of reactive oxygen intermediates and proteolytic enzymes. The purpose of this study was the analysis of cell-biochemical parameters of granulocytes by flow cytometry and the use of the multifunctional parameter pattern for the prediction of sepsis- and trauma-related pulmonary and cardiovascular organ failure.

Materials and Methods

Buffy coat leukocytes were prepared from 236 samples of heparinized (10 U/ml) venous blood obtained serially from 55 patients of an intensive care unit. The leukocytes were sedimented at the erythrocyte/plasma interface by centrifugation at 200 g and 4 °C for 10 min. The surface layer of cells was carefully removed and resuspended in the supernatant plasma to a final concentration of 3.5×10^7 leukocytes/ml.

A suspension of 7×10^9 *E. coli* K12 bacteria (Sigma, Deisenhofen, FRG) in HEPES-buffered saline (HBS) (0.15 *M* NaCl, 5 m*M* HEPES, Serva, Heidelberg, FRG, pH 7.35) was prepared as described earlier [1]. One hundred microliters of the leukocytes suspended in autologous plasma were incubated with 10 µl of the *E. coli* suspension at 37 °C. Controls were incubated with HBS alone. Aliquots of 30 µl were taken at 15, 30, and 60 min respectively, diluted with 3 ml cold HBS, and stored on ice.

The phagocytic samples and control samples were each divided into five samples and incubated with different stains. Stock solutions of all dyes were made in *N,N*-dimethylformamide (DMF) (Merck, Darmstadt, FRG). Phagocytosis and degradation of bacterial DNA were measured as described in [1] after staining of the samples for 15 min at 4 °C in the presence of 8 µg/ml acridine orange (AO) (stock solution 0.4 mg/ml, Sigma). Intracellular pH and esterase activity were measured following 30 min incubation of the samples at 4 °C in the presence of 82 µ*M* 1,4-diacetoxy-2,3-dicyanobenzene (ADB) (stock solution 4.1 m*M*, Paesel, Frankfurt, FRG), which is cleaved intracellularly by esterases to the pH indicator 2,3-dicyano-hydroquinone (DCH) and acetate [2]. Cytosolic-free calcium was measured after 30 min incubation at 37 °C with INDO-1 AM (stock so-

* This work was supported by DFG SFB 0207, project G6.

Immune Consequences of
Trauma, Shock and Sepsis
Eds. Faist/Ninnemann/Green

lution 1 m*M*, Calbiochem, Frankfurt, FRG) at a final concentration of 2 μ*M* [3]. The phagosomal peroxidase-mediated hydrogen peroxide metabolism was measured after staining for 15 min at 37 °C in the presence of 10 μ*M* 2′,7′-dichlorfluorescein diacetate (stock solution 10 m*M*, Serva, Heidelberg, FRG), which following cleavage is oxidized intracellularly to 2′,7′-dichlorfluorescein (DCF) [4]. NADPH oxidase activity was measured through the intracellular oxidation of hydroethidine (HE) (stock solution 63.5 m*M*, Polyscience, St. Goar, FRG) to ethidium bromide (EB) after incubation for 15 min at 37 °C at a concentration of 160 μ*M* HE [5].

For the analysis of maximal achievable respiratory burst activity 10 μl of the leukocyte suspension was diluted with 1 ml HBS, prestained for 15 min at 37 °C in the presence of 10 μ*M* DCFH-DA and/or 160 μ*M* hydroethidine, and stimulated for an additional 30 min at 37 °C with 150 n*M* phorbol 12-myristate 13-acetate (PMA) (stock solution 1.5 m*M* in DMF, Sigma).

Propidium iodide (PI) (Sigma) was added at a final concentration of 60 μ*M* 3 min prior to the flow-cytometric measurement to counterstain the DNA of dead cells.

The electrical cell volume and two fluorescences of each cell were measured simultaneously with a Fluvo-Metricell flow cytometer (HEKA-Elektronik, Lambrecht/Pfalz, FRG). The electrical cell volume was determined in a hydrodynamically focused cylindrical sizing orifice 80 μm in diameter and 80 μm in length at an electrical current of 0.15 mA using HBS as the sheath fluid. Fluorescence was excited with a HBO-100 high-pressure mercury arc lamp (Osram, Augsburg, FRG). DCH and INDO-1 fluorescence were excited between 340 and 400 nm and emission collected between 420 and 450 nm and above 500 nm. The fluorescences of AO, DCF, and EB were excited between 450 and 500 nm and measured between 500 and 530 nm and above 590 nm. The list-mode data were evaluated by the DIAGNOS1 program system for calculation, display, and databasing of flow cytometric data [6]. Between 12 and 24 parameters were automatically calculated for each measurement and transferred to a self-learning data base.

The prospectively identified patients were classified for each day of the study on the basis of pulmonary and/or cardiovascular organ failure of infectious or traumatic origin into four categories: (T) post-traumatic organ failure within 6 days following a trauma with a mean trauma score >21 [7], (S) septic organ failure according to the definition of Montgomery et al. [8] (in addition either an infectious focus or a positive blood culture was present), (M) transition state, or (N) stable pulmonary and cardiovascular function after recovery from organ failure. The significance of the differences between groups was evaluated using the nonparametric Kruskal-Wallis one-way analysis of variance. A discriminant analysis based on the stepwise reduction of Wilks' lambda was calculated using the SPSS/PC+ package (SPSS, Chicago, USA).

Results and Discussion

Twenty-three of the 55 patients of this study developed at least one septic episode and 15 of the patients had post-traumatic organ failure in the absence of bacterial

Table 1. Functional parameters of phagocytosing and phorbol-ester-stimulated granulocytes as determined by flow cytometry

Parameters	Min	Stimulant	Clinical classification of the patients			Significance
			Normal ($n=146$)	Sepsis ($n=28$)	Trauma ($n=22$)	
Cell volume (% of control)	30	*E. coli*	139.2 ± 1.8[b]	140.5 ± 3.5	158.9 ± 7.8	0.037**
	90	*E. coli*	126.4 ± 1.6	129.0 ± 4.0	140.3 ± 7.3	0.313
AO green fluorescence (% of control)	30	*E. coli*	123.4 ± 2.3	122.2 ± 5.0	125.4 ± 4.9	0.783
	90	*E. coli*	134.5 ± 2.0	130.4 ± 5.1	135.1 ± 6.0	0.754
Internal pH	30	–	7.53 ± 0.02	7.64 ± 0.05	7.46 ± 0.06	0.059
	30	*E. coli*	7.47 ± 0.03	7.60 ± 0.05	7.35 ± 0.07	0.017**
Dead cells (% of leukocytes)	30	–	11.9 ± 0.7	11.3 ± 1.4	17.8 ± 3.8	0.040**
	30	*E. coli*	12.8 ± 0.9	11.5 ± 1.3	16.6 ± 4.2	0.443
Granulocytes (% of leukocytes)	0	–	66.2 ± 1.1	73.6 ± 1.9	76.8 ± 2.4	0.000**
			Normal ($n=27$)	Sepsis ($n=5$)	Trauma ($n=2$)	
Internal Ca^2 (F1/F2 ratio)	30	–	14.1 ± 0.2[b]	14.9 ± 0.6	15.5 ± 0.1	0.110
	30	*E. coli*	14.5 ± 0.2	15.5 ± 0.6	16.2 ± 0.6	0.049**
DCF fluorescence (% of control)	15	*E. coli*	401.0 ± 36.6	280.3 ± 50.7	153.4 ± 19.1	0.049**
	30	PMA	698.4 ± 66.4	723.0 ± 112.0	249.8 ± 9.5	0.061
EB fluorescence (% of control)	15	*E. coli*	174.0 ± 9.6	150.4 ± 9.9	176.8 ± 9.1	0.442
	30	PMA	333.2 ± 10.4	361.3 ± 16.3	371.6 ± 21.6	0.222

** $P<0.05$; Kruskal-Wallis one-way analysis of variance.
[a] Classification as described in "Methods." Groups (M) and (N) are combined.
[b] ±SEM.

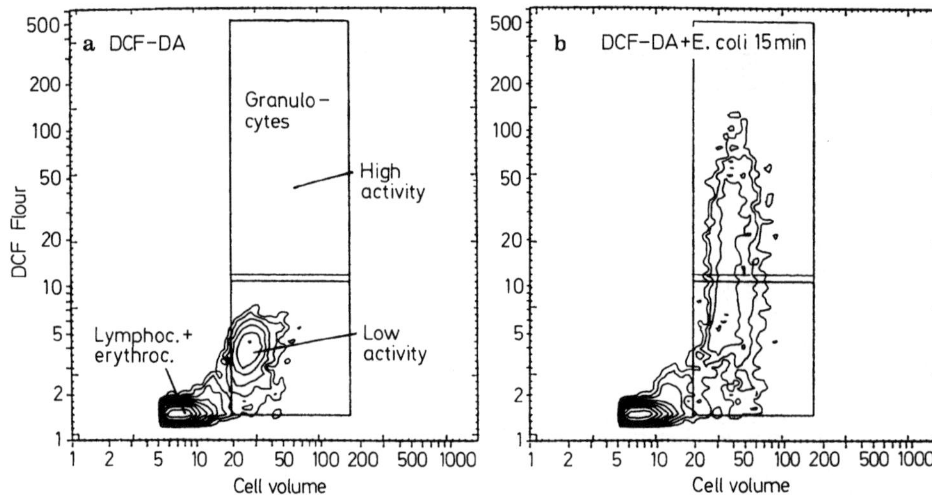

Fig. 1 a, b. Cell volume versus 2′,7′-dichlorfluorescein-fluorescence of buffy coat leukocytes after 15 min incubation at 37 °C in the absence **a** or presence **b** of *E. coli*. The phagosomal peroxide level is increased after phagocytosis of bacteria. Dead cells are excluded from the display through gating on the simultaneously measured red fluorescence of DNA stained with PI

infection. Four patients developed sepsis following post-traumatic organ failure. Thirty-three of the 236 samples were obtained during septic episodes and 24 samples were obtained during post-traumatic organ failure.

Twenty-two of the 49 parameters of granulocyte function obtained by processing the flow-cytometric list mode with the DIAGNOS1 program system showed significant differences between samples obtained from septic patients, patients with post-traumatic organ failure, and patients in stable condition after recovery from organ failure. Granulocytes from post-traumatic patients were discriminated by increased phagocytosis of *E. coli* as measured by increased cell volume during incubation with *E. coli* and increased green fluorescence due to the ingested bacterial DNA (Table 1). The intracellular pH of the granulocytes was more acidic and more cells died during phagocytosis. The cytosolic-free calcium concentration was increased and peroxidase activity was decreased during phagocytosis (Fig. 1) and after stimulation with PMA (Fig. 2) despite unchanged NADPH oxidase activity. Granulocytes from septic patients had an alkaline pH but the mean uptake of bacteria was unchanged. NADPH oxidase activity and peroxidase activity were both depressed in phagocytosing but not in PMA-stimulated cells, which may reflect a defect in the activation cascade of the respiratory burst during sepsis.

Three canonical discriminant functions derived from stepwise variable selection based on the reduction of Wilks' lambda were used for the classification of granulocytes according to this functional pattern. Ninety percent of the post-traumatic samples and 78% of the septic samples were correctly classified by this procedure, the remainder being misclassified as transition state. No samples from patients in the (N) state were misclassified as septic or post-traumatic. This dis-

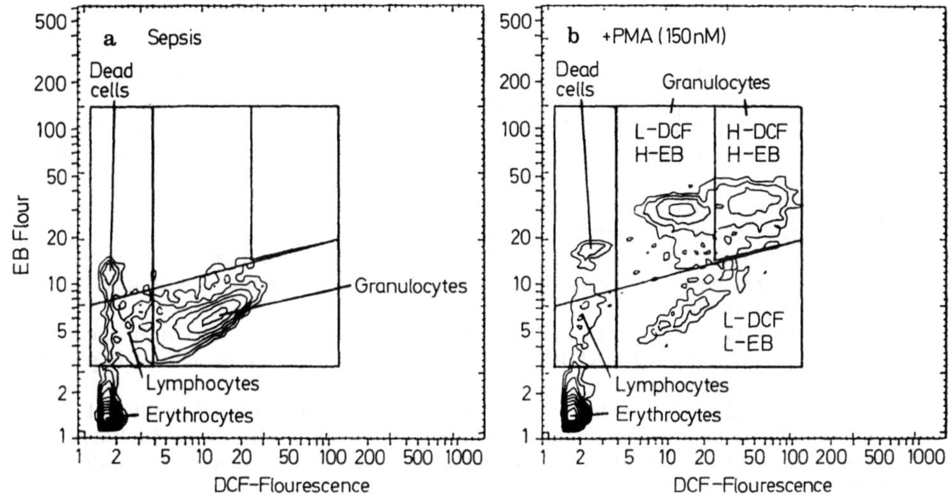

Fig. 2 a, b. 2′,7′-Dichlorfluorescein fluorescence versus ethidium bromide fluorescence of buffy coat leukocytes of a septic patient incubated with 2′,7′-dichlorfluorescein diacetate and hydroethidine without **a** or with **b** 150 n*M* PMA. More than 95% of the leukocytes are granulocytes. The simultaneous measurement of phagosomal H_2O_2 and NADPH oxidase activity reveals three subpopulations of granulocytes with different activity upon PMA stimulation

Table 2. Automated 3-day advance classification of intensive care patients using flow cytometric parameters of granulocyte function

Clinical diagnosis 3 days later	*n*	diagnosis/SPSS classification			
		Post-traumatic organ failure	Septic organ failure	Transition state	Normal
Post-traumatic organ failure	8	**100.0%**	0.0%	0.0%	0.0%
Septic organ failure	12	0.0%	**91.7%**	8.3%	0.0%
Transition state	94	1.1%	7.4%	**87.2%**	4.3%
Normal	23	0.0%	4.3%	0.0%	**95.7%**

Classification by three canonical discriminant functions based on stepwise minimization of Wilks' lambda. Clinical diagnosis as described in "Methods."

crimination was even improved when the discriminant analysis was run against the clinical classification on the 3rd day after the analysis of granulocyte function. One hundred percent of the episode could be predicted 3 days in advance on the basis of flow-cytometric parameters (Table 2).

The multifunctional analysis of cell-biochemical parameters by flow cytometry revealed significant early alterations of granulocyte function in septic and post-traumatic patients. The pattern of granulocyte function had a high predictive value for the progress of the disease and should be of value for the analysis of early effects of medical intervention on granulocyte function.

References

1. Rothe G, Valet G (1989) Phagocytosis, intracellular pH and cell volume in the multi-functional analysis of granulocytes by flow cytometry. Cytometry 9(4): in press
2. Valet G, Raffael A, Moroder L, Wünsch E, Ruhenstroth-Bauer G (1981) Fast intracellular pH determination in single cells by flow-cytometry. Naturwissenschaften 68:265–266
3. Valet G, Raffael A, Rüssmann L (1985) Determination of intracellular calcium in vital cells by flow-cytometry. Naturwissenschaften 72:600–602
4. Bass DA, Olbrantz P, Szejda P, Seeds MC, Mc Call CE (1986) Subpopulations of patients with increased oxidative product formation in blood of patients with infection. J Immunol 136:860–866
5. Rothe G, Valet G (1989) Use of hydroethidine and 2,7-dichlorfluorescein for the flow-cytometric measurement of NADPH-oxidase activity and peroxidase activity in phagocytes. Submitted for publication
6. Valet G, Warnecke HH, Kahle H (1987) Automated diagnosis of malignant and other abnormal cells by flow-cytometry using the DIAGNOS1 program system. In: Burger G, Ploem JS, Goerttler K (eds) Clinical cytometry and histometry. Academic, London, pp 58–65
7. Oestern HJ, Sturm JA, Tscherne H (1983) Die Klassifizierung der Verletzungsschwere. Hefte Unfallheilkde 156:171–177 ff
8. Montgomery AB, Stager MA, Carrico CJ, Hudson L (1985) Causes of mortality in patients with the adult respiratory distress syndrome. Am Rev Respir Dis 132:485–489

Cellular and Humoral Reactions of the Nonspecific Immune System of Polytraumatized Patients with and without the Adult Respiratory Distress Syndrome *

A. Dwenger, G. Regel, G. Schweitzer, M. Funck, J. A. Sturm, and H. Tscherne

Introduction

Several lines of evidence suggest that an imbalance of the humoral-phagocytic immune system conclusively contributes to the development of the adult respiratory distress syndrome (ARDS) (Zimmerman 1983; Solomkin 1985; Lanser 1986, Dwenger 1986a). The most important cells of this system, polymorphonuclear neutrophilic leukocytes (PMNLs), are ambivalent cells in that they manage the host defense by intracellular processing of microorganisms and debris on one hand, and liberate inflammation mediators on the other hand, e.g., by frustrated phagocytosis, thus initiating and enhancing destructive processes in their environment (Dwenger 1986a–c; Regel 1987). After being stimulated intravascularly, neutrophils adhere to the capillary endothelium, preferably in the lung microvasculature, and pass across the blood/air barrier into the alveolar space, hereby releasing inflammatory mediators like arachidonic acid metabolites, reactive oxygen agents, and lysosomal enzymes (Worthen 1983), which initiate and/or amplify the destruction of endothelial, interstitial, and epithelial structures (Smedley 1986) and ARDS development.

So far it has not been clear whether and how humoral and/or cellular alterations of the humoral-granulocytic system appear after trauma and whether such alterations are pathophysiologically interrelated with lung tissue injuries and ARDS.

Methods

Citrated venous blood (9 vol blood +1 vol 3.13% sodium citrate solution) was obtained from 34 multiply traumatized patients with ARDS predisposition (Injury Severity Score >30) up to 14 days after trauma, 19 of them without (group A) and 15 of them with (group B) an increase of extravascular lung water (EVLW) above 10 ml/kg body wt. and with a pulmonary arterial wedge pressure <15 mmHg, as a sign of ARDS. Seventy-four blood donors served as a control group.

Plasma was separated by centrifugation and PMNLs were isolated by two-step discontinuous Percoll gradient centrifugation (Dwenger 1986b). By different

* Supported by the Deutsche Forschungsgemeinschaft, Project II B6.

Immune Consequences of
Trauma, Shock and Sepsis
Eds. Faist/Ninnemann/Green

modifications of chemiluminescence (CL) probing techniques (Dwenger 1986a, c, 1987) the humoral-granulocytic immune system in toto as well as single components of this system were monitored.

1. The nonopsonized zymosan-induced and luminol-enhanced whole blood CL response, which reflects the reactivity of the complete humoral-granulocytic immune system, was measured by the following test composition (volumes of blanks in brackets): 500 μl (520 μl) minimal essential medium (MEM), 10 μl luminol (22.6 mmol/liter, containing triethylamine, 40 mmol/liter, 20 μl (0 μl) nonopsonized zymosan A suspension (100 mg/ml), 40 μl citrated blood.
2. The CL response of isolated PMNLs, which represents their metabolic capacity or oxygenation activity, was measured according to the schema: 495 μl (515 μl) MEM, 10 μl luminol, 20 μl plasma (standard or autologous), 20 μl (0 μl) zymosan, 25 μl patient PMNL suspension (25000 cells).
3. The patient plasma opsonic capacity, which reflects the total mediator effects between zymosan and PMNLs of all plasma opsonins, was measured by: 495 μl (515 μl) MEM, 10 μl luminol, 20 μl plasma (patient or standard), 20 μl (0 μl) zymosan, 25 μl isolated normal PMNL suspension (25000 cells).
4. The patient plasma inhibitory potency to half-maximally reduce the latex-induced, complement-independent and nonspecific CL response of normal PMNLs was determined as follows: 300 μl MEM, 40 μl standard plasma, 10 μl luminol, 10 μl latex (Unisphere latex 22, 0.777 μm diameter, 10%, Serva, Heidelberg), 0–150 μl patient plasma, 185–35 μl sodium chloride solution (0.9%), 25 μl isolated normal PMNL suspension (25000 cells); the half-maximal CL response reduction was calculated by graphical methods from measurement with different plasma dilutions and expressed as the plasma volume to produce this effect (${}^{\varkappa}l_{1/2}$). Peak maximum values of photon emission measured by employment of a six-channel Biolumat LB 9505 (Berthold, FRG) were used for calculations.

Results

As a result of experiments according to (1), the time courses of the whole blood CL exhibited a decline from 1.7 to $0.7 \cdot 10^6$ cpm/$2 \cdot 10^5$ PMNLs below normal values ($1.22 \pm 0.09 \cdot 10^6$ cpm/$2 \cdot 10^5$ PMNLs, $\bar{x} \pm$ SEM, $n = 74$) within the first posttraumatic day for both patient groups, followed by a complete recovery until day 2 (Fig. 1). Beginning with days 3–4 after trauma a clear dissociation of the CL behavior could be seen, in that group A showed a nearly five fold increase of the stimulatory response, whereas the reactivity of group B was generally reduced to only slightly above normal values. The stimulatory response of isolated PMNLs demonstrated higher than normal values ($3.07 \pm 0.17 \cdot 10^6$ cpm/$2.5 \cdot 10^4$ PMNLs, $\bar{x} \pm$ SEM, $n = 43$) for both groups during 14 days; group B values were found still higher (between 3.6 and $12.5 \cdot 10^6$ cpm/$2.5 \cdot 10^4$ PMNLs) in comparison to group A (between 4.5 and $6.8 \cdot 10^6$ cpm/$2.5 \cdot 10^4$ PMNLs) (Fig. 2). From the common results of Figs. 1 and 2 an opsonin defect and/or a plasma CL inhibitor could be assumed. Measuring the opsonic capacity of the patient plasma according to (3) a reconstitution of initially below normal opsonin concentrations was observed

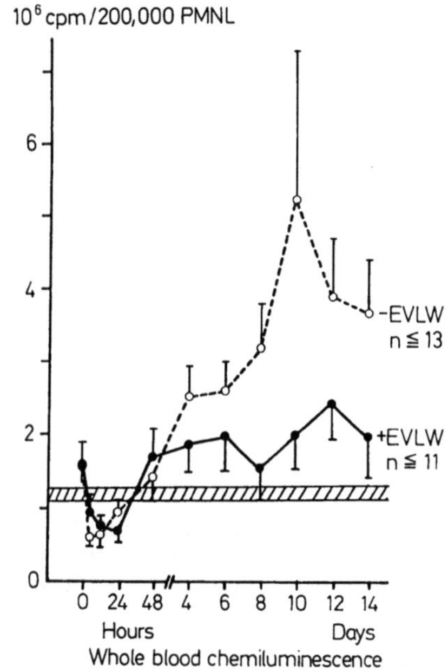

Fig. 1. Whole blood chemiluminescence response after zymosan A stimulation. ---, group A ($n = 13$) without EVLW increase; —, group B ($n = 11$) with EVLW increase; normal range ($\bar{x} \pm$ SEM, $n = 74$)

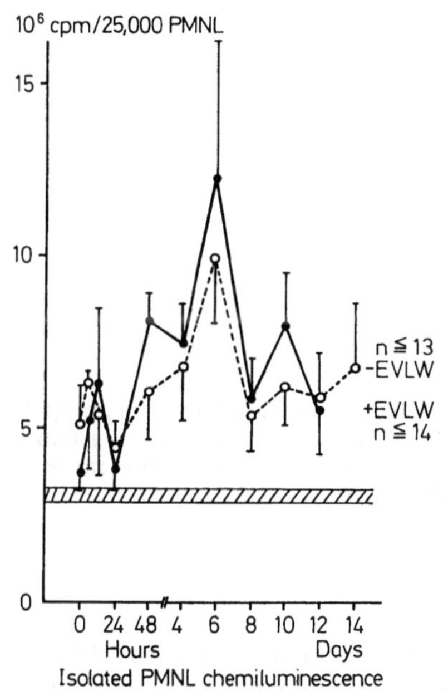

Fig. 2. Chemiluminescence response of isolated neutrophils after zymosan A stimulation, ---, group A ($n = 13$) without EVLW increase; —, group B ($n = 14$) with EVLW increase; normal range ($\bar{x} \pm$ SEM, $n = 43$)

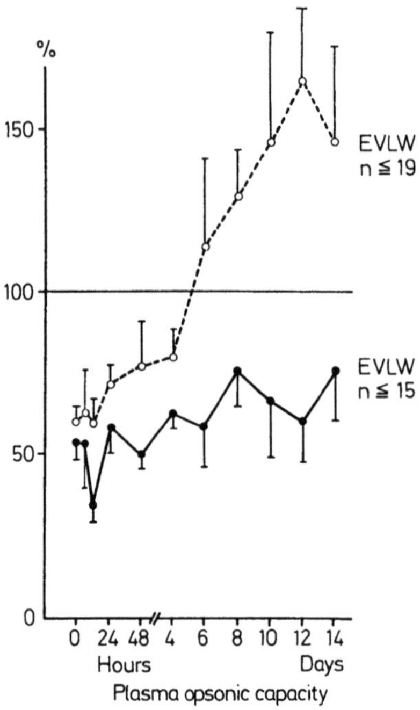

Fig. 3. Plasma opsonic capacity (standard plasma = 100%). ---, group A ($n=19$) without EVLW increase; —, group B ($n=15$) with EVLW increase

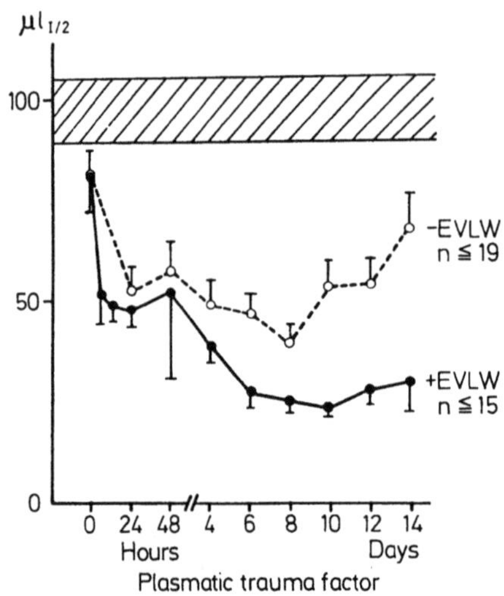

Fig. 4. Plasmatic trauma factor. ---, group A ($n=19$) without EVLW increase; —, group B ($n=15$) with EVLW increase; normal range ($\bar{x} \pm$ SEM, $n=16$)

at day 5 for group A (100% of normal) with a further increase (up to 170% of normal after 12 days), whereas group B remained far below normal values (70% of normal) during the complete post-traumatic course (Fig. 3). As could be seen by the test procedure (4) a CL-suppressing trauma-related factor was synthesized immediately after the traumatic event, which increased continuously for group B, whereas group A demonstrated the disappearance of this factor beginning with days 7–8 after trauma (Fig. 4).

Discussion

From the above results, alterations of humoral as well as cellular components of the nonspecific immune system could be supposed to be involved in ARDS pathogenesis. The observed differences in whole blood CL response between patients without and with extravascular lung water (EVLW) increases were only caused by humoral components. A plasma opsonin defect could be detected, especially for group B patients with EVLW increase, and these patients also demonstrated a continuous synthesis of a trauma factor that suppressed CL responses and presumably also phagocytosis and killing functions of PMNLs in blood (Lanser 1986), hereby predisposing this patient group to inflammation/ sepsis and inflammation/ sepsis-associated and -amplified ARDS development. Such an inhibition factor has been described in septic patients (Lanser 1986), but our results demonstrated that this factor seemed always to be rapidly synthesized after a traumatic event irrespective of septicemia. As a consequence, the increased endogenous respiratory burst potential of ARDS neutrophils (Zimmerman 1983), presumably produced by priming effects (Guthrie 1984), leads to an amplified toxic attack of PMNLs on the endothelial wall after increased attachment (Dwenger 1988; Jonas 1988). Furthermore, this increased destructive potential of PMNLs will become effective after the neutrophil has left the capillary and has entered the alveolar space, no longer being kept in check by the plasma trauma factor and then liberating the complete set of inflammation mediators for lung structure damage. In conclusion, the post-traumatic development of ARDS seemed to be related to a blood-borne increased respiratory burst activity of alveoli-invaded neutrophils in association with their host defense suppression in blood by a stimulation-inhibiting humoral trauma factor and by an opsonin deficiency, predisposing multiply traumatized patients to inflammation-, or sepsis-, amplified EVLW increase and ARDS development.

References

Dwenger A, Schweitzer G, Regel G (1986a) Bronchoalveolar lavage fluid and plasma proteins, chemiluminescence response and protein contents of polymorphonuclear leukocytes from blood and lavage fluid in traumatized patients. J Clin Chem Clin Biochem 24:73

Dwenger A, Regel G, Neumann C, Schweitzer G (1986b) Pathomechanisms of the adult respiratory distress syndrome (ARDS): elastase contents of polymorphonuclear leukocytes and elastase release during passage across the blood/air barrier. Fresenius Z Anal Chem 324:359

Dwenger A, Regel G, Schweitzer G (1986c) Pathomechanisms of the adult respiratory distress syndrome (ARDS): chemiluminescence analysis of polymorphonuclear leukocytes. Fresenius Z Anal Chem 324:360

Dwenger A, Lindena J, Schweitzer G, Neumann C, Regel G (1987) Bioluminescence and chemiluminescence, new perspectives. In: Schölmerich J, Andreesen R, Kapp A, Ernst M, Wood WG (eds) Proceedings of the IVth international bioluminescence and chemiluminescence symposium. Wiley, Chichester, p 41

Dwenger A, Schweitzer G, Funck M (1988) Lipopolysaccharide-dependent enhancement of adherence-mediated chemiluminescence response of polymorphonuclear leukocytes. J Biolum Chemilum 2:35

Guthrie LA, McPhail LC, Henson PM, Johnston RB Jr (1984) Priming of neutrophils for enhanced release of oxygen metabolites by bacterial lipopolysaccharide. Evidence for increased activity of the superoxide-producing enzyme. J Exp Med 160:1656

Jonas E, Dwenger A, Lueken B (1988) Chemiluminescence response and endothelial cell damage following lipopolysaccharide priming of polymorphonuclear leukocytes. Fresenius Z Anal Chem 330:421

Lanser ME, Brown GE, Mora R, Coleman W, Siegel JM (1986) Trauma serum suppresses superoxide production by normal neutrophils. Arch Surg 121:157

Regel G, Dwenger A, Seidel J, Nerlich ML, Sturm JA, Tscherne H (1987) Die Bedeutung der neutrophilen Granulozyten bei der Entstehung des posttraumatischen Lungenversagens. Unfallchirurg 90:99

Smedley LA, Tonnesen MG, Sandhaus RA, Haslett C, Guthrie LA, Johnston RB Jr (1986) Neutrophil-mediated injury to endothelial cells. Enhancement by endotoxin and essential role of neutrophil elastase. J Clin Invest 77:1233

Solomkin JS, Cotta LA, Satoh PS, Hurst JM, Nelson RD (1985) Complement activation and clearance in acute illness and injury: evidence for C5a as a cell-directed mediator of the adult respiratory distress syndrome in man. Surgery 97:668

Worthen GS, Henson PM (1983) Clin Lab Med 3:601

Zimmerman GA, Renzetti AD, Hill HR (1983) Am Rev Respir Dis 127:290

Granulocyte Adherence in Patients Undergoing Cardiac Surgery Under Cardiopulmonary Bypass *

P. Kinnaert, N. Van Geertruyden, B. Bournonville, J. Bastenier, and J. L. Leclerc

Inflammation is the first line of defense of the body against infection. Granulocyte adherence (GA) is an important component of inflammatory reactions. It is profoundly altered by complement activation. Therefore, it seemed interesting to study GA in patients undergoing cardiac surgery under cardiopulmonary bypass (CPB), a procedure known to activate the complement cascade.

Materials and Methods

Adult patients undergoing valvular replacement or coronary bypass surgery were bled at various times before, during, and after CPB. The surgical procedures were performed with the patient under standardized stress-free anesthesia using fentanyl, droperidol, pancuronium, and endotracheal intubation. A bolus injection of 30 mg/kg body weight of methylprednisolone was given 20–30 min before the beginning of CPB. Heparin was administered at the dose of 3 mg/kg body weight. Protamine was given as needed after restoration of the normal circulation. CPB was performed with a roller pump and a membrane oxygenator (COBE-CML) primed with 1400 ml Haemaccel, 0.3 g/kg mannitol, and 60 ml HCO_3 Na. The GA index, which is the percentage of adhering cells to nylon fibers, was measured according to the technique of MacGregor et al. [2], and the actual number of adhering granulocytes/mm^3 was calculated taking into account the variations in total granulocyte counts.

In a second series of tests, plasma was obtained from patients with an 0 Rh+ blood group preoperatively and 45 min post-CPB. These samples were stored at −30 °C. Cell fractions from other 0 pos patients bled preoperatively or after CPB were isolated by low-speed centrifugation. The cells were washed three times and resuspended either in preoperative or post-CPB plasma. The GA index of the resulting cellular suspension was measured.

Results

None of the studied parameters varied significantly between the preoperative period and the beginning of CPB. When compared with pre-CPB values, the GA index dropped during CPB and a further decrease was observed 45 min after res-

* This work was supported by grant No. 3-4526-88 from the Fonds de la Recherche Scientifique Médicale and by the Fondation David et Alice van Buuren, Université Libre de Bruxelles.

Immune Consequences of
Trauma, Shock and Sepsis
Eds. Faist/Ninnemann/Green

Table 1. Values of GA index, granulocyte counts, actual number of adhering cells/mm³, and hematocrit immediately before CPB, 10 and 30 min after its start and 45 min after restoration of normal circulation

	Pre-CPB	CPB		45′ post-CPB
		10′	30′	
Granulocyte adherence index (%)	75.7 ± 2.5	50.0 ± 3.7**	50.0 ± 5.5**	39.3 ± 3.4*
Granulocytes/mm³	3707 ± 401	1923 ± 377**	2184 ± 390**	10024 ± 1771**
Adhering granulocytes/mm³	2749 ± 238	950 ± 187**	1047 ± 163**	3529 ± 492
Hematocrit	34.5 ± 1.6	23.7 ± 4.2**	23.5 ± 2.4**	27.1 ± 4.0*

** $P < 0.001$ compared with pre-CPB values.

Table 2. Granulocyte adherence index in various combinations of preoperative and post-CPB cells and preoperative and post-CPB plasma

		Plasma	
		Preoperative	Post-CPB
Cells	Preoperative	85.8 ± 2.0	81.3 ± 2.6
	Post-CPB	79.8 ± 1.8	68.4 ± 4.0*

toration of the normal circulation (Table 1). Granulocyte counts were very low during CPB. This was not simply due to hemodilution because circulating granulocytes reached 52% of the pre-CPB value while the hematocrit dropped only to 68% of its initial value. Moreover after cessation of CPB, granulocyte counts increased markedly while the hematocrit remained low. The actual number of adhering cells decreased during CPB and was slightly higher than normal although not significantly so after restoration of the normal circulation.

The relative effect of plasma factors and cell alterations on the variations of cell adherence was studied by mixing preoperative and post-CPB plasma with preoperative and post-CPB cells and measuring the GA index of the resulting cellular suspension. Table 2 shows that it was different from the preoperative value only when post-CPB plasma was mixed with post-CPB cells.

Discussion

MacGregor et al. [2] demonstrated a correlation between adherence of granulocytes to nylon fibers and to endothelial cells [3]. Therefore the GA index has been used as a parameter of the immune status of surgical patients [1]. The present data show, however, that GA index does not reflect the total capacity of adherence of the pool of circulating granulocytes. Indeed, after CPB the actual number of adhering cells was back to normal while the GA index showed a further decrease. This discrepancy was due to the increased blood granulocyte counts. Moreover, our in vitro studies show that plasmatic alterations [presence of inhibitor(s) or lack of factor(s) required for normal adherence] were not sufficient to explain the post-CPB reduction of GA. The GA index was not significantly modified when preoperative cells were resuspended in post-CPB plasma. The drop was only observed when post-CPB cells were mixed with post-CPB plasma. Consequently, alterations of circulating granulocytes induced by the procedure also play a role.

The nature of these plasmatic and cellular changes remains to be determined. Alterations in granulocyte counts and the GA index presumably result from a combination of various factors such as: complement activation, high doses of steroids, perhaps other plasma factors (TNF, prostaglandins, priming fluids, etc.), sequestration of leukocytes in tissues, variations of marginal and circulating leukocyte pools, and eventually modifications of cell surfaces. Further studies are needed to evaluate the role of these various factors. One possible explanation for leukopenia and decrease of GA index observed during CPB could be that complement activation induced by the tubing and oxygenator provokes trapping of the leukocytes in the various tissues and a shift from the circulating to the marginal pool. Only the less adherent cells would remain in the circulation.

References

1. Christou NV, Meakins JL (1979) Neutrophil function in anergic surgical patients: neutrophil adherence and chemotaxis. Ann Surg 190:557–564
2. Mac Gregor RP, Spagnuolo PJ, Lentnek AL (1974) Inhibition of granulocyte adherence by ethanol, prednisone and aspirin measured with an assay system. N Engl J Med 291:642–646
3. Mac Gregor RP, Marcarak EJ, Kefalides NA (1978) Comparative adherence of granulocytes to endothelial monolayers and nylon fibers. J Clin Invest 61:687–702

Studies on the Release of Lipoxygenase Products from Granulocytes of Severely Burned Patients *

M. Köller, W. König, J. Brom, W. Schönfeld, G. Erbs, and F. E. Müller

Introduction

In recent years major interest has been addressed to the functional behavior of polymorphonuclear granulocytes (PMNs) in patients suffering from severe burns. It was observed that serious PMN dysfunctions were associated with acquired immunological abnormalities including impairment of chemotaxis, phagocytosis, and bacterial killing (Arturson 1985; Deitch et al. 1984). Granulocytes are not only involved in host defense against microbial infections, but also as effector cells in inflammatory reactions. One of the early responses after their stimulation is the release of biologically active mediators such as the leukotrienes (Bray 1986). Leukotrienes represent a family of hydroxy fatty acids which were generated from arachidonic acid by the activity of a 5-lipoxygenase. The enzymatic conversion of LTA_4 leads to the formation of LTB_4, which is a chemotactic and chemokinetic agent for granulocytes, monocytes, and macrophages. A further hydroxylation of LTB_4 leads to metabolites with minor biological activities, e.g., omega-oxidation products (Hansson et al. 1981). The leukotrienes C_4, D_4, and E_4 (together constituting the slow-reacting substance, SRS) are potent constrictors of smooth muscles and lead to an increase in vasopermeability. In addition, the involvement of leukotrienes in the regulation of cell-mediated reactions has recently been demonstrated (Rola-Pleszczynski 1987). The purpose of the present study was to analyze the generation of leukotrienes in vitro from granulocytes of severely burned patients in comparison to the granulocytes of normal healthy donors.

Materials and Methods

Materials

Synthetic leukotrienes (LTs) B_4, C_4, D_4, and E_4 as well as the omega-oxidation products 20-OH-LTB_4 and 20-COOH-LTB_4 were a generous gift from Dr. J. Rokach (Merck Frosst, Pointe-Claire/ Dorval, Québec, Canada). The leukotriene B_4 isomers 6-*trans*-LTB_4 and 12-epi-6-*trans*-LTB_4 were kindly provided by Dr. P. Borgeat (University Laval, Québec, Canada). Ca-ionophore A23187 and arachidonic acid were obtained from Sigma (Munich, FRG).

* Supported by the Bundesamt für Zivilschutz.

Immune Consequences of
Trauma, Shock and Sepsis
Eds. Faist/Ninnemann/Green

Analytical HPLC System

High-performance liquid chromatography was performed on reversed-phase columns (4 × 250 mm) packed with Nucleosil (C_{18}) 5-µm particles (Macherey-Nagel, Düren) as described elsewhere (Köller et al. 1988). Identification and quantitation of leukotrienes were performed as has been described (Köller et al. 1985).

Preparation and Stimulation of Cells

Polymorphonuclear granulocytes were separated from 40 ml heparinized blood (15 U/ml) on a Ficoll-metrizoate gradient followed by dextran sedimentation. The stimulation of the cells was performed as has been described (Köller et al. 1988). Part of the incubations were performed in the presence of exogenously added arachidonic acid (64 µ*M*).

Patient Population

Ten patients admitted to the intensive burn care unit of the Universitätsklinik Bergmannsheil, Bochum (Abteilung für Verbrennungsbehandlung, Plastische Chirurgie und Handchirurgie, Leitung: Prof. Dr. Dr. Müller), were included in this study. The data obtained from six patients are summarized in this paper: patient A: male, 28 years old, 45% total burned surface area (TBSA), inhalation injury (I), artificially ventilated (V); patient B: female, 22 years old, 26% TBSA, I, V; patient E: male, 36 years old, 36% TBSA, V, diabetes mellitus; patient F: male, 36 years old, 42% TBSA; patient G: male, 44 years old, 30% TBSA, I, V; patient H: male, 18 years old, 75% TBSA, V.

Results and Discussion

The patient PMNs were stimulated with the Ca-ionophore (7.3 µ*M*). Leukotriene composition and concentration of the resulting supernatants were then analyzed by reversed-phase HPLC. As shown in Fig. 1, an overall decrease in leukotriene B_4 generation from the patients' granulocytes was observed as compared with the cells of healthy donors (broken line). Figure 1 includes three patients (A, B, E) who finally recovered from their injuries. It is shown that the granulocytes lost their responsiveness toward ionophore stimulation during the 2nd and 3rd week postburn. In the later phases the responsiveness of the granulocytes increased in this patient group. The granulocytes of patients who finally succumbed to their injuries showed poor responsiveness over the total period (data not shown). Thus, our data confirmed the reported results of Braquet et al. (1984).

The LTC_4 generation of the patients' PMNs exhibited a similar profile to that in the LTB_4 generation. However, two patients revealed elevated LTC_4 generation especially in the later phases postburn. This increase in LTC_4 generation correlated to an increase in the eosinophil cell count within the cell preparation (data not shown).

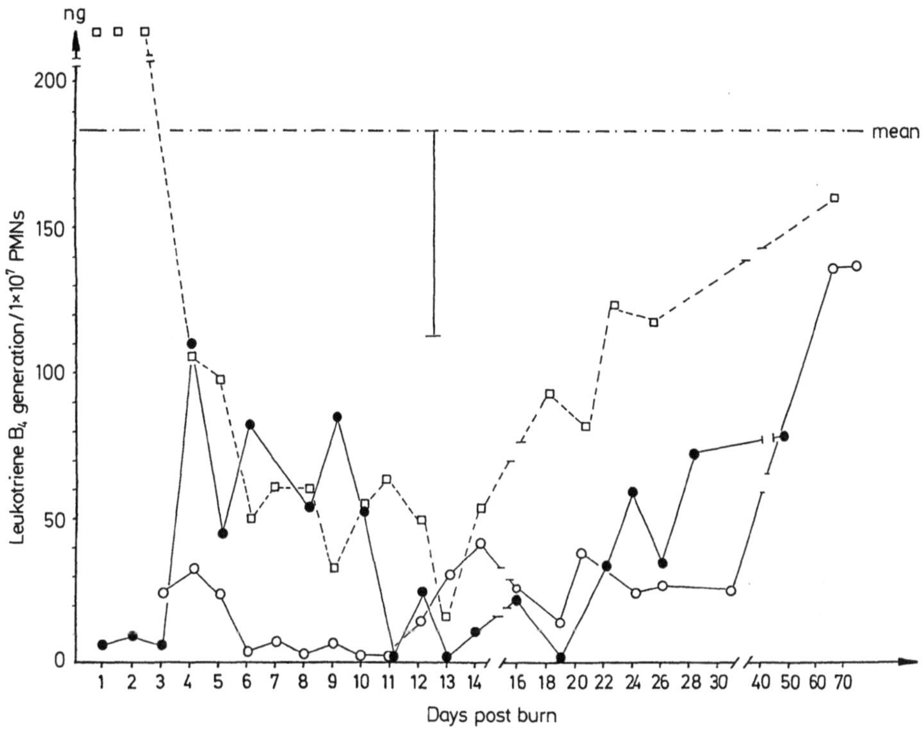

Fig. 1. LTB_4 generation fromPMNs (1×10^7) after ionophore A23187 stimulation (7.3 μM). ○——○, patient A; ●——●, patient B; □---□, patient E. Mean value ±SD from PMNs of healthy donors ($n = 8$)

All patients showed a shift to immature PMNs (mainly band cells). This shift was observed approximately 3 days postburn. The cellular composition of the PMNs only returned to a normal distribution when the patients survived. As we observed there was no correlation between the cell count of mature granulocytes and leukotriene generation especially in the later phases postburn. Therefore, we conclude that the decreased leukotriene release from granulocytes of burned patients is not solely due to changes in the cellular composition; it rather reflects an impairment in the functional properties of these granulocytes.

Since LTB_4 is metabolized to omega-oxidated products by granulocytes, we additionally analyzed the functional characteristics of the patients' cells. It became apparent that the patient's granulocytes induced an increased metabolism of LTB_4 (Fig. 2). As is shown, the generation of omega-oxidated products increased in the later phases postburn. Among them the generation of 20-carboxy-LTB_4 was clearly enhanced. The capacity of the cells to generate and metabolize LTB_4 returned to normal levels in the later phases postburn. These data were confirmed by incubating the patients' granulocytes with tritium-labeled LTB_4 (data not shown; Brom et al. 1987). In addition, a decreased generation of omega-oxidated products was observed between days 6–9 postburn, which apparently reflects a lack of metabolizable substrate. A similar stimulation profile as was

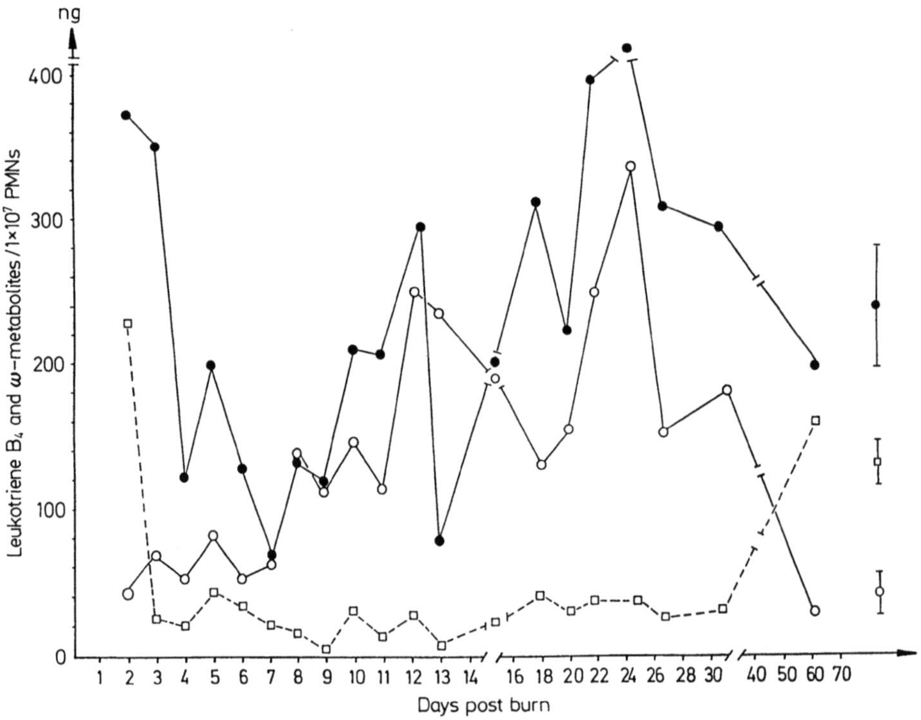

Fig. 2. Generation of omega-oxidated products from LTB_4 (□---□); patient E; ●—●, 20-OH-LTB_4; ○—○, 20-COOH-LTB_4. Mean values ±SD of healthy donors ($n=8$) are depicted at the right margin

shown for the ionophore was obtained when opsonized zymosan was used as stimulus (data not shown). These results suggest that the decreased generation of LTB_4 from the patients' granulocytes is the net result of two concomitant mechanisms which are due to a decreased LTB_4 generation and further to an increased metabolism of LTB_4.

In order to elucidate the decrased LTB_4 generation the patients' granulocytes were stimulated in the presence of exogenous arachidonic acid, which is the parent molecule of the leukotrienes. As is demonstrated by Fig. 3 an enhanced leukotriene generation in the presence of exogenous arachidonic acid (closed circles) was observed. In Fig. 3 the sum of LTB_4 and of the respective omega-oxidated products were plotted. These data were obtained from a patient (G) of the survivors' group.

The curve which indicates the release of leukotrienes in the presence of exogenous arachidonic acid (closed circles) shows a parallel pattern when compared with the release characteristics of cells from normal healthy donors. Even when a decreased leukotriene generation was measured, e.g., day 7 postburn, the enhancement of leukotriene generation with the presence of the exogenous arachidonic acid was comparable to release quantities obtained from cells of the later phase postburn. These results led us to suggest that the decreased leukotriene gen-

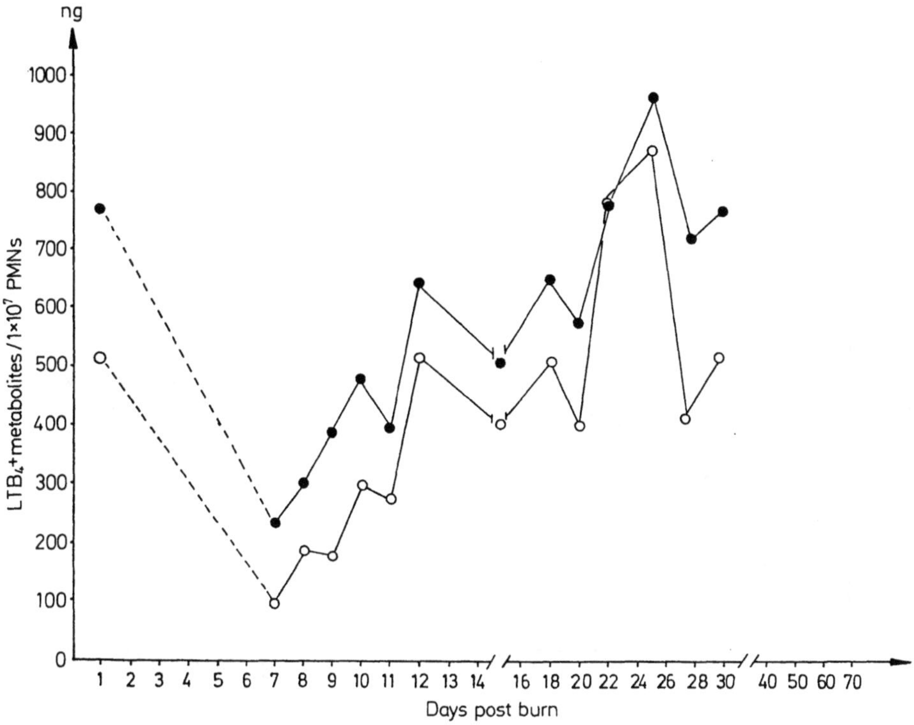

Fig. 3. Generation of LTB_4 and LTB_4 metabolites from PMNs (patient G) after ionophore A23187 stimulation (7.3 μ*M*) in the presence (●——●) or absence (○——○) of exogenously added arachidonic acid (64 μ*M*)

eration from PMNs of severely burned patients may be due to the fact to what degree arachidonic acid becomes available. Therefore the defect is related to the release of arachidonic acid from the phospholipid structures of the cellular membranes. These results were only valid for the patients within the survivors' group. We next quantitated the differences of leukotriene release, which was obtained from cells in the presence and absence of exogenous arachidonic acid (Fig. 4). With the cells of the surviving patients (E, F) similar differences were obtained, i.e., the degree of enhancement did not change. No enhancement was observed for one nonsurviving patient (H; with 75% burns TBSA and an early onset of burn wound sepsis); even in the presence of exogenous arachidonic acid the leukotriene release decreased.

Finally the quantitative bacterial analysis of the respective biopsy specimen indicates that the decreased capacity to generate leukotrienes by PMNs preceded and/or accompanied the invasive bacterial infections (data not shown). The presented results demonstrated a significant decrease in leukotriene generation by PMNs from severely burned patients. The decreased LTB_4 release was accompanied by an enhanced LTB_4 metabolism into omega oxidated products which exert minor biological activities (Hansson et al. 1981). These functional alterations led to a decrease in chemotactic capacity of PMNs from burned patients. In addition,

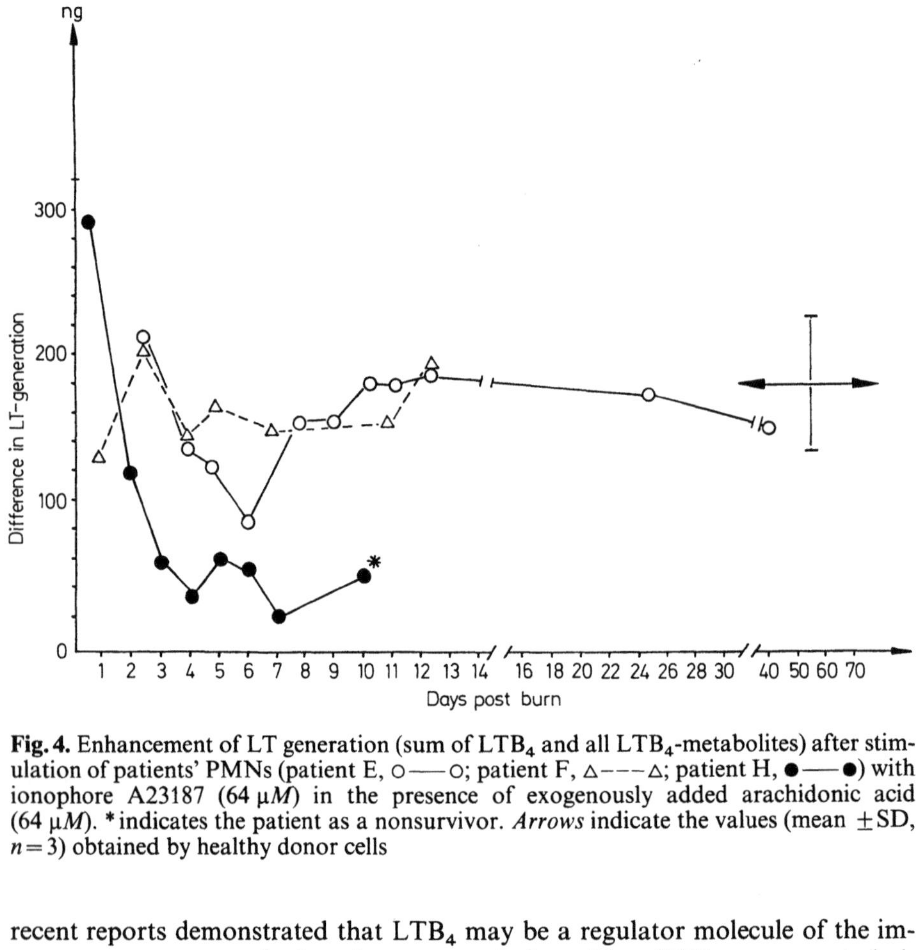

Fig. 4. Enhancement of LT generation (sum of LTB_4 and all LTB_4-metabolites) after stimulation of patients' PMNs (patient E, ○—○; patient F, △---△; patient H, ●—●) with ionophore A23187 (64 μ*M*) in the presence of exogenously added arachidonic acid (64 μ*M*). * indicates the patient as a nonsurvivor. *Arrows* indicate the values (mean ±SD, $n=3$) obtained by healthy donor cells

recent reports demonstrated that LTB_4 may be a regulator molecule of the immune responses, e.g., for lymphocyte populations. Thus LTB_4 may counterbalance the multiple trauma-induced suppressive cell-mediated immune functions (Goodwin et al. 1986; Rola-Pleszczynski et al. 1987).

References

Arturson G (1985) Neutrophil granulocyte functions in severely burned patients. Burns Incl Therm Inj 11:309–319

Braquet M, Ducousso R, Garay R, Guilbaud J, Carsin H, Braquet P (1984) Leukocyte leukotriene B secretion precedes anergy in burn-injured patients. Lancet 8409:976–977

Bray MA (1986) Leukotrienes in inflammation. Agents Actions 19:87–99

Brom J, König W, Köller M, Groß-Weege W, Erbs G, Müller FE (1987) Metabolism of leukotriene B4 by polymorphonuclear granulocytes of severely burned patients. Prostaglandins Leukotrienes Med 27:209–225

Deitch EA, Gelder F, McDonald JC (1984) Sequential prospective analysis of the nonspecific host defense system after thermal injury. Arch Surg 119:83–89

Goodwin JS, Atluru D, Sierakowski S, Lianos EA (1986) Mechanism of action of glucocorticoids. J Clin Invest 77:1244–1250

Hansson G, Lindgren JA, Dahlén S-E, Hedqvist P, Samuelsson B (1981) Identification and biological activity of novel ω-oxidized metabolites of leukotriene B4 from human leukocytes. FEBS Lett 130:107–112

Köller M, König W, Brom J, Bremm KD, Schönfeld W, Knöller J (1985) Functional characteristics of leukotriene C4- and D4-metabolizing enzymes (γ-glutamyl transpeptidase, dipeptidase) within human plasma. Biochim Biophys Acta 836:56–62

Köller M, König W, Brom J, Raulf M, Gross-Weege W, Erbs G, Müller FE (1988) Generation of leukotrienes from human polymorphonuclear granulocytes of severely burned patients. J Trauma 28:6

Rola-Pleszczynski M, Bouvrette L, Gingras D, Girad M (1987) Identification of interferon-γ as the lymphokine that mediates leukotriene B4-induced immunoregulation. J Immunol 139:513–517

Section 4

Endotoxin, Prostaglandin, and other Triggers of Trauma-Induced Immunosuppression

Immune Modulation by Microorganisms

H. Friedman, W. Cruse, T. Klein, J. Djeu, and S. Pross

Introduction

Infection by opportunistic and ubiquitous microorganisms is a major cause of mortality in patients with extensive trauma, including burns [1–4]. Microbial infection is considered a leading cause of death following major injuries and it is now known that increased susceptibility to infection exists over and above that associated merely with the loss of a skin barrier. It is also now known that traumatic injury, including burn injury, results in markedly altered immune competence of the injured individual. Besides the generalized physiological alterations which develop in burned individuals, important immune dysfunctions become evident at both the humoral and cellular levels [5–7]. Many model systems with experimental animals as well as clinical studies have shown numerous immunological alterations in burn patients. Nevertheless, it is still not clear whether such immunological dysfunctions, especially T-lymphocyte deregulation, are a direct result of the injury or an indirect one due factors associated with cellular elements responding to the injury or possibly even to the microorganisms which may rapidly colonize burned tissue.

Many investigators believe that infectious agents, especially gram-negative bacteria, are markedly immunomodulatory and may contain immunostimulatory or immunosuppressive substances which are pharmacologically quite active in altering the immune response of an individual [8–10]. All microorganisms, including both pathogenic and nonpathogenic bacteria, as well as fungi, viruses, and single or multicellular parasites, contain potent antigenic determinants which, when recognized by the immune system of an individual, elicit a strong immune response. Such responses are the result of a complex series of cellular and molecular interactions following stimulation of lymphoid cells by specific antigenic determinants, culminating in the release of a wide variety of molecules by lymphoid cells, such as antibodies, lymphokines, and monokines. Thus, antigenic stimulation results in a cascade phenomenon resulting in what is considered a specific active immune response. The immune system, in turn, is a complex network of interacting cells and their products and usually develops to protect the individual from exogenous challenges, especially those associated with opportunistic or pathogenic microorganisms.

Studies in the past decade or so have begun to focus attention on examining the ability of microorganisms and their products to affect negatively the immune response in order to develop better rationale for therapeutic approaches to alleviating the consequences of microbial challenges to the immune system [8, 9].

Immune Consequences of
Trauma, Shock and Sepsis
Eds. Faist/Ninnemann/Green

Since microorganisms contain a variety of pharmacologically active components that have the capacity to affect the immune system, it has become necessary to utilize purified microbial components to dissect the specific cellular and molecular mechanisms whereby these components exert their immunomodulatory activity. Furthermore, the utilization of in vitro immune assays has also facilitated the ability to understand the mechanisms by which such components exert activity. Thus, the combination of purified microbial components and in vitro systems has provided an opportunity to examine the effects of microbes and/or their products on the immune system, and more specifically to determine precisely by what mechanisms a microorganism or its product exerts an immunomodulatory activity.

In general, it is widely recognized that infectious agents influence individual specific immune responses to the microorganism itself, as well as affecting nonspecific resistance to a wide variety of other microbes and the integrity of the immune system itself. In this regard, the effects of a given microbe or its products may be on the afferent phase of the immune response (i.e., sensitization phase). In contrast, an effect may also be on the effector phase. In the case of burn victims, microbes infecting the area of damage include not only pathogenic bacteria, fungi, and viruses, but also microorganisms which are considered opportunistic pathogens or normal flora which cause disease only after a damaging event or defect to an immune mechanism, either local or systemic [1–3]. In turn, such infecting organisms may exert a continuing influence on the immune response, usually in a negative manner. It is often difficult, however, to ascertain which phase of the immune system is involved and frequently both afferent and efferent phases may be influenced by a microorganism. Also, a specific mechanism of alteration of the immune system may be difficult to ascertain. Thus, in the case of the sensitization phase (disposition or processing of a specific antigen) in which an individual response may be altered, the change may be a direct effect on any one of a number of cells participating in immune reactions, i.e., macrophages, T-lymphocytes, B-lymphocytes, etc. [1–4, 11].

In the effector phase of the immune response, qualitative changes may occur in antibody function or reactivity, alterations and activation of classic versus alternative complement pathways, or changes in the release, as well as action, of pharmacological mediators. In regard to cell-mediated immunity, the effector cells, i.e., lymphocytes or macrophages, as well as their products, may be affected [1–4]. The possible relationship of such alterations of immune functions by microbial agents in a burn or trauma patient is of major concern since therapeutic approaches aimed at reversing immunosuppression by the microbe are considered by some to be an important aspect of treatment.

Mechanisms of Immunity

Much is currently known about the immune system at present and how the various components may be affected by microorganisms such as bacteria, fungi, or viruses [1, 2, 12]. Macrophages are considered an essential nonspecific cell in the immune system [12, 13]. Macrophages may be antigen-presenting cells and in this way may directly interact with antigen-specific lymphocytes, especially T-lymphocytes. The activation of T-lymphocytes involves the recognition of antigen, as well as the recognition of a major histocompatibility complex antigen [14]. Following antigen presentation to the T-lymphocyte, the macrophage is also induced to produce the cytokine interleukin 1 (IL-1). The simultaneous recognition of antigen plus histocompatibility class II antigen in combination with IL-1 initially induces the T-lymphocytes to express IL-2 receptors on their surface. Expression of this receptor is followed by the T-lymphocyte-producing IL-2. Subsequent to IL-2 secretion, other lymphokines, such as gamma-interferon or other interleukins, may be produced. These soluble factors elaborated by the activated cell are capable of augmenting the immune response to activation and/or differentiation of other lymphoid cell populations, including cytotoxic T cells, natural killer cells, lymphokine-activated killer cells and macrophages, as well as other T- and B-lymphocytes [12, 4].

Besides activation of B-lymphocytes resulting in antibody synthesis, which is dependent on the participation of soluble factors produced by activated T-helper cells, B-lymphocytes can also be directly activated by antigens which are considered thymus independent and most of these antigens are derived from gram-negative bacterial components, such as lipopolysaccharide antigens. Thus, bacterial components may often function as immunomodulatory agents by exerting their activity directly on cells or to induction of soluble mediators that affect other cells resulting in overall modulation of the immune response [8, 12].

Bacterial- and Fungal-Induced Immunoderegulation

There are many bacteria which have been studied in detail concerning their effects on the immune response, including immunosuppressive effects (Table 1). Although immune mechanisms in a normal host function by inducing soluble molecules, it is now recognized that gram-negative bacteria stimulate mainly IgM and this may serve as a complement-complexing antibody against gram-negative microorganisms. Such bacteria can also be markedly immunosuppressive [3, 8]. Various components and factors derived from gram-negative bacteria have also been shown to be immunomodulatory. Several other bacteria, including myobacteria and corynebacteria, are also known to be immunostimulatory as well as immunosuppressive and various factors derived from such bacteria have been identified as important in immunomodulation. In addition, a number of gram-positive bacteria, especially gram-positive cocci, many of which are considered to be opportunistic in nature, have been shown to be immunomodulatory, i.e., they may suppress the immune response as well as often enhance the response. Immune suppression is usually nonspecific and not directed at the microorganism itself. Various factors have been identified as directly responsible for the immunomodulatory effects of these bacteria (Table 2). Fungi have also been shown to be immunomodulatory [3]. Although antibody responses are often found in many fungi, both systemic and opportunistic in man and experimental animals, it is now thought that cell-mediated immunity is most important in controlling fungal infections in man. Many fungi and/or their products, including capsular polysac-

Table 1. Microbial factors affecting immune responses

Bacterial class	Factor
Gram-negative bacilli	
Enterobacteriae, Vibrios, Pertussis	Lipopolysaccharides, cell wall components
Other bacteria	
Mycobacteria	Cell wall, cord factor
Corynebacteria	Peptidoglycans, muramyl dipeptide
Gram-positive cocci	
Staphylococci	Capsule, clumping factor, protein A and B, teichoic acid
Streptococci	Lipoteichoic acid, membrane enzymes, pyogenic exotoxin, peptidoglycans
Pneumococci	Capsule, cell wall
Gram-negative cocci	Cell wall, exotoxins
Neisseria	
Fungi	
Candida	Glycans, polysaccharides
Cryptococci	Capsular polysaccharides

Table 2. Microbial-derived products and their reported immunomodulatory activity

Product	Mechanism of action
Bacterial membranes	
lipopolysaccharide/lipid A	MØ induction of IL-1, B-cell activation
Peptidoglycan	MØ induction of IL-1, B-cell activation
Muramyl dipeptide	MØ induction of IL-1
Mucoid exopolysaccharides	Induction of IL-1, B-cell activation
Bacterial toxins	
Staphylococcal enterotoxins	T-cell induction of IL-2, Induction of IFN-γ, Induction of T_s
Toxic shock syndrome toxin	MØ induction of IL-1, T-cell induction of IL-2
Streptococcal pyrogenic exotoxin	T-cell induction of IFN-γ, Induction of IL-1
Pertussis toxin	MØ induction of IL-1, T-cell induction of IL-2, Induction of IFN-γ
Pseudomonas exotoxin A	T-cell induction of T_s, Activation
Other microbial products	
Mycoplasma soluble products	B-cell-induced differentiation

IL-1, interleukin; IFN-γ, gamma interferon; MØ, macrophage.

charides, are now known to be immunomodulatory, i.e., they either enhance or suppress the immune response by several mechanisms. Effects of the fungi and their products on macrophages, T-lymphocytes, and B-lymphocytes are well known and it is now recognized that lymphokines and soluble factors are involved in the immunomodulation induced by fungi.

Virus-Induced Immunoderegulation

Many viral infections are also known to affect one or more components of the immune defense system [10, 15]. Which components are affected and to what extent depends upon many variables including the type and strain of virus as well as the state of activation of the immune system itself. Mechanisms whereby immune alteration occurs following virus infection are still ill-defined and probably highly diversified, but studies from many laboratories with various model systems, both in vivo and in vitro, have allowed some generalizations to be made. In most, if not all, instances, where insights into the mechanisms have been obtained, immunological impairment appears due to functional alterations of immunocompetent cells (Tables 3,4). In turn these effects may be caused by direct interaction of immunocompetent cells with the virus and less frequently by substances produced by the cells as a consequence of virus infection. Indeed, available data accumulating from many laboratories have indicated that viruses may be endowed with direct immunosuppressive properties as well as possibly immunostimulatory activities [10, 15, 16].

Because of the functional complexity of the immune system, viruses may affect immunity at various levels. Numerous alterations of immunocompetent cell functions can occur. Such fundamental alterations do not necessarily presuppose extensive damage to the lymphoid tissue. In fact hyperplastic changes may occur. Nevertheless, some viral infections of lymphoid tissue show lesions, usually limited in extent, which may resemble the cytopathogenic characteristic of the infecting virus in vitro. However, it should be noted that structural integrity of lymphoid tissue does not prevent immunocompetent cells from expressing profound manifestations of a functional deficiency. A typical defect is reduced in vitro blastogenic responses of lymphocytes to specific antigens, mitogens, or alloantigens during many viral infections [15, 16]. Among other modifications are those of lymphoid cell migration activities. Modifications of lymphocyte traffic are well

Table 3. Parameters of immunological responsiveness suppressed during viral infections

Virus infection	Immune parameter
Cytomegalovirus, influenza, measles, parainfluenza	Resistance to superinfection
Dengue virus	Graft-versus-host induction
Junin	Antibody-dependent hypersensitivity
Lactic dehydrogenase virus	Lymphocyte and antigen trapping by spleen
Lymphocytic choriomeningitis	Immunological maturation
Murine cytomegalovirus Marek's disease virus	Skin allograft rejection
Polio, Coxsackie B, mumps, measles, Epstein-Barr virus	Contact sensitivity, cell-mediated hypersensitivity
Selected retroviruses	T-cell-mediated cytotoxicity
Reovirus, selected retroviruses	Circulating autoantibody
Rubella	Ig levels in serum
Venezuelan equine encephalitis, lymphocytic choriomeningitis	Tolerance induction

Table 4. Viruses which replicate in immunocompetent virus cells

Adenovirus	L+
Coxsackie B	L+
Cytomegalovirus	MØ; LB
Dengue	MØ; LB, LT*
Echo	MØ; L*
Epstein-Barr	LB
Herpes simplex	MØ; LT*; LB*
Influenza	MØ; LT (aboritive infection)
Lymphocytic choriomeningitis	MØ
Measles	MØ; LT*; LB
Mumps	L+
Parainfluenza	MØ/LT; LB
Poliomylitis	MØ L*
Rubella	MØ; LT
Vaccinia	MØ; L*
Varicella zoster	MØ
Yellow fever	MØ; LT

MØ, macrophages; LT*, lymphocytes not characterized; LB, B-lymphocytes; LT, T-lymphocytes; *, viral replication is possible, or is substantially potentiated, if cells have been specifically or unspecifically stimulated.

documented and have been attributed to cell surface changes which subsequently reduce the ability of these cells to interact with vascular endothelial cells. Altered cell traffic patterns during virus infection may account for fluctuation of the peripheral lymphocyte count which occurs in many viral diseases and which so far remains unexplained [3].

It appears likely that the major mechanisms whereby immunocompetent cell alteration occurs in viral infections are associated either with the direct activity of the virus or an indirect one mediated by soluble factors, including lymphokines induced by activation of various lymphoid cells by virus infection [3, 10, 15, 16]. Direct action of the virus may occur during an acute phase of infection when the virus can be isolated from peripheral blood leukocytes. It seems likely, however, that interaction between a virus and immunocompetent lymphoid cells depends upon the metabolic state of the cells. Thus, macrophages often restrictive for many viruses may undergo changes and susceptibility when nonspecifically activated to signals emitted by lymphocytes. In turn, lymphocytes, if placed in contact with a virus while in a quiescent state, may often result in abortive infection followed by incomplete synthesis of virus components with little or no production of infectious progeny. On the other hand lymphocytes can often be induced to replicate larger amounts of virus by blastogenic stimulation induced by reaction with appropriate antigens or mitogens. It is important to know, however, that it has now been well established that a number of viruses can cause unsensitized lymphocytes to undergo rapid polyclonal activation or blastogenesis. This effect does not appear to be an experimental artifact because lymphocytes from a subject in an acute phase of a viral infection and cultured in vitro often show a high degree of spontaneous proliferation.

It should also be noted that some of the infections associated with virus-induced immunomodulation may be related to an autoimmune phenomenon in which viral antigens are expressed on the infected lymphoid cell surfaces [3]. These antigens may then be recognized by the immunocompetent cells which then react against the particular lymphoid cell bearing the virus antigen. Such cells, even though functioning normally despite the virus infection or expression of viral antigen, may then be destroyed or inactivated by other lymphoid cells responding to the viral antigens, resulting in a net loss of immunocompetent cells and their immunological deregulation. It is apparent that many viral infections can readily alter the immune response, often in a negative manner. There are a number of viruses which are now known to be markedly immunosuppressive, including human cytomegalovirus, other herpesviruses, as well as the retroviruses. Indeed, the acquired immune deficiency syndrome (AIDS), which has now been recognized as the major pandemic of man in the last half decade or so, is caused by an immunosuppression induced by infection of lymphoid cells directly by the retrovirus (human immunodeficiency virus, HIV) [17], but also is related to infection of other cells by the virus including neurological cells, etc. Thus, immunosuppressive effects resulting from altered physiological parameters in the host including effects on the CNS and endocrine system, which are modulated by the CNS, may indirectly affect the immune response.

Discussion and Conclusions

Burns are a major contributing factor to the altered susceptibility of individuals to infection by microorganisms [12]. The mechanisms should be understood in order to approach the complication of immune suppression in burn patients not only by the use of antibiotics, but in those cases where antibiotics are not effective, i.e., fungal and viral infection, by the use of immunotherapeutic agents. Infections by a wide variety of what are now considered to be opportunistic microorganisms, including fungi and viruses, are a significant cause of additional morbidity and, indeed, mortality in burned and traumatically injured individuals. There are many studies showing that altered immune responses accompany burns. Among these are alterations in humoral immune components, including antibody, complement, and soluble mediators of immune function such as lymphokines [2, 3]. In general, altered antibody formation at the cellular level as well as altered cell-mediated immune responses have been consistently noted in a wide variety of clinical and experiment studies concerning burn injury. It is now generally believed that such altered immune responses after severe or even moderate burn injury may make an individual highly susceptible to opportunistic microorganisms.

Burned tissue itself may become rapidly colonized and infected by microbial flora which in turn may further alter the immune responses of the host [3]. Thus, an important question which still remains unanswered is whether the putative defect in immune responses in a burn-injured patient is a primary cause for the increased susceptibility to infection, or alternatively, whether the organism which is colonizing burned tissue may in turn cause further physiological and immunological alterations, depressing lymphoid function and activities, resulting further in increased susceptibility to either the same or other infectious agents. The interaction of a microorganism with the host is a two-way system in that the host attempts to respond to the microbe by preventing colonization and eventually infection. In turn, the microbe attempts to subvert the defense mechanism of the host in order to establish a foothold.

Over the eons, natural selection of healthy individuals and their parasites has resulted in a symbiotic relationship in which most microorganisms after establishing themselves do not appear to cause untoward effects. Much of the responsiveness of the host to microorganisms may be beneficial, especially in regards to the normal stimulation of the immune system development and maturation. Individuals become immunologically competent after constant exposure to normal flora from birth onwards. Any alteration in this normal host-parasite relationship, including the disease process related to an organism, abuse of drugs, and accidents such as burns or trauma, may alter or influence the outcome of such a carefully balanced system. Microorganisms can interact with normal immune mechanisms to avoid complement- and antibody-associated lysis, and thus utilize nutritional factors of the host for their own benefit. The host may resist invasion by a microorganism even after colonization has occurred by mobilization of bone-marrow-derived lymphoid cells necessary for immune defenses, as well as inflammatory and chemotactic reactions to the invading organism, opsonization of the microbe by humoral antibody and complement, phagocytosis by macrophages and other lymphoid cells, and, finally, intracellular killing of those microbes which had penetrated into the host proper and intracellular milieu. This normal chain of events, however, is influenced by injuries such as burns, which permit establishment of large numbers of organisms, which in turn may have a detrimental effect on the host immunity.

Thus, an understanding of the nature or interaction of microorganisms and their products with the immune system in not only normal, but also burned, individuals will permit development of new strategies whereby immunostimulatory properties of various agents, including even possibly microbial products, may be used to restore immunocompetence. In addition, an understanding of the nature and mechanism of cellular versus humoral immune systems in normal individuals will permit development of methods for reversing immune defects in burned individuals. "Natural" immunostimulating factors such as interleukins, cytokines, neurohormones, and neuropeptides that have been tested in immunosuppressed individuals, especially those with cancer and AIDS, may also be quite useful in burned individuals. Study of the effects of these agents on the immune system of the burned individual, especially those with microbial infection, should make it possible in the near future to determine whether known mediators of normal immune responses are useful in burned individuals.

References

1. Ninnemann JL (ed) (1983) Traumatic injury: infection and other immunologic sequelae. University Park Press, Baltimore
2. Ninnemann JL (ed) (1981) The immune consequences of thermal injury. Williams and Wilkins, Baltimore
3. Antonacci AC, Friedman H, Mannick JA (1984) How do immunomodulators affect host defense in the burn patient? J Trauma 24:[Suppl]101–117
4. Winkelstein A, Ninnemann J (1984) What are the immunological alteration induced by burn injury? J Trauma 24[Suppl]72–83
5. Alexander JW, Ogle CK, Stinnet JD et al. (1978) A sequential prospective analysis of immunologic abnormalities and infection following severe thermal injury. Ann Surg 188:809–816
6. Bjornson AB, Attemeier WA, Bjornson HS (1977) Changes in humoral components of host defense following burn trauma. Ann Surg 186:88–95
7. Munster AM, Eurenius K, Katz RM et al. (1973) Cell mediated immunity after thermal injury. Ann Surg 177:139–143
8. Friedman H, Klein TW, Szentivanyi A (1981) Immunomodulation by bacteria and their products. Plenum, New York
9. Yamamura Y, Kotani S, Azuma T, Koda A, Shiba T (1982) Immunomodulation by microbial products and related synthetic components. Excerpta Medica, Amsterdam
10. Friedman H, Specter S, Farber P, Ceglowski W (1979) Interactions of viruses with lymphoid cells. In: Quastel M (ed) Cell biology and immunology of leukocyte function. Academic, New York, pp 783–802
11. Antonacci AC, Good RA (1982) T cell subpopulations following thermal injury. Surg Gynecol Obstet 155:1–8
12. Paul WE (ed) (1984) The immune system: an introduction in fundamental immunology. Raven, New York
13. Van Furth R (1982) Current view on the mononuclear phagocyte system. Immunobiology 161:178–185
14. Janeway CA Jr, Cone RE, Owen FL (1984) T lymphocyte receptor. In: Paul WE (ed) Fundamental immunology. Raven, New York
15. Friedman H, Specter S (1981) Virus induced immunomodulation. In: Hadden J, Chedid L, Muller P, Sprecifico F (eds) Advances in immunopharmacology. Pergamon, New York, pp 91–100
16. Specter S, Friedman H (1978) Viruses and the immune response. Pharmacol Ther (A) 2:595–622
17. Gallo RC, Sarin PS, Gelmann EP et al. (1983) Isolation of human T-cell leukemia virus in acquired immune deficiency syndrome (AIDS). Science 220:865–868

References

Endotoxin-Induced Impairment of Host Defenses

E. A. Deitch

Introduction

The cell walls of gram-negative bacteria are composed of three layers which include outer and inner membranes that enclose an electron dense peptidoglycan backbone [1]. The outer membrane is a trilamellar structure which has a different chemical composition than the inner cytoplasmic membrane and contains the lipopolysaccharide moiety. Lipopolysaccharide is unique in nature and is found only in gram-negative bacteria. Although the terms endotoxin and lipopolysaccharide are frequently used interchangeably, the two terms are not always identical, since endotoxin contains protein as well as the lipopolysaccharide moiety. In fact, the term endotoxin is a misnomer, left over from the era when toxins were classified as either toxins synthesized and excreted by viable organisms (exotoxin) or intracellular toxins released only upon lysis of the organism (endotoxin).

Endotoxin consists of three regions: polysaccharide side chains, core lipopolysaccharide, and a lipid A component that consists of a glucosamine backbone to which are linked long chain fatty acids. Lipid A is considered by most investigators to be primarily responsible for the toxicity of endotoxin and its structure appears to be constant among the different genera of gram-negative bacilli. The core polysaccharide is similar within groups of the Enterobacteriacae, while the side-chain polysaccharides containing the somatic 0 antigens vary greatly. However, neither the presence of the 0 side chains nor the core polysaccharide are necessary for toxicity. Since lipid A appears to be responsible for the toxic properties of endotoxin and its structure is constant, considerable effort has been directed towards producing vaccines against lipid A. The topic of vaccines and immunotherapy will be discussed in detail later in this chapter.

The concept that endotoxin mediates the pathophysiological changes associated with sepsis is based on extensive in vivo animal studies. These studies document that many of the effects observed when endotoxin is injected into experimental animals are similar to those observed in septic man. Although both septic man and endotoxin treated animals display fever, shock, and dissemenated intravascular coagulation, there is no longer a universal consensus that endotoxin is the direct mediator of disease caused by gram-negative bacteria. Instead, it has become clear that endotoxin exerts its toxic effect by triggering the release of endogenous factors produced by the host [2]. Endotoxin, as well as many other microbial products, induce the production, synthesis, and secretion of a variety of endogenous mediators and cytokines, as well as exerting profound effects on diverse organ systems in addition to the immune and cardiovascular systems.

Immune Consequences of
Trauma, Shock and Sepsis
Eds. Faist/Ninnemann/Green

Before discussing the effects of endotoxin on the immune system, it is important to realize that the exact in vivo effects of endotoxin depend on the route of administration, the dose, timing, and frequency of administration, the parameter measured, and the experimental species tested. For example, multiple small doses of intravenously administered, but not intradermally injected, endotoxin will induce a state of endotoxin tolerance. Similarly, endotoxin can augment or suppress the host's ability to withstand a septic challenge. For example, animals receiving sublethal doses of endotoxin are more resistant to bacterial challenge than control animals when tested 24–48 h after receiving endotoxin. In contrast, endotoxin-treated animals are less resistant to the same bacterial challenge when tested shortly after receiving endotoxin. Lastly, it is important to remember that the response to endotoxin varies greatly between species. Certain species, such as the rodent, are much more resistant to endotoxin than man, while other species, such as the dog, show major differences in their hemodynamic response to an endotoxin challenge.

With these caveats in mind, the remainder of this chapter will focus on the effect of endotoxin on host defenses.

Endotoxin-Elicited Mediators

Hemodynamic, metabolic, and immunologic disturbances have all been documented after endotoxin challenge and endotoxin shock remains a clinically common cause of death. Recently, it has become clear that the toxicity of endotoxin is dependent upon the production of endogenous factors by the host [3]. The classic experiments establishing the role of the macrophage in the lethal effects of endotoxin were carried out in two strains of mice, one that is endotoxin sensitive (C3H/HeN) and the other that is endotoxin resistant (C3H/HeJ). In these studies, lethally irradiated C3H/HeJ mice reconstituted with macrophages from C3H/HeN donors resulted in the production of endotoxin-sensitive radiation chimeras. Conversely, irradiated endotoxin-sensitive C3H/HeN mice became endotoxin resistant when reconstituted with macrophages from endotoxin resistant C3H/HeJ mice. Furthermore, macrophages from endotoxin-sensitive mice exposed to endotoxin in vitro produced factor(s) that were capable of killing endotoxin resistant mice. In addition to activating macrophages, endotoxin also activates the coagulation and complement cascades resulting in the production of other biologically active factors. Since the length of this chapter is limited, only a brief discussion of each mediator will be possible.

In vitro, endotoxin activates both the classical and alternate pathways of complement. The lipid A region of endotoxin can activate the classical pathway, in the absence of specific antibody, by directly binding to C1. Activation of the alternate pathway appears to be due to the polysaccharide moiety. Once activated, the anaphylatoxins C3a and C5a are produced, which have vasodilatory properties and may contribute to endotoxin shock. Furthermore, complement breakdown products may modulate neutrophil and lymphocyte activity, since these cells have been recently documented to have complement receptors. Although in some experimental models complement has been shown to play a role in endotoxin shock, the role of complement in clinical endotoxemia is controversial. Gram-negative bacteremia and activation of the alternate complement pathway has been documented by some investigators [4] but not others [5].

Arachidonic acid metabolites produced by endotoxin-activated macrophages appear to play a role in endotoxin mediated disease. This conclusion is based on the fact that endotoxin can elicit the production of prostaglandins and leukotrienes and that inhibitors or antagonists of these metabolites can modulate physiologic effects of endotoxin. Other macrophage products have also been shown to be induced by endotoxin. These include interleukin-1 (IL-1), tumor necrosis factor (TNF) or cachectin, colony stimulating factor (CSF), and interferon. Each of these factors alone or in combination can have profound effects on multiple homeostatic systems including immune integrity. However, at this point in time, it appears that TNF is responsible for most of endotoxin's systemic effects, including the induction of endotoxin shock [2].

Clinical and experimental endotoxemia is associated with diffuse microvascular thrombosis and activation of the coagulation system. The coagulation system can be activated directly by endotoxin activation of Hageman's factor (factor XII) or indirectly by endotoxin stimulated secretion of tissue factor by macrophages [3].

Another potential mediator of endotoxin shock is platelet activation factor (PAF). PAF is produced by many cells, including macrophages, neutrophils, platelets, and endothelial cells and its biologic effects include increased vascular permeability, hypotension, and death. Furthermore, endotoxin-induced hypotension is temporally associated with detectable levels of plasma PAF and PAF antagonists reverse endotoxin-induced shock. Determination of the exact role of these endotoxin-induced mediators and cytokines in endotoxin shock is compounded by the fact that these mediators appear to interact synergistically.

The role of endogenous opiates as mediators of endotoxin shock has been proposed on the basis that naloxone, a potent opiate antagonist, improves survival in a variety of endotoxin and septic shock models. Unfortunately, clinical trials have not shown that naloxone improves survival in gram-negative sepsis. Nonetheless, endotoxin can induce the synthesis of immunoreactive endorphins and these and other neuropeptides have been shown to have immunoregulatory activity [6].

Thus, endotoxin shock appears to be due to the activation of endogenous host systems and cells, especially the macrophage/monocyte system. In fact, as stated by Thomas [7], the lethal effects of endotoxin appear to be due to the fact that "our arsenals for fighting off bacteria are so powerful and involve so many defense mechanisms, that we are in more danger from them than from the invaders." If the host survives the early lethal hemodynamic effects of endotoxin, then the other effects of endotoxin on host defense systems become manifest, including alterations in host defenses.

Endotoxin-Mediated Alterations in Host Defenses

In addition to endotoxin's direct effect, many of the same mediators that potentiate endotoxin shock also can alter neutrophil, lymphocyte, and macrophage function. The effect of endotoxin on neutrophil function is variable and depends on the species tested, the assay measured, and whether the effect of endotoxin is tested in vivo or in vitro. There is general agreement that neutrophils exposed to endotoxin in vitro have increased hexose monophosphate shunt (HMPS) activity, glycolysis, degranulation, and nitro blue tetrazolium (NBT) reduction [8]. However, the effects of endotoxin on oxygen consumption and bactericidal activity is not clear, since different investigators have reported that neutrophil oxygen consumption in the presence of endotoxin is either normal, increased, or decreased. Proctor [8] has concluded, based on elegant in vitro studies of human neutrophils, that endotoxin in doses ranging from 10–100 μg dissociates glucose metabolism from oxygen consumption and bactericidal activity. That is, endotoxin depressed neutrophil bactericidal activity while increasing HMPS activity and glycolysis. They propose that the toxicity of endotoxin on neutrophil bactericidal activity is related to the production of oxidants or due to membrane alterations. The effect of endotoxin appears to be dose dependent, since Guthrie et al. [9] documented that human neutrophils incubated with endotoxin at concentrations ranging from 10 to 100 ng were primed and had an increased response to subsequent stimuli. Many investigators believe that endotoxin affects neutrophil function primarily through activated soluble mediators, such as products of the complement cascade. Recently, Moore et al. [10] reported that the infusion of endotoxin (20 U/kg) into healthy volunteers would activate neutrophils directly in the absence of complement activation. These results indicate that endotoxin can activate neutrophils directly, as well as through soluble mediators, and that the exact effect on neutrophil function is dose dependent.

Regardless of how the neutrophils are activated, it is clear that activated neutrophils produce a multitude of products that can potentiate the inflammatory response and may, in fact, lead to local tissue injury. Conclusions on the ultimate clinical significance of endotoxin as a mediator of tissue injury and multiple organ failure, as well as its effect on neutrophil bactericidal activity, will require further study.

The specific immune system appears to have evolved to help vertebrate species cope with bacterial and viral pathogens. In fact, bacteria and endotoxin are among the most powerful antigens in nature. Under normal circumstances, the immune response to a bacterial or endotoxin challenge can be beneficial. B cells are activated to produce antibodies, macrophages are activated to become more efficient phagocytes, granulocytes are released from the bone marrow, and the reticuloendothelial system (RES) is primed to clear more efficiently the circulation of circulating bacteria or debris. Endotoxin's effect on B-cell activation, in contrast to most antigens, is not T-cell dependent. Although endotoxin has no direct effect on T cells, it can modulate the T-cell response to other antigens that are T-cell dependent.

Endotoxin's modulating effects on T-cell proliferation and the host's immune response vary from complete suppression to immune enhancement and increased resistance to an infectious challenge. Based on in vivo studies, it appears that endotoxin administered 24 h prior to an antigenic or infectious challenge suppresses the host's response. However, this period of increased susceptibility is limited, since if the animals are challenged 24–48 h after receiving endotoxin their responses are enhanced. Furthermore, the administration of endotoxin simultaneously with or shortly after an antigenic or infectious challenge frequently bolsters rather than suppresses the host's immune response. Thus, endotoxin will modulate the host's immune response to antigens distinct from those associated with the endotoxin molecule, and its specific immunomodulating effect is related to the temporal relationship between endotoxin administration and the antigenic challenge.

The ability of endotoxin to modulate T-cell activity appears to be mediated to a large extent by cytokines produced by activated macrophages. In fact, enhancement of macrophage and reticuloendothelial system (RES) activity was one of the earliest documented effects of endotoxin on host defenses. Endotoxin-induced macrophage activation is associated with complex alterations in macrophage metabolism and activated macrophages display enhanced microbicidal and tumoricidal capacities. Depending upon which cytokines are produced by the activated macrophages the immune response can be enhanced or suppressed. Endotoxin-mediated immune enhancement appears to be associated with the preferential production and secretion of IL-1 by activated macrophages, while suppression is associated with prostaglandin E_2 (PGE_2) release. Thus, endotoxin appears to induce a stimulatory circuit that is associated with increased macrophage bactericidal activity and the secretion of IL-1, or a suppressive circuit associated with PGE_2 secretion. In the suppressive circuit, PGE_2 down regulates macrophage activity as well as other effector cells via a feedback suppression loop. In fact, Faist [11] has recently documented that increased production of PGE_2 by monocytes prevents IL-2 synthesis in trauma patients.

Thus, endotoxin has a wide range of immunologic activities. On the positive side, endotoxin stimulates B-lymphocyte proliferation, and when administered simultaneously with a test antigen, it exerts a strong adjuvant effect on the subsequent antibody response to that test antigen. Additionally, it can activate macrophages and the RES, as well as induce granulocytosis, increase serum complement levels, and promote an inflammatory response. On the other hand, depending on the dosage and the timing of its administration, endotoxin can induce suppressor T-cell activity and PGE_2 secretion by macrophages, and decrease the resistance of experimental animals to an infectious challenge. Thus, endotoxin initiates a complex series of events leading to the production of numerous mediators many of which, such as IL-1, TNF, CSF, PGE_2, and the interferons, have their own immunomodulating effects. Therefore, in considering the effects of endotoxin on the immune response, it is important to keep in mind the fact that endotoxin, in addition to its direct effects on the immune system, also induces the production and release of numerous cytokines and inflammatory mediators, all of which induce their own cascade of effects.

Bacterial Translocation, Gut Failure, and Endotoxemia

My own work has concentrated primarily on the relationship between bacteremia, endotoxemia, and gut failure. The impetus for this work was based on the results of epidemiologic and clinical studies suggesting that the gut can be a reservoir for bacterial infections and can leak endotoxin into the systemic circulation in immunocompromised patients [12]. To work out the mechanisms by which gut failure and the subsequent translocation (escape) of bacteria from the gut into systemic tissues occurs we developed and employed multiple animal models. Based on the study of these models, it appears that gut failure and bacterial translocation can occur when: (1) the normal ecology of the gut flora is disrupted resulting in bacterial overgrowth of gram-negative enteric bacilli, (2) the host is immunosuppressed, or (3) the epithelial physical barrier is disrupted.

Since endotoxin increases gut permeability, alters host immune defenses, and is relatively common in patients at increased risk of developing infections with gut-associated microorganisms, we investigated whether nonlethal doses of endotoxin would promote bacterial translocation from the gastrointestinal tract. Endotoxin promoted bacterial translocation in a dose-dependent fashion and the incidences of bacterial translocation were similar whether the endotoxin was administered intramuscularly or intraperitoneally. Additionally, the incidences and magnitudes of endotoxin-induced bacterial translocation were similar between CD-1 and C3H/HeJ (endotoxin hyporesponsive) mice, indicating that bacterial translocation is not prevented by genetic resistance to endotoxin. Furthermore, the combination of endotoxin with either a nonlethal thermal injury [13] or a protein malnourished state [14] resulted in the development of lethal systemic infections originating from the gut. Endotoxin appears to induce bacterial translocation primarily by injuring the gut mucosa. Furthermore, the mechanism by which endotoxin injures the gut mucosa appears to be through oxidants generated by xanthine oxidase.

Thus, it appears that under some circumstances, endotoxemia may become self-sustaining, since systemic endotoxin promotes the absorption of intestinal endotoxin and the systemic translocation of bacteria from the gut. The exact role of gut failure and the translocation of bacteria and endotoxin insepticemia and multiple organ failure is currently under study.

Therapy

Conceptually, there are several general approaches that can be taken to reduce the risk or biologic consequences of systemic endotoxemia. These include attempts to prevent the development of endotoxemia. Drugs or vaccines can be used to neutralize the deleterious effects of endotoxin, either by binding directly to the endotoxin molecule, by preventing release, or blocking the activity of endogenous mediators. And, lastly, agents to bolster normal host defenses can be used.

Endotoxemia generally originates from the gut or from areas of localized infection, such as an intraabdominal abscess or an infected burn wound. Thus, to prevent endotoxemia we must concentrate on methods to maintain the gut antibacterial barrier and to prevent or treat infections. The judicious use of broad-spectrum antibiotics to reduce the risk of disruption of the normal gut flora, the use of enteral nutrition to prevent gut mucosal atrophy, and the avoidance of intestinal ischemia appear to be critical elements in maintaining gut integrity. Prompt drainage of abscesses, early resection of necrotic tissue, optimal nutritional and physiologic support, and good infection control policies all play a role in the prevention or limitation of infectious complications. It is clear that the prevention of uncontrolled endotoxemia is superior to attempts at its treatment.

In general, therapeutic manuevers to neutralize endotoxin have concentrated on the use of vaccines, monoclonal antibodies, or drugs, such as polymyxin B. All these therapeutic agents share one characteristic property: they bind directly to the endotoxin molecule and neutralize its biologic activity. Although many vaccines and monoclonal antibodies have been shown to be effective against endotoxin and bacteria in experimental animals, the majority of the human studies reported to date have used a vaccine developed against the J5 mutant of *E. coli* 0111:B4. In a multicenter randomized controlled trial [15], patients with suspected gram-negative sepsis received either immune serum or preimmune serum from the same donors. The patients receiving the immune serum had half the mortality rate of the control group, indicating that antisera directed against the J5 mutant improves survival in patients with gram-negative sepsis. Recently, Munster [16] has evaluated the use of prophylactically administered polymyxin B to neutralize endotoxin in burn patients. Although the results of this study are not conclusive, this concept is appealing.

The use of specific drugs to block or neutralize endotoxin induced mediators from activated macrophages is in its infancy. However, this approach may be more widely used in the future. For example, Revhaug et al. [17], have recently documented that inhibition of cyclooxygenase activity with ibuprofen will attenuate the metabolic response to intravenous endotoxin in healthy human volunteers. Further work in this field is needed to determine if specific inhibitors or antibodies to endogenous mediators, such as TNF or PAF, will be clinically beneficial.

The role of immunomodulators in the treatment of endotoxemia is not clear, since experimentally drugs, such as *C. parvum,* that activate macrophages may predispose the host to endotoxic shock. Nonetheless, Bertok [18] has published some exciting work indicating that radiodetoxified endotoxin will booster host defenses and improve survival in a variety of experimental conditions. Unfortunately, there is not adequate information available at present to reach any conclusions about the clinical efficacy of immunomodulators in the treatment of endotoxemia in humans.

Conclusion

Endotoxin exerts a bewildering array of biologic effects on the normal host, which vary depending upon the dose, timing, and frequency of administration. The fact that different species respond differently to a similar endotoxin challenge hinders the translation of experimental studies in animals to man. Hopefully, as more information is obtained clarifying the molecular mechanisms by which endotoxin exerts it effects, it should be possible to devise therapeutic strategies to prevent the deleterious effects of endotoxemia.

References

1. Stephen J, Pietrowski RA (1986) Cell-associated toxins. In: Stephen J, Pietrowski RA (eds) Bacterial toxins. American Society for Microbiology, Washington D.C., chap 8, pp 105–144
2. Beutler B, Cerami A (1987) The endogenous mediator of endotoxic shock. Clin Res 35:192–197
3. Morrison DC, Ryan JL (1987) Endotoxins and disease mechanisms. Annu Rev Med 38:417–432
4. Fearson DT, Ruddy S, Schur PH, McCabe WR (1975) Activation of the properdin pathway of complement in patients with gram-negative bacteremia. N Engl J Med 292:937–940
5. Shatney CH, Benner C (1985) Sequential serum complement (C3) and immunoglobulin levels in shock/trauma patients developing acute fulminant systemic sepsis. Circ Shock 16:9–17
6. Adler R (1981) Psychoneuroimmunology. Academic, Orlando
7. Thomas L (1974) The lives of a cell: notes of a biology watcher. Viking, New York
8. Proctor RA (1979) Endotoxin in vitro interactions with human neutrophils; depression of chemiluminescence, oxygen consumption, superoxide production, and killing. Infect Immun 25:912–921
9. Guthrie LA, McPhail PM, Johnson RB (1984) Priming of neutrophils for enhanced release of oxygen metabolites by bacterial lipopolysaccharide. J Exp Med 160:1656–1671
10. Moore FD Jr, Moss NA, Revhaug A et al. (1987) A single dose of endotoxin activates neutrophils without activating complement. Surgery 102:200–205
11. Faist E, Mewes A, Baker CC et al. (1987) Prostaglandin E_2-dependent suppression of interleukin (IL-2) production in patients with major trauma. J Trauma 27:837–848
12. Deitch EA, Berg R (1987a) Bacterial translocation from the gut: a mechanism of infection. J Burn Care Rehabil 8:475–482
13. Deitch EA, Berg R (1987b) Endotoxin but not malnutrition promotes bacterial translocation of the gut flora in burned mice. J Trauma 27:161–166
14. Deitch EA, Winterton J, Ma L, Berg R (1987c) The gut as a portal of entry for bacteremia; the role of protein malnutrition. Ann Surg 205:681–692
15. Ziegler EJ, McCutchan JA, Fierer J, Glauser MP, Sadoff JC, Douglas H, Braude AI (1982) Treatment of gram-negative bacteremia and shock with human antiserum to a mutant *Escherichia coli*. N Engl J Med 307:1255–1230
16. Munster AM, Winchurch RA, Thupari JN, Ernst CB (1986) Reversal of postburn immunosuppression with low-dose polymyxin. Br J Trauma 26:995–998
17. Revhaug A, Michie HR, Manson JM et al. (1988) Inhibition of cyclo-oxygenase attenuates the metabolic response to endotoxin in humans. Arch Surg 123:162–170
18. Bertok L (1980) Radio-detoxified endotoxin as a potent stimulator of nonspecific resistance. Perspect Biol Med 24:61–66

Prostaglandins and Leukotrienes in Monocyte/ T Cell Function in Stress and Trauma

J. L. Ninnemann

Introduction

Prostaglandins (PGs) and leukotrienes (LTs) are products of arachidonic acid metabolism and are produced by many types of mammalian cells. These versatile compounds participate in a variety of normal physiological processes, including the maintenance of blood pressure and body temperature, protection of organs from damage caused by disease, and the regulation of parturition. It is now also clear that the PGs (particularly PGE_2) and the LTs (particularly LTB_4) are important in the normal regulation of the immune response. Conversely, shifts in the balance of arachidonic acid metabolite production have been implicated in shock, and a wide variety of disease states, including arthritis, malignancy, and the allergic disorders (reviewed by Ninnemann 1988).

Three substrate fatty acids are thought to be the primary precursors of PGs and LTs. Of these, cis-5,8,11,14-eicosatetraenoic acid (arachidonic acid) is considered to be the most important. Arachidonic acid is metabolized, subsequent to its release from membranes, enzymatically (via a family of lipoxygenase enzymes or cyclooxygenase) or nonenzymatically (via ultraviolet light irradiation or O_2-generating systems), to form oxidation products.

The sequential biosynthesis of the PGs is carried out by two membrane-bound enzymes, cyclooxygenase and endoperoxide isomerase, and by the soluble enzyme, peroxidase. The bioactive PGs are formed very quickly from their corresponding precursors, but are then quickly converted to metabolites with much weaker activities (Oates et al. 1980).

The enzymatic metabolism of arachidonic acid by 5-lipoxygenase results in the formation of 5-hydroperoxyeicosatetraenoic acids (5-HPETE). The 5-HPETEs can be metabolized to either their analogous alcohols via peroxidase, or to the leukotrienes (Bach 1983).

Eicosanoids and Macrophage Activity

The products of arachidonic acid metabolism are important regulators of macrophage activity, and of macrophage-lymphocyte cooperation. For example, PGE_2 has been shown to have a profound inhibitory effect on human macrophage lysosomal hydrolase release, and on macrophage locomotion, shape change and phagocytosis (Bonta and Parnham 1982). These changes are associated with an increase in cyclic AMP levels, however in some cases, functional changes seem to result directly from PGE-membrane interactions (Oropeza-Rendon et al. 1980).

Immune Consequences of
Trauma, Shock and Sepsis
Eds. Faist/Ninnemann/Green

Not only are macrophages affected by the presence of cyclooxygenase and lipoxygenase products, they are also clearly a major source of immunologically active eicosanoids (Morley et al. 1979; Goldyne and Stobo 1979; Kennedy et al. 1980). The identification of the monocyte as the primary human peripheral blood mononuclear cell responsible for PG production (specifically PGE) was largely the result of work by Bankhurst et al. (1981). Just as macrophage response to the presence of eicosanoids is related to the state of cell differentiation, macrophage production of these metabolites is also activation dependent (Humes et al. 1977). Stimulated macrophages produce PGE, and are active in down-regulating the immune response through induction of suppressor T cells, direct interaction with lymphocytes in culture, and by acting as mediators or carriers of T-cell suppressor factors (Humes et al. 1977).

Macrophages which function in this capacity are sometimes called *suppressor macrophages*. Their activity can be reversed in culture by the addition of cyclooxygenase inhibitors such as indomethacin (Ninnemann 1988). Stimulated macrophages are also able to synthesize and release 5-lipoxygenase products such as LTB_4 and LTC_4 (Williams et al. 1984; Neill et al. 1985) and it is thought that the release of these compounds acts as a counterbalance to the effects of PGE_2 synthesis.

Prostaglandins, Leukotrienes, and Lymphocyte Response

While it is now almost certain that lymphocytes do not themselves produce cyclooxygenase or lipoxygenase products of arachidonic acid metabolism, it is clear that they bear receptors for PGE_2 (Goodwin et al. 1979) and are profoundly suppressed by the presence of this metabolite. Recent studies have shown that physiological concentrations of PGE_2 will suppress antibody production by B cells (Simkin et al. 1987) as well as many T-cell functions including mitogen responsiveness (Goodwin et al. 1978), clonal proliferation (Bockman 1979), antigenic stimulation (Gorski et al. 1982), erythrocyte-rosette formation (Enteu et al. 1980), lymphokine production (Gordon et al. 1976; Rappaport and Dodge 1982), generation of cytotoxic cells (Darrow and Tomar 1980), and lymphocyte migration (Van Epps 1981). Recent studies have suggested that several products of lipoxygenase activity also control cellular immune responses, including 15-HPETE (Goodman and Weigle 1980), and LTB_4 (Payan and Goetzl 1983).

In addition, various products of arachidonic acid metabolism (particularly PGE_2) participate in the induction of nonspecific suppressor T-lymphocyte activity (Fischer et al. 1981). Kaszubowski and Goodwin (1982) showed that monocyte-produced PGE_2 (3×10^{-6} *M*) induced Fc_{gamma} receptor expression on human T cells, and that these cells were responsible for in vivo suppressor activity. Supportive results have been reported by Rappaport and Dodge (1982) and by Chouaib et al. (1984) who found that when cell separation was performed after PGE_2 incubation, OKT8(+) lymphocytes were responsible for most of the observed suppression (68%) with little contribution from OKT4(+) lymphocytes (15%), whereas unincubated cells had less activity in the OKT8(+) fraction (58%) and more in the OKT4(+) fraction (27%). While PGE_2 treatment of peripheral blood lymphocytes induced suppressor T-cell activity, Chouaib found that PGE_2 incubation did not alter the distribution of T-cell subsets.

Rappaport and Dodge found that exogenous PGE was capable of inhibiting interleukin 2 (IL-2) production by normal human peripheral blood lymphocytes (1982). The removal of glass-adherent cells from mononuclear cell populations, on the other hand, led to an increase in IL-2 production by nonadherent cells, and the addition of PG synthetase inhibitors raised IL-2 production to supranormal levels. In addition to regulating the production of IL-2 by T lymphocytes, there is now evidence that PGE_2 can suppress the expression of IL-2 receptors, and the response of lymphocytes to the addition of exogenous IL-2 (Teodorczyk-Injeyan et al. 1987; Ninnemann 1987).

Eicosanoids and Immune Depression Following Injury

There has been increasing concern about the immunological depression that is unavoidably acquired as a result of major accidental or operative injury in an otherwise normal host. As a result, the question of how the immunological depression in the injured patient is mediated has received a great deal of attention. Experimental studies have shown that the general circulation of patients after injury or a major operation, often contains factors affecting vascular permeability, causing hemolytic changes in red blood cells, depressing cardiac output and renal function, causing profound immunosuppression, and, in some cases, precipitating multiple organ failure.

That at least some of these mediators are eicosanoids is indicated both by biochemical attempts to characterize immunosuppression, and by the constellation of immunological changes which take place as a result of injury. Just as has been found in the above cited studies, injury is often accompanied by strong, suppressor macrophage activity, a profound decrease in IL-2 production and response, and nonspecific T-suppressor cell generation with little increase in OKT8(+) cell numbers (reviewed by Ninnemann 1988). Furthermore, it appears that at least in certain circumstances, injury induced suppression can be mitigated by the use of cyclooxygenase inhibitors (Faist et al. 1986).

The pathophysiology of injury is often characterized by a strong inflammatory response which includes the release of the products of arachidonic acid metabolism. This is particularly well characterized for burn injuries, which can be considered a model for the study of all types of trauma. Experiments by Anggard et al. (1970) showed that a scald burn of the dog paw was followed by an eflux of prostaglandins (primarily PGE_2) in the lymphatic fluid draining the paw. This finding suggested increased PGE_2 biosynthesis as a result of injury. Guinea-pig studies verified this effect of thermal damage to the skin, and demonstrated an increased excretion of urinary 5-beta,7-alpha-dihydroxy-11-ketotetranor-prostanoid acid, a major metabolite of PGE (Hamberg and Jonsson 1973). Lipid extracts of guinea-pig skin, excised 2 h after injury, contained PG-like material at 20–40 times the concentration found in the lipid extracts of skin excised immediately, indicating a local, rather than systemic increase in PG biosynthesis as a result of injury. Heggers et al. (1980) confirmed the direct release of large quantities of PGs from skin cells as a result of thermal injuries. Ninnemann and Stockland (1984) also found that the concentrations of PGE in the circulation of patients with greater than 40% body surface area burns was 1000–3000 pg/ml, and that these same samples were often significantly suppressive to in vitro lymphocyte responsiveness. Ninnemann and Stockland found that both delipidation and the addition of rabbit anti-PGE_2 significantly reduced the lymphocyte suppressive activity of low molecular weight fractions of burn serum.

Grbic et al. (1985) found that burn-patient lymphocytes are particularly sensitive to the suppressive effects of PGE_2. This effect is similar to an earlier observation by Goodwin et al. (1981) who showed that physical stress of various types increased the sensitivity of lymphocytes to suppression by PGE_2, suggesting that eicosanoid production may be hormonally moderated.

Rodrick et al. (1985) reported that burn serum was capable of suppressing IL-2 synthesis, and Wood et al. (1986) showed that the suppression of IL-2 production in an animal model of thermal injury was related to PG synthesis. Wood hypothesized that reduced IL-2 levels reflected a reduction in IL-2-producing OKT4(+) helper cells, however, a direct confirmation of this concept could not be made. Likewise, while an increase in OKT8(+) suppressor cell activity is also suggested, shifts in the actual available numbers of these cells do not appear to occur as a result of injury.

Teodorczyk-Injeyan et al. (1986) found that there were significant differences between patients who survived major burn injuries and those who did not survive, in terms of IL-2 (Tac) receptor expression by lymphocytes, lymphocyte response levels, and IL-2 production. This group of investigators later showed that the impaired expression of IL-2 (Tac) receptors in burn patients was mediated by PGE_2, and that this defect could be duplicated in culture via the addition of burn serum (1986). Ninnemann also reported that the exposure of normal lymphocytes to PGE_2 or burn serum resulted in their inability to respond to exogenous IL-2 stimulation (1987).

Therapeutic Reversal of Eicosanoid Suppression

There is some indication that postinjury eicosanoid effects can be manipulated to patient advantage. Heggers et al. (1980), for example, showed that early cooling of burn injuries in an animal model prevented conversion of partial-thickness injuries to full-thickness injuries. This effect was due to temperature-dependent suppression of cyclooxygenase activity in the damaged tissue, providing a persuasive argument for cautious cooling in the case of certain injuries. It also appears that injury-associated deterioration of the cell-mediated immune response, can also be remediated by blocking or reducing prostanoid production. Hansbrough et al. (1984) demonstrated that the cellular immune response could be restored in burn-injured animals by means of treatment with various pharmacological agents, including the cyclooxygenase inhibitors ibuprofen and indomethacin. Faist et al. (1986) have demonstrated the improvement of trauma-patient lymphocyte phytohemagglutinin (PHA) responses as a result of indomethacin treatment. Clearly, more work is needed in this area.

Summary and Conclusions

It is becoming clear that the products of arachidonic acid metabolism can act as mediators in both normal and abnormal immunological responses. There is compelling evidence, for example, that the release of PGE_2 by activated macrophages regulates T-lymphocyte responsiveness by limiting IL-2 production and response through activation of a nonspecific suppressor-cell subpopulation. This sequence may be of particular clinical importance in the case of injured patients, whose immune depression makes them inordinately susceptible to opportunistic infection.

References

Anggard E, Arturson G, Jonsson CE (1970) Efflux of prostaglandins in lymph from scalded tissues. Acta Physiol Scand 80:46A

Bach MK (1983) The leukotrienes; their structure, actions, and role in diseases. Current concepts series. Upjohn, Kalamazoo

Bankhurst AD, Hastain E, Goodwin JS, Peake GT (1981) The nature of the prostaglandin-producing mononuclear cell in human peripheral blood. J Lab Clin Med 97:179–186

Bockman RS (1979) PGE inhibition of T lymphocyte colony formation. J Clin Invest 64:812–821

Bonta IL, Parnham MJ (1982) Immunomodulatory-antiinflammatory functions of E-type prostaglandins. Minireview with emphasis on macrophage mediated effects. Int J Immunopharmacol 4:103–109

Chouaib S, Chatenoud L, Klatzmann D, Fradelizi D (1984) The mechanism of inhibition of human IL-2 production. II. PGE2 induction of suppressor T lymphocytes. J Immunol 132:1851–1857

Darrow TL, Tomar RH (1980) Prostaglandin-mediated regulation of the mixed lymphocyte culture and generation of cytotoxic cells. Cell Immunol 65:172–178

Enteu U, Enre T, Cavdar AO, Turker RK (1980) An in vitro study on the effect of prostaglandin E2 and F2 alpha on E-rosette forming activity of normal lymphocytes. Prostaglandins Leukotrienes Med 5:255–261

Faist E, Kupper TS, Baker CC, Chaudry IH, Dwyer J, Baue AE (1986) Depression of cellular immunity after major injury. Arch Surg 121:1000–1005

Fischer A, Durandy A, Griscelli C (1981) Role of prostaglandin E2 in the induction of nonspecific T lymphocyte suppressor activity. J Immunol 126:1452

Goldyne ME, Stobo JD (1979) Synthesis of prostaglandins by subpopulations of human peripheral blood monocytes. Prostaglandins 18:687–695

Goodman MG, Weigle WO (1980) Modulation of lymphocyte activation. I. Inhibition by an oxidation product of arachidonic acid. J Immunol 125:593–600

Goodwin JS, Messner RP, Peake GT (1978) Prostaglandin suppression of mitogen-stimulated lymphocytes in vitro. J Clin Invest 62:753–760

Goodwin JS, Wiik A, Lewis M, Bankhurst AD, Williams RC (1979) High affinity binding sites for prostaglandin E on human lymphocytes. Cell Immunol 43:150–159

Goodwin JS, Bromberg S, Staszak C, Kaszubowski PA, Messner RP, Neal JF (1981) Effect of physical stress on sensitivity of lymphocytes to inhibition by prostaglandin E2. J Immunol 127:518–522

Gordon D, Bray M, Morley J (1976) Control of lymphokine secretion by prostaglandins. Nature 262:401–407

Gorski A, Graciong Z, Dupont B (1982) Enhanced colonability of human T lymphocytes causes by their culturing in vitro. Immunology 44:617–622

Grbic JT, Wood JJ, Jordan A, Rodrick ML, Mannick JA (1985) Lymphocytes from burned patients are more sensitive to suppression by prostaglandin E2. Surg Forum 108–110

Hamberg M, Jonsson CE (1973) Increased synthesis of prostaglandins in guinea pig following scalding injury. 87:240
Hansbrough J, Petersonn V, Zapata-Sirvent R, Claman HN (1984) Postburn immunosuppression in an animal model. II. Restoration of cell-mediated immunity by immunomodulating drugs. Surgery 95:290–295
Heggers JP, Loy GL, Robson MC, DelBeccaro EJ (1980) Histological demonstration of prostaglandins and thromboxanes in burned tissue. J Surg Res 28:110–117
Humes JL, Bonney RW, Pelus L, Dahlgren ME, Sadowski SS, Kuehl FA, Davies P (1977) Macrophages synthesize and release prostaglandins in response to inflammatory stimuli. Nature 269:159
Kaszubowski PA, Goodwin JS (1982) Monocyte-produced prostaglandin induces Fc gamma receptor expression on human T cells. Cell Immunol 68:343–348
Kennedy MS, Stobo JD, Goldyne ME (1980) In vitro synthesis of prostaglandins and related lipids by populations of human peripheral blood mononuclear cells. Prostaglandins 20:135–145
Morley J, Bray MA, Jones RW, Nugteren DH, VanDorp DA (1979) Prostaglandins and thromboxanes production by human and guinea pig macrophages and leukocytes. Prostaglandins 17:729–736
Neill MA, Henderson WR, Klebanoff SJ (1985) Oxidative degradation of leukotriene C4 by human monocytes and monocyte-derived macrophages. J Exp Med 162:1634–1644
Ninnemann JL (1987) PGE regulates lymphocyte stimulation by Il-2. Proc Am Burn Assoc 19:10
Ninnemann JL (1988) Prostaglandins, leukotrienes, and the immune response. Cambridge University Press, New York
Ninnemann JL, Stockland AE (1984) Participation of prostaglandin E in immunosuppression following thermal injury. J Trauma 24:201–207
Oates JA, Roberts LD, Sweetman BJ, Maas RL, Gerkens JF, Tabber DF (1980) Metabolism of the prostaglandins and thromboxanes. Adv Prostaglandin Thromboxane Leukotriene Res 6:35–41
Oropeza-Rendon RL, Bauer HC, Fischer H (1980) Effect of prostaglandin E1 on the level of cAMP in bone marrow macrophages. Inhibition of phagocytosis and cell shape changes. J Immunopharmacol 2:133–147
Payan DG, Goetzl EJ (1983) Specific suppression of human T lymphocyte function by leukotriene B4. J Immunol 131:551–553
Rappaport RS, Dodge GR (1982) Prostaglandin E inhibits the production of human interleukin 2. J Exp Med 155:943–948
Rodrick ML, Saporoschetz IB, Wood JJ, Davis CF, Mannick JA (1985) Serum suppression of interleukin-2 (IL-2) production and IL-2 action in thermal injury. Surg Forum 98–99
Simkin NJ, Jelinek DF, Lipsky PE (1987) Inhibition of human B cell responsiveness by prostaglandin E2. J Immunol 138:1074–1081
Teodorczyk-Injeyan J, Sparkes BG, Mills GB, Peters WJ, Falk RE (1986) Impairment of T cell activation in burn patients: a possible mechanism of thermal injury-induced immunosuppression. Clin Exp Immunol 65:570–581
Teodorczyk-Injeyan JA, Sparkes BG, Peters WJ, Gerry K, Falls RE (1987) Prostaglandin E-related impaired expression of interleukin 2 receptor in the burn patient. Adv Prostaglandin Thromboxane Leukotriene Res 17:151–154
VanEpps D (1981) Suppression of human lymphocyte migration by PGE2. Inflammation 5:81–87
Williams JD, Czop JK, Austen KF (1984) Release of leukotrienes by human monocytes on stimulation of their phagocytic receptor for particulate activators. J Immunol 132:3034–3040
Wood JJ, Rodrick ML, Grbic JT, Mannick JA (1986) Suppression of interleukin-2 (IL-2) production in an animal model of thermal injury is related to prostaglandin synthesis. Proc Surg Infect Soc:33

Serum Mediators and the Generation of Immune Suppression

A. N. Ozkan

Introduction

Trauma is one of the most serious health care problems in the United States. It is the leading cause of mortality in the 1–40 year age group with more than 50 million injuries per year. In 1982 alone there were over 165 000 trauma deaths resulting in an economic impact of more than $88 billion.

Mortality associated with traumatic injuries has been described as having a trimodal pattern [1]. The first category of mortality has been classified as immediate death consisting of death due to laceration of the spinal cord, brain or brain stem. The second category is early death which occurs minutes to hours following injury from hemorrhage or internal bleeding. The last is late death occurring 3–10 days post injury and generally associated with sepsis and/or multiple organ failure. It is with late death and the factors which contribute to the septic outcome associated with late death that this article is concerned.

There is considerable clinical evidence for immune depression in trauma. Among clinical changes associated with injury are: (1) increased infection rates, (2) altered skin test reactivity (delayed type hypersensitivity response), and (3) numerous serum protein abnormalities. Immunologic changes described in trauma include: (1) depressed neutrophil function, (2) depressed natural-killer cell function, (3) depressed lymphocyte function, and (4) altered cytokine biosynthesis.

Immunosuppression in Trauma: The Search for Peptide Mediators

Peptide Mediators of Unknown Origin

The occurrence of circulating or serum-borne immunosuppressive peptides generated following traumatic injury has been widely documented. The majority of the early work involving the search for immunosuppressive factors in trauma has focused on burn injuries. One of the first reports on the existence of serum-borne factors was in 1974 by Warden, Mason and Pruitt [2]. It was demonstrated that normal neutrophils incubated in serum or plasma from thermally injured patients could be suppressed to a degree similar to that in neutrophils isolated directly from the patient.

The isolation of circulating factors began shortly thereafter. Constantian and coworkers [3] reported on the isolation of a low molecular weight peptide from

Immune Consequences of
Trauma, Shock and Sepsis
Eds. Faist/Ninnemann/Green

serum of operative and accidental trauma patients. The molecular mass of this peptide was determined to be $< 10\,000$ daltons and to be present in trauma patient serum at concentrations 5–10 times greater than in noninjured controls. This peptide was found to suppress T cell blastogenesis, inhibit phagocytosis, prolong skin allografts and inhibit the delayed type hypersensitivity response (DTH). The mode of action of this material was found to be elicited via a noncytotoxic pathway. Column chromatography of trauma serum yielded a protein fraction, identified as fraction I, whose specific activity paralleled the severity and duration of the clinical course. The origin of this peptide has not been fully elucidated. It has been suggested that this peptide is a feedback regulator of T cell-mediated immunity, and may be produced by suppressor lymphocytes during immune stimulation.

Also in 1977, Hakim [4] reported on the isolation and partial characterization of a low molecular weight ($< 10\,000$) peptide from the albumin-rich fraction of serum from thermally injured patients. This noncytotoxic peptide was found to inhibit the migration of guinea pig peritoneal macrophage and peripheral blood leukocytes from burn patients. The mitogenic response of phytohemagglutinin (PHA) on normal lymphocytes was also suppressed by the immunosuppressive peptide. Again the origin of this factor was not determined.

A similar factor to that described by Hakim was isolated and characterized by Christou and Meakins [5]. This peptide was found to be present in serum from anergic patients and correlated with clinical outcome. The molecular mass of the inhibitor was calculated to be approximately 8000 daltons. Activity of the peptide could be reversed by heat treatment of the sample or by the addition of 10 m*M* levamisole hydrochloride. The presence of this inhibitor at low concentrations in control serum was reported. It was postulated that following surgical or accidental trauma the inhibitor concentration could rise in the serum leading to episodes of immune suppression. Additionally it was suggested that a "piggyback" effect of this small inhibitor on a larger serum protein may be occurring.

In 1985 our group reported the isolation and partial characterization of a low molecular weight immunosuppressive peptide from burn-patient plasma [6]. This peptide given the acronym SAP (suppressor active peptide) was capable of suppressing T and B lymphocyte blastogenesis, inhibiting neutrophil migration, and lysing human erythrocytes. The physicochemical characteristic of the peptide have been previously reported and include: (1) heat resistance at 56 °C for 30 min but sensitivity to boiling, (2) high concentrations of glucosamines with activity dependent on a sialic acid moiety, (3) resistance to RNAse, DNAse, and trypsin with sensitivity to pronase, and (4) a molecular mass of $< 10\,000$ daltons [8]. Recent studies have found that SAP levels correlate with clinical outcome in the trauma patient [9]. Additionally, in a collaborative study with Jane Shelby at the University of Utah it was determined that SAP is a potent inhibitor of the in vivo DTH response as measured by sensitivity to dinitrofluorobenzene (DNFB). The origin of SAP has not been clearly elucidated, however, based on preliminary studies using an anti-SAP monoclonal antibody affinity column it is likely that the peptide is a degradation product of a larger molecular weight serum protein, or may have a "piggyback" effect on a larger molecular weight protein as proposed by Christou and Meakins [5].

Peptide Mediators of Known Origin

Recently several peptide mediators of known origin have been identified and characterized. In many instances these peptides are derived from larger molecular weight serum-borne proteins. Figure 1 represents a potential scheme for the generation of peptides following traumatic injury. It is likely that the peptide mediators which follow in this discussion are generated in a similar fashion.

The first of these peptides is fibrinogen. In 1977 Krzystyniak et al. [10] reported on the suppressive effect of low molecular weight fibrinogen degradation products on human and rat lymphocytes. Further studies by Edgington, Curtiss and Plow [11, 12] localized the suppressive peptides to the alpha chain of fibrinogen. These peptides were found to suppress both T and B lymphocyte blastogenesis via a noncytotoxic mechanism. It was hypothesized that since the localization of fibrinogen, conversion to fibrin, and subsequent proteolytic degradation is a prominent event in DTH reactions, the role of these peptides serves to limit the localized reactions and promote resolution of the lesions.

Immunological activity in fibronectin has also been reported. Low molecular weight plasmin digested fibronectin peptides were found to depress phagocytic activity of rat peritoneal macrophages in vitro [13]. In vivo studies demonstrated significantly reduced hepatic phagocytosis after injection of fibronectin peptides and delayed clearance of injected test particles. It was suggested by Ehrlich that the role of fibronectin peptides as a systemic phagocytic inhibitor might be of greatest significance during fibronectin depletion, that is, at a time when fibronectin degradation products are at high concentration and the beneficial effects of the intact molecule are at a minimum. Additional research on fibronectin peptides was reported by Easter et al. [14] and Hoyt et al. [15] in which a fibronectin peptide from the gelatin binding domain was demonstrated to be suppressive to T cell blastogenesis and to neutrophil migration. This peptide, having a molecular mass

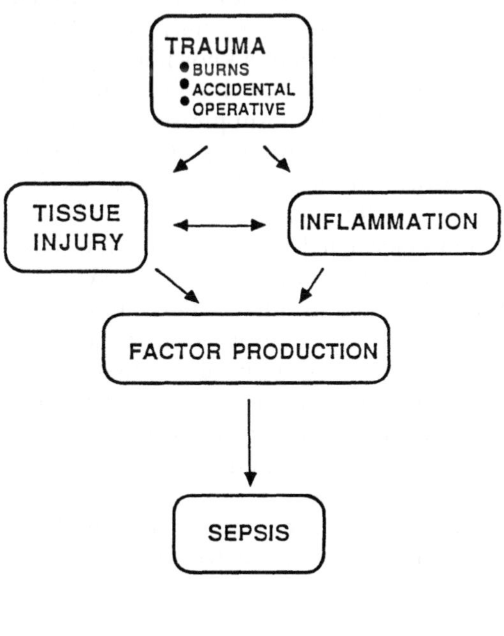

Fig. 1. Scheme for the generation of immunosuppressive factors following trauma

of less than 15 000 daltons elicited its effects via a noncytotoxic mechanism. It was suggested that the fibronectin peptide may compete with the whole molecule for fibronectin binding sites on the cell membrane thereby inhibiting activity of the cell.

Additional structural proteins possessing immunological activity are the collagens. In 1982 Dayer et al. [16] found that heat or protease digests of types II and III collagen readily and potently stimulated the biosynthesis of mononuclear cell factor (MCF) and prostaglandin E_2 (PGE_2) from human monocytes. Biosynthesis of PGE_2 or MCF was not reduced by the addition of polymyxin B or fibronectin depleted serum, suggesting that neither endotoxin nor fibronectin were responsible for their biosynthesis. Activity was localized to the alpha chains of collagen. In 1985 we demonstrated the activity of low molecular weight collagen peptides generated from heat or elastase digested calf skin collagen [17]. These peptides were found to inhibit the migration of neutrophils via a noncytotoxic mode of action. T lymphocytes were not suppressed by the collagen peptides.

The last peptide mediator that will be addressed in this discussion is an interleukin 1 (IL-1) peptide fragment described by Clowes et al. [18]. This peptide was identified in plasma from septic or trauma patients and found to stimulate muscle proteolysis. The low molecular weight peptide given the acronym PIF (proteolysis inducing factor) was found to be glycosylated as demonstrated by sensitivity to sialidase as well as heat and trypsin stable. A potential mode of action of PIF was determined to be stimulation of PGE_2 from monocytes. Interestingly this factor was found to enhance T lymphocyte activity.

Immunosuppression in Trauma: Pathways of Action

The mediators of immunosuppression following trauma have been widely documented, as have the effects elicited by these factors. The molecular and cellular mechanisms behind the observed changes are only now being elucidated. An example of potential mechanisms and pathways of action of a known immunosuppressive peptide, SAP, previously described is presented here. It is likely that other trauma or inflammation induced mediators with immunosuppressive activity exert their effects in similar fashion. The results presented represent early preliminary studies and are part of an ongoing investigation into the molecular mechanisms of SAP supported by the Office of Naval Research.

One of the first mechanisms of action determined for the suppressor active peptide was the ability of SAP to enhance the stimulation of PGE_2 biosynthesis in monocytes and amnion cells [19]. SAP was found to enhance PGE_2 biosynthesis by as much as 425% compared to controls. The addition of polymyxin B to cultures did not abrogate the enhanced PGE_2 production suggesting that prostaglandin stimulation was not due to endotoxin. In an effort to determine whether SAP induced suppression of T cell blastogenesis was due solely to enhanced biosynthesis of PGE_2, the addition of indomethacin or anti-PGE_2 antisera to mixed lymphocyte cultures (MLC) exposed to SAP was assessed. It was found that the addition of these agents did not reduce the activity of the suppressive peptide indicating the existence of additional noncyclooxygenase mediated pathways of action.

The next phase of our investigation into mechanisms led to analysis of IL-2 biosynthesis in peripheral blood mononuclear cells (PBMC) exposed to SAP. Previous reports of inhibition of IL-2 biosynthesis following traumatic injury have been published; however, the factor(s) responsible for this have not been identified [20, 21]. Our study demonstrated the ability of SAP to markedly inhibit the biosynthesis of IL-2 from concanavalin A stimulated PBMC [22]. SAP at concentrations of 100 n*M* inhibited IL-2 synthesis up to 95%. Inhibitory activity was not reduced by addition of indomethacin, anti-PGE_2 antibody or polymyxin B to cultures but was reduced by the addition of an anti-SAP monoclonal antibody or calcium ionophore A23187. Knowing that SAP could inhibit the production of IL-2, a key signal in T lymphocyte activation, exogenous IL-2 was added to mixed lymphocyte cultures exposed to SAP. Activity of these cultures was only partially restored, suggesting that the defect elicited by SAP is not simply due to depressed IL-2 signal [23]. The next series of experiments involved the interaction of SAP and calcium influx in PBMC following mitogen activation. Extracellular calcium influx into cells was inhibited up to 46% in suppressor peptide exposed cultures. This inhibition was partially reversible by the addition of calcium ionophore to the culture media. The mobilization of intracytosolic calcium influx of SAP exposed cells is currently underway.

One of the better characterized calcium transport proteins is calmodulin. This protein is an intracellular calcium receptor protein which regulates a wide variety of enzymatic processes in eukaryotic cells. It is known that the immunosuppressive drug cyclosporin exerts its biological activity in part by inhibiting calcium-calmodulin binding [24, 25].

In an attempt to determine whether SAP, like cyclosporin, was capable of inhibiting calcium-calmodulin interaction, the binding of calcium-45 to calmodulin-agarose in the presence or absence of the suppressor was assessed. At SAP concentrations above 150 n*M* significant inhibition of calcium-calmodulin binding was noted. We suggest from these preliminary results that a key mechanism in the immunosuppressive mode of action elicited by SAP is via interference in calcium-calmodulin binding. Inhibition of this interaction could lead to suppression of several key enzyme systems involved with cellular activation. These systems include: (1) calmodulin-dependent and calcium-activated kinases required for transferrin and IL-2 receptor expression and lymphokine biosynthesis, (2) phosphodiesterase which regulates cAMP levels, (3) calcium ATPase which regulates calcium movement out of erythrocytes. These findings help to explain many of the immunological manifestations presented by SAP, including (1) inhibition of IL-2 biosynthesis, (2) inhibition of cell membrane receptors such as IL-2 receptor and transferrin receptor, (3) inhibition of neutrophil migration, and (4) lysis of erythrocytes.

Summary

The generation of immunosuppressive serum-borne mediators following traumatic injuries has been widely documented. Several low molecular weight immunosuppressive factors of unknown origin have been reported by several groups.

Based on the similarities in physicochemical and immunological properties many of these mediators may stem from a common source. It is likely that these peptides are derived from larger molecular weight serum or tissue proteins and are elicited from proteases released with inflammation following trauma [26, 27]. It is known that several of the immunologically active peptide mediators of known origin are generated via this pathway. These factors include degradation products from fibrinogen, fibronectin, collagen, complement, and interleukin.

Determination of the pathways of action of several of these mediators is currently underway. Using preliminary data from our laboratory, several key sites in the sequence of T cell activation are likely acted on by SAP, leading to an inhibition of these cells [28]. We have demonstrated that SAP stimulates production of PGE_2 from monocytes, however this is not the sole mode of action of this peptide since addition of indomethacin or anti-PGE_2 to cultures does not restore full activity. Inhibition of IL-2 biosynthesis of concanavalin A activated PBMC exposed to SAP has also been demonstrated. Biosynthesis of IL-2 can be partially restored by the addition of calcium ionophore A23187. Addition of exogenous IL-2 to SAP exposed MLC only partially restores the blastogenic response of cells, leading to the conclusion that suppression is not due to lack of IL-2 signal alone. Additional studies indicate that the suppressor active peptide is capable of inhibiting calcium mobilization and of interfering with the interaction of calcium and calmodulin. This then could potentially lead to inhibition of several key enzymes required in T cell activation.

We hypothesize that SAP exerts its effect on calcium-calmodulin dependent enzymes involved in the breakdown of membrane polyphosphoinositides (PPI) to inositol 1,4,5 trisphosphate (IP3), which leads to calcium release from intracellular stores, and diacylglycerol (DAG), which activates protein kinase C. Both IP3 and DAG, along with IL-1, are prerequisites for transcription of lymphokine genes and cellular activation [29]. Current studies are underway to determine more precisely the sites of action of SAP on the T cell activation cascade and to determine potential means of restoring activity to SAP exposed cells.

References

1. Walker RI (1984) The pathophysiology of combined injury and trauma. In: Walker RI, Gruber DF, MacVittie TJ, Conklin JJ (eds) The pathophysiology of combined injury and trauma. Bethesda, Armed Forces Radiobiology Research Institute, pp 3–8
2. Warden GD, Mason AD, Pruit BA (1974) Evaluation of leukocyte chemotaxis in vitro in thermally injured patients. J Clin Invest 54:1001–1004
3. Constantian MB, Menzoian JO, Nimberg RB et al. (1977) Association of a circulating immunosuppressive polypeptide with operative and accidental trauma. Ann Surg 185:73–79
4. Hakim AA (1977) An immunosuppressive factor from serum of thermally traumatized patients. J Trauma 17:908–919
5. Christou NV, Meakins JL (1983) Partial analysis and purification of polymorphonuclear neutrophil chemotactic inhibitors in serum from anergic patients. Arch Surg 118:156–160
6. Ozkan AN, Ninnemann JL (1985) Circulating mediators in thermal injuries: isolation and characterization of a burn-injury induced immunosuppressive serum component. J Burn Care Rehabil 6:147–151

7. Ozkan AN, Ninnemann JL (1985) Suppression of in vitro lymphocyte and neutrophil responses by a low molecular weight suppressor active peptide from burn patient sera. J Clin Immunol 5:221–228
8. Ozkan AN, Ninnemann JL (1986) Progress in the characterization of an immunosuppressive glycopeptide from patients with major thermal injuries. J Burn Care Rehabil 7:388–397
9. Ozkan AN, Ninnemann JL (1987) Reversal of suppressor active peptide induced immunosuppression and SAP detection by a monoclonal antibody. J Trauma 27:123–126
10. Krzystyniak K, Stacharska J, Ryzewski K et al. (1978) Suppressive effect of low molecular weight fibrinogen degradation products on human and rat lymphocytes. Thromb Res 12:523–530
11. Edgington TS, Curtiss LK, Plow EF (1985) A linkage between the hemostatic and immune systems embodied in the fibrinolytic release of lymphocyte suppressive peptide. J Immunol 134:471–477
12. Plow EF, Edgington TS (1986) Lymphocyte suppressive peptides from fibrinogen are derived predominantly from the A alpha chain. J Immunol 137:1910–1915
13. Ehrlich MI, Krushell JS, Blumenstock FA et al. (1981) Depression of phagocytosis by plasmin degradation products of plasma fibronectin. J Lab Clin Med 98:263–271
14. Easter DW, Hoyt DB, Ozkan AN (1988) Immunosuppression by a peptide from the gelatin binding domain of human fibronectin. J Surg Res (in press)
15. Hoyt DB, Ozkan AN, Easter DW (1988) Isolation of an immunosuppressive trauma peptide and its relationship to fibronectin. J Trauma 28:1–7
16. Dayer JM, Trentham DE, Krane SM (1982) Collagens act as ligands to stimulate human monocytes to produce mononuclear cell factor and prostaglandins. Coll Relat Res 2:523–540
17. Ozkan AN, Ninnemann JL (1985) Burn-associated suppressor active peptide: relationship to tissue collagen. Proc Am Burn Assoc 15:50
18. Clowes GH, George BC, Villee CA et al. (1983) Muscle proteolysis induced by a circulating peptide in patients with sepsis or trauma. N Engl J Med 308:545–552
19. Ozkan AN, Hoyt DB, Mitchell MD et al. (1988) Trauma peptide mediated prostaglandin E2 biosynthesis: a potential mechanism for trauma-induced immunosuppression. Immunol Lett 17:79–83
20. Rodrick ML, Wood JJ, O'Mahony JB et al. (1986) Mechanisms of immunosuppression associated with severe nonthermal traumatic injuries in man. Production of interleukin-1 and -2. J Clin Immunol 6:310–318
21. Wood JJ, O'Mahony JB, Rodrick ML et al. (1986) Abnormalities of antibody production after thermal injury: an association with reduced interleukin 2 production. Arch Surg 121:108–115
22. Tompkins SD, Gregory S, Hoyt DB et al. (1988) Inhibition of IL-2 biosynthesis by a trauma-induced glycopeptide. FASEB J 2:8978
23. Pinney E, Hoyt DB, Ozkan AN (1988) The effect of a trauma-induced immunosuppressive peptide on phorbol ester activated T lymphocyte. FASEB J 2:8974
24. Colombani PM, Robb A, Hess AD (1985) Cyclosporin a binding to calmodulin: a possible site of action on T lymphocytes. Science 19:337–339
25. Le Grue SJ, Munn CG (1986) Comparison of the immunosuppressive effects of cyclosporin, lipid soluble anesthetics and calmodulin antagonists. Transplantation 42:679–685
26. Ozkan AN, Hoyt DB, Ninnemann JL (1987) Generation and activity of suppressor peptides following traumatic injury. J Burn Care Rehabil 8:527–530
27. Ozkan AN, Pinney E, Hoyt DB et al. (1988) Protease and suppressor active peptide activity following burn injury. J Trauma (in press)
28. Mary D, Aussel C, Ferrua B et al. (1987) Regulation of interleukin 2 synthesis by cAMP in human T cells. J Immunol 139:1179–1184
29. Imboden JB (1988) The regulation of intracellular signals during lymphocyte activation. Immunol Today 9:17–18

Trauma Peptide T-Cell Suppression: Mechanisms of Action

D. B. Hoyt, E. Pinney, and A. N. Ozkan

Introduction

Immunosuppression in trauma patients has been well documented by several groups. The causes of this suppression are at both the humoral and cellular level. Many of the described immunosuppressive effects can be induced in normal cells by coincubation with trauma serum, suggesting the presence of circulating immunosuppressive factors. The isolation and partial characterization of a low molecular weight peptide from the serum of trauma patients have been previously described [1].

Previous reports have demonstrated the isolation of a low molecular weight immunosuppressive glycopeptide that: (1) suppresses T-cell mitogenesis in phytohemagglutinin- and concanavalin A-activated peripheral lymphocytes, (2) suppresses T-cell blastogenesis in the mixed lymphocyte reaction, (3) inhibits polymorphonuclear chemotaxis, (4) induces production of prostaglandin E_2 in monocytes and amnion cells, (5) induces multiple changes in T-cell marker expression [2–5]. Changes documented to occur following trauma include both humoral and cellular alterations in severely injured patients. Among these is a small, but significantly increased elevation of interleukin-2 (IL-2) receptor positive T-cells, increased prostaglandins, and numerous serum protein abnormalities. Mannick et al. have reported inhibited IL-2 production and suppressed responsiveness in lymphocytes isolated from trauma patients [6]. Impaired expression of IL-2 receptors has been reported [7].

The immunological effects of suppressive peptides have been established, with high levels documented in trauma patients. Our study was undertaken to better define the molecular and cellular mechanisms involved in trauma-induced immunosuppression. Specifically, the purpose of this study was to better define the cellular mechanisms of action of this glycopeptide on T-lymphocyte suppression.

Methods and Materials

T-Lymphocyte Isolation

T-lymphocytes were isolated using the nylon wool adherence method. Whole blood was collected in heparinized tubes and sedimented by addition of 10% Dextran 70 (v/v) (Flow Labs., Inc., McLean, VA) at room temperature (RT) for 1 h. A nylon wool column was packed by adding 2 gm nylon wool (Travenol Labs,

Immune Consequences of
Trauma, Shock and Sepsis
Eds. Faist/Ninnemann/Green

Deerfield, IL) into a 50 cc syringe barrel with a stopcock to regulate flow rates. The column was equilibrated by washing 3 × with prewarmed RPMI 1640 supplemented with 10% fetal calf serum. The column was incubated with the medium after the third wash for 15 min at RT. The cell suspension was prepared by removing the plasma layer from the dextran-sedimented blood and the cell concentration was adjusted to 5 million cells/ml in prepared medium. The column was allowed to run dry and sealed. The cell suspension was added to the column and the cells were allowed to run into the column. Enough medium was added to cover the nylon wool in the column and the column was covered and incubated at RT for 45 min. Nonadherent cells were collected by washing the column with 60 ml of medium. The eluted cells were washed, counted, and diluted to the desired concentration.

Activation of T-Lymphocytes

Enriched T-lymphocytes were diluted to 2 million cells/ml in RPMI 1640 supplemented with *l*-glutamine (2 m*M*), penicillin (100 U/ml), streptomycin (100 µg/ml), 50 µ*M* 2-mercaptoethanol, 10% fetal calf serum, and 20 n*M* phorbol myristate acetate (PMA). Cells were incubated for 72 h in the PMA-RPMI medium. After 72 h a portion of both PMA-stimulated and non-PMA-stimulated cells were harvested and quantitated for TAC (IL-2) receptor expression by fluorescence activated cell sorter (FACS) analysis.

One-Way Mixed Lymphocyte Reaction

A modified, one-way, mixed lymphocyte reaction was used in this assay. The methods used have been previously described [4]. Briefly, 100 µl IL-2 R(+) cells or IL-2 R(−) (responder cells) at a concentration of 2 million cells/ml were added to the wells of a 96-well tissue culture plate (Costar, Cambridge, MA). To each well 200000 mitomycin-treated peripheral blood mononuclear cells were added (antigen-presenting cells), as well as 200000 mitomycin-treated GM 3105 (stimulator cells). To triplicate wells 2, 4, 8, or 20 µl peptide or sample buffer was added, and the standard MLR incubation, pulsing, and harvesting times were carried out.

Isolation

Suppressive active peptide (SAP) was isolated by ion exchange chromatography using an SP Sephadex C-25 column attached to a Pharmacia Fast Protein Liquid Chromatography unit (Pharmacia, Piscataway, NJ). The condition gradients and buffers used have been previously described [1].

Suppression and Addition of Modulators with Suppressive Active Peptide

In an attempt to determine potential mechanisms of action of SAP, the addition of the following modulations to the MLR was assessed: (1) indomethacin at a final concentration of 1 μg/ml, (2) anti-PGE 10 μl (10 mg protein/ml), (3) IL-2 at 50 units/ml final concentration, (4) calcium ionophore A23187 (500 n*M*).

Results

Table 1 shows the results of IL-2 positive cells, both resting cells and PMA-activated cells at 48 h, as determined by FACS analysis. Table 2 shows results of one-way mixed lymphocyte response and expresses the mean suppression (negative) or stimulation (positive) for resting and activated T-lymphocytes in the presence of SAP alone, SAP plus indomethacin, SAP plus anti-PGE2, SAP plus IL-2, and SAP plus the calcium ionophore A23187. A dose response at 2, 4, 8, and 20 μl, which corresponds to 19, 38, 75, and 200 n*M* final concentration, is demonstrated.

It is clear that significant suppression follows the dose-dependent gradient for both resting and activated cells. The presence of indomethacin and anti-PGE2 does not reverse this suppression. The addition of exogenous IL-2 appears to decrease SAP-induced suppression in activated cells and, to a much greater degree, addition of the calcium ionophore A23187 reverses the suppression induced by SAP in activated cells.

Table 1. $\bar{X}$ PMA activation (% IL-2+ cells): FACS analysis

Resting	4%
Activated	33%

Table 2. MLR response: mean percentage suppression (−) or stimulation (+)

	SAP (1)	SAP alone	SAP/ indo.	SAP/ AN-PG 32	SAP/ IL-2	SAP/ Ca2+
Rest	2	+ 7.3	−23	−23	− 0.4	+ 7
	4	+ 1.3	−19	−15	+ 4.0	−11
	8	−37	−44	−38	−30	−83
	20	−63	−87	−98	−99	−99
ACT	2	−23	− 5	−13	+ 2	+ 6
	4	−29	−40	−20	− 6	+47
	8	−59	−72	−50	−16	+68
	20	−94	−98	−98	−99	−99

Discussion

From the above data one can suggest that SAP suppression is greater in activated cells (IL-2-receptor-positive cells) at low peptide concentrations than in nonactivated cells. SAP suppression of blastogenesis appears to be independent of prostaglandin-mediated suppression. PMA-activated cells (IL-2 receptor positive) are less suppressed by SAP when treated with exogenous IL-2. Calcium ionophore reverses SAP inhibition of blastogenesis in activated cells, suggesting that the pathophysiologic mechanism by which SAP works is in part due to interference with cytosolic calcium mobilization and inhibition of IL-2 synthesis. IL-2 appears only partially to resuscitate SAP-suppressed activated cells, indicating that SAP-induced suppression is not due to a lack of an IL-2 signal alone.

References

1. Ozkan AN, Ninnemann JL (1985) Suppression of an in vitro lymphocyte and neutrophil responses by a low molecular weight depressive active peptide from burn patient sera. J Clin Immunol 5:172
2. Hoyt DB, Ozkan AN, Ninnemann JL et al. (1988) Trauma peptide induction of lymphocyte changes predictive of sepsis. J Surg Res 45:342–348
3. Ozkan AN, Pinney E, Hoyt DB et al. (1983) Elastase and suppressor active peptide activity following injury. J Trauma 28:207–210
4. Ozkan AN, Hoyt DB, Tompkins S et al. (1988) Immunosuppressive effects of a trauma induced suppressor active peptide. J Trauma 28:589–592
5. Ozkan An, Hoyt DB, Ninnemann JL et al. (1988) Trauma peptide mediated prostaglandin E2 biosynthesis: a potential mechanism for trauma induced immunosuppression. Immunol Lett 17:79
6. Rodrick ML, Wood JJ, O'Mahony JB et al. (1986) Mechanisms of immunosuppression associated with severe nonthermal traumatic injuries in man: production of interleukin 1 and 2. J Clin Immunol 6:310
7. Teodorczyk-Injeyan JA, Sparkes BG, Mills GB et al. (1987) Impaired expression of interleukin-2 receptor (IL2R) in the immunosuppressed burned patient: reversal by exogenous IL2. J Trauma 27:180

Role of Platelet-Activating Factor and Structurally Related Alkyl Phospholipids in Immune and Cytotoxic Processes

P. Braquet, D. Hosford, and M. Braquet

Introduction

Alkyl phospholipids are a diverse chemical species characterized structurally by the presence of an ether bond at the *sn*-1 position of the glycerol moiety. This ether linkage confers unique pharmacological properties upon this group of molecules and distinguishes them from other phospholipids, which usually possess an ester linkage at this position. In this review we consider the role of two different classes of these compounds, platelet-activating factor (PAF) and the structurally related alkyl lysophospholipids (ALP), in modulating the complex system of host defenses, in particular the direct effects of PAF on cellular interactions in the immune response and the tumoricidal activity of ALP.

Direct Effects of PAF on the Cellular Immune Response

Lymphocyte Proliferation, Interleukin-2-Production, and Surface Antigen Expression

When PAF is added to human peripheral blood lymphocyte cultures (containing 5%–10% monocytes) stimulated with the mitogens phytohemagglutinin (PHA) or concanavalin A (Con A), a concentration-dependent inhibition of lymphocyte proliferation is observed (Rola-Pleszczynski et al. 1987a). The IC_{50} ranges between 1 p*M* and 0.1 n*M* and inhibition is observed when PAF is added within the first 3 h of a 72-h culture period. Addition of PAF at a later time has no significant effect on lymphocyte proliferation. The inhibition is not accompanied by cell toxicity and a similar suppression of lymphocyte proliferation is observed with 2-ethoxy-PAF, a nonhydrolysable PAF analogue (Pignol et al. 1987a). PAF-induced inhibition of lymphocyte proliferation is prevented by the PAF receptor antagonist, BN 52021. A similar effect of PAF and 2-ethoxy-PAF is observed when production of interleukin 2 (IL 2) by human lymphocytes is measured. In both cases suppression of IL 2 production is reversed by BN 52021 (Pignol et al. 1987a; Rola-Pleszczynski et al. 1987a). Recently, Dulioust et al. (1987) have reported that the mediator also suppresses CD4+ T-cell proliferation. However, this effect is apparent at higher concentrations of PAF or when the mediator is added late during the culture cycle. In addition, this PAF effect is not associated with an alteration in IL 2 production. In contrast to these results, Behrens and Goodwin (1987) have reported that PAF stimulates CD4- T-cell proliferation but has no effect on CD8+ T cells.

Immune Consequences of
Trauma, Shock and Sepsis
Eds. Faist/Ninnemann/Green

Recent preliminary data indicate that the ginkgolide mixture BN 52063 (which contains BN 52020, BN 52021, and BN 52022, molar ratio 2:2:1) may also modulate the CD4+/CD8+ T-cell ratio in vivo. A randomized double-blind pilot study on six male healthy volunteers showed a dose-related reduction in the CD4+/CD8+ cell ratio in individuals treated with BN 52063 for 15 days but no change in the control group. With 240 mg BN 52063/day there was a 43% decrease in the CD4+/CD8+ T-cell ratio at day 15, a 17.5% decrease with 80 mg/day of the drug, and a 2.5% decrease with the placebo (calculated relative to the ratio on day 0 in each case). The CD4+/CD8+ T-cell ratio returned to normal values after the end of treatment (P. Guinot, unpublished).

Since inhibition of lymphocyte proliferation and IL 2 production may be due to the activation of T-suppressor cells, studies have been conducted on lymphocytes preincubated with PAF for 3–18 h, washed, added to fresh autologous lymphocytes, and the cells then stimulated with a mitogen. This coculture assay demonstrated that PAF activates suppressor cells which subsequently inhibit lymphocyte proliferation in the absence of any further contact with the mediator (Rola-Pleszczynski et al. 1987b). This induction of suppressor cells is accompanied by an increase in the CD8+ T/CD4+ T-cell ratio after 18–48 h. The PAF antagonists BN 52021 and WEB-2086 also generate some suppressor cell activity, although to a lesser extent than PAF itself (Rola-Pleszczynski et al. 1987b).

In a different system, PAF and two nonhydrolysable PAF analogues have been shown to increase the proliferation of IL 2-stimulated human lymphoblasts, whereas some antagonists (CV-3988 and L-652, -731), but not WEB 2086 and BN 52021) are inhibitory (Barrett et al. 1986). This effect of the antagonists is observed even when the drugs are added 48 h after the beginning of a 72-h culture period, suggesting interference with a late event in T-cell activation. It is possible that endogenously produced PAF may be involved in some step(s) of IL 2-induced proliferation of T-lymphoblasts. This is indicated by the inhibition of this process by the PAF synthesis inhibitor, L-648,611 (Barrett et al. 1986). An important corrobation of some of the in vitro effects outlined above has been provided by the in vivo instillation of PAF into rats via subcutaneously implanted osmotic minipumps connected to the jugular vein (Pignol et al. 1988a). In this system, after 7 days of instillation, PAF-treated rat splenocytes show enhanced IL 2 production in response to Con A.

Interleukin 1 (IL 1) Production

A biphasic response is observed when increasing concentrations of PAF are added to lipopolysaccharide (LPS)-stimulated human monocytes (Pignol et al. 1987b). Low concentrations of PAF (1 p*M* to 0.1 n*M*) significantly enhance IL 1 production while high concentrations (10 n*M* to 1 μ*M*) are markedly inhibitory. These effects are more pronounced when platelets are added (10–30:1) to the monocyte cultures. All these effects of PAF on IL 1 production are blocked by the PAF receptor antagonist BN 52021. In addition, Barrett et al. (1987) have demonstrated that (R) PAF and a less hydrolysable synthetic racemic analogue, PR1501, can induce IL 1-like activity from LPS-stimulated and unstimulated human monocyte-macrophage cell cultures, with optimum production of IL 1-like activity being observed with 30–300 p*M* PAF.

In ex vivo experiments using minipumps loaded with PAF or solvent alone, placed under the back skin of rats and connected to the jugular vein, Pignol et al. (1988a) demonstrated that monocytes from animals receiving 1, 4.5, or 9 μg PAF for 7 days exhibit increased capacity to produce IL 1. In contrast, with 28 μg PAF/7 days, IL 1 production by the monocytes is markedly decreased.

Lymphocyte Cytotoxicity

The PAF antagonist BN 52021 potentiates alloantigen recognition in primary and secondary mixed lymphocyte cultures and enhances the generation of cytotoxic lymphocytes in vitro (Gebhardt et al. 1988), its presence throughout the duration of culture period having the greatest enhancing effect on the proliferative capacity of the cells. Similar effects are observed in the mixed cultures employed to generate cytotoxic T-lymphocytes; indeed, removal of BN 52021 up to 24 h after culture initiation eliminates the enhancing effect of the antagonist on cell-mediated cytotoxicity (Gebhardt et al. 1988).

Recently Farkas et al. (1988a) have examined the protective effect of BN 52021 (300 μ*M*) on in vitro rat splenic lymphocyte-induced cytotoxicity of Langerhans islets. When the islets are pretreated with BN 52021, almost total inhibition of cellular destruction relative to the control is observed, a direct effect of BN 52021 on the target cells. Using BN 52021-pretreated splenic lymphocytes the inhibition is significant with respect to the control cytotoxicity, but sightly lower than that in the above circumstances. The protective effect of BN 52021 is dose dependent since at a concentration of 10 μ*M* inhibition of cytotoxicity is only transient.

In further studies on the same system (Farkas et al. 1988b) the cytotoxic reaction is inhibited by BN 52021 (30 and 100 μ*M*), and the somatostatin analogues BIM 23014 and BIM 23026 (0.1 μ*M*) when these drugs are added individually. A concentration of 10 μ*M* BN 52021 is ineffective alone, but when combined with either somatostatin analogue a synergistic protective effect on the destruction of Langerhans islets by cytotoxic splenic lymphocytes is observed.

Natural Killer Cells

Natural killer (NK) cell-mediated lysis of the erythroleukemic target cell line K562 is markedly enhanced by picomolar concentrations of PAF (reviewed in Braquet and Rola-Pleszczynski 1987). Preincubation of NK cells with PAF prior to culture with K562 target cells, or delayed addition of PAF, also produces enhanced NK activity, an effect than BN 52021 is unable to block. In contrast, without PAF addition, the NK-mediated cytotoxicity of rat and human lymphocytes against YAC-1 or K562 target cells, respectively, is significantly diminished by BN 52021. Target cell lysis is reduced while the binding of target cells to effector cells is unaffected. Furthermore, pretreatment of K562 cells with the PAF antagonist produces greater inhibition than pretreatment of the effector cells (Mandi et al. 1988).

Mandi and colleagues have evaluated the effects of BN 52021, BN 52024 (a ginkgolide devoid of PAF antagonistic activity), and WEB 2086 (an antagonist of PAF belonging to the triazolobenzodiazepine series) and the somatostatin analogue BIM 23026 on the lysis of K562 target cells by human NK cells. Lysis is decreased when either BN 52021 or BIM 23026 is introduced into the system at concentrations of 10 μ*M* to 0.1 m*M* or 10 n*M* to 0.1 μ*M*, respectively. In contrast, BN 52024 is almost ineffective and WEB 2086 (0.1–0.5 μ*M*) exerts intermediate effects. BIM 23026 (1 μ*M*–10 μ*M*) not only inhibits NK cytolysis but exhibits a synergistic effect with BN 52021 (1 μ*M*). Both substances block an early event in the lytic process, a decrease in lysis only being observed when the drugs are added within the 1st h of the assay (Farkas et al. 1988 b).

Natural cytotoxic cells and macrophages mediate their cytotoxic activities, at least in part, through synthesis and release of tumor necrosis factor (TNF). When preincubated, or coincubated with PAF, LPS-treated human monocytes and mouse peritoneal macrophages produce significantly higher quantities of TNF (Bonavida and Braquet 1988). In addition, large granular lymphocytes, which comprise the effector NK cells responsible for lysis of K562 target cells, generate PAF under certain conditions (Malavasi et al. 1986). Thus it appears that endogenous PAF may assist in the regulation of NK cell functions.

Alkyl Lysophospholipid-Induced Tumor Necrosis

While considerable attention has been focussed on PAF as an immunomodulator, the studies of Munder and colleagues (reviewed in Munder et al. 1981; Berdel 1982, 1987) have led to the recognition that other closely related alkyl phospholipids may play an important role in various immune and cytotoxic processes. In 1966, Munder et al. noted that, after phagocytosis by macrophages, phospholipase A_2 is activated, which degrades cellular phosphatidylcholine and phosphatidylethanolamine to the corresponding lyso compounds, 2-lysophosphatidylcholine (2-LPC) and 2-lysophosphatidylethanolamine (2-LPE), with the concomitant release of free fatty acids (Munder et al. 1969, 1976). These workers hypothesized that the accumulation of lyso compounds in cell membranes might represent an endogenous principle in the host defense mechanisms. While naturally occurring 2-LPC is rapidly metabolized by a lysophospholipase (Hill and Lands 1970), analogues of 2-LPC have been synthesized which are not substrates for this enzyme and possess an increased half-life in the organism (Weltzien and Westphal 1967).

These synthetic alkyl lysophospholipids (ALPs) exhibit strong prophylactic and therapeutic effects on the growth of animal tumors and thus may provide a new approach to cancer therapy (reviewed in Andreesen 1988). In vitro these compounds exert cytostatic effects on mouse methylcholantrene-induced fibrosarcoma cells (Modollel et al. 1979), human leukemic cells (Andreesen et al. 1978; Tidwell et al. 1981), and cells from various solid human malignomas such as hypernephromas (Berdel et al. 1981 a), and urologic (Berdel et al. 1981 b) and gynecologic (Runge et al. 1980) tumors. Apart from direct cytostatic activity, ALPs are also able to enhance the tumoricidal capacity of macrophages (Berdel et al. 1980). Unlike most antitumoral agents, ALPs do not appear to have a direct effect on DNA synthesis or function and are nonmutagenic.

Direct Cytotoxic Effects of ALP

A number of derivatives of ALP have been synthesized, such as 1-hexadecylthio-2-methoxymethyl-*rac*-glycero-3-phosphocholine (BM-14-440) (Herrmann 1987), SRI 62-834 and analogues (Houlihan 1987), 1-octadecyl-2-methyl-*rac*-glycero-3-phosphocholine (ET-18-OCH_3) (Storme et al. 1985), and various *rac*-(2-alkoxy-alkyl)-phosphocholines (Bonjouklian et al. 1986). The presence of acetamine or methoxy substituents at the *sn*-2 position of ALP enhances the selective antitumor activity of these compounds (Hoffman et al. 1984). The methoxy analogue of PAF, ET-18-OCH_3, one of the most effective ALPs, abolishes [^{3}H]thymidine incorporation in various tumor cells and causes cell death.

A characteristic feature of the cytotoxic action of ALP on tumor cells is that of membrane disruption. Neoplastically transformed cells possess numerous microvilli, membrane ruffles, and blebs indicative of an actively moving membrane and transient surface alterations (Winslow et al. 1978; Spence and Coates 1981). When human brain tumor cells are incubated for 24 h with ET-18-OCH_3, these features are reduced in size and number and changes in the adherent properties of these cells are also detected (Berdel et al. 1984). A decrease in surface activity and membrane discontinuity is also observed in ET-18-OCH_3-incubated esophagus carcinoma cells (Maistry et al. 1980), while cells of an acute myelomonocytic leukemia suffer membrane rupture when treated with this compound (Munder et al. 1979).

These observations imply direct cytotoxic surface activity by ALP; however, there is a striking difference in cytotoxicity between the potent lysophospholipids possessing an ether linkage at the *sn*-1 position of the glycerol and those almost rendered inactive by the presence of an ester linkage; both these chemical species exhibit identical surface activity (Berdel et al. 1980). Furthermore, ALPs are bound to albumin and lipoproteins and are only exchanged slowly with cellular phospholipids, producing an extremely low concentration of ALPs at the cell surface (Munder et al. 1981). Both of these facts tend to invalidate the theory of direct surface activity as the primary mechanism of direct ALP cytotoxicity.

A more likely explanation of direct ALP action stems from the presence of the ether linkage. Neoplastic tissues do not contain the *O*-alkyl-cleavage enzyme required for ALP degradation, while this enzyme is present in normal cells, enabling ALP metabolism to take place. This enzymatic difference was originally thought to account for the selectivity of their action (Snyder and Wood 1969) and allow the accumulation of ether-linked lipids in tumor cells blocking vital pathways of the phospholipid metabolism. In addition, the severe membrane damage inflicted was attributed to these compounds acting as antimetabolites of the synthesis of phosphatidylcholine (Modollel et al. 1979). Indeed, this mechanism of ALP-mediated tumor cell destruction is supported by the fact that the ester-linked analogue, 2-LPC, exhibits no cytotoxicity and by data demonstrating that pretreatment of ET-18-OH with an *O*-alkyl-cleavage enzyme preparation abolishes its cytotoxic effect (Berdel et al. 1983).

However, it appears that the mechanism of direct ALP action is more complex than initially thought and cannot be solely attributed to the enzymatic difference between normal and malignant cells. While it is certain that neoplastic cells adsorb more ALP than normal cells, normal lymphoblasts which possess high levels of the cleavage enzyme are also susceptible to ALP cytotoxicity (Andreesen et al. 1979). Furthermore, due to substrate specificity of the *O*-alkyl-cleavage enzyme, some ALPs substituted at the *sn*-2 position are not subject to degradation (Lee et al. 1981). Thus, the disruption of phospholipid metabolism may result from metabolic alterations caused by ALP interaction with acetyl transferase (Bador et al. 1983) and/or protein kinase (Helfman et al. 1983) possibly initiated by ALP-induced formation of diacylphosphatidyl-choline and 1-*O*-octadecyglycerol (Fleer et al. 1987) rather than intracellular accumulation of ALPs per se.

Immunomodulated Cell Necrosis

The antitumor activity of ALPs also appears to be mediated by the generation of highly tumoricidal immunocompetent cells from the monocyte/macrophage lineage (Munder et al. 1981). Intraperitoneal injection of 2-LPC or ALPs in mice induces temporary ascites, which contain 60%–70% macrophages, the remainder being lymphocytes and a few granulocytes (Bausert 1978). These peritoneal cells significantly protect the animal from metastasis of syngeneic 3-LL cells when reinjected intravenously after the excision of the primary tumor (Berdel et al. 1980). If macrophages are removed from the peritoneal cell suspension, the remaining lymphocytes and granulocytes are rendered ineffective. Furthermore, pure syngeneic bone marrow macrophages treated in vitro with ALPs afford significantly higher protection against metastasis in mice than untreated cells (Berdel et al. 1980). Macrophages can also be activated by incubation with ALPs to induce in vitro necrosis of 3-LL syngeneic tumor cells (Berdel et al. 1980), methylcholanthrene-induced sarcomas (Munder et al. 1976), and cells from human hypernephromas (Berdel et al. 1981 a) and lung carcinomas (Berdel et al. 1980). It is interesting to note that only alkyl-analogues are capable of generating macrophage cytotoxicity. The efficacy of ALPs in this process is positively correlated with the number of carbon atoms in the alkyl chain at the *sn*-1 position, while removal of the substituent at the *sn*-2 position renders the compound virtually ineffective (Munder et al. 1981). The process of macrophage activation is still unclear, but a stimulation of IL 1 production by ALPs is possible (Pignol et al. 1987 a).

In addition, ALPs induce the release of arachidonic acid metabolites (Leser et al. 1981) and restore the capacity of human monocyte-derived macrophages to respond to endotoxin with the secretion of large amounts of IL 1-like material (Andreesen and Giese 1987). Human macrophage activation by ALPs seems to synergize with endotoxin (Andreesen and Giese 1987) and it may be that minute amounts of endotoxin need to be present in the culture system in order to facilitate the response of macrophages to ALPs.

Finally, it is interesting to note that the uptake of PAF or its methoxy analogue by HL 60 cells is not inhibited by the PAF antagonists BN 52021 and kadsurenone (Record et al. 1986), suggesting that the uptake of ether lipids is not mediated by PAF receptors. Indeed, PAF and related agonists are poor antitumor agents and an inverse relationship appears to exist between alkyl phospholipids exhibiting PAF activity (i.e., those being hypotensive, inflammatory, and involved in allergic reactions) and those possessing selective antitumor properties.

References

Andreesen R (1988) Ether lipids in the therapy of cancer. In: Braquet P, Mangold HK, Vargaftig BB (eds) Biologically active ether lipids. Karger, Basel, pp 118–132 (Progress in biochemical pharmacology, vol 22)

Andreesen R, Giese V (1987) Differential effects of ether lipids on the activity and secretion of interleukin-1 and interleukin-2. Lipids 22:836–841

Andreesen R, Modolell M, Weltzien HU, Eibl H, Common HH, Löhr GW, Munder PG (1978) Selective destruction of human leukemic cells by alkyl-lysophospholipids. Cancer Res 38:3894–3899

Andreesen R, Modolell M, Weltzien HU, Munder PG (1979) Alkyllysophospholipid induced suppression of human lymphocyte response to mitogens and selective killing of lymphoblasts. Immunobiology 156:498–508

Bador H, Morelis R, Louisot P (1983) Biochemical evidence for role of alkyl-lysophospholipids on liver sialyltransferase. Int J Biochem 15:1137–1142

Barrett ML, Lewis GP, Ward S, Westwick J (1986) Platelet-activating factor modulates interleukin-2induced proliferation of human T-lymphoblasts. Br J Pharmacol 89:505P

Barrett ML, Lewis GP, Ward S, Westwick J (1987) Platelet-activating factor induces interleukin 1 production from human adherent macrophages. Br J Pharmacol 90:113P

Bausert W (1978) Der Einfluß von synthetischen Lysolecithin Analoga auf das Wachstum experimenteller Tumoren der Maus. PhD Thesis, University of Freiburg, Freiburg

Behrens T, Goodwin JS (1987) Platelet-activating factor enhances proliferation of human OKT4(+) T lymphocytes. Clin Res 35:893

Berdel WE (1982) Antineoplastic activity of synthetic lysophospholipid analogs. Blut 44:71–78

Berdel WE (1987) Ether lipids and analogs in experimental cancer therapy. A brief review of the Munich experience. Lipids 22:970–973

Berdel WE, Bausert WR, Weltzien HU, Modolell ML, Widmann KH, Munder PG (1980) The influence of alkyl-lysophospholipids and lysophospholipid-activated macrophages on the development of metastasis of Lewis lung carcinoma. Eur J Cancer 16:1199–1204

Berdel WE, Fink U, Egger B, Reichert A, Munder PG, Rastetter J (1981 a) Alkyl-lysophospholipids inhibit the growth of hypernephroid carcinomas in vitro. J Cancer Res Clin Oncol 101:325–330

Berdel WE, Fink U, Egger B, Reichert A, Munder PG, Rastetter J (1981 b) Inhibition by alkyl-lysophospholipids of tritiated thymidine uptake in cells of human malignant urologic tumors. J Natl Cancer Inst 66:813–817

Berdel WE, Greiner E, Fink U, Stavrou D, Reichert A, Rastetter J, Hoffman DR, Snyder F (1983) Cytotoxicity of alkyl-lysophospholipid derivatives and low-alkyl-cleavage enzyme activities in rat brain tumor cells. Cancer Res 43:541–545

Berdel WE, Greiner E, Fink U, Zänker KS, Stavrou D, Trappe A, Fahlbusch R, Reichert A, Rastetter J (1984) Cytotoxic effects of alkyl-lysophospholipids in human brain tumor cells. Oncology 41:140–145

Bonavida B, Braquet P (1988) Effect of platelet-activating factor (PAF) on monocyte activation and production of tumour necrosis factor (TNF). Prostaglandins 35:802A

Bonjouklian R, Phillips ML, Kuhler KM, Grindey GB, Poore GA, Chultz RM, Altom MG (1986) Studies of the antitumor activity of (2-alkoxyalkyl)- and (2-alkoxyalkeny)-phosphocholines. J Med Chem 29:2472–2477

Braquet P, Rola-Pleszczynski M (1987) Platelet-activating factor and cellular immune responses. Immunol Today 8:345–352

Dulioust A, Vivier E, Salem P, Derynckz S, Benveniste J, Thomas Y (1987) Inhibition of human T4$^+$ cell proliferation by PAF-acether (platelet-activating factor). Fed Proc 46:2731

Farkas G, Mandi Y, Koltai M, Braquet P (1988 a) Graft protective effect of BN 52021, a specific PAF antagonist in an in vitro Langerhans islet-splenic lymphocyte model. In: Braquet P (ed) The ginkgolides: chemistry, pharmacology and clinical perspectives. Prous, Barcelona, pp 737–748

Farkas G, Mandi Y, Belali I, Koltai M (1988 b) The effect of platelet-activating factor (PAF) antagonists and somatostatin analogues on lymphocyte and natural killer (NK) cell cytotoxicity. Prostaglandins 35:804A

Fleer EAM, Unger C, Kim DJ, Eibl H (1987) Metabolism of ether lipids and analogs in neoplastic cells. Lipids 22:856–861

Gebhardt PB, Bazan HEP, Braquet P, Bazan NG (1988) Platelet-activating factor suppresses cell mediated immune reactions in vivo. In: Braquet P (ed) Platelet-activating factor and cell immunology. Karger, Basel pp 99–107 (New trends in lipid mediators research, vol 1)

Helfman D, Barnes K, Rinkade J, Vogler W, Shojl M, Kuo J (1983) Phospholipid-sensitive Ca^{2+}-dependent protein phosphorylation system in various types of leukemic cells from human patients and in human leukemic cell lines HL60 and K562, and its inhibition by alkyl-lysophospholipids. Cancer Res 43:2955–2961

Herrmann DBJ, Besenfelder E, Bicker U, Pahlke W, Böhm E (1987) Pharmacokinetics of the thioether phospholipid analogue BM 41.440 in rats. Lipids 22:952–954

Hill EE, Lands WEM (1970) Phospholipid metabolism. In: Wakil SJ (ed) Lipid metabolism. Academic, New York, p 185

Hoffman DR, Stanley JD, Berchtold R, Snyder F (1984) Cytotoxicity of ether-linked phytanyl phospholipid analogs and related derivatives in human HL-60 leukemia cells and polymorphonuclear neutrophils. Res Commun Chem Pathol Pharmacol 44:293

Houlihan WJ, Lee ML, Munder PG, Nemecek GM, Handley DA (1987) Antitumor activity of SRI 62-834, a cyclic ether analog of ET-18-OCH_3. Lipids 22:884–890

Lee RC, Blank ML, Fitzgerald V, Snyder F (1981) Substrate specificity in the biocleavage of the O-alkyl bond: 1-alkyl-2-acetyl-*sn*-glycero-3-phosphocholine (a hypotensive and platelet-activating lipid) and its metabolites. Arch Biochem Biophys 208:353–357

Leser HG, Barlin E, Weltzien HU, Gemsa D (1981) Die Wirkung von Lysolezithin-analoga (LLA) auf den Arachidonsäuremetabolismus von Makrophagen. Verh Dtsch Ges Inn Med 87:757–760

Maistry L, Robinson KM, Evers P, Munder PG, Andreesen R (1980) Morphologic effects of an antitumor agent on human esophagal carcinoma cells in vitro. Scan Electron Micros 3:109–114

Malavasi F, Tetta C, Funaro A, Bellone G, Ferrero E, Franzone AC, Dellabona P, Rusci R, Matera L, Camussi G, Caligaris-Cappio F (1986) Fc receptor triggering induces expression of surface activation antigens and release of platelet-activating factor in large granular lymphocytes. Proc Natl Acad Sci USA 83:2443–2447

Mandi Y, Farkas G, Koltai M, Braquet P, Beladi L (1988) The effect of BN 52021, a PAF-acether antagonist, on natural killer activity. In: Braquet P (ed) Platelet-activating factor and cell immunology. Basel, Karger, pp 76–88 (New trends in lipid mediators research, vol 1)

Modollel M, Andreesen R, Pahlke W, Brugger U, Munder PG (1979) Disturbance of phospholipid metabolism during the selective destruction of tumor cells induced by alkyl-lysophospholipids. Cancer Res 39:4681–4686

Munder PG, Modolell M, Ferber E, Fischer H (1966) Phospholipide in quarzgeschädigten Makrophagen. Biochem 344:310

Munder PG, Ferber E, Modolell M, Fischer H (1969) The influence of various adjuvants on the metabolism of phospholipids in macrophages. Int Arch Allergy 36:117

Munder PG, Weltzien HU, Modolell M (1976) Lysolecithin analogs: a new class of immunopotentiators. In: Miescher PA (ed) VII. international symposium on immunopathology. Schwabe, Basel, pp 411–424

Munder PG, Modolell M, Andreesen R, Weltzien HU, Westphal O (1979) Lysophosphatidylcholine (lysolecithin) and its synthetic analogues, immune modulating and other biologic effects. Springer Semin Immunopathol 2:187–203

Munder PG, Modolell M, Bausert W, Oettgen HF, Westphal O (1981) Alkyl-lysophospholipids in cancer therapy. In: Hersh EM (ed) Augmenting agents in cancer therapy. Raven, New York, pp 411–458

Pignol B, Henane S, Mencia-Huerta JM, Braquet P, Rola-Pleszczynski M (1987 a) Platelet-activating factor (PAF-acether) inhibits interleukin 2 (IL2) production and proliferation of human lymphocytes. Australia 10th international congress of pharmacology, Sydney, 3–5 September 1987

Pignol B, Henane S, Mencia-Huerta JM, Rola-Pleszczynski M, Braquet P (1987 b) Effect of PAF-acether (platelet-activating factor) and its specific antagonist, BN 52021, on interleukin 1 (IL 1) synthesis and release by rat monocytes. Prostaglandins 33:931–939

Pignol B, Henane S, Sorlin B, Rola-Pleszczynski M, Mencia-Huerta JM, Braquet P (1988 a) Effect of long-term in vivo treatment with platelet-activating factor on interleukin 1 and interleukin 2 production by rat splenocytes. In: Braquet P (ed) Platelet-activating factor and cell immunology. Karger, Basel, pp 38–43 (New trends in lipid mediators research, vol 1)

Pignol B, Henane S, Pirotzky E, Mencia-Huerta JM, Braquet P (1988 b) Potentiation of immunosuppressive action of cyclosporine by platelet-activating factor antagonists: an aproach of the mechanism of action of these drugs in graft rejection. Transplant Proc 20:259–265

Record M, Wagner M, Snyder F (1986) A kinetic study of the uptake and subcellular distribution of an antitumor PAF-analog ([^{3}H]alkyl-2-methoxy-GPC) in HL-60 cells (abstract). In: Second international conference on platelet-activating factor and structurally related alkyl ether lipids. Gatlinburg, Tennessee, 26–29 October 1986, p 52

Rola-Pleszczynski M, Pignol B, Pouliot C, Braquet P (1987 a) Inhibition of human lymphocyte proliferation and interleukin 2 production by platelet-activating factor (PAF-acether): reversal by a specific antagonist, BN 52021. Biochem Biophys Res Commun 142:754–760

Rola-Pleszczynski M, Pouliot C, Pignol B, Braquet P (1987 b) Platelet-activating factor induces human suppressor cell activity. Fed Proc 46:743

Runge MH, Andreesen R, Pfleiderer A, Munder PG (1980) Destruction of human solid tumors by alkyl-lysophospholipids. J Natl Cancer Inst 64:1301–1306

Snyder F, Wood R (1969) Alkyl and alkyl-l-enyl ethers of glycerol in lipids from normal and neoplastic human tissues. Cancer Res 29:251–257

Spence AM, Coates PW (1981) Scanning and transmission electron microscopy of cloned rat astrocytoma cells treated with dibutyryl cyclic AMP in vitro. J Cancer Res Clin Oncol 100:51–58

Storme G, Berdel WE, Blitterswije WJ von, Bruyneel EA, De Bruyne GK, Mareel MM (1985) Anti-invasive effect of racemic-1-octadecyl-2-methoxy-glycero-3-phosphocholine and other lysophospholipid analogs on MO4 mouse fibrosarcoma cells in vitro. Cancer Res 45:351–357

Tidwell T, Guzman G, Volgler WR (1981) The effects of alkyllysophospholipids on leukemic cell lines. I. Differential action on two human leukemic cell lines, HL 60 and K 562. Blood 57:794–797

Weltzien HU, Westphal O (1967) Synthesen von Cholinphosphatiden. IV. O-methylierte und O-acetylierte Lysolecithine. Justus Liebigs Ann Chem 709:240–243

Winslow DP, Roscoe JP, Rowles PM (1978) Changes in surface morphology associated with ethylnitrosurea-induced malignant transformation of cultured rat brain cells studied by scanning electron microscopy. Br J Exp Pathol 59:530–539

Regulatory Role of Platelet-Activating Factor on Cytokine Production

B. Pignol, S. Henane, J. M. Mencia-Huerta, and P. Braquet

Introduction

Platelet-activating factor (PAF) is a potent mediator of inflammatory processes produced by platelets, polymorphonuclear leukocytes, and macrophages (reviewed in [1, 2]). Several antagonists of PAF have been described [3], among which some are extracted from *Ginkgo biloba* leaves [4]. These substances, namely BN 52020, BN 52021, and 52022, inhibit PAF-induced platelet aggregation, the most potent one being BN 52021 (ginkgolide B) [5]. Stimulated macrophages released both PAF [2] and interleukin (IL)1 [6]. The involvement of IL1 in many aspects of the immune response suggests that this mediator is also an important regulatory molecule of the inflammatory reactions [6]. However, the possible link between the generation of PAF and IL1 has not yet been considered.

In this review, we focus on the possible role of PAF in the regulation of IL1 and IL2 production both in vitro and ex vivo from rat splenocytes. The interference of the specific PAF antagonist, BN 52021, with the effects of the mediator in such processes is also analyzed.

Materials and Methods

Reagents

Phytohemagglutinin P (PHA) (Difco Laboratories, Detroit, USA), concanavalin A (ConA) (Sigma, St Louis, USA), PAF (Novabiochem, Cleryen-Vexin, France), and lipopolysaccharide (LPS) (Sigma) were obtained as noted. BN 52021 was supplied by IHB (Le Plessis-Robinson, France).

Minipump Preparation and Implantation

Minipumps were loaded with either defined quantities of PAF in solution in 10% ethanol in 0.15 *M* NaCl or solvent alone. After 4 h equilibration in warm 0.15 *M* NaCl solution, the minipumps were connected to the jugular vein of Sprague Dawley rats and placed unter the skin of the back. The rats received over a 7-day period a total amount of 1, 4.5, 9, or 28 μg PAF. As a control group, animals were implanted with minipumps loaded with 10% ethanol solution in 0.15 μ NaCl. In selected experiments, rats were implanted with PAF-containing minipumps and were given 5 mg/kg BN 52021 intraperitoneally twice a day for 7 days prior to determination of IL1 and IL2 production.

Immune Consequences of
Trauma, Shock and Sepsis
Eds. Faist/Ninnemann/Green

Lymphocyte and Monocyte Preparations

Spleen mononuclear cells from Sprague Dawley rats or human peripheral blood mononuclear leukocytes (PBMLs) were isolated by centrifugation at 200 × g for 30 min on Ficoll-Hypaque gradients. The cells at the interface were collected and washed twice by centrifugation in a phosphate-buffered saline solution (PBS) for 10 min at 200 × g.

For the assessment of IL2 production and lymphocyte proliferation, mononuclear cells were resuspended in RPMI 1640 supplemented with 10% fetal calf serum (FCS). IL2 production or lymphocyte proliferation was initiated or not by the addition of ConA. Cultures were incubated at 37 °C for 24 h before the cell-free supernatants were harvested. For the assessment of IL1 production, monocytes were separated by adherence on plastic petri dishes for 60 min at 37 °C under a 5% CO_2/95% air atmosphere. Monolayers were washed with PBS and the cells were detached with a rubber policeman. IL1 production was initiated or not by the addition of LPS. When indicated, defined concentrations of PAF were added during the culture period.

IL1 and IL2 Assays

The released and cell-associated IL1 activity in the samples was assessed using the mouse thymocyte proliferation assay [7]. The IL2 activity in the cell-free supernatants from spleen lymphocytes was determined by the proliferation assay using the IL2-dependent murine cytotoxic lymphocyte line (CTLL) cell line [8].

Cell Proliferation

Lymphocyte proliferation was measured by the uptake of [^{3}H]thymidine (Amersham, Les Ulis, France) at the end of a 72-h culture in the presence of PHA.

Results and Discussion

In Vitro Studies

Platelet-activating factor markedly altered in a dose-dependent fashion the in vitro IL1 production by rat monocytes stimulated with LPS. When added at a concentration ranging from 1 f*M* to 1 n*M* to LPS-stimulated adherent monocytes, PAF enhanced the release and synthesis of IL1, whereas concentrations above 10 n*M* decreased them. In Table 1 are presented the results obtained with 1 p*M* and PAF 0.1 μ*M* PAF, respectively, representative of such increases and decreases. The antagonist, BN 52021 (10 μ*M*), reversed the increase in LPS-induced IL1 release and synthesis evoked by 1 p*M* PAF. In addition, the decrease in IL1 release and synthesis by 0.1 μ*M* PAF was markedly reduced in the presence of BN 52021. No direct action of BN 52021 on the IL1 production or in the IL1 assay on thymocyte was noted (data not shown).

Table 1. Effects of PAF with or without BN 52021 (10 μ*M*) on LPS-induced IL1 release and synthesis from rat spleen adherent monocytes

PAF	Released IL1	Cell-associated IL1
1 p*M*	6460±2076*	4838±250***
1 p*M*+BN 52021	2858+ 80	2538±101
0.1 μ*M*	1301± 361*	1207±242*
0.1 μ*M*+BN 52021	2332± 161	2164± 83
None	2697± 550	2624±538

Results are expressed as means ± SEM of five experiments.
* $P<0.05$; *** $P<0.005$.

Table 2. Dose-dependent inhibition by PAF of IL2 production in vitro by PBMLs in response to PHA and reversal by BN 52021 (10 μ)

PAF	Units of IL2/ml	
	Without BN 52021	With BN 52021
None	5.00±0.52	4.85±0.78
1 μ*M*	2.00±0.31**	3.9 ±0.52
0.1 μ*M*	1.55±0.21***	3.8 ±0.36
10 n*M*	1.25±0.15***	3.3 ±0.21*

Results are expressed as mean ± SEM of three experiments.
* $P<0.05$; ** $P<0.01$; $P<0.005$.

Table 3. Effect of in vivo administration of PAF on the LPS-induced IL1 production from rat-adherent spleen cells

Treatment of the rats	[^{3}H] Thymidine incorporation (cpm) % variation in cytokine production over control		
	n	IL1	IL2
Vehicle alone	12	100%	100%
PAF 1 μg	5	+ 0.8± 0.2	+236.0±71.4**
PAF 4.5 μg	2	+ 52.4±13.2	+139 ±56*
PAF 9 μg	5	+ 91.2±15.6	+ 50 ±28
PAF 28 μg	10	− 61.8±13.7**	+ 34 ±22

Results are expressed as means±SEM of the indicated number of experiments.
* $P<0.05$; $P<0.01$.

The present data demonstrated that PAF may play a critical role in the regulation of IL1 production by monocytes. The opposite effects of the mediator on the IL1 production suggests that PAF may either act on two different monocyte populations or on two receptor classes present on the same or different cells. In the absence of LPS stimulation, PAF did not affect the IL1 production. This result is in contradiction to that of Barret et al. [9], who demonstrated a direct

IL1 secretory effect of PAF, but the observed difference may be related to species variation.

As assessed using the IL2-dependent CTLL cell line, PAF significantly reduced IL2 production by peripheral blood mononuclear leukocytes (PBMLs) following PHA stimulation (Table 2). BN 52021 at 10 μ*M* had no effect by itself but reversed the inhibition induced by PAF.

Ex Vivo Studies

Monocytes from rats treated for 7 days with 4.5 or 9 μg PAF exhibited no alteration of the LPS-induced IL1 release and synthesis. When the rats were administered with 28 μg PAF, a marked and significant decrease in the LPS-induced IL1 production was observed (Table 3). As compared with ConA-stimulated spleen lymphocytes from untreated animals, those from rats receiving 1 or 4.5 μg PAF exhibited an increased capability to produce IL2 (Table 3).

In another set of experiments, the rats were treated with either 28 or 1 μg PAF to assess the effect of BN 52021 on the alterations of IL1 and IL2 production induced by the lipid mediator. Administration of BN 52021 during treatment with 28 μg PAF fully reversed the inhibitory effect of the mediator on the IL1 production. In addition, treatment of the PAF-infused rats with BN 52021 reversed by 81% the stimulatory effect of 1 μg PAF on the IL2 production.

In conclusion, the present data demonstrate that PAF might play an in vivo immunoregulatory role since it markedly alters cytokine production and thus may be critical in various immune processes. That BN 52021 almost totally abolished the action of PAF is suggestive of the presence of specific high-affinity binding sites for the autacoid on immunocompetent cells.

References

1. Braquet P, Touqui L, Shen TY, Vargaftig BB (1987) Perspectives in platelet-activating factor research. Pharmacol Rev 39:97–145
2. Braquet P, Rola-Plesczcynski M (1979) The role of PAF in immunological responses. Immunol Today 9:409
3. Braquet P, Godfroid JJ (1986) PAF specific binding sites: 2. Design of specific antagonists. Trends Pharmacol Sci 397
4. Braquet P (1985) Treatment or prevention of PAF disorders provoked by a new series of highly specific inhibitors. G.B. Patent. 84/18 424, 1984. BE 901, 915 (See CA 103:189808d)
5. Braquet P (1987) The ginkgolides: potent platelet-activating factor antagonists isolated from *Ginkgo biloba L.*: chemistry, pharmacology and clinical applications. Drugs Future 12:643–699
6. Dinarello CA (1984) Interleukin-1 and the pathogenesis of the acute-phase response. N Engl J Med 311:1413
7. Mizel SB, Oppenheim JJ, Rosenstreich DL (1978) Characterization of lymphocyte-activating factor (LAF) produced by a macrophage cell line, P 388 D1. Biochemical characterization of LAF-induced by activated T cells and LPS. J Immunol 120:1504
8. Gillis S, Ferm M, Ou W, Smith KA (1978) T cell growth factor: parameters of production and a quantitative microassay for activity. J Immunol 120:2027
9. Barrett ML, Lewis GP, Ward S, Westwick J (1987) Platelet-activating factor induces interleukin 1 production from adherent macrophages. Br J Pharmacol 90:113

Potential Role for Platelet-Activating Factor and Tumor Necrosis Factor in the Immune Impairments in Shock and Trauma

D. Hosford and P. Braquet

Introduction

Endotoxic shock, burn, and sepsis are major pathological manifestations associated with high morbidity that are refractory to classical treatments. The clinical symptoms are characterized by profound hemodynamic alterations such as systemic hypotension associated with a decrease in peripheral vascular resistance, cardiac failure, pulmonary hypertension, bronchoconstriction, and lung edema (Gilbert 1960). In addition there are marked alterations in immune functions. For example, thermal injury is accompanied by anergy comprising a fall in CD4+/CD8+ ratio (Braquet et al. 1984a), reduced mitogen-induced interleukin 2 (IL 2) production, and depressed natural killer (NK) cell and lymphocyte activity (Braquet 1986). In shock states reduction in the number and function of circulating platelets and leukocytes also contributes to circulatory disorders. The increase in vascular permeability is a determinant for the prognosis and evolution of endotoxemia since it leads to hypovolemia that enhances cardiac and pulmonary failure.

Although the pathophysiology of endotoxemia and gram-negative sepsis is unclear, Morrisson and Ulevitch (1978) have suggested that septic shock probably relates more to the host defense of the organism than from aggression by the bacteria itself. Thus, the pathogenesis of endotoxemia probably involves various humoral and cellular components leading to the final release of inflammatory mediators such as histamine, kinins, serotonin, arachidonic acid metabolites, and complement-derived peptides. Indeed, there is considerable evidence implicating these mediators in the early phase of endotoxic shock (Jacobs 1985). In this paper we will consider the role of two such mediators, platelet-activating factor (PAF) and tumor necrosis factor (TNF) in endotoxemia and examine their potential relationship with the immunological modifications which occur in the shock state.

Platelet-Activating Factor in Various Shock States

Three lines of evidence suggest the involvement of PAF in shock: (1) infusion of PAF in animals mimics the shock state, (2) increased levels of PAF are generated during shock, and (3) specific antagonists of PAF inhibit or alleviate shock induced by various mechanisms.

Immune Consequences of
Trauma, Shock and Sepsis
Eds. Faist/Ninnemann/Green

Platelet-Activating Factor-Induced Shock

MacManus et al. (1980) showed that PAF infused into rabbits at very low concentrations produced death of the animals. In this model, the pathology induced is similar to that of systemic shock, and activation of platelets by PAF appears to play a central role in the process, since the mortality rate is significantly reduced by platelet depletion (Pinckard et al. 1979). PAF also induces the signs of shock in guinea pigs, i.e., hypotension, bronchoconstriction, thrombocytopenia, and death (Vargaftig et al. 1980; Kenzora et al. 1984). In dogs the mediator induces hypotension, myocardial contractility impairment, decreased coronary artery flow, systemic and pulmonary vascular changes, renal dysfunction, hemoconcentration, and metabolic acidosis (Bessin et al. 1983; Handley et al. 1984; Sybertz et al. 1985). Leukopenia and thrombocytopenia have also been observed in conscious dogs. Portal vein pressure rises during the 1st min following a PAF injection, suggesting a crucial role of blood maldistribution in this form of shock (Bessin et al. 1983). Hypovolemia is a well-known typical feature of the shock state, characterized during anaphylaxis in monkeys (Smedegard et al. 1979) and rats (Carlson et al. 1975) by a significant rise of hematocrit associated with plasma loss, decreased blood volume, and increased plasma extravasation. These vascular permeability impairments have also been reported in septic shock in dogs (Wedmore and Williams 1981; Van Lambalgen et al. 1984). PAF induces hemoconcentration, plasma extravasation into interstitial space, and edema formation in rats (Sanchez-Crespo et al. 1982) and guinea pigs (Hwang et al. 1986). Locally injected, PAF induces plasma extravasation in guinea pigs (Morley et al. 1983) and rabbit skin, and intense plasma leakage and sludge in the rabbit retina (Braquet et al. 1984b). Further evidence for this involvement of PAF in shock comes from its ulcerogenic effects, these being similar to gastrointestinal impairments obtained after endotoxin administration (Rosam and Wallace 1986).

Generation of PAF During Shock

The first description of the presence of PAF in the blood from rabbits with systemic anaphylaxis was reported by Pinckard et al. (1977), who inactivated serum acetyl hydrolase to allow the isolation and assay of PAF. Further evidence has been provided by Inarrea et al. (1985), who showed that in mice a PAF-like substance appears in the liver and spleen of the animals after challenge with IgG. Furthermore, the appearance of this substance precedes the blood volume reduction due to plasma extravasation. Previous treatment of the animals with mepacrine, BN 52021, or depletion of mononuclear phagocytes by total irradiation lead both to the disappearance of the extravasation induced by the aggregates and reduction of PAF generation by the spleen and the liver. Indeed, soluble aggregates of immunoglobulin G initiate a number of responses in experimental animals which mimic the pathophysiology of the shock state and which are also potent in vitro triggers for the generation of PAF (Mencia-Huerta and Benveniste 1981; Sanchez-Crespo et al. 1980). This suggests PAF might be an endogenous mediator of the physiological responses initiated by soluble aggregates of immunoglobulin G (Inarrea et al. 1985).

Platelet-activating factor also appears in rat blood samples after intravenous injection of *Salmonella enteritidis,* while it is not present in control animals (P. Braquet, unpublished data). Similar results have been obtained by Buxton et al. (1984, 1986) using in situ perfused rat livers challenged with soluble IgG aggregates. Under these conditions a compound similar to PAF was found in the effluent, which, interestingly, initiated glycogenolysis by the hepatic cells.

Platelet-Activating Factor Antagonists and Inhibition of Shock

A wide range of specific PAF antagonists are capable of alleviating various pathologies of the shock state. The ginkgolide BN 52021 inhibits the hemodynamic changes induced by intravenous injection of human IgG aggregates in rats (Sanchez-Crespo et al. 1985, 1986). Whereas a sustained hypotension appears in the control animals, no variation in arterial pressure is observed in the treated rats. This protection is accompanied by a significant inhibition in the associated lethality and plasmatic extravasation. In shock induced by *S. enteriditis* endotoxin (Etienne et al. 1985; Adnot et al. 1986), a significant dose-dependent inhibition of the lethality is also observed with BN 52021, total protection being provided by the highest doses of the antagonist (Etienne et al. 1985). This effect is associated with a reduced increase in body temperature, suggesting that BN 52021 has an effect on the release of the interleukin 1 (IL 1).

In guinea pigs injected with *S. typhimurium* endotoxin, a similar protection is also afforded by ginkgolide B and other PAF antagonists including CV 3988 (Terashita et al. 1985), kadsurenone (Doebber et al. 1985), L-652,731 (Inerrea et al. 1983), SRI 63-072 and SRI 63-441 (Handley et al. 1986), ONO 6240 (Miyamoto et al. 1985), and WEB 2086 (Casals-Stenzel et al. 1986). In platelet-depleted animals, BN 52021 affords total protection against the drop in arterial pressure, suggesting that platelets contribute to hypotension by releasing an unknown factor, not inhibited by ginkgolide B (Adnot et al. 1986). Recently, Touvay et al. (1988) have also shown that lung parenchymal strips from guinea pigs treated with endotoxin exhibit specific desensitization to PAF, an effect not observed in animals also administered with BN 52021 and indicating PAF production in endotoxemia.

In a similar model using *E. coli* endotoxin, BN 52021 inhibits the endotoxin-induced tracheal hyperreactivity to histamine in the guinea pig, suggesting that PAF may be important in inducing this process (Nijkamp et al. 1988). Hyperreactivity may result from platelet infiltration in the lung. Indeed, pretreatment of guinea pigs with BN 52021, CV-3988, or brotizolam results in a dose-related inhibition of *E. coli* endotoxin-induced pulmonary platelet recruitment. In contrast, no inhibition is recorded with indomethacin at doses known to inhibit cyclooxygenase (Beijer et al. 1988). Interestingly, PAF antagonists inhibit the oliguric acute renal failure with decreased renal blood flow (RBF) and glomerular filtration rate (GFR) induced by endotoxin in the rat (Ha et al. 1987). Since PAF injection in the rat induces a rapid and significant increase in plasma protease activity, part of the benefical effect of PAF antagonists may result from the indirect inhibition of this process. Indeed, as demonstrated by Etienne et al. (1987), BN 52021 inhibits both the PAF- and endotoxin-induced plasma protease activity.

Furthermore, BN 52021 also protects against impairments induced by myotoxin injection in rats. At a dose of 5–15 mg/kg i.v., BN 52021 prolongs the survival of animals exposed to a highly lethal dose of trichothecenes (Feuerstein et al. 1987). Finally, PAF may also be involved in acute immune pancreatitis since BN 52021 reduces by approximately 50% the increase in vascular permeability and the associated release of leukotrienes (Jancar et al. 1988).

Tumor Necrosis Factor and Shock

The administration of endotoxin to animals can prompt severe metabolic and physiological disturbances which lead to shock and death by multi-organ system failure (Gilbert et al. 1960; Fry et al. 1980). Recently, it has become apparent that endotoxin does not injure the host directly but via inducing the release of endogenous mediators (Beutler et al. 1985). Indeed, the injection of endotoxin is associated with extensive production of TNF and there is much evidence indicating that this substance is also one of the internal vectors in endotoxin-induced shock.

For example, rabbits given a lethal dose of endotoxin are estimated to produce several milligrams of TNF per kilogram of body weight (Abe et al. 1985). Mice injected with recombinant human (rh)-TNF, free of contaminating endotoxin, develop piloerection of the hair, develop diarrhea, become withdrawn, and die if sufficient amounts are given (Tracey et al. 1986). When TNF is administered to rats the animals become mildly hypotensive and tachypneic, and die of sudden respiratory arrest (Tracey et al. 1986), before which severe metabolic acidosis, marked hemoconcentration, and biphasic changes in blood glucose concentration are apparent. Pathological surveys of animals dying of TNF poisoning have revealed severe leukostasis in the lungs, hemorrhagic necrosis in the adrenals, pancreas, and other organs, and tubular necrosis of the kidney (reviewed in Cerami and Beutler 1988).

All the above changes are prevented if the animals are pretreated with a neutralizing monoclonal antibody against TNF (Tracey et al. 1986). The role of TNF in endotoxin-induced shock is further evidenced by the fact that early passive immunization of mice with rabbit anti-mouse TNF antibodies significantly prevents mortality after subsequent injection with lethal doses of endotoxin (Beutler et al. 1985).

Thus, although some pathological changes that occur in shock are undoubtedly evoked by the release of other secondary mediators, such as prostaglandins and leukotrienes, a major role can be attributed to PAF and TNF. There is also accumulating evidence that these two substances are important modulators of the immune response, suggesting that they may elicit detrimental effects on this system during trauma and shock.

Effects of Platelet-Activating Factor on the Immune Response

An increasing number of studies have indicated that PAF is a potent modulator of the immune system (reviewed in Braquet and Rola-Pleszczynski 1987). PAF inhibits in vitro both the proliferation of human lymphocytes and the production of IL 2, in a BN 52021- and indomethacin-sensitive process. In addition, when the lymphocyte preparation is depleted in monocytes, higher inhibition is reached in an indomethacin-insensitive mechanism. In contrast, ex vivo experiments using minipumps loaded with PAF or solvent alone, placed under the back skin of rats and connected to the jugular vein, have shown that lymphocytes from animals receiving 9, 4.5, or 1 μg PAF/7 days exhibit increased capacity to produce IL 2. This effect is prevented by treating the animals with BN 52021.

Added at 1 p*M* to adherent cell monolayers stimulated with LPS, PAF induces an increase in IL 1 synthesis and release, whereas at 0.1 μ*M* PAF a decrease in both these parameters is observed. In the same minipump model IL 1 is also increased following ex vivo stimulation of lymphocytes from PAF-treated animals. BN 52021 (10 μ*M*) reverses by more than 70% the increase and inhibition of LPS-induced synthesis and release of IL 1 induced by 1 p*M* and 0.1 μ*M* PAF, respectively. PAF also induces an increase in the number of both CD^4+ and CD^8+ lymphocytes, the suppressive effect of the autacoid being more apparent. PAF increases NK cell activity, and BN 52021 reduces it, a result in keeping with the protective role of the latter drug in graft rejection and prevention of killing of Langerhans islets by cytotoxic lymphocytes. At the picomolar range, PAF acts on B-lymphocytes by increasing the number of immunoglobulin-producing cells. Finally, PAF stimulates TNF production from macrophages and TNF primes PAF-induced superoxide anion generation by polymorphonuclear leukocytes, two processes likely to play a role in endotoxemia (see "Relationship Between PAF, TNF, and Immune Impairments in Shock" below).

Tumor Necrosis Factor as an Immunomodulator

Several studies suggest that TNF can modulate the response of cells of the immune system. T-helper cell differentiation factor, which was once thought to be distinct from TNF-α, has now been found to be identical to TNF-α based on purification and amino acid sequence determinations (Takeda et al. 1986). Whether TNF-β also displays similar activities is not known at present. TNF-α has also been shown to activate macrophages for the production of IL 1, GM-CSF, and prostaglandins (Dinarello et al. 1986; Munker et al. 1986). The production of interferon-γ (INF-γ) by lymphocytes also appears to be modulated by TNF-α (Wong and Goeddel 1986). The exposure of neutrophils to both TNF-α and TNF-β causes the production of superoxide radicals, induces a phagocytic response, and enhances antibody-dependent cell cytotoxicity (Shalaby et al. 1987). The differentiation of hematopoietic stem cells has also been reported to be suppressed by TNF-α and TNF-β (Murphy et al. 1986). The expression of HLA-DR antigens and high-affinity IL 2 receptors on human T cells is also increased by TNF-α (Scheurich et al. 1987). Thus, overall from several in vitro studies it appears that TNF may play a major role in the modulation of the immune system.

Relationship Between PAF, TNF, and Immune Impairments in Shock

The evidence presented above indicates that in vivo PAF induces a TNF-mediated-like shock syndrome; thus we determined whether PAF activates peripheral blood-derived monocytes to produce TNF (Bonavida and Braquet 1988). Monocyte activation was measured by direct cytotoxicity against sensitive target cells, the release in the supernatant of cytotoxic factors, and the secretion of TNF as assessed by a sensitive radioimmunoassay. The addition of various concentrations of PAF (1–30 μ*M*) to monocyte cultures for 24 h did not result in any significant enhancement of cytotoxicity. Supernatants derived from these preparations were only slightly cytotoxic to target cells, but did contain TNF. In these supernatants, concentration of TNF as determined by RIA was dependent on the dose of PAF added and reached levels equivalent to those found from INF-γ-stimulated monocytes. BN 52021 inhibited the PAF-induced TNF release (Table 1). The kinetics of TNF production were rapid and significant, TNF being produced in the 2 h following exposure to PAF (Fig. 1). The cytotoxic activity in the supernatant was present initially but declined after 24 h. These results suggest that PAF induces TNF release from monocytes but that the cytotoxic activity is masked by the presence of inhibitor or is partially denatured. These findings also suggest that PAF-induced shock may be the result of monocyte activation and TNF production. Preliminary experiments have also demonstrated that PAF at very low doses (1 p*M* to 10 n*M*) significantly amplifies the LPS-induced production of TNF. This is in accordance with the phenomenon discussed above concerning IL 1 generation induced by PAF. Further studies are currently in progress to examine the effect of anti-TNF antibody on PAF- and LPS-induced activation in vivo and in vitro.

The amplification or enhancement of a PMN response to a given stimulus by prior exposure of the cell to different agonists has been referred to as "priming." Enhanced PMN responses to thrombin and FMLP have been reported following pre-exposure to PAF (Vercelotti et al. 1988); similarly, TNF has also been shown to prime PMN to various agonists (Berkaw et al. 1986). Interestingly, while PAF per se at low doses is not able to produce superoxide generation, a preincubation of the same PMN system with TNF results in a significant amplification of O_2^-

Table 1. Effect of BN 52021 (1 μ*M*) on PAF-induced TNF production by human monocytes

	BN	TNF (ng/ml)[a]
–	–	0
–	+	0
γ-IFN	–	3.18 ± 0.57
PAF 10 μ*M*	–	1.37 ± 0.43
PAF 10 μ*M*	+	0.47 ± 0.21
PAF 20 μ*M*	–	3.25 ± 0.67
PAF 20 μ*M*	+	1.17 ± 0.17

[a] Radioimmunoassay, mean ± SEM, $n = 7$.

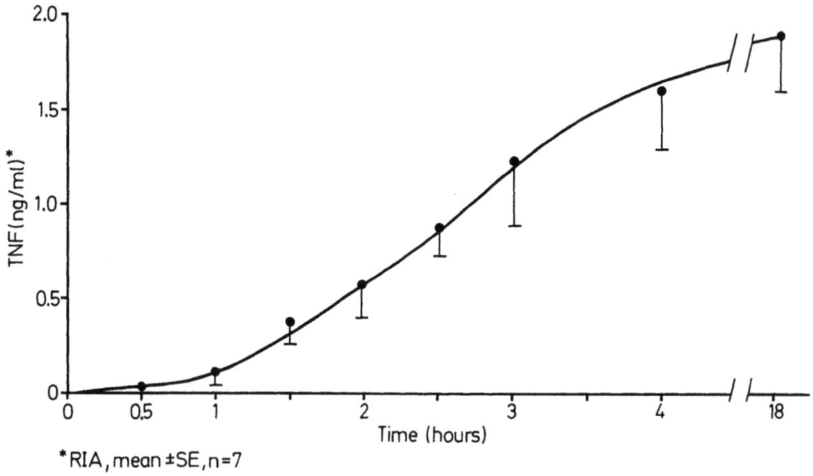

Fig. 1. Effect of PAF (1 μ*M*) on kinetics of TNF production by human monocytes

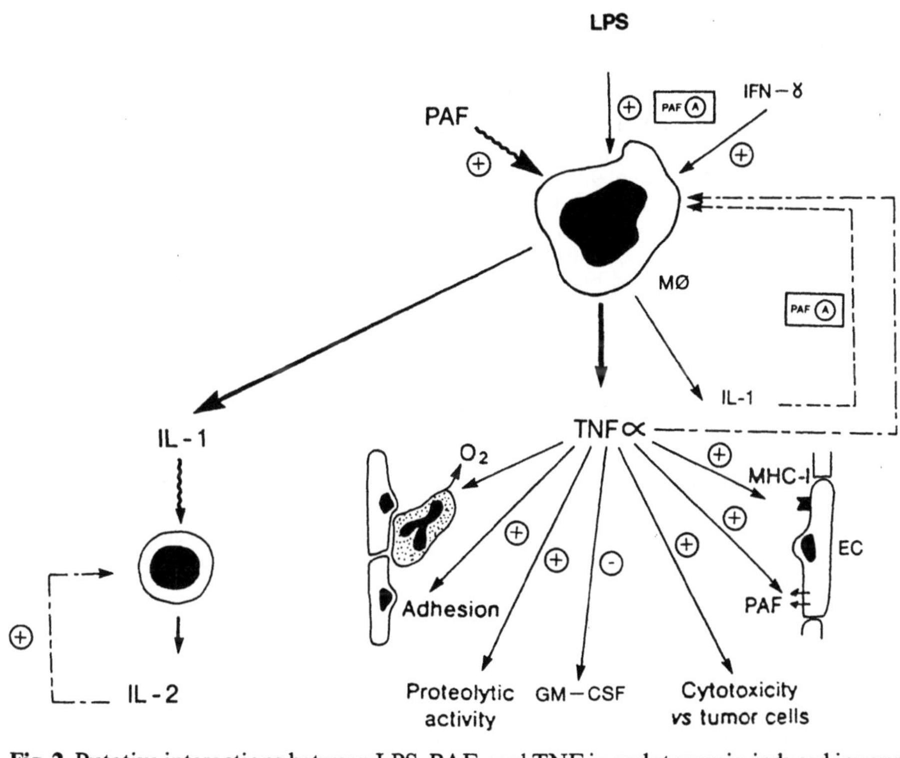

Fig. 2. Putative interactions between LPS, PAF, and TNF in endotoxemia-induced immune impairments

production (Braquet et al. 1988). This phenomenon is inhibited by various PAF antagonists and appears to be impaired after thermal injury. Since PAF is synthesized and present on surfaces of endothelial cells under TNF stimulation, the ether lipid may produce an amplification feedback involving marginated PMNs that eventually becomes damaging to the PAF-synthesizing endothelium itself.

Conclusion

These preliminary data allow us to speculate on the relationship between PAF and TNF. The potential interactions between these two substances and the immune impairments resulting from endotoxemia are presented in Fig. 2. Further experiments are required to more clearly define the role of these mediators in the pathology of shock and trauma.

References

Abe S, Gatanaga T, Yamazaki M, Soma G, Mizuno D (1985) Purification of tumor necrosis factor. FEBS Lett 180:203

Adnot S, Lefort J, Lagente V, Braquet P, Vargaftig BB (1986) Interference of BN 52021, a PAF-acether antagonist with endotoxin-induced hypotensin in the guinea-pig. Pharmacol Res Commun 18:197–200

Beijer L, Botting J, Crook P, Oyekan AO, Page CP, Rylander R (1988) The involvement of platelet activating factor in endotoxin-induced pulmonary platelet recruitment in the guinea-pig. Br J Pharmacol 92:803–808

Berkaw RL, Wang D, Larrich JW, Howard TH (1986) Recombinant tumor necrosis factor augments human neutrophil superoxide production. Blood 68:80A

Bessin P, Bonnet J, Appfel D, Soulard C, Desgroux L, Pelas I, Benveniste J (1983) Acute circulatory collapse caused by platelet-activating factor (PAF-acether) in dogs. Eur J Pharmacol 86:403–413

Beutler B, Milsark IW, Cerami AC (1985) Passive immunisation against cachectin/tumor necrosis factor protects mice from lethal effects of endotoxin. Science 229:869–871

Bonavida B, Braquet P (1988) Effect of platelet-activating factor (PAF) on monocyte activation and production of tumor necrosis factor (TNF). Prostaglandins 35:802

Braquet M (1986) Nature and origin of burn immunologic alteration. Transplant Proc 18(5):83–90

Braquet P, Rola-Pleszczynski M (1987) Platelet-activating factor and the immune response. Immunology Today 8:345–352

Braquet M, Ducousso R, Garay R, Guilbaud J, Carsin H, Braquet P (1984a) Leukocyte leukotriene B^4 secretion precedes anergy in burn-injured patients. Lancet II (8409):976–977

Braquet P, Vidal RF, Braquet M, Hamard H, Vargaftig BB (1984b) Involvement of leukotrienes and PAF-acether in the increase microvascular permeability of the rabbit retina. Agents Actions 15:82–85

Braquet P, Paubert-Braquet M, Bessin P, Vargaftig BB (1987) Platelet-activating factor, a potential mediator of shock. In: Samuelsson B, Paoletti R, Ramwell P (eds) Advances in prostaglandin, thromboxane and leukotriene research, vol 17. Raven, New York, pp 822–827

Braquet M, Longchamp MO, Koltz PL, Guilbaud J (1988) Tumor necrosis factor (TNF) primes neutrophil (PMN) platelet-activating factor (PAF)-induced superoxide generation in thermal-injured (TI) patients: consequences in promoting PMN-mediated endothelial cell (EC) damages. Prostaglandins 35:803

Buxton D, Hanaham DJ, Olson MS (1984) Stimulation of glycogenolysis and platelet-activating factor production by heat aggregated immunoglobulin G in the perfused rat liver. J Biol Chem 259:13758–13761
Buxton DB, Fisher RA, Hanahan DJ, Olson MS (1986) Platelet-activating factor-mediated vasoconstriction and glycogenolysis in the perfused rat liver. J Biol Chem 261:644–649
Carlson RW, Schaeffer RC, Whigham H, Michaels S, Russel FE, Weil MH (1975) Rattlesnake venom shock in the rat: development of a method. Am J Physiol 229:1658–1674
Casals-Stenzel J, Muacevic G, Hueer H (1986) Inhibition of platelet-activating factor (PAF) induced effects in vitro and in vivo by WEB 2086, a new and specific PAF antagonist. In: Second international conference on platelet activating factor and structurally related alkyl ether lipids. Gatlinburg, Tennessee, 26–29 October 1986, p 107
Cerami A, Beutler B (1988) The role of cachectin/TNF in endotoxic shock and cachexia. Immunol Today 9:28–31
Dinarello C, Cannon J, Wolff SM, Bernheim H, Beutler B, Cerami A, Figari I, Palladino MA, O'Connor JW (1986) Tumor necrosis factor (cachectin) is an endogenous pyrogen and induces production of interleukin 1. J Exp Med 163:1433–1450
Doebber TW, Wu MS, Robbins JC, Choy BM, Chang MN, Shen TY (1985) Platelet activating factor (PAF) involvement in endotoxin-induced hypotension in rats. Studies with PAF receptor antagonist kadsurenone. Biochem Biophys Res Commun 127:799–808
Etienne A, Hecquet F, Soulard C, Spinnewyn B, Clostre F, Braquet P (1985) In vivo inhibition of plasma protein leakage and *Salmonella enteridis*-induced mortality in the rat by a specific PAF acether antagonist: BN 52021. Agents Actions 17:368–370
Etienne A, Hecquet F, Guilmard C, Soulard C, Braquet P (1987) A potential link between platelet-activating factor and plasma protease activity in endotoxemia. Int J Tissue Reac 9:19–26
Feuerstein G, Leader P, Siren AL, Braquet P (1987) Protective effect of a PAF antagonist, BN 52021, in trichothecene toxicosis. Toxicol Lett 38:271–274
Fry DE, Pearltein RL, Fulton HC, Polk Jr (1980) Multiple system organ failure. The role of uncontrolled infection. Arch Surg 115:136
Gilbert RP (1960) Mechanism of the hemodynamic effects of endotoxin. Physiol Rev 40:245–279
Ha B, Tolins JP, Vercellotti G, Jacob HS, Raij L (1988) The role of platelet-activating factor in endotoxemic acute renal failure in the rat. Kidney Int 33:358
Handley DA, Van Valen RG, Melden MK, Saunders RN (1984) Evaluation of dose and route effects of platelet activating factor-induced extravasation in the guinea-pig. Thromb Haemost 52:34–46
Handley DA, Van Valen RG, Saunders RN (1986) Vascular responses of platelet-activating factor in the *Cebus apella* primate and inhibitory profile of antagonists SR 63-072 and 63-119. Immunopharmacology 11:175–182
Hwang SB, Lam MH, Lee CL, Shen TY (1986) Release of platelet activating factor and its involvement in the first phase of carrageenan-induced rat foot edema. Eur J Pharmacol 120:33–41
Inarrea P, Alonso F, Sanchez-Crespo M (1983) An effector substance of the vasopermeability changes induced by infusion of immune aggregates in the mouse. Immunopharmacology 6:7–14
Inarrea P, Gomez-Cambronero J, Pascual J, Ponte MC, Hernando L, Sanchez-Crespo M (1985) Synthesis of PAF-acether and blood volume changes in gram-negative sepsis. Immunopharmacology 9:45–52
Jacobs ER (1985) Overview of mediators affecting pulmonary and systemic vascular changes in endotoxemia. In: Hinshaw JB (ed) Handbook of endotoxin. Elsevier, Amsterdam, pp 1–15
Jancar S, De Giaccobi G, Mariano M, Sirois P, Braquet P (1988) Involvement of platelet-activating factor in acute immune-complex-induced pancreatitis. In: Braquet P (ed) The role of platelet-activating factor in immune disorders. New trends in lipid mediators research. Karger, Basel, pp 194–198

Kenzora JL, Perez JE, Bergman SR, Lange LG (1984) Effects of acetyl glyceryl ether phosphorylcholine (platelet-activating factor) on ventricular preload, afterload and contractility in dogs. J Clin Invest 74:1193–1203

MacManus LM, Hanahan DJ, Demopoulos CA, Pinckard RN (1980) Pathobiology of the intravenous infusion of acetyl-glyceryl-ether phosphorylcholine (AGEPC) a synthetic platelet-activating factor (PAF) in the rabbit. J Immunol 124:2919–2924

Mencia-Huerta JM, Benveniste J (1981) Platelet-activating factor and macrophages. II: Phagocytosis-associated release of PAF from rat peritoneal macrophages. Cell Immunol 57:281–292

Miyamoto T, Ohno H, Yano T, Okada T, Hamanaka N, Nawasaki A (1985) A new potent antagonist of platelet-activating factor. In: Hayaishi O, Yamamot S (eds) Advances in prostaglandin, thromboxane and leukotriene research, vol 15. Raven, New York, pp 719–720

Morley J, Page CP, Paul W (1983) Inflammatory actions of platelet-activating factor (PAF-acether) in guinea-pig skin. Br J Pharmacol 80:503–509

Morrisson DC, Ulevitch RJ (1978) The effects of bacterial endotoxins on host mediation systems. A review. Am J Pathol 93:525–618

Munker R, Gasson J, Ogawa M, Koeffler HP (1986) Recombinant human TNF induces production of granulocyte-monocyte colony-stimulating factor. Nature 323:79–82

Murphy M, London R, Kobayashi M, Trinchieri G (1986) Interferon and lymphotoxin released by activated T-cells synergise to inhibit granulocyte/monocyte colony formation. J Exp Med 164:263–279

Nijkamp FP, Braquet P, Van Heuven-Nolsen (1988) BN 52021 inhibits the endotoxin-induced tracheal hyperactivity to histamine in the guinea-pig but not the increased response to histamine in the heart and coronary vessels. In: 1st International congress on the immune consequences of trauma, shock and sepsis, Munich, March 3–5, 1988

Pinckard RN, Halonen M, Palmer DJ, Butler C, Shaw JO, Henson PM (1977) Intravascular aggregation and pulmonary sequestration of platelets during IgE-induced systematic anaphylaxis in the rabbit: abrogation of lethal anaphylatic shock by platelet depletion. J Immunol 119:2185–2191

Pinckard RN, Farr RS, Hanahan DJ (1979) Physiochemical and functional identity of rabbit platelet-activating factor (PAF) released in vivo during IgE anaphylaxis with PAF released in vitro from sensitized basophils. J Immunol 123:84–90

Rosam AC, Wallace JL, Whittle BJ (1986) Potent ulcerogenic actions of platelet activating factor on the stomach. Nature 319:54–56

Sanchez-Crespo M, Alonso F, Egido J (1980) Platelet-activating factor anaphylaxis and phagocytosis. I. Release from human peripheral polymorphonuclears and monocytes during the stimulation of ionophore A23187 and phagocytosis but not from degranulating basophils. Immunology 10:645–655

Sanchez-Crespo M, Alonso F, Inarrea P, Alvarez V, Egido J (1982) Vascular actions of synthetic PAF-acether (a synthetic platelet activating factor in the rat): evidence for a platelet independent mechanism. Immunopharmacology 4:173–185

Sanchez-Crespo M, Fernandez-Gallardo S, Nieto ML, Baranes J, Braquet P (1985) Inhibition of the vascular actions of IgG aggregates by BN 52021, a highly specific antagonist of PAF-acether. Immunopharmacology 10:69–75

Sanchez-Crespo M, Fernandez Gallardo S, Nieto ML, Braquet P (1986) Effect of a series of ginkgolides on the processing and the pathophysiological responses initiated by soluble aggregates of immunoglobulin G. In: 6th International conference on prostaglandins. 3–5 June 1986, Florence

Scheurich P, Thoma B, Ucer U, Pfizen-Maier K (1987) Immunoregulatory activity of recombinant human tumor necrosis factor (TNF)-alpha: induction of TNF receptors on human T cells and TNF-alpha mediated enhancement of T cell responses. J Immunol 138:1786–1790

Shalaby MR, Palladino MA, Hirabashi SE, Eessalu TE, Lewis GD, Shepard HM, Aggarwal BB (1987) Receptor binding and activation of polymorphonuclear neutrophils by tumor necrosis factor-alpha. J Leukocyte Biol 41:196–204

Smedegard G, Revenas B, Argors KE (1979) Anaphylaxis in the monkey: hemodynamics and blood flow distribution. Acta Physiol Scand 106:191–198

Sybertz EJ, Watkins RW, Baum T, Pula K, Rivelli M (1985) Cardiac, coronary and peripheral vascular effects of acetyl glyceryl ether phosphorylcholine in anesthetized dogs. J Pharmacol Exp Ther 232:156–162

Takeda K, Iwamoto S, Sugimoto H, Takuma T, Kawatami N, Noda M, Masaki M, Morise H, Arimura H, Konno K (1986) Identification of differentiation inducing factor and tumor necrosis factor. Nature 323:338–340

Terashita Z, Imura Y, Nishikawa K, Sumida S (1985) Is platelet activating factor (PAF) a mediator of endotoxin shock? Eur J Pharmacol 109:257

Touvay C, Vilain B, Carré C, Mencia-Huerta JM, Braquet P (1988) Role of platelet-activating factor (PAF) in the bronchopulmonary alterations induced by endotoxin. Effects on beta-adrenoceptors. In: Braquet P (ed) The ginkgolides: chemistry, biology, pharmacology and clinical perspectives. Prous, Barcelona, pp 477–486

Tracey KJ, Beutler B, Lowry SF, Merryweather J, Milsark IW, Hariri RJ, Fahey TJ, Zentella A, Albert JD, Shires T, Cerami A (1986) Shock and tissue injury induced by recombinant human cachectin. Science 234:470

Van Lambalgen AA, Bronsweld W, Van Den Bos GC, Thus LG (1984) Distribution of cardiac output, oxygen consumption and lactate production in canine endotoxic shock. Cardiovasc Res 18:195–205

Vargaftig BB, Lefort J, Chignard M, Benveniste J (1980) Platelet-activating factor induces a platelet-dependent bronchoconstriction unrelated to the formation of prostaglandin derivatives. Eur J Pharmacol 65:185–192

Vercellotti GM, Yin HQ, Gustafson KS, Nelson RD, Jacob HS (1988) Platelet-activating factor primes neutrophil responses to agonists: role in promoting neutrophil-mediated endothelial damage. Blood 71:1100–1106

Wedmore CV, Williams TJ (1981) Platelet-activating factor (PAF), a secretory product of polymorphonuclear leucocytes, increases vascular permeability in rabbit skin. Br J Pharmacol 916P–917P

Wong GM, Goeddel DV (1986) Tumor necrosis factor α and β inhibit virus replication and synergise with interferons. Nature 323:819–822

[illegible]

Suppression of Endotoxin-Induced Monokine Release by Human Serum Fractions

W. A. Flegel and H. Northoff

Introduction

Minute amounts of endotoxin (lipopolysaccharide, LPS) will induce monocytes concomitantly to release interleukin 1 (IL1), tumor necrosis factor (TNF), and interleukin 6 (IL6). This mechanism was shown (Lehmann et al. 1987; Freudenberg et al. 1986) to be central in mediating the in vivo toxicity of LPS. Therefore, the mediator release by human monocytes upon stimulation with LPS is a suitable and sensitive in vitro model for investigating the toxic effects of LPS. Inhibition of LPS to induce mediator release in this in vitro model by different means might have implications for diminished in vivo toxicity of endotoxin.

Binding of LPS to a variety of serum proteins and the subsequent impairment of endotoxin detection in the limulus assay was shown by several authors (for review see Obayashi 1984). Others (Ulevitch et al. 1979; Freudenberg et al. 1980) described the binding of LPS to lipoproteins, especially the high-density lipoproteins. Little is known as to whether this interaction of physiological serum components and endotoxin changes the toxicity of LPS. We approached this question using the mediator release by human monocytes as a redout. We found that serum from healthy donors could inhibit a certain amount of LPS. This "LPS-neutralizing capacity" is shown to reside exclusively in the lipoprotein fraction. We report results of lipoprotein subfractions and were able to exclude the influence of naturally occurring anti-LPS antibodies and complement.

Materials and Methods

Enriched adherent cells were prepared starting from buffy coats of normal blood units as described earlier (Northoff et al. 1987). Cells were then counted and seeded along with LPS from *Salmonella typhi* in medium supplemented with serum, serum fractions, or mixtures of serum fractions to be tested. The final concentration of serum or fractions was the equivalent of 10% normal serum. LPS was either added at the start or incubated with the serum/fractions 24 h prior to culture. Fractionation of serum was accomplished by KBr density gradient ultracentrifugation according to standard techniques. Sera used in the above-described procedures had tested negative for endotoxin in a combined interleukin 1 production and assay system (IPAS) as described elsewhere (Northoff et al. 1986). The supernatants were transferred to secondary plates 24 h later, titrated, and measured by use of the C3H/HeJ thymocyte costimulator assay. Serum fractions

Immune Consequences of
Trauma, Shock and Sepsis
Eds. Faist/Ninnemann/Green

tested were extensively dialysed prior to use. Interleukin 1 units were calculated by comparison with the international standard (NBS, Oxford) using a computer-based program (Biostat Vers. 1.1., Hochgeladen, Neu Ulm).

Results

First we determined whether exogenous endotoxin was still able to induce interleukin 1 release by human monocytes after interacting with normal human serum. When graded amounts of LPS were incubated with medium containing 10% serum prior to contact with monocytes, about 0.1–1 ng LPS/ml serum could be inhibited. When LPS was added at the start of culture, normal IL1 release was observed (Fig. 1 a). Here it should be mentioned that monocytes can respond to as little as 1 pg LPS/ml when this is added at the start of culture (Northoff et al. 1987). The LPS-neutralizing capacity of normal serum resides entirely in the lipoprotein fraction. This is demonstrated by the fact that removal of lipoproteins from serum by ultracentrifugation resulted in a total loss of its neutralizing capacity (Fig. 1 b). Readdition of the lipoprotein fraction restored the LPS-neutralizing capacity of lipoprotein-free serum (Fig. 1 c).

Lipopolysaccharide-neutralizing capacity could be shown for all of seven LPS species and one lipid A component tested (Table 1). We asked which subfraction of lipoproteins might neutralize the LPS. So far we have found that the effect is due to low (LDL) and high-density lipoproteins (HDL) (data not shown). None

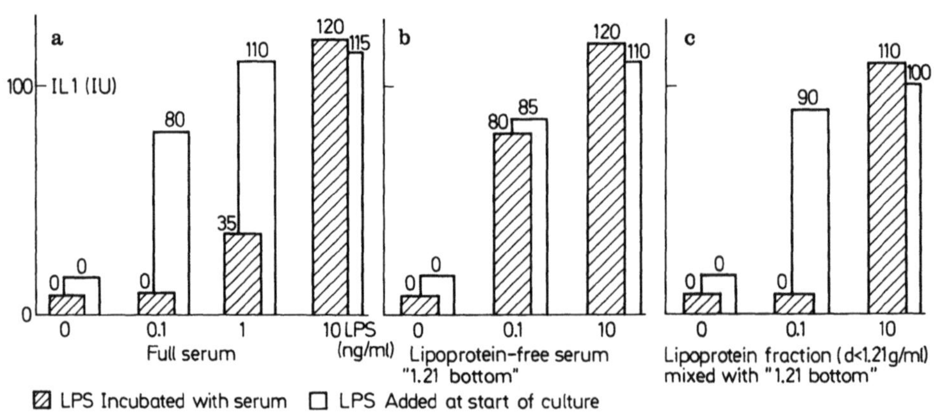

Fig. 1 a–c. Human monocytes were cultured for 24 h in the presence of 10% full serum or serum fractions and serial log 10 dilutions of LPS as indicated. This LPS was either added at the start of the monocyte culture (*open columns*) or incubated with the serum or serum fractions for 24 h at 37 °C before the start of the monocyte culture (*filled columns*). In a second step, the IL1 generated was biologically assayed with the C3H/HeJ thymocyte costimulator assay. **a** Full serum (10% concentration) inhibits 100 pg LPS/ml completely after 24 h incubation and 1 ng/ml partially. **b** Lipoprotein-free serum with a specific density $d > 1.21$ g/ml in ultracentrifugation ("1.21 bottom") exhibits no neutralizing of LPS. **c** Readdition of the lipoprotein fraction ($d > 1.21$ g/ml) into the "1.21 bottom" reconstituted the neutralizing effect, as shown for full serum

Table 1. Lipopolysaccharide-neutralizing capacity of serum from healthy donors as defined in the text could be shown for all seven LPS species and one lipid A component used

Lipopolysaccharide derived from	*E. coli* 0128:B12
	0127:B 8
	0111:B 4
	055:B 5
	026:B 6
	S. abortus equi
	S. typhi
Lipid A derived from	*S. minnesota* Re 595

of the other serum proteins of healthy donors showed the capacity to neutralize LPS in our system. We also determined that nutritive lipids have no discernible effect, since lipemic sera had no apparent enhanced capacity for neutralizing LPS. We have evidence that the neutralization of LPS by serum is not related to inactivation of complement. Finally we tested whether naturally occurring anti-LPS antibodies might play a role in our system. We compared 10 high-titer and 10 low-titer antisera (upper and lower 10% of 200 sera, tested by ELISA). They showed no significant difference in capacity to neutralize LPS in our system (data not shown).

Discussion

The importance of lipoproteins in binding, transporting, and serum kinetics of LPS is well established (Freudenberg et al. 1982; Munford et al. 1981). So far the effect of LPS-lipoprotein interaction on endotoxin-induced mediator release has not been thoroughly investigated. Here we show that interaction of LPS with lipoproteins from human serum leads to an inactivation of limited amounts of endotoxin. This endotoxin was not only neutralized by HDL but by LDL to at least the same extent, which is depicted schematically in Fig. 2.

Other serum components of normal human serum including naturally occurring anti-LPS antibodies, complement, and nutritive lipids had no significant in-

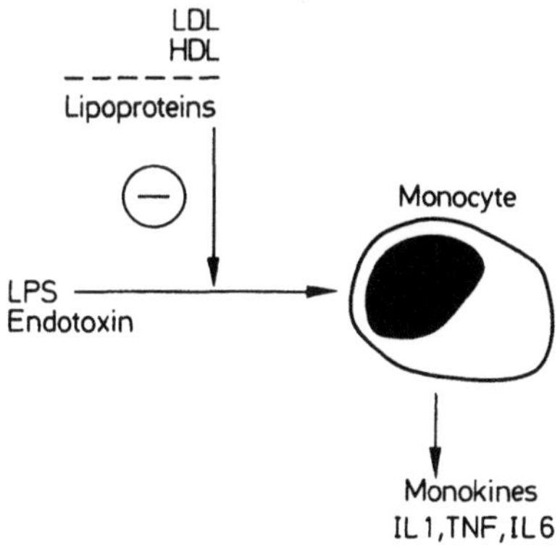

Fig. 2. Lipopolysaccharide-neutralizing capacity is due to the lipoproteins. Both LDL and HDL can inhibit the endotoxin-induced monokine release, which is relevant for mediating the toxicity of lipopolysaccharide/endotoxin

fluence on neutralization of LPS. The observation that lipoprotein-free serum has no LPS-neutralizing capacity at all provides a means of testing various manipulations designed to reduce LPS toxicity.

It has been shown (Ulevitch et al. 1979) that large amounts of LPS can be bound by lipoproteins, especially HDL. Compared with this figure, which is in the microgram range, the amount of LPS which can be neutralized in our system seems relatively small. We therefore conclude that binding cannot necessarily mean detoxification. On the other hand, neutralization of 1–10 ng LPS/ml full serum may be quite significant, given the fact that monocytes can respond to picogram amounts of LPS. LPS concentrations in endotoxemia are described in the range of nanograms/ml (Fink et al. 1981). The fact that HDL and LDL can both neutralize LPS is striking and unexpected based on the data reported for LPS binding. It may be, however, a significant finding since changes in levels and composition of lipoproteins during acute-phase response have been described and may contribute to an enhanced detoxification of LPS in man.

References

Fink PC, Lehr L, Urbaschek RM, Kozak J (1981) Limulus amebocyte lysate test for endotoxemia. Klin Wochenschr 59:213–218

Freudenberg MA, Bøg-Hansen TC, Back U, Galanos C (1980) Interaction of lipopolysaccharides with plasma high-density lipoprotein in rats. Infect Immun 28:373–380

Freudenberg MA, Freudenberg N, Galanos C (1982) Time course of cellular distribution of endotoxin in liver, lungs and kidneys of rats. Br J Exp Pathol 63:56–65

Freudenberg MA, Keppler D, Galanos C (1986) Requirement for lipopolysaccharide-responsive macrophages in galactosamine-induced sensitization to endotoxin. Infect Immun 51:891

Lehmann V, Freudenberg MA, Galanos C (1987) Lethal toxicity of lipopolysaccharide and tumor necrosis factor in normal and *d*-galactosamine-treated mice. J Exp Med 165:657–663

Munford RS, Andersen JM, Dietschy JM (1981) Sites of tissue binding and uptake in vivo of bacterial lipopolysaccharide-high density lipoprotein complexes. J Clin Invest 68:1503–1513

Northoff H, Kabelitz D, Galanos C (1986) Interleukin 1 production for detection of bacterial polysaccharide in fetal calf sera and other solutions. Immunol Today 7:126–127

Northoff H, Glück D, Wölpl A, Kubanek B, Galanos C (1987) Lipopolysaccharide-induced elaboration of interleukin 1 by human monocytes: use for detection of lipopolysaccharide in serum and the influence of serum-lipopolysaccharide interactions. Rev Infect Dis 9:S599–S601

Obayashi T (1984) Addition of perchloric acid to blood samples for colorimetric limulus test using chromogenic substrate: comparison with conventional procedures and clinical applications. J Lab Clin Med 104:321–330

Ulevitch RJ, Johnston AR, Weinstein DB (1979) New function for high density lipoproteins. J Clin Invest 64:1516–1524

Role of Corticosteroids in the Pathogenesis of Post-traumatic Thymic Involution

M. Čolić and A. Dujić

Introduction

Thymic involution is a constant finding during the general response of the organism to various kinds of trauma (Selye 1936). It has previously been shown that thymic involution in mice subjected to mechanical injury (Čolić and Dujić 1983) or thermal injury (Čolić and Dujić 1984) is a consequence of massive thymocyte pyknosis and destruction, mainly in the cortical zone of the thymus. Similar findings were demonstrated after exogenous administration of glucocorticoids (Cowan and Sörenson 1964), indicating that these hormones could be one of the main etiopathogenetic factors involved in post-traumatic thymic involution. Following this hypothesis we studied thymic changes in bilaterally adrenalectomized mice subjected to experimental thermal injury (TI).

Materials and Methods

Experiments were done on male BALB/c mice, 6–7 weeks old, bred at the Military Medical Academy Farm for Experimental Animals, Belgrade. Sublethal TI (scalding of the back, 15% body surface area in 80 °C hot water bath, 5 s) was performed as described by Arthurson (1964), on bilaterally adrenalectomized mice (A-T) under short ether anesthesia, 10 days after the operation. The control group consisted of sham-operated and then scalded animals (SO-T). A group of either adrenalectomized (A-C) or sham-operated mice (SO-C) received corticosterone (25 mg/kg, i.p.).

Mice were killed 1 and 2 days after TI or corticosterone administration. The following parameters were measured: (1) thymic mass and cellularity; (2) relative and absolute numbers of thymocyte subpopulations determined by anti-Thy1.2, anti-Ly2.2 (CD8) and anti-L3T4 (CD4) monoclonal antibodies (kindly donated by M. Lukić, Medical Faculty, Belgrade), and species-specific secondary antibodies conjugated with FITC (Amersham International) using a flow cytometer (EPICS C, Coulter); (3) proliferation of thymocytes in vivo determined by [^{3}H]thymidine uptake, 1 h after i.v. administration (60 μCi/kg) and expressed as proliferative index (cpm radioactivity/10^6 thymocytes); and (4) plasma concentrations of corticosterone using a radioimmunoassay for cortisol (Biodata).

Immune Consequences of
Trauma, Shock and Sepsis
Eds. Faist/Ninnemann/Green

Results

In SO-T mice acute thymic involution occurred in the first 2 days, followed by a decrease in thymic mass (Fig. 1) and cellularity (not shown). Similar changes were seen in both SO-C and A-C mice. In contrast, TI did not affect thymic mass and cellularity in adrenalectomized mice. These results are in correlation with plasma corticosterone concentrations (Fig. 2). In SO-T mice values of corticosterone in plasma were increased up to 6 h followed by a normalization at 24 h after TI. No changes in corticosterone concentrations in A-T mice from basal levels were seen.

Results presented in Fig. 3 show that TI or corticosterone treatment caused similar changes of thymocyte subpopulations in mice with intact adrenal glands (SO-T and SO-C mice). In both groups of animals the percentage of Thy1.2$^+$ cells was unimpaired, although an enrichment of Thy1.2^{low+} cells (see histograms of fluorescence) and a decrease of absolute numbers of Thy1.2$^+$ cells were seen. In addition, a decrease of relative and absolute numbers of CD4$^+$ as well as CD8$^+$ thymocytes occurred. The changes were more pronounced in CD8$^+$ cell subsets.

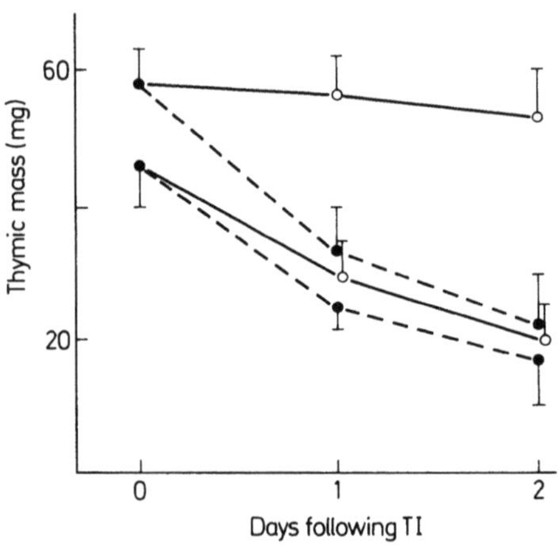

Fig. 1. Thymic mass in mice subjected to TI or corticosterone treatment. Values are given as $\bar{X} \pm SD$ for five to six mice in a group. ·— (A-T); ·--- (A-C); ○— (SO-T); ○--- (SO-C). All differences, except A-T, are significant ($P < 0.005$) compared with values of corresponding A or SO mice

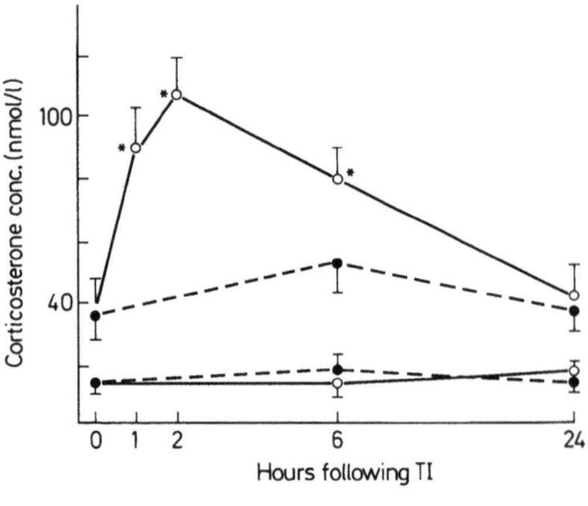

Fig. 2. Plasma corticosterone concentrations in mice subjected to TI. Values are given as $\bar{X} \pm SD$ for six animals in a group. ·--- (SO); ·— (SO-T); ○--- (A); ○— (A-T); *$P < 0.005$ compared with values in SO mice

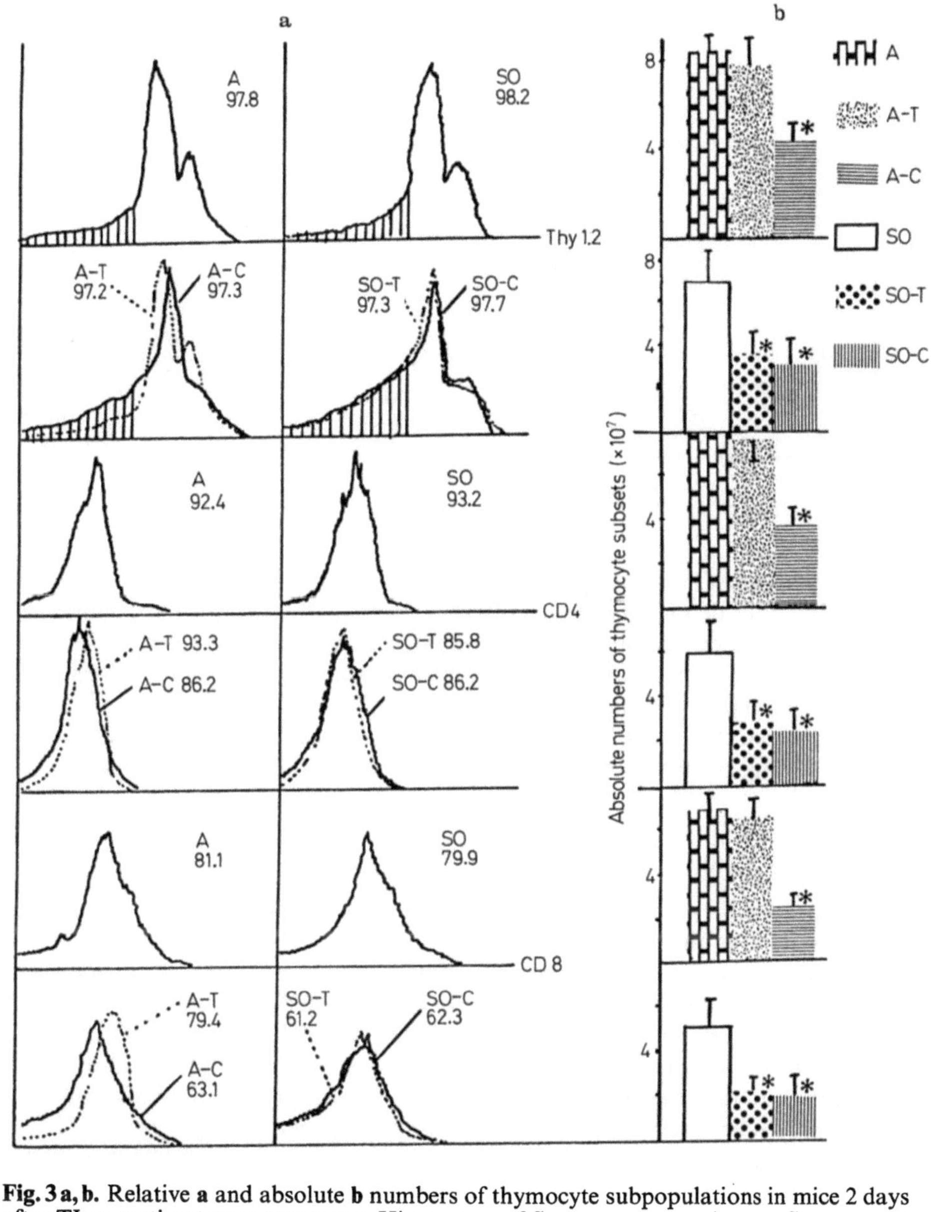

Fig. 3 a, b. Relative **a** and absolute **b** numbers of thymocyte subpopulations in mice 2 days after TI or corticosterone treatment. Histograms of fluorescence are given as fluorescence intensity (au) (x-axis) and numbers of thymocytes (5000) (y-axis). The percentages of thymocyte subsets show representative values from three pooled thymuses in each group. Absolute numbers of thymocyte subsets are given as $\bar{X} \pm SD$ for five to six animals in a group. $^{*}P<0.001$ compared with values in corresponding nontraumatized (nontreated) mice. *Dashed areas on histograms* represent Thyl.2^{low+} cells

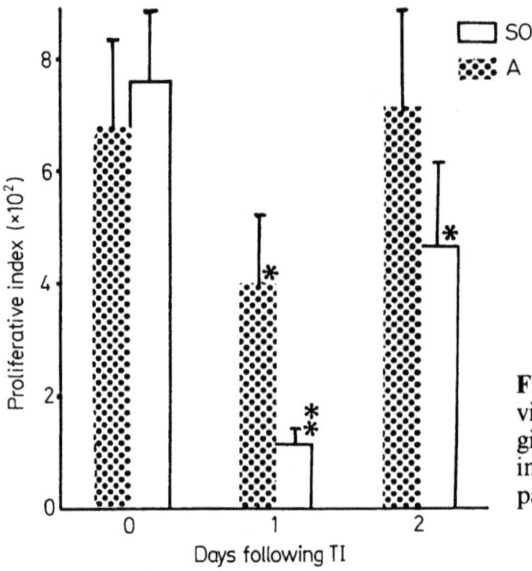

Fig. 4. Proliferative index of thymocytes in vivo in mice subjected to TI. Values are given as $\bar{X} \pm SD$ for five to seven animals in a group. $*P<0.005$; $**P<0.001$ compared with values in nontraumatized mice

Figure 3 also shows that no significant differences in any of the thymocyte subpopulations and their histograms of fluorescence were seen in A-T mice compared with values in adrenalectomized-nontraumatized (A) animals. In contrast, corticosterone treatment in the A-C group of mice produced similar thymocyte subset changes as in mice with intact adrenal glands.

TI decreased thymocyte proliferation in vivo, 24 h after injury in adrenalectomized mice (Fig. 4). However, suppression was much higher in SO-T mice.

Discussion

In this work we present evidence of the dominant role of corticosteroids in postburn thymic involution. It is concluded from the findings that sublethal TI increases plasma corticosterone levels and causes similar effects to those seen after administration of corticosterone (25 mg/kg), manifested as a decrease of thymic mass, cellularity, number of thymocytes in different subsets, and their proliferation in vivo. In contrast, bilateral adrenalectomy prevents all these alterations following TI except the suppression of thymocyte proliferation, indicating that corticosteroids are probably not the only etiopathogenetic factor involved.

It is difficult to define additional factors acting independently or synergistically with corticosteroids. Of all the adrenal hormones, glucocorticoids possess the most potent immunosuppressive properties (Claman 1972). In the thymus they cause apoptosis and destruction of immature, cortical thymocytes, which are rapidly cycling cells (Cohen and Duke 1984). It could be hypothesized that lower thymocyte proliferation in A-T mice is a consequence of either reduction in numbers of these cells or a decrease in their proliferation rates.

A possible additional factor could be the catecholamines. It is known that these hormones possess immunosuppressive activities, their secretion is increased following thermal injury (Vujnov et al. 1982), and they are partly removed by adrenalectomy. In our previous studies (Čolić 1987) we administrated labelatol (alpha- and beta-adrenergic blocker) (10 mg/kg) to mice 30 min before scalding but we did not confirm their effect.

Many immunosuppressive factors have been isolated from sera of burned patients such as endotoxin, burn toxin, prostaglandins, and gamma-interferon (Ninnemann et al. 1982), but their actions on the thymus are not sufficiently known. Endotoxin has been shown to cause thymic involution but it probably acts through glucocorticoids (Gad and Clark 1968). One of the candidates for the suppression of thymocyte proliferation could be the prostaglandins. It is known that burn trauma is followed by an increase in their levels partly as a consequence of interleukin 1 (IL-1) stimulation (Ninnemann et al. 1982). Immunoregulatory feedback between IL-1 and glucocorticoids (Besedovsky et al. 1986) is probably altered in adrenalectomized mice. The absence of inhibitory effects of glucocorticoids in these animals on IL-1 and prostaglandin production and synthesis could result in suppression of thymocyte proliferation. However, these explanations are hypothetical and need further investigation.

Summary

The hypothesis implicating corticosteroids as the main etiopathogenetic factor in post-traumatic thymic involution was studied in adrenalectomized mice subjected to sublethal thermal injury (TI) or corticosterone treatment. The following findings confirm this hypothesis: (1) adrenalectomy prevented thymic involution after TI as judged by thymic mass, cellularity, and number of thymocytes in different subsets; (2) TI caused an increase of plasma corticosterone concentrations in mice with intact adrenal glands; (3) exogenous administration of corticosterone to both adrenalectomized or sham-operated mice caused similar thymic changes to thermal injury in animals with intact adrenal glands. As adrenalectomy did not totally prevent a decrease of thymocyte proliferation in vivo following TI, this suggests that corticosteroids are probably not the only etiopathogenetic factor involved in the pathogenesis of postburn thymic involution.

References

Arturson G (1964) The infliction and healing of large standard burn in rats. Acta Pathol Microbiol Immunol Scand 61:353–364

Besedovsky H, del Rey A, Sorkin E, Dinarello AC (1986) Immunoregulatory feedback between interleukin 1 and glucocorticoid hormones. Science 233:652–654

Claman HN (1972) Corticosteroids and lymphoid cells. N Engl J Med 287:388–397

Cohen JJ, Duke RC (1984) Glucocorticoid activation of a calcium-dependent endonuclease in thymocyte nuclei leads to cell death. J Immunol 132:38–42

Cowan WK, Sorenson DG (1964) Electron microscopic observations of acute thymic involution produced by hydrocortisone. Lab Invest 13:353–370

Čolić M, Dujić A (1983) Ultrastructural alterations of the thymus in mice subjected to mechanical trauma. Period Biol 85 [Suppl 3]:47–50

Čolić M, Dujić A (1984) Uticaj traume, egzogenog hidrodortizona i adrenalektomije na histološku gradju timusa miša. Vojnosanit Pregl 41:356–363

Čolić M (1987) Morphological and functional characteristics of thymic cells in mice subjected to combined radiation injury. Doctoral thesis, University of Belgrade

Gad P, Clark SL (1968) Involution and regeneration of the thymus in mice induced by bacterial endotoxin and studied by quantitative histology and electron microscopy. Am J Anat 122:573–606

Ninnemann JL, Condie JT, Stanley E, Davis BA, Crockett RA (1982) Isolation of immunosuppressive serum components following thermal injury. J Trauma 22:837–844

Selye H (1936) Thymus and adrenals in the response of the organism to injuries and intoxications. Br J Pathol 17:234–248

Vujnov S, Savić J, Pantelić D (1982) Functional changes in the sympatho-adrenal system in rats submitted to non-lethal thermal injury. Yugosl Physiol Pharmacol Acta 18(2):163–169

Section 5

Immunology of the Skin and Wound Healing

Immunology of Skin

T. S. Kupper

Human skin is a complex organ composed of a stratified squamous epithelium (the epidermis), containing bone-marrow-derived and neural crest symbionts, which overlies a richly vascular matrix of connective tissue (dermis) and subcutaneous fat. The role of skin (and particularly the epidermis) in host defense has long been considered a passive one, and the production of keratins and lipids by the epidermal keratinocyte and of collagen and elastin by the dermal fibroblast were considered to be the most important functions of this organ.

The appreciation that Langerhans cells (once thought to represent otiose melanocytes) were intimately involved with the processing of antigen and its presentation to T cells in an immunogenic form led to a modification of the role of the skin in host defense [1]. Subsequently, it was found that keratinocytes could produce cytokines with immunologic and proinflammatory activities, and that keratinocyte cytokine gene expression was linked to injurious stimuli to the epidermis [2]. Most recently, the appreciation that a novel class of dendritic T-lymphocytes resides within (and may differentiate in) epidermis has led to the perception that the epidermis is an integrated and immunologically important tissue [3]. Such a role is well suited to a tissue which provides the primary interface between host and environment. The following treatise will emphasize the role of the epidermis in host defense.

Langerhans cells are bone-marrow-derived dendritic cells which first appear in epidermis at roughly 10 weeks gestational age. Such cells have been presumed to belong to the monocyte/macrophage family, and have been defined (primarily in a murine system) by their constitutive expression of class II MHC antigens, Fc receptors, and C3b receptors and their high level of ATPase. In man, the definition of a Langerhans cell has remained ultrastructural, and the presence of Birbeck granules in the cytoplasm of cells is considered a sufficient criterion for their identification. More recently, CD1a (previously T6) has been used as a marker for Langerhans cells. Murine Langerhans cells, when cultured in the presence of keratinocytes or another source of exogenous granulocyte macrophage colony-stimulating factor, are capable of presenting antigen to T-lymphocytes in a highly efficient fashion. This has been attributed to their high level of class II expression and their capacity to process antigen. It is presumed that Langerhans cells produce IL-1 and thus can provide the "second signal" required for T-cell activation, but formal proof of this is still lacking.

Keratinocytes comprise the principal cellular mass of the epidermis. These cells produce IL-1 alpha and beta in vitro, and it appears that under normal conditions biologically significant amounts of IL-1 reside within viable as well as ter-

Immune Consequences of
Trauma, Shock and Sepsis
Eds. Faist/Ninnemann/Green

minally differented keratinocytes in the epidermis [4]. The contiguity of the dendrites of Langerhans cells with keratinocytes, coupled with the observation that keratinocytes contain IL-1 in a membrane-associated compartment, has led to the concept of the Langerhans cell/keratinocyte antigen-presenting unit [3].

Keratinocytes, like many other cells, bear high-affinity receptors for IL-1 alpha and beta [5]. The expression of these receptors appears to be tightly regulated; confluent cultures of keratinocytes bear few IL-1 receptors, while activated keratinocytes bear tens of thousands of IL-1 receptors. Expression of keratinocyte IL-1 receptors parallels responsiveness of keratinocytes to exogenous IL-1. IL-1 stimulation of receptive keratinocytes induces gene expression of multiple cytokines, including GM-CSF, IL-6, G-CSF, M-CSF, and chemotactic factors for granulocytes, monocytes, and T cells [3]. In addition, proliferation and type IV collagen production are also induced, enabling keratinocytes to recreate in intact epithelium and basement membrane during the reepithelialization phase of wound healing [3].

Since normal epidermis contains significant quantities of preformed IL-1, it might be anticipated that trauma or injury would lead to release of this IL-1 within the epidermis and dermis [6]. This event provides a signal to the host that injury has occurred. Wound healing is preceded by a brisk inflammatory response which may be mediated by keratinocyte cytokines and designed to "sterilize" the cutaneous defect by activating local bactericidal defenses. To a large extent, the release of preformed IL-1 by injury allows this process to ensue. The consequences of IL-1 release in the epidermis include the release of factors from epidermal keratinocytes and dermal fibroblasts which attract and activate granulocytes (MNCF, GM-CSF, G-CSF, and TNF alpha), T cells (ELCF, GM-CSF, IL-6), monocytes (TGF beta, GM-CSF, M-CSF), and B cells (IL-6). Furthermore, the enhancement of Langerhans cell antigen-presenting function by GM-CSF [7], as well as the T-cell stimulatory factor activity provided by IL-6 [8], places the IL-1-activated keratinocyte at the center of this process. The role of cytokines in the reparative response of wound healing is less well understood.

Recently, a novel population of dendritic T cells was identified in murine epidermis. These cells are CD3+, but bear neither CD4 nor CD8 and express a T-cell receptor composed of a gamma/delta heterodimer [9]. Congenitally athymic (nude) mice have dendritic Thy-1+ cells in their epidermis, while T-cell-deficient SCID mice (which possess a recombinase deficiency resulting in absence of mature T cells) do not. These observations have led to the suggestion that these dendritic T cells mature and differentiate in the epidermal microenvironment, which may resemble that of the thymus. Such cells can be activated in vitro to proliferate and produce lymphokines, including IL-2, IL-3, IL-4, GM-CSF, and gamma-interferon. Though the biological role of such cells in vivo remains obscure, release of lymphokines by activated dendritic T cells will have profound effects on keratinocyte and Langerhans cells in situ.

We and others have been able to identify a population of CD2+ CD3+ dendritic T cells in human epidermis, some of which appear to bear gamma/delta heterodimers. Such observations have led to difficulties with nomenclature. While in the murine system, Langerhans cells are defined both functionally (antigen presentation to T cells) and morphologically, and human Langerhans cells are defined morphologically based upon Birbeck granules and CD1 expression (see above). Since we are able to see T-cell markers on a subpopulation of Birbeck granule-positive and CD1-positive cells, it is likely that what we now call Langerhans cells are actually a heterogeneous population composed of dendritic T cells and dendritic cells of the monocyte lineage ("true" Langerhans cells).

While the role of such dendritic T cells is unknown, their presence in other tissues which form an interface with the environment (gut, bronchial epithelium, eye, and placenta) suggests a primary role in host defense. It is likely that the function of such cells can be modified by the products of both epithelial cells and Langerhans cells, and that lymphokines produced by such cells upon activation have reciprocal activities. Studies are underway to dissect the activation requirements and the antigenic specificity of such cells.

Far from being a passive organ with regard to immunity, the skin (and particularly the epidermis) contains multiple immunologically active cells which interact in a complex fashion, resulting in a formidable first line of defense against pathogens. The loss of large areas of skin (as in burn injury) is thus a primary immune insult, and the immunocompromised state of such patients may reflect the absence of this important immunological organ.

References

1. Katz SI, Tamaki K, Sachs DH (1979) Epidermal Langerhans cells are derived from cells originating in bone marrow. Nature 282:324
2. Kupper TS (1988) Interleukin 1 and other keratinocyte cytokines: functional and molecular characterization. Adv Dermatol 3:293
3. Kupper TS (1988) The role of epidermal cytokines. In: Shevach E, Oppenheim J (eds) The immunophysiology of cells and cytokines. Oxford University Press
4. Kupper TS, Ballard D, Chua AO et al. (1986) Human keratinocytes contain mRNA indistinguishable from monocyte interleukin 1 mRNA. J Exp Med 164:2095
5. Kupper TS, Dower S, Birchall N, Clark S, Lee F Interleukin 1 binds to specific receptors on human keratinocytes and induces granulocyte macrophage colony stimulating factor mRNA and protein: a potential autocrine role for IL-1 in epidermis (submitted for publication)
6. Kupper TS, Chua AO, Flood P, McGuire J, Gubler U (1987) Interleukin 1 gene expression in cultured human keratinocytes is augmented by ultraviolet irradiation. J Clin Invest 80:430
7. Witmer-Pack M, Oliveier W, Valinsky J, Schuler G, Steinman R (1987) Granulocyte/macrophage colony-stimulating factor is essential for the viability and function of cultured murine epidermal Langerhans cells. J Exp Med 166:1484
8. Kupper TS, Mizutani H, Birchall N, May L, Sehgal P (1989) Beta 2 interferon/BSF-2/interleukin 6 synergizes with interleukin 1 in the induction of T cell proliferation. (submitted for publication)
9. Stingl G, Koning F, Yamada H et al. (1987) Thy-1+ dendritic epidermal cells express T3 antigen and the T cell receptor gamma chain. Proc Natl Acad Sci USA 84:4586

Immune Regulation of Wound Healing

A. Barbul

Introduction

Wound healing is a complex cascade of biochemical, cellular, and biological events which interact to achieve restoration of tissue integrity following injury (Fig. 1). A lot has been learned about the individual events that comprise this cascade, but still we know little about their interweaving, spatially or temporally, and how one biological event sets the stage for subsequent observed phenomena.

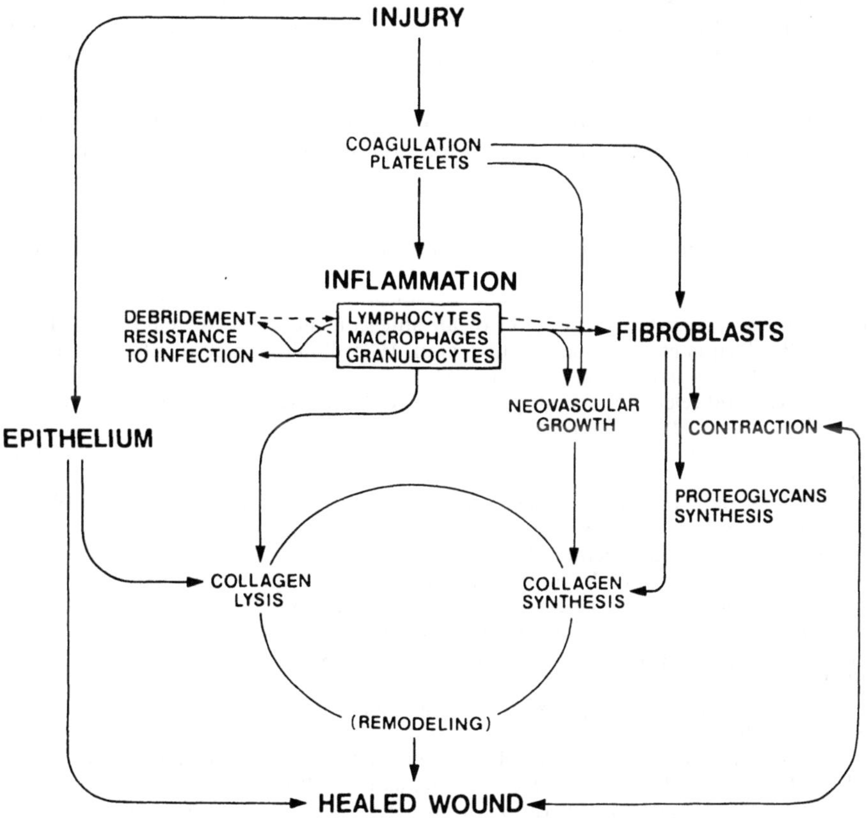

Fig. 1. Schematic representation of key events in wound healing (By permission from Dr. T.K. Hunt)

Immune Consequences of
Trauma, Shock and Sepsis
Eds. Faist/Ninnemann/Green

During the past few years it has become evident that the cellular immune system plays a major role in the successful completion of various phases of wound healing. Although we have much to learn about the interaction of the immune system with the healing wound, the explosion of knowledge in the field of growth factors and, more specifically to this topic, of monokines and lymphokines, has generated new knowledge which greatly increases our understanding of the wound healing phenomenon. Since there is little evidence that B lymphocytes play a role in fibroplasia, in this exposition we will restrict our definition of the cellular immune system to macrophages and T lymphocytes, as both have been demonstrated to greatly influence wound healing.

Macrophages and Wound Healing

Macrophages appear in wounds within 48–96 h postwounding. Their first role is to participate in the inflammatory and debridement phase that has to take place prior to the fibroblastic phase. Macrophages then become the predominant cell prior to fibroblast migration and replication. It is during these phases of wound healing that macrophages play a major role in the events leading to successful wound repair.

The crucial role of macrophages in wound healing was first demonstrated in vivo. Leibovich and Ross (1975) showed that guinea pigs treated with antimacro-

Table 1. Effects of monokines on cultured endothelial cells. (Adapted and updated from Harlan 1987)

Induce synthesis and surface expression of an adhesion molecule for leukocytes (IL-1, TNF-α) (Bevilacqua et al. 1986a; Gamble et al. 1985; Pohlmann et al. 1986; Schleimer and Rutlege 1986; Cavender et al. 1986, 1987)
Induce synthesis and release of hematopoietic growth factors (IL-1, TNF-α) (Broudy et al. 1986; Munker et al. 1986; Bagby et al. 1986)
Induce synthesis and release of endogenous IL-1 (TNF-α) (Nawroth et al. 1986; Libby et al. 1986)
Induce synthesis and expression of class I MHC antigens (TNF-α) (Collins et al. 1986)
Induce synthesis and surface expression of a neoantigen (IL-1, TNF-α) (Pober et al. 1986)
Stimulate chemotaxis (Leibovich et al. 1987)
Inhibit proliferation (IL-1, TNF-α) (Norioka et al. 1987; Stolpen et al. 1986)
Induce synthesis of platelet-activating factor and prostacyclin (IL-1, TNF-α) (Bussolino et al. 1986; Rossi et al. 1984; Kawakami et al. 1986)
Induce release of platelet-derived growth factor (IL-1, TNF-α) (Libby et al. 1985; Hajjar et al. 1987)
Induce synthesis and surface expression of tissue factor (IL-1, TNF-α) (Bevilaqua et al. 1984; Nawroth and Stern 1986a)
Induce synthesis and release of tissue plasminogen activator-inhibitor (IL-1) (Nachman et al. 1986; Emeis and Kooistra 1986; Bevilacqua et al. 1986b)
Suppress cell surface-dependent activation of protein C (IL-1, TNF-α)(Nawroth and Stern 1986; Nawroth et al. 1986b)
Reorganize endothelial cytoskeleton (IL-1, TNF-α) (Stolpen et al. 1986; Montesano et al. 1985)
Increase superoxide release (IL-1) (Matsubara and Ziff 1986)

phage serum plus steroids (to remove circulating monocytes) had impaired wound debridement and fibroplasia. Subsequently, injection of wound macrophages into rabbit corneas was shown to induce angiogenesis and scar formation (Clark et al. 1976), while intradermal injections increased collagen synthesis and breaking strength in 8-day rat skin wounds (Casey et al. 1976).

The major monokines released by activated macrophages are interleukin-1 (IL-1) and tumor necrosis factor-α/cachectin (TNF-α). These monokines have been shown to have a variety of biological effects on endothelial cells in vitro (Table 1) and thus affect two of the earliest phases of wound healing, i.e., inflammation and angiogenesis. Recently, TNF-α has been confirmed to be the angiogenic principle secreted by wound macrophages (Frater-Schroeder et al. 1987; Leibovich et al. 1987), even though it has been shown to be cytostatic for endothelial cells in vitro (Stolpen et al. 1986). This points out some of the difficulties in translating in vitro data to the in vivo situation. Nevertheless, the in vitro activities of IL1 and TNF-α on endothelial cells are so diverse that it seems highly likely that they play a role in wound healing in vivo.

Macrophage secretory products have also been shown to influence in vitro fibroblast chemotaxis, proliferation, and collagen synthesis (Table 2). Most of

Table 2. Monokines which regulate fibroblast growth and function. (Adapted and updated from Wahl 1985)

Fibroblast function	Monokine (M_r)	Ref.
Chemotaxis		
Stimulation	Fibronectin	Tsukamoto et al. (1982)
	MDCF-F mu (<10000)	Diegelmann et al. (1986)
Proliferation		
Stimulation	IL-1 hu (10–15000)	Schmidt et al. (1982)
	AMDGF hu (18000)	Bitterman et al. (1982)
	MDGF mu (56000)	Estes et al. (1984)
	mu (≧100000)	Martin et al. (1981)
	mu (46–57000)	Wyler et al. (1984)
		Wyler et al. (1984)
	FAF gp (40–60000)	Wahl et al. (1979)
	PDGF	Shimokado et al. (1985)
Inhibition	IFN-β	Kohase et al. (1986)
Collagen synthesis		
Stimulation	–[a]	Wahl et al. (1979)
	IL-1 hu	Kahari et al. (1987)
	TNF-α	Amento and Granstein (1987)
Inhibition	–[a]	Jimenez et al. (1979)
	IL-1 hu	Bhatnager et al. (1986)
Collagenase and PGE_2 synthesis	IL-1	Mizel et al. (1980)
	TNF-α	Dayer et al. (1985)

[a] Not characterized.

AMDGF, alveolar macrophage-derived growth factor; MDGF, macrophage-derived growth factor; FAF, fibroblast-activating factor; IL-1, interleukin-1; hu, human; mu, murine; gp, guinea pig.

these monokines have not been fully characterized or sequenced, although recent evidence suggests that macrophage-derived growth factor may be a PGDF-like molecule (Shimokado et al. 1985). Furthermore, antagonistic effects have been ascribed to the same molecule as in the case of IL-1, which has been shown to both stimulate and inhibit collagen synthesis in fibroblast cultures. The conditions under which one or the other effect may predominate have not been characterized.

So far no monokine has been shown to influence wound healing in vivo. However, such data are sure to become available soon, given the diversity of in vitro effects of these various monokines.

Lymphocytes and Wound Healing

Not so long ago it was commonly stated that lymphocytes do not participate in wound healing. This has been totally reversed by recent in vitro and in vivo evidence demonstrating that lymphocytes are major modulators of cells involved in wound healing and fibroplasia.

T lymphocytes migrate into wounds following the influx of inflammatory cells and macrophages. The ratio of T-helper to T-suppressor lymphocytes at the wound site is less than one, much decreased in comparison to peripheral blood and lymph node subpopulation ratios (Fishel et al. 1987). Lymphokines, products of activated lymphocytes, have varied effects on vascular endothelial cells (Table 3). The best characterized lymphokine, inferferon-γ (IFN-γ), has mainly an immune modulatory effect on endothelial cells, affecting major histocompatibility antigen expression of both class I and II type. Transforming growth factor β (TGF-β) has in vivo angiogenic properties (Roberts et al. 1986). However, TGF-β as well as IFN-γ inhibit in vitro endothelial-cell proliferation. This is simi-

Table 3. Effects of lymphokines on cultured endothelial cells. (Adapted and updated from Harlan 1986)

Interferon-γ
Increases class I and induces class II MHC antigen expression (Pober et al. 1983; Collins et al. 1984)
Confers antigen-presenting capability on EC (Geppert and Lipsky 1985)
Induces neoantigen expression (Duijvestijn 1986)
Increases adhesivity for lymphocytes (Yu et al. 1985; Masuyama et al. 1986)
Reorganizes cytoskeleton (Stolpen et al. 1986)
Increases superoxide anion release (Matsubara and Ziff 1986)
Inhibits proliferation (Stolpen et al. 1986)
Transforming growth factor-β
Inhibits proliferation (Baird and Durkin 1986; Frater-Schroder et al. 1986; Heimark et al. 1986)
Lymphokine-containing supernatants
Enhances plasminogen activator synthesis (Tiku and Tomasi 1985)
Enhances proliferation and motility (Watt and Auerbach 1986; Groenewegen et al. 1985)
Inhibit migration (Cohen et al. 1982)

lar to the action of TNF-α, which is also angiogenic in vivo but inhibits proliferation in vitro, suggesting that angiogenic stimulation may somehow require a concomitant growth inhibitory signal.

A variety of lymphokines have been shown to both inhibit and stimulate fibroblast recruitment at the healing site (Table 4). TGF-β is a potent fibroblast chemotactic molecule (Postlethwaite et al. 1987). In addition, TGF-β induces monocyte chemotaxis and secretion of fibroblast growth factors, including IL-1 (Wahl et al. 1987). TGF-β, which is also secreted by platelets and monocytes, is present in large quantities at the wound site (Cromack et al. 1987) and, as stated above, can modulate fibroblast activity directly or via its effect on monocyte function and growth-factor secretion.

Following recruitment, lymphokines can lead to an increase in the number of fibroblasts present by inducing proliferation. Fibroblast activating factor (FAF), which stimulates fibroblast proliferation, has been described in humans and in guinea pigs and is a product of activated T lymphocytes. On the other hand, IFN-γ is a potent inhibitor of fibroblast proliferation. Once fibroblasts have been recruited and have increased in number, their synthesis of collagenous protein can be stimulated by lymphokines, such as TGF-β and lymphotoxin (LT). Lymphokines that inhibit collagen synthesis have also been described, most notably IFN-γ, which blocks constitutive as well as growth-factor-induced collagen syn-

Table 4. Lymphokines which regulate in vitro fibroblast growth and function. (Adapted and updated from Wahl 1985)

Fibroblast function	Lymphokine (M_r)	Ref.
Migration		
Stimulation	TGF-β	Postlethwaite et al. (1987)
Inhibition	FIF (28–34000)	Rola-Pleszczynski et al. (1982)
Proliferation		
Stimulation	FAF gp (40000)	Wahl et al. (1978)
	gp (50000)	Neilson et al. (1982)
	hu (40000)	Wahl and Gately (1983)
	gp (10–15000)	Neilson et al. (1982)
	IFM-γ	Brinckerhoff and Guyre (1985)
	LT	Hofsli et al. (1987)
Inhibition	IF	Neilson et al. (1982)
	IFN-γ	Duncan and Berman (1985)
Collagen synthesis		
Stimulation	CPF (100–170000)	Postlethwaite et al. (1984)
	TGF-β hu	Roberts et al. (1985)
	FAF	Agelli et al. (1987)
	LT	Amento and Gramstein (1987)
Inhibition	– (55000)	Postlethwaite et al. (1984)
	IFN α and γ	Jimenez et al. (1984)

FIF, fibroblast migration inhibitory factor; FAF, fibroblasts-activating factor; CPF, collagen production factor; IF, inhibitor of fibroblast proliferation; IFN, interferon; LT, lymphotoxin; TGF, transforming growth factor; gp, guinea pig; hu, human.

thesis. It is evident that lymphokines can exert both stimulatory and inhibitory signals on all aspects of fibroblast activity and there seems to be a well-defined balance between these effects. Our knowledge is scant regarding how this balance is achieved; however, it is clear that an imbalance could result in wound failure or conversely in excessive fibrosis. This has been elegantly demonstrated by Wahl (1985) who showed that continued presence of an antigenic stimulus at the healing site leads to excessive fibrosis, presumably because of continued activation of T lymphocytes with unchecked production of fibroblast activating factors (FAF).

The only lymphokines used in vivo so far have been TGF-β and IFN-γ. Subcutaneous injection of 800 ng of TGF-β into newborn mice resulted in increased formation of granulation tissue (Roberts et al. 1986), while application to linear incisions in rats led to increased wound-breaking strength and collagen deposition with a concomitant increase in mononuclear cell and fibroblast infiltration (Mustoe et al. 1987). On the other hand, implantation of subcutaneous osmotic pumps containing IFN-γ into mice resulted in decreased thickness and collagen content of the fibrous capsule that forms around the pumps (Granstein et al. 1987).

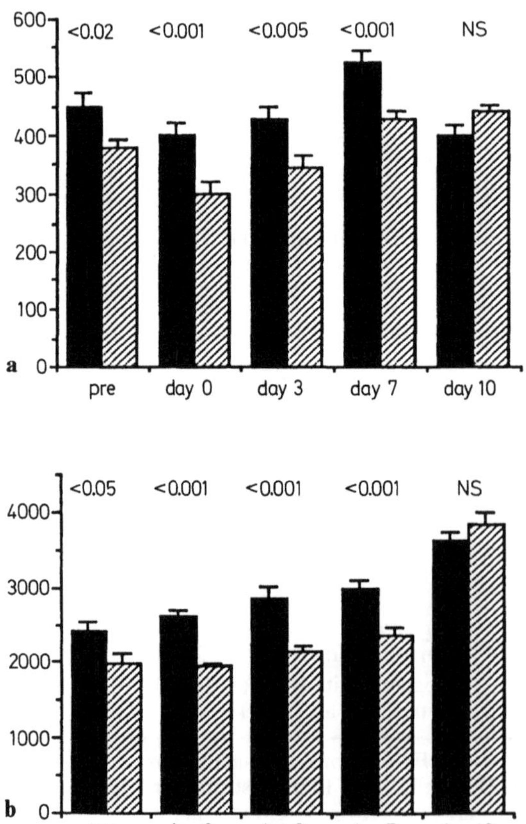

Fig. 2 a, b. Effect of T-lymphocyte depletion on wound healing. **a** Wound-breaking strength (g ± SEM); **b** hydroxyproline content of subcutaneously implanted polyvinyl alcohol sponges (µg ± SEM/100 mg sponge). Days on the *abscissa* represent the start of the T-lymphocyte depletion in relation to the day of wounding (day 0). ■, control; ▨ 30H12

In our laboratory we have studied the effect of T-lymphocyte depletion on wound healing in vivo. Using the monoclonal antibody 30H12, a rat antimouse antibody against the Thyl1.2 determinant of the IgG2b type (cytotoxic in vivo), we showed that mice depleted of T lymphocytes prior to wounding have decreased wound breaking strength and reparative collagen synthesis (Peterson et al. 1987). Subsequently, we have shown that starting T-lymphocyte depletion even 1 week postwounding results in impaired wound healing and collagen deposition, as assessed four weeks postwounding (Fig. 2). We are now in the process of determining which T-lymphocyte subset is responsible for normal wound repair. All of the foregoing clearly demonstrate that T lymphocytes play a major modulatory role in wound healing.

Conclusions

Mononuclear cells which infiltrate wounded tissue prior to fibroblast migration play a major role in the expansion of the fibroblast population and their subsequent synthesis of collagen and other extracellular matrix proteins. Since monokines and lymphokines which stimulate or inhibit fibroblast function have been described, a balance must exist that leads to regulated and successful tissue repair. Conversely, an imbalance in the production and/or activity of these factors could lead to wound failure or abnormal fibrosis. Therefore, an understanding of the role of these cytokines in normal wound healing would provide a biochemical tool for correcting disorders of repair.

Acknowledgements. Supported in part by NIH grant no. 1R29 6M 38650-01.

References

Agelli M, Sobel ME, Wahl SM (1987) Mononuclear cell modulation of fibroblast collagen synthesis. Fed Proc 46:924

Amento EP, Granstein RD (1987) Effects of immune cytokines (IL1, TNF, LT and IFN-γ) on fibroblasts. 2nd international symposium on tissue repair. 13–17 May 1987, Tarpon Springs, Fla

Bagby GC, Dinarello CA, Wallis P et al. (1986) Interleukin-1 stimulates granulocyte macrophage colony stimulating activity release by vascular endothelial cells. J Clin Invest 78:1316–1323

Baird A, Durkin T (1986) Inhibition of endothelial cell proliferation by type β-transforming growth factor: interactions with acidic and basic fibroblast growth factor. Biochem Biophys Res Commun 138:4167–4171

Bevilacqua MP, Pober JS, Majeau GR et al. (1984) Interleukin 1 (IL-1) induces biosynthesis and cell surface expression of procoagulant activity in human vascular endothelial cells. J Exp Med 160:618–623

Bevilacqua MP, Pober JS, Wheeler ME et al. (1986) Interleukin-1 acts on cultured human vascular endothelium to increase the adhesion of polymorphonuclear leukocytes, monocytes, and related leukocyte cell lines. J Clin Invest 76:2003–2011

Bevilacqua MP, Schleef RR, Gimbrone MA Jr et al. (1986a) Regulation of the fibrinolytic system of cultured human vascular endothelium by interleukin 1. J Clin Invest 78:587–591

Bhatnagar R, Penfornis H, Mauviel A et al. (1986) Interleukin-1 inhibits the synthesis of collagen by fibroblasts. Biochem Int 13:709–720

Bitterman PB, Rennard SI, Hunninghake GW et al. (1982) Human alveolar macrophage growth factor for fibroblasts. Regulation and partial characterization. J Clin Invest 70:806–822

Brinckerhoff CE, Guyre PM (1985) Increased proliferation of human synovial fibroblasts treated with recombinant immune interferon. J Immunol 134:3142–3146

Broudy VC, Kaushansky K, Segal GM et al. (1986) Tumor necrosis factor-α stimulates human endothelial cells to produce granulocyte/macrophage colony-stimulating factor. Proc Natl Acad Sci USA 83:7467–7471

Bussolino F, Breviario F, Tetta C et al. (1986) Interleukin 1 stimulates platelet-activating factor production in cultured human endothelial cells. J Clin Invest 77:2027–2033

Casey WJ, Peacock EE Jr, Chvapil M (1976) Induction of collagen synthesis in rats by transplantation of allogenic macrophages. Surg Forum 27:53

Cavender D, Haskard DO, Joseph B et al. (1986) Interleukin 1 increases the binding of human B and T lymphocytes to endothelial cell monolayers. J Immunol 136:203–207

Cavender D, Saegusa Y, Ziff M (1987) Stimulation of endothelial cell binding of lymphocytes by tumor necrosis factor. J Immunol 139:1855–1860

Clark RA, Stone RD, Leung DYK et al. (1976) Role of macrophages in wound healing. Surg Forum 27:16

Cohen MC, Picciano PT, Douglas WJ et al. (1982) Migration inhibition of endothelial cells by lymphokine-containing supernatants. Science 215:301–303

Collins T, Korman AJ, Wake CT et al. (1984) Immune interferon activates multiple class II major histocompatibility complex genes and the associated invariant chain gene in human endothelial cells and dermal fibroblasts. Proc Natl Acad Sci USA 81:4917–4921

Collins T, Capierrer LA, Fiers W et al. (1986) Recombinant human tumor necrosis factor increases mRNA levels and surface expression of HLA-A,B antigens in vascular endothelial cells and dermal fibroblasts in vitro. Proc Natl Acad Sci USA 83:446–450

Cromack DT, Sporn MB, Roberts AB et al. (1987) Transforming growth factor β levels in rat wound chambers. J Surg Res 42:622–628

Dayer JM, Beutler B, Cerami A (1985) Cachectin/tumor necrosis factor stimulates collagenase and prostaglandin E_2 production by human synovial cells and dermal fibroblasts. J Exp Med 162:2163–2168

Diegelmann RF, Schuller-Levis G, Cohen IK et al. (1986) Identification of a low molecular weight, macrophage-derived chemotactic factor for fibroblasts. Clin Immunol Immunopathol 41:331–341

Duncan MR, Berman B (1985) γ-Interferon is the lymphokine and β-interferon the monokine responsible for inhibition of fibroblast collagen production and late but not early fibroblast proliferation. J Exp Med 162:516–527

Emeis JJ, Kooistra T (1986) Interleukin 1 and lipolysaccharide induce an inhibitor of tissue-type plasminogen activator in vivo and in cultured endothelial cells. J Exp Med 163:1260–1266

Estes JE, Pledger WJ, Gillespie GY (1984) Macrophage-derived growth factor for fibroblasts and interleukin-1 are distinct entities. J Leukocyte Biol 35:115–129

Fishel RS, Barbul A, Beschorner WE et al. (1987) Lymphocyte participation in wound healing: morphologic assessment using monoclonal antibodies. Ann Surg 206:25–29

Frater-Schroder M, Muller G, Birchmeier W et al. (1986) Transforming growth factor-beta inhibits endothelial cell proliferation. Biochem Biophys Res Commun 137:295–302

Frater-Schroder M, Risau W, Hallmann R et al. (1987) Tumor necrosis factor type α, a potent inhibitor of endothelial cell growth in vitro, is angiogenic in vivo. Proc Natl Acad Sci USA 84:5277–5281

Gamble JR, Harlan JM, Klebanoff SJ et al. (1985) Stimulation of the adherence of neutrophils to umbilical vein endothelium by human recombinant tumor necrosis factor. Proc Natl Acad Sci USA 82:8667–8671

Geppert ID, Lipsky PE (1985) Antigen presentation by interferon-gamma-treated endothelial cells and fibroblasts: differential ability to function as antigen presenting cells despite comparable Ia expression. J Immunol 135:3750–3762

Granstein RD, Murphy GF, Margolis RJ et al. (1987) Gamma-interferon inhibits collagen synthesis in vivo in the mouse. J Clin Invest 79:1254–1258

Groenewegen G, Buurman WA, van der Linden CJ (1985) Lymphokines induce changes in morphology and enhanced motility of endothelial cells. Clin Immunol Immunopathol 36:378–385

Hajjar KA, Hajjar DP, Silverstein RL et al. (1987) Tumor necrosis factor-mediated release of platelet-derived growth factor from cultured endothelial cells. J Exp Med 166:235–245

Harlan JA (1987) Consequences of leukocyte-vessel wall interactions in inflammatory and immune reactions. Semin Thromb Hemost 13:434–444

Heimark RL, Twardzik DR, Schwartz SM (1986) Inhibition of endothelial regeneration by type-beta transforming growth factor from platelets. Science 233:1078–1980

Hofsli E, Austgulen R, Nissen-Meyer J (1987) Lymphotoxin-induced growth stimulation of diploid human fibroblasts in the presence and absence of gamma interferon. Scand J Immunol 26:585–588

Jimenez SA, McArthur W, Rosenbloom J (1979) Inhibition of collagen synthesis by mononuclear cell supernates. J Exp Med 150:1421–1431

Jimenez SA, Freundlich B, Rosenbloom J (1984) Selective inhibition of human diploid fibroblast collagen synthesis by interferons. J Clin Invest 74:1112–1116

Juijvestijn AM, Butcher EC (1986) Indication that high endothelium is controlled by immune regulatory products released in a local immune reactivity. 4th international symposium on biology of the vascular endothelial cell. Noordwijkerhout, The Netherlands, August 1986

Kahari V-M, Heino J, Vuorio E (1987) Interleukin-1 increases collagen production and mRNA levels in cultured skin fibroblasts. Biochim Biophys Acta 929:142–147

Kawakami M, Ishibashi S, Ogawa H et al. (1986) Cachectin/TNF as well as interleukin-1 induces prostacyclin synthesis in cultured vascular endothelial cells. Biochem Biophys Res Commun 141:482–487

Kohase M, Henriksen-DeStefano D, May LT et al. (1986) Induction of beta2-interferon by tumor necrosis factor: a homeostatic mechanism in the control of cell proliferation. Cell 45:659–666

Leibovich SJ, Ross R (1975) The role of the macrophage in wound repair. A study with hydrocortisone and antimacrophage serum. Am J Pathol 78:71–91

Leibovich SJ, Polverini PJ, Shepard MH et al. (1987) Macrophage-induced angiogenesis is mediated by tumour necrosis factor-α. Nature 328:630–632

Libby P, Janicka MW, Dinarello CA (1985) Interleukin 1 promotes production by human endothelial cells of activity that stimulates the growth of arterial smooth muscle cells. Fed Proc 44:1908a (abstract)

Libby P, Ordovas JM, Auger KR et al. (1986) Endotoxin and tumor necrosis factor induce interleukin-1 gene expression in adult human vascular endothelial cells. Am J Pathol 124:179–185

Martin BM, Gimbrone MA Jr, Unanue ER et al. (1981) Stimulation of nonlymphoid mesenchymal cell proliferation by a macrophage-derived growth factor. J Immunol 126:1510–1515

Masuyama JI, Minato N, Kano S (1986) Mechanisms of lymphocyte adhesions to human vascular endothelial cells in culture. T lymphocyte adhesion to endothelial cells through endothelial HLA-DR antigens induced by gamma interferon. J Clin Invest 77:1596–1605

Matsubara T, Ziff M (1986) Increased superoxide anion release from human endothelial cells in response to cytokines. J Immunol 137:3295–3298

Mizel SB, Dayer JM, Krane SM et al. (1980) Stimulation of rheumatoid synovial cell collagenase and prostaglandin production by partially purified lymphocyte activating factor (Interleukin 1). Proc Natl Acad Sci USA 78:2474–2477

Montesano R, Orci L, Vassalli P (1985) Human endothelial cell cultures: phenotypic modulation by leukocyte interleukins. J Cell Physiol 122:424–434

Munker R, Gasson J, Ogawa M et al. (1986) Recombinant human tumor necrosis factor induces production of granulocyte-monocyte colony-stimulating factor. Nature 323:79–82

Mustoe TA, Pierce GF, Thomason A et al. (1987) Accelerated healing of incisional wounds in rats induced by transforming growth factor-β. Science 237:1333–1336

Nachman RL, Hajjar KA, Silverstein RL et al. (1986) Interleukin-1 induces endothelial cell synthesis of plasminogen activator inhibitor. J Exp Med 163:1595–1600

Nawroth PP, Stern DM (1986) Modulation of endothelial cell hemostatic properties by tumor necrosis factor. J Exp Med 163:740–745

Nawroth PP, Bank I, Handley D et al. (1986a) Tumor necrosis factor/cachectin interacts with endothelial cell receptors to induce release of interleukin 1. J Exp Med 163:1363–1323

Nawroth PP, Handley DA, Esmon CT et al. (1986b) Interleukin 1 induces endothelial cell procoagulant while suppressing cell-surface anticoagulant activity. Proc Natl Acad Sci USA 83:3460–3464

Neilson EG, Phillips SM, Jimenez S (1982) Lymphokine modulation of fibroblast proliferation. J Immunol 128:1484–1486

Norioka K, Hara M, Kitani A et al. (1987) Inhibitory effect of human recombinant interleukin-1 α and β on growth of human vascular endothelial cells. Biochem Biophys Res Commun 145:969–975

Peterson JM, Barbul A, Breslin RJ et al. (1987) Significance of T lymphocytes in wound healing. Surgery 102:300–305

Pober JS, Gimbrone MA, Cotran KS et al. (1983) Ia expression by vascular endothelium is inducible by activated T cells and by human gamma-interferon. J Exp Med 157:1339–1353

Pober JS, Bevilacqua MP, Mendrick DL et al. (1986) Two distinct monokines, interleukin 1 and tumor necrosis factor, each independently induce biosynthesis and transient expression of the same antigen on the surface of cultured human vascular endothelial cells. J Immunol 136:1680–1687

Pohlman TH, Stanness KA, Beatty PG et al. (1986) An endothelial cell surface factor(s) induced in vitro by lipopolysaccharide, interleukin-1, and tumor necrosis factor-α increases neutrophil adherence by a CDw18-dependent mechanism. J Immunol 136:4548–4553

Postlethwaite AE, Smith GN, Mainardi CL et al. (1984) Lymphocyte modulation of fibroblast function in vitro: stimulation and inhibition of collagen production by different effector molecules. J Immunol 132:2470–2477

Postlethwaite AE, Keski-Oja J, Moses HL et al. (1987) Stimulation of the chemotactic migration of human fibroblasts by transforming growth factor β. J Exp Med 165:251–256

Roberts AB, Sporn MB, Assoian RK et al. (1986) Transforming growth factor type β: rapid induction of fibrosis and angiogenesis in vivo and stimulation of collagen formation in vitro. Proc Natl Acad Sci USA 83:4167–4171

Rola-Pleszczynski M, Lieu H, Hamel J et al. (1982) Stimulated human lymphocytes produce a soluble factor which inhibits fibroblast migration. Cell Immunol 74:104–110

Rossi V, Breviario F, Ghezzi P et al. (1984) Prostacyclin synthesis induced in vascular cells by interleukin-1. Science 229:174–176

Schleimer RP, Rutledge BR (1986) Cultured human vascular endothelial cells acquired adhesiveness for neutrophils after stimulation with interleukin 1, endotoxin and tumor-promoting phorbol diesters. J Immunol 136:649–654

Schmidt JA, Mizel SB, Cohen D et al. (1982) Interleukin 1, a potential regulator of fibroblast proliferation. J Immunol 128:2177–2182

Shimokado K, Raines EW, Madtes DK et al. (1985) A significant part of macrophage-derived growth factor consists of at least two forms of PDGF. Cell 43:277–286

Stolpen AH, Guinan EC, Fiers W et al. (1986) Recombinant TNF and immune interferon act singly and in combination to reorganize human vascular endothelial cell monolayers. Am J Pathol 123:16–24

Tiku M, Tomasi TB (1985) Enhancement of endothelial plasminogen activator synthesis by lymphokines. Transplantation 40:293–298

Tsukamoto Y, Helsel WE, Wahl SM (1982) Macrophage production of fibronectin, a chemoattractant for fibroblasts. J Immunol 127:673–678

Wahl SM, Wahl LM, McCarthy JB (1978) Lymphocyte mediated activation of fibroblast proliferation and collagen production. J Immunol 121:942–946

Wahl SM, Wahl LM, McCarthy JB (1979) Macrophage activation by mycobacterial water soluble compounds and synthetic muramyl dipeptide. J Immunol 122:2226–2731

Wahl SM, Gately CL (1983) Modulation of fibroblast growth by a lymphokine of human T cell and continous T cell line origin. J Immunol 130:1226–1230

Wahl SM (1985) Host immune factors regulating fibrosis. Ciba Found Symp 114:175–195

Wahl SM, Hunt DA, Wakefield LM et al. (1987) Transforming growth factor type β induces monocyte chemotaxis and growth factor production. Proc Natl Acad Sci USA 84:5788–5792

Watt SL, Auerbach R (1986) A mitogenic factor for endothelial cells obtained from mouse secondary mixed leukocyte cultures. J Immunol 136:197–202

Wyler DJ, Stadecker MJ, Dinarello CA et al. (1984) Fibroblast stimulation in schistosomiasis. V. Egg granuloma macrophages spontaneously secrete a fibroblast-stimulating factor. J Immunol 132:3142–3148

Yu CL, Haskard DO, Cavender D et al. (1985) Human gamma interferon increases the binding of T lymphocytes to endothelial cells. Clin Exp Immunol 62:554–560

[illegible]

Aspects of Immunological Control of Compensatory Organ Growth *

B. Radosevic-Stasic, M. Cuk, M. Segon, M. Susa, and D. Rukavina

Regulatory processes that control growth and differentiation of cells are of fundamental biological importance. During embryogenesis they ensure the regular and synchronized development of tissue units and organs, while during adulthood they maintain steady state and morphostasis, maintaining the balance between cell proliferation and cell death.

Among the theories of growth control, some postulate the existence of a centrally located physiological mechanism that regulates cell mitosis and maintains the balance among all the tissues in the body. According to Burwell [1] and Burch [2], this fundamental biological function is performed by the lymphoid system, which, due to its widespread distribution, mobility, and ability to distinguish between its own and foreign tissue, is very well suited to coordinate the overall growth of the organism. This theory emphasizes that lymphoid cells have other functions besides those known as immunological. During the past several years, it has become clear that lymphokines as multifunctional lymphoid cell products profoundly regulate the activation, growth, and differentiation not only of T- and B-lymphocytes but also of many other cell types [3]. The findings that some of these cytokines are very similar to the mediators typical for the neuroendocrine system [4] led to the hypothesis that lymphocytes act as a general, mobile, sensory organ which share with neuroendocrine system a similar set of peptide signals and receptors [5]. Since it is known that most genetically determined cellular functions are regulated by the neuroendocrine system, it seems very likely that the lymphatic system also plays a role in this control.

Indirectly this evidence supports the previously established hypothesis of the central role of lymphatic tissue in the control of normal growth, but the direct experimental proofs for this are still very scanty. The most convincing results have been obtained in the experiments in which morphostasis has been suddenly interrupted by tissue damage or surgical removal of an organ, or its part. Most of the earlier data about the participation of the lymphatic system in regenerative growth and wound healing, that follow after such procedures, are reviewed by Burch [2], and more recently by Babaeva [6]. According to Babaeva (1985), removal or resection of an organ leads to the decrease of organ-specific antigens. Owing to the disturbance of balance between these antigens and lymphatic tissue, the activity of T-suppressor cells diminishes. As a further step the activation of T- and B-lymphocytes occurs, which through the action of lymphokines and

---

* This study was supported by grant 2.05.01.05.04 from the Republic of Croatia Research Fund, Zagreb.

Immune Consequences of
Trauma, Shock and Sepsis
Eds. Faist/Ninnemann/Green

autoantibodies results in the stimulation of mitosis and growth of the remaining part of the resected organ. So lymphocytes activated by partial hepatectomy (Hx) or unilateral nephrectomy (UNx) gain the capacity to transfer "regenerative information" and perform their morphogenetic functions [6–10]. The effects of such "primed" lymphocytes have been found always to be organ specific: Hx-lymphocytes affected the liver, UNx-lymphocytes the kidney, those after jejunectomy provoked mitoses in the intestinal cripts, while those stimulated by hypoxia or anemia stimulated the production of reticulocytes (see [6]).

The effects were also dependent on stimulus intensity and on time elapsed from the operation. Thus splenocytes obtained from donors in which one-third Hx was performed were less effective than those from donors with two-thirds Hx. The greatest morphogenetic capacity is assumed by lymphocytes at an early period after disturbance of morphostasis (4th–17th h – see [6]), while later even suppressive effects can be obtained, especially with the transfer of splenocytes. A similar time-dependent relationship has been noticed when the effect of supernatant of the bone marrow from Hx mice was tested on DNA synthesis of intact BM and spleen cells [11]. It is reported also that later after Hx (5th–15th day) augmentation of K cells and NK activity in spleen occur that lead to the development of cytotoxicity to the syngeneic lymphoblasts in vitro [12].

Besides these in vivo obtained proofs for the activation of the lymphatic system by partial Hx, it was possible also in vitro to activate the syngeneic lymphocytes [13] or splenocytes [14] by the regenerating liver cells. In our experiments [14] the most potent stimulators were hepatic cells obtained 2 days after partial Hx. Moreover, in cultures where Hx-liver cells were mixed with Hx-lymphocytes or splenocytes signs of secondary immune reaction were obtained, suggesting that lymphatic cells were "primed" by Hx in vivo [13, 14]. In the primary syngeneic MLR the responder cells were mostly Lyt 1^+, but in the secondary MLR they were Lyt 1^-2^+ [15]. All these findings suggest that in the process of organ regeneration various types of activated lymphatic cells perform the autoregulatory function.

Since it is known that a crucial role for the cellular recognition of foreign antigens and induction and regulation of the immune response is played by class II MHC antigens, we started our next investigation with the analysis of tissue distribution and quantification of Ia molecules in the regenerating liver tissue [16, 17]. It was found that partial Hx induces good expression of Ia molecules on the vascular endothelium, bile duct epithelium, and mostly on previously W3/25^+ but Ia^- cells. Since, according to Steiniger et al. [18], these cells are phagocytic Kupffer's cells, we speculated [16], that after Hx they became phenotypically new, as activated cells, or that the number of dendritic cells in regenerating liver had increased, owing to greater immigration of these cells from the BM. Peaks of hyperplasia in BM noticed in the partially hepatectomized animals [19], support the latter hypothesis. In any case, as antigen-presenting cells these cells probably expose new antigens to the lymphatic system, such as α-fetoproteins or other fetal enzymes, that are released during the process of retrodifferentiation in the regenerating liver. The finding that Ia molecules, in fact, do not have the fine specificity for recognition between self- and non-self-molecules, but function as a carrier system that protects even autologous peptides from catabolism and transports them to the surface of cell [20], supports the hypothesis that through class II molecules activation of the lymphatic system occurs also after the disturbance of morphostasis. Greater presence of Ia molecules in the regenerating liver tissue might be, however, connected also with the action of γ-interferon released from the activated lymphatic cells.

It is obvious that many of the described events are the same as those thought to exist in the development of an autoimmune disease, but represent the regulated form of the breakdown of previously maintained tolerance to self-tissue. The greater appearance of class II molecules in the foci of lymphocytes in filtration and tissue damage [21, 22] might therefore be not only the consequence of an immunological autoagressive attack, but also the sign of tissue repair that follows after tissue lesion. For the present, most of these basic questions related to the eventual physiological role of lymphatic tissue are completely unsolved.

References

1. Burwell RG (1963) The role of lymphoid tissue in morphostasis. Lancet 2:69–74
2. Burch PRJ (1976) Is normal growth regulated by a central system? In: The biology of cancer – a new approach. MTP Press, Lancaster, pp 17–39
3. Dinurello CA, Mier JW (1987) Lymphokines. N Engl J Med 317:940–945
4. Morley JE, Kay NE, Solomon GF, Plotnikoff NP (1987) Neuropeptides: conductors of the immune orchestra. Life Sci 41:527–544
5. Blalock JE (1984) The immune system as a sensory organ. J Immunol 132:1067–1070
6. Babaeva IG (1985) Regeneration and the system of immunogenesis. Medicina Moscow (in Russian)
7. Pliskin ME, Prehn RT (1975) Stimulation of liver regeneration and compensatory kidney hyperplasia by passive transfer of spleen cells. RES J Reticuloendothel Soc 17:290–299
8. Fox M, Wahman GE (1968) Etiology of the compensatory renal response: observation on the role of the lymphoid system. Invest Urol 5:521–538
9. Radosevic-Stasic B, Cuk M, Rukavina D (1979) Cellular and humoral mediators in the compensatory renal growth. Period Biol 81:149–150
10. Radosevic-Stasic B, Cuk M, Rukavina D (1980) The role of lymphatic tissue in the compensatory renal growth. Adv Physiol Sci 11:141–145
11. Pierpaoli W, Balakrishnan J, Sache E, Choay J, Maestroni GJM (1986) Neuroendocrine and bone marrow factors for control of marrow transplantation and tissue regeneration. Ann NY Acad Sci 496:27–39
12. Ono M, Tanaka N, Orita K (1984) Activation of NK activity and autoreactive cytotoxicity after hepatectomy. Acta Med Okayama 38:207–213
13. Miyahara S, Yokomuro K, Takahashi H, Yoshitami K (1983) Regeneration and the immune system. I. In vitro and in vivo activation of lymphocytes liver regeneration and the role of Kupffer cells in stimulation. Eur J Immunol 13:878–883
14. Susa M, Radosevic-Stasic B, Segon M, Rukavina D (1987) In vitro and in vivo activation of syngeneic splenocytes by the liver cells obtained from the hepatectomized donors. Period Biol 89[Suppl 1]:187
15. Yokomuro K, Miyahara S, Takahashi H, Kimura Y (1983) Regeneration and the immune system. II. Suppressor activities of lymphocytes activated in vivo by liver regeneration and their genetic control. Eur J Immunol 13:883–889
16. Jonjic S, Radosevic-Stasic B, Cuk M, Jonjic N, Rukavina D (1987) Class II antigens induction in the regenerating liver of rats after partial hepatectomy. Transplantation 44:165–168

17. Segon M, Radosevic-Stasic B, Jonjic N, Cuk M, Susa M, Jonjic S, Rukavina D (1987) The role of class II MHC molecules in the regulation of normal growth. Period Biol 89[Suppl 1]:187
18. Steiniger B, Klempnaur J, Wonigeit K (1984) Phenotype and histological distribution of interstitial dendritic cells in the rat pancreas, liver, heart and kidney. Transplantation 38:169–175
19. Cuk M, Radosevic-Stasic B, Milin C, Kirigin M, Rukavina D (1986) Lymphoid system as a regulator of morphostasis and hormonal modulation of these functions. Ann NY Acad Sci 496:104–108
20. Unanue ER, Allen PM (1987) The basis for the immunoregulatory role of macrophages and other accessory cells. Science 236:551–557
21. Bovo P, Mirakian R, Merigo F, Angelini G, Cavallini R, Rizzini P, Bottazzo GF, Scuro LA (1987) HLA molecule expression on chronic pancreatitis specimens: is there a role for autoimmunity? A preliminary study. Pancreas 2:350–356
22. Todd I, Pujol-Borrell R, Abdul-Karim AS, Hammond LJ, Feldmann M, Bottazzo GF (1987) HLA-D subregion expression by thyroid epithelium in autoimmune thyroid diseases and induced in vitro. Clin Exp Immunol 69:532–542

Section 6

Impact of Therapeutic Regimen on Immune Function

Relationship Between Immune Function and Posttrauma Morbidity and Mortality

N. V. Christou

Introduction

Trauma in any form has been shown to alter the capacity of the host to resist infection. The reason for this is believed to be reduced host defense capability towards microbial organisms following blunt, penetrating, thermal, or operative trauma. Host defense can be subdivided into a humoral or antibody component, a specific cellular component, a nonspecific inflammatory component and complement. This division is suitable for discussion and study, but in reality all components of host defense interact in a predefined manner in order to contain and resolve an infectious process. In this section we will review the abnormalities in each component of host defense produced by trauma and relate these to the clinical outcome of the host.

Specific Immune Response after Trauma: Humoral and Cell-Mediated Immunity

Alexander and Moncrief [1] were able to show that the primary response to a new antigen, alligator erythrocytes, was depressed following burns whereas the secondary response to tetanus toxoid was enhanced. Support for an intact secondary response has been presented by Balch [2]. Data by Volenec et al. [3] indicate that immediately following a burn injury, there are immature mononuclear cells released in the circulation and the numbers of B lymphocytes are decreased in nonsurvivors. Miller and Trunkey found decreased ability to generate de novo antibody-forming cells in vitro in mice receiving 10% scald burns, further supporting this thesis [4]. Immunoglobulin levels of all five classes are not different between trauma patients who survive or die, but nearly all trauma patients have elevated acute-phase proteins as measured by C-reactive protein [5]. Such static studies may not be valid in the acutely traumatized patient due to the need for aggressive hemodynamic support with crystalloids, plasma and blood, which may change the in vivo "native" values of these substances. Studies by Nohr et al. of the secondary or anamnestic response indicate that there is a defect in antibody synthesis to protein antigens in bluntly traumatized man [6] and thermally injured rats (C. W. Nohr, personal communication). This reduction is more severe and more frequent in anergic trauma patients (see below). Similar work from Boston has shown an abnormality in antibody production to tetanus toxoid from burn patients [7]. Because most bacterial antigens are not protein, but polysaccharides,

Immune Consequences of
Trauma, Shock and Sepsis
Eds. Faist/Ninnemann/Green

the humoral immune response to such antigens is more clinically relevant. We studied in vivo and in vitro antibody responses to a relatively T-cell-independent polysaccharide antigen, 23 valent pneumococcal vaccine (PPS) [8]. There was no difference in vivo anti-PPS production between laboratory controls or injured anergic patients. There was also a good correlation of in vivo and in vitro specific antibody responses. The data imply that a T-cell defect is responsible for reduced humoral immunity to protein antigens. Also, active immunization of surgical patients with bacterial vaccines may produce effective immunity.

A means of globally assessing host defense was introduced 13 years ago by MacLean et al. [9]. They used the delayed type hypersensitivity (DTH) skin test response to recall antigens [10] as a predictor of clinical outcome in surgical patients. Anergic patients (those with no response to any antigen) had a higher sepsis and mortality rate than reactive patients ($\geqq 5$ mm induration to 2 or more antigens at 24–48 h posttest). This work has been confirmed by others [11–19], though there are some contrary views [19]. Even this group of researchers, who categorically state that DTH responses are not useful in the clinical setting, have shown mortality rates of 35% in anergic patients, compared to 0% in the reactive patients. Table 1 shows the relationship between the DTH skin test response and clinical outcome in a group of bluntly traumatized patients studied at our institution [20].

Thermal injury, if severe enough, will cause profound suppression of cell-mediated immune response, including the DTH response. Table 2 illustrates the effect of burn on the DTH response and clinical outcome. Sepsis refers to a clinically detectable bacteremia.

Alterations in cell-mediated immune responses after trauma have been attributed to serum inhibitors of T-cell function [21], alterations in the helper/suppressor lymphocyte ratio [22], or inappropriate lymphokine production. Several studies have tried to relate the abnormal T-cell function to clinical outcome. None have been able to better the prediction provided by the DTH response. This test

Table 1. The effect of blunt trauma on the DTH response and clinical outcome in 176 patients

DTH response	Number	Sepsis-related mortality (%)
Reactive	58	5
Relative anergy	44	14
Anergy	73	26

Table 2. The effect of thermal trauma on the DTH response and clinical outcome in 27 patients

DTH response	Number	% Burn	Sepsis (%)	Mortality (%)
Reactive	3	35 ± 8	0	0
Relative anergy	6	44 ± 10	50	17
Anergy	18	55 ± 11	72	61

requires an intact specific immune response (memory T-cell recognition of the antigen, specific lymphokine release, amplification) and nonspecific immune capability (recruitment of nonspecific lymphocytes, monocytes and polymorphonuclear leukocytes) in order to produce the measured induration. Failure at any of these steps will result in a reduced or absent DTH response. Thus, this simple test provides a global assessment of host defense.

In contrast to thermal injury, few patients sustaining blunt trauma show consistent in vitro T-cell defects. In vitro lymphocyte studies from anergic patients show normal mixed lymphocyte culture reactions, normal response to lymphokines, normal generation of cytotoxic T cells, and normal proliferative reactions to mitogens and antigens. The in vitro lymphocyte proliferative reaction to PPD is normal despite in vivo anergy to PPD skin tests. These plus other observations in our laboratory, indicate that the failure to obtain a DTH is due to a suppressive "anergic environment" in the host, preventing in vivo lymphocyte activation [23]. Using a skin-window correlate of the DTH response we found that in anergic patients, a negligible cell delivery without "additives" to the window was seen to be corrected by injection of antigen and lymphokine [24], supporting the hypothesis of an in vivo block to immune function.

Nonspecific Immune Response

In contrast to specific immunity discussed above, nonspecific immunity does not discriminate on the basis of antigen-antibody specificity. It is directed against a wide variety of "invaders." For example a macrophage will phagocytose and kill an *E. coli* organism, just as easily as it will kill a *Staphylococcus,* or a fungus, without regard to surface antigen expression other then appropriate opsonization. This system guards against bacterial invasion of the body through the four most common portals of entry: the skin, the respiratory tract, the genitourinary tract, and the peritoneal cavity. Once the environmental or mechanical barrier of the skin or the intact bowel mucosa is damaged, bacteria gain access to the subcutaneous space or the peritoneal cavity. The phagocytes in the skin and the peritoneal cavity, together with circulating humoral factors such as antibodies and the complement system, provide the first line of defense.

Patients with anergy seen immediately following trauma, major surgery or severe sepsis are different from those with anergy seen in elective surgical patients who walk into the hospital with no focus of infection, a condition we term "walk-in anergy." The first group, in addition to anergy, have stickier polymorphonucleocytes (PMNs) determined from in vitro adherence measurements to nylon fiber. The in vitro chemotaxis of such PMNs is always reduced, measured both in filter-type assays or under agarose. The reduced PMN chemotaxis is inversely related to the adherence, i.e., the cells are stickier and they move more slowly than controls in in vitro studies [25]. These in vitro abnormalities have in vivo significance in that the accumulation of PMNs to Rebuck-type window chambers over a skin abrasion is much reduced in anergic patients with increased adherence and decreased chemotaxis compared to laboratory controls or reactive patients with normal PMN function [26]. In some patients there is divergence of anergy and local nonspecific host defense. Some patients who remain reactive following trauma show abnormalities in local nonspecific host defense, albeit or lesser magnitude compared to those with anergy [27]. The reverse does not occur. Anergic patients after trauma always have abnormal local nonspecific host defense. Patients with walk-in anergy have normal adherence and chemotaxis and cannot be distinguished from laboratory controls on the basis of these measurements [28]. Furthermore, delivery of PMNs to skin windows in these walk-in anergic patients is not reduced compared to reactive patients. In the postoperative period the walk-in anergic patients (along with the reactive patients) develop increased adherence, decreased chemotaxis and decreased delivery of PMNs to skin windows, i.e., they demonstrate decreased local nonspecific host defense in addition to decreased DTH.

Like the T-cell defects, these abnormalities in local nonspecific host defense are due to an in vivo "suppressive environment": there are factors in the plasma of patients with increased PMN adherence that increase the adherence of normal control PMNs following treatment in vitro; in the case of PMN the decreased chemotaxis is mediated by factors in the serum [29]. Cell transfer experiments with burned rats have confirmed this suppressive environment effect on local nonspecific host defense, in particular PMN localization. Normal unburned PMNs injected into burned rats accumulate in inflammatory sites at the same rate as burned PMNs in burned rats. Burned rat PMNs injected into unburned rats accumulate in inflammatory sites at the same rate as unburned PMNs into normal rats [30].

Predicting Sepsis-Related Mortality in Surgical Patients

The various components of the immune system are elegantly integrated in vivo and along with local nonspecific host defense provide for control of bacterial infections. One can study how some of these components interact in the trauma host by multivariate logistic regression analysis. Sepsis-related mortality is a good dependent variable. DTH expressed as a skin test score (the sum of the diameters of induration of each of the individual five antigens), PMN function, serum albumin, hemoglobin, sex, and age were used as independent variables in such an analysis which showed that DTH score, age, and serum albumin were the variables statistically associated with sepsis-related mortality [31]. The following equation can be used to calculate the probability of sepsis-related mortality of any patient given his preoperative DTH score, age, and serum albumin:

$$P|\text{death}| = 1 - \{1 + \exp(1.343 - 1.372(\text{albumin}) - 0.173(\log[\text{DTH score}]) + 0.026(\text{age})\}^{-1}$$

This equation can give an *objective measure* of a trauma patient's risk for a post-trauma adverse outcome. It has been tested in a prospective manner and the predicted and expected mortalities are similar.

The strong contribution of the serum albumin to predicting sepsis-related mortality is an interesting observation. Thought it is tempting to attribute this to malnutrition in the traumatized host, this may not be the case. A variable such as the Acute Physiology Score which measures the degree of physiologic stress on the host displaces the albumin from the predictive model. This does not occur with preoperative patients. The reduced albumin may reflect a condition of "physiologic stress" that exists in the host. This "stress" results in a redirection of protein synthesis by the liver, with suppression of albumin synthesis in favor of acute phase proteins which may be needed for survival. The mediator may be IL-1, which together with its breakdown product proteolysis inducing factor (PIF), is present in the host undergoing any form of stress such as trauma or sepsis [32]. Tumor necrosis factor is another candidate. In fact this observation may indicate a possible modulating control of macrophages on the immune system, at both the specific and local nonspecific host defense levels. We found that rats who had their Kuppfer cells activated by an intraportal injection of bacteria exhibited suppressed DTH responses in the skin, whereas when Kuppfer cells were ablated with intraportal carageenan there was an enhancement of the DTH response [33].

References

1. Alexander JW, Moncrief JA (1966) Alterations of immune response following severe thermal injury. Arch Surg 93:75–80
2. Balch HH (1955) The effect of severe battle injury and post-operative renal failure on resistance to infection. Ann Surg 142:145–147
3. Volenec FJ, Wood GW, Mani MM, Robinson DW, Humphrey LJ (1979) Mononuclear cell analysis of peripheral blood from burn patients. J Trauma 19:86–90
4. Miller CL, Trunkey DD (1977) Thermal injury: defects in immune response induction. J Surg Res 22:621–626
5. Christou NV, McLean APH, Meakins JL (1980) Host defense in blunt trauma: interrelationships between kinetics of anergy and depressed neutrophil function, nutritional status and sepsis. J Trauma 20:833–837
6. Nohr CW, Christou NV, Broadhead M, Meakins JL (1983) Failure of humoral immunity in surgical patients. Surg Forum 34:127–129
7. Wood JJ, O'Mahony ML, Rodrick R, Eaton R, Demling RH, Manick JA (1986) Abnormalities of antibody production following thermal injury. An association with reduced interleukin 2 production. Arch Surg 121:108–115
8. Nohr CW, Latter DA, Meakins JL, Christou NV (1986) In vivo and in vitro humoral immunity in surgical patients: antibody response to pneumococcal polysaccharide. Surgery 100:229–238
9. MacLean LD, Meakins JL, Taguchi K, Duignan J, Dhillon KS, Gordon J (1975) Host resistance in sepsis and trauma. Ann Surg 182:207–211
10. Zinsser H (1921) Delayed hypersensitivity. J Exp Med 34:495–497
11. Johnson WC, Ulrich F, Meguid MM et al. (1979) Role of delayed hypersensitivity in predicting postoperative morbidity and mortality. Am J Surg 137:536–539
12. Adami GF, Terrizzi A, Vita M et al. (1980) The assessment of skin tests in surgery. Surgery in Italy 10:297–301
13. Tasseau F, Gaucher L, Nicolas F (1982) Cell-mediated immunity studied by skin tests in patients receiving intensive care. Prognostic value of repeated tests. Study of some factors predisposing towards anergy. Sem Hop (Paris) 58:781
14. Gertner MH, Mullen JL, Buzby GP, Goodhart GL, Rosato EF (1979) Implications of malnutrition in the surgical patient. Arch Surg 114:121–125
15. Morath MA, Miller SF, Finley RK (1981) Nutritional indicators of postburn bacteremic sepsis. JPEN 5:488–491

16. Harvey KB, Moldawer LL, Bistrian BR, Blackburn GL (1981) Biological measures for the formulation of a hospital prognostic index. Am J Clin Nutr 34:2013–2022
17. Casey J, Flinn WR, Yao JS, Fahey V, Pawlowski J, Bergan JJ (1983) Correlation of immune and nutritional status with wound complications in patients undergoing vascular operations. Surgery 93:822–827
18. Kienlen J, Chardon P, Nury G, Lubrano JF, Messmer JC, du Cailar J (1981) Study of delayed skin hypersensitivity using the multitest in an intensive care unit. Ann Anesthesiol Fr 22:285–291
19. Brown R, Bancewicz J, Hamid J, Patel NJ, Ward C, Farrand RJ, Pamphrey RSH, Irving M (1982) Failure of delayed hypersensitivity skin testing to predict post-operative sepsis and mortality. Br J Surg 284:851–853
20. Christou NV, McLean APH, Meakins JL (1980) Host defense in blunt trauma: interrelationships of kinetics of anergy and depressed neutrophil function, nutritional status, and sepsis. J Trauma 20:833–841
21. Munster AM (1984) Immunologic response of trauma and burns. An overview. Am J Med 76:142–145
22. Christou NV, Mannick JA, West MA, Kasper DL (1987) Lymphocyte macrophage interactions in the response to surgical infections. Arch Surg 122:239–251
23. Rode HN, Christou NV, Bubenik O, Superina R, Gordon J, Meakins JL, MacLean LD (1981) Lymphocyte function in anergic patients. Clin Exp Immunol 47:155–159
24. MacPhee MJ, Rode H, Broadhead M, Christou NV, Meakins JL, Gordon J (1987) Skin window chambers, a novel method for recovering the cells involved in delayed-type hypersensitivity. J Immunol Methods 103:267–273
25. Christou NV (1985) The delayed hypersensitivity response, granulocyte function and sepsis in surgical patients. JBCR 6:157–166
26. Morris JS, Meakins JL, Christou NV (1985) In vivo neutrophil delivery to inflammatory sites in surgical patients: correlation with in vitro neutrophil chemotaxis and adherence. Arch Surg 120:205–209
27. Christou NV, McLean APH, Meakins JL (1980) Host defense in blunt trauma: interrelationships of kinetics of anergy and depressed neutrophil function, nutritional status, and sepsis. J Trauma 20:833–841
28. Christou NV, Rode HN, Larson D, Loose L, Broadhead M, Meakins JL (1984) The walk-in anergic patient: how best to assess the risk following elective surgery. Ann Surg 199:438–444
29. Christou NV, Meakins JL (1979) Neutrophil function in surgical patients: two inhibitors of granulocyte chemotaxis associated with sepsis. J Surg Res 26:355–364
30. Tchervenkov JI, Latter DA, Psychogios J, Christou NV (1988) Altered leukocyte delivery to specific and nonspecific inflammatory skin lesions following burn injury. J Trauma (in press)
31. Christou NV (1986) Predicting septic related mortality of the individual surgical patient based on admission host defense measurements. Can J Surg (in press)
32. Clows GHA Jr, George BC, Villee CA, Salaris CA (1983) Muscle proteolysis induced by a circulating peptide in patients with sepsis or trauma. N Engl J Med 308:545–552
33. Marshall JC, Christou NV, Meakins JL (1988) Immunomodulation of altered GI flora: the effects of orally administered *Pseudomonas aeruginosa* on specific and non-specific immunity. Arch Surg (in press)

Immunological Alterations Following Simple Hemorrhage

I. H. Chaudry, R. N. Stephan, J. M. Harkema, and R. E. Dean

Introduction

Trauma is considered to be the leading cause of death during the first three decades of life in the USA (Shires 1985; Trunkey 1982, 1983) ranking overall as the fourth leading cause of death. Accidental injury accounts for approximately 165000 deaths each year (Trunkey 1982). Furthermore, sepsis is the major nonneurologic cause of death after trauma, thermal injury, and major surgery. It carries an overall mortality rate of 60% (Baker et al. 1980). Numerous studies have been carried out exploring the causal relationships between the traumatic insults to the organism and its predisposition to develop septic complications and generalized septicemia (Alexander et al. 1979; Baker et al. 1985; Bjornson et al. 1978; Christou et al. 1980). Earlier studies indicated that patients with significant thermal and soft tissue injuries showed a marked tendency for multiple organ failure usually observed in association with persistent septicemia (Baue and Chaudry 1980; Miller et al. 1982). Efforts were therefore directed towards the eradication of septic foci by surgical procedures, antibiotic coverage, and overzealous fluid and nutritional therapy. However, the prognosis of such complications in the setting of major traumatic injuries has remained grim, mostly because of uncontrollable sepsis leading to severe homeostatic derangements and cellular dysfunction.

Intensive investigations were launched which dealt with the effect of trauma on the immune system (Antonacci 1986; Faist et al. 1986, 1987, 1988; Keane et al. 1983a, b; Kupper et al. 1984; Kupper and Green 1984; Ninneman and Stockland 1984; O'Mahony et al. 1984). Based on those findings, it is now widely accepted that extensive trauma results in a markedly altered immunocompetency and increases the susceptibility to infection. A large number of studies have demonstrated that a wide variety of abnormal immunological reactions develop within a predictable time pattern according to the type of injury and its severity. Studies dealing with burns and soft tissue destruction have shown that in the immediate phase following the burn, neutrophil chemotaxis and macrophage function are severely impaired (Alexander et al. 1978; Deitch et al. 1982; Kupper et al. 1985). This is followed by a decrease in the immunoresponsiveness of the specific immune system, i.e., the cell-mediated immunity (CMI) (Kupper and Green 1984b; Munster 1976; Wang et al. 1980; Wolfe et al. 1981). It appears that injury activates the suppressor system which in turn triggers a specific cellular response such as a decrease in helper T lymphocytes (McIrvine et al. 1982; O'Mahony et al. 1984), decrease in immunoglobulin production, and impaired reticuloendothe-

Immune Consequences of
Trauma, Shock and Sepsis
Eds. Faist/Ninnemann/Green

lial system (RES) function (Chaudry et al. 1982; Saba 1986). As a consequence of the RES depression, the capacity to handle and phagocytize antigen is depressed, resulting in a defective antigen presentation to the T helper cells (Kupper et al. 1985). This may have some serious consequences since antigen presentation plays a central role in the activation of T helper cells (Unanue et al. 1984).

Hemorrhage is a prevalent complication in trauma patients arising from soft tissue and bony injuries causing life-threatening blood loss. Hemorrhage is also frequently encountered during complex surgical procedures. Although the improved resuscitation of such patients has resulted in increased short-term survival, late septic complications continue to be a major problem.

Numerous studies concerning the etiology of immunosuppression following thermal and mechanical trauma are being carried out, however, there has not been any systematic investigation addressing the question whether hemorrhage which occurs in conjunction with other accidental injuries as well as a separate pathophysiological entity plays any major role in producing immunosuppression. Should pure hemorrhage lead to depressed immunity, one would expect an additive suppressive effect in situations where hemorrhage occurs in conjunction with injuries to different organ systems. In this regard, recent studies of Abraham and Chang (1985) have shown that mitogen-induced proliferation of lymphocytes was depressed as early as 30 min after hemorrhage and was even more depressed at 2.0 h after hemorrhage in rats. Furthermore, they suggested that there is a hemorrhage-induced serum factor(s) which inhibit(s) lymphocyte proliferation (Abraham and Chang 1986). Although the above studies clearly indicate that host defense mechanisms are altered, they do not provide any information on whether CMI is altered during such conditions. Moreover, the time course studies of generation of such a factor(s) have not been conducted even in a rat model of hemorrhage. Thus, it becomes necessary to investigate in detail whether such serum factor(s) are at all relevant to the observed immunosuppressive effects of hemorrhage in an immunologically well characterized species. Since there appear to be no other laboratories examining the effects of hemorrhage on CMI, the work described below is exclusively from our laboratory. Appropriate references to the work of others are, however, provided.

Aims of Our Studies

The aims of our studies were to determine: (1) whether simple hemorrhage (without significant tissue trauma) suppresses CMI, alters peritoneal macrophages (PM0) and splenic adherent cell antigen presentation (AP) function, produces perturbation in lymphokine production, and increases susceptibility to sepsis and (2) whether the use of immunomodulators following hemorrhage have any beneficial effects on those processes.

Species for Hemorrhage Studies

In order to determine the immunological consequences of hemorrhage, it is necessary to use a species which is well characterized immunologically. For these purposes, the use of a mouse hemorrhage model is well suited. Standardized immunological assays using lymphoid cells from mice are readily available, and therefore the mouse hemorrhage model allows an in-depth evaluation of different aspects of immunological function in a systematic and reliable manner.

Mouse Hemorrhage Model

Adult C3H/HEJ mice were lightly anesthetized with ether and using a gentle and minimal dissection technique, both femoral arteries were cannulated with polyethylene (PE) 10 tubing. The animals were then heparinized (100 U/kg), restrained in a supine position, and allowed to awaken. One of the catheters was used for monitoring blood pressure continuously and the other cannula was used for bleeding the animals. As soon as the animals were awake, they were bled rapidly to a mean blood pressure of 35 mmHg and maintained at that level for 1 h. This was followed by reinfusion of the shed blood along with Ringer's lactate, two times the shed blood volume. Following resuscitation, the catheters were removed and the groin incisions were closed. The mice were then returned to their cages and food and water was allowed ad lib. There was no significant mortality with this model. Control animals underwent the same procedure but hemorrhage was not induced (Stephan et al. 1987a).

Immunological and Other Parameters Measured

On days 1 through 10 after resuscitation, the mice were sacrificed and the proliferative responses of splenocytes to concanavalin A were measured. In addition, allogeneic mixed lymphocyte reaction (MLR) was performed. Since interleukin-2 (IL-2) is required for clonal T-cell proliferation and activation of specific and nonspecific cytotoxic effector systems, IL-2 production by splenic cells following hemorrhage and resuscitation was also measured. Moreover, since AP by macrophages (MO) plays a critical role in antigen-specific activation process of T-helper cells, we investigated whether the function of the MO as an AP cell is altered following hemorrhage. In addition, the effect of hemorrhage on subsequent susceptibility to sepsis was also investigated. Lastly, the effects of ATP-$MgCl_2$ as an immunomodulator were examined. Details of these various measurements are not provided here, since they have been published (Stephan et al. 1986, 1987a, b, 1988a, b).

The results indicated that on day 1 following hemorrhage, the proliferative responses of spleen cells to concanavalin A stimulation was markedly impaired and the responses were only 18% of control (Stephan et al. 1987a). There was, however, a slow and steady increase in the proliferation on the subsequent days. On day 10 following hemorrhage, proliferative responses of spleen cells from posthemorrhage mice returned to control levels. Using the MLR, it was found that a profound depression was also evident on days 1 and 2 following hemorrhage. This depression was not apparent on day 9 following hemorrhage and resuscitation (Stephan et al. 1987a).

Additional experiments were conducted to determine the effect of hemorrhage on AP by splenic and PMO cells. For these studies, immediately following hemorrhage and resuscitation, the mice were sacrificed and PMO as well as splenic adherent cells were harvested. AP function of these cells was tested by co-culturing different numbers of PMO and splenic adherent cells with D10.G4.1 cells in the presence of conalbumin. This cell clone, D10.G4.1, proliferates in the presence of Ia^k-bearing MO and specific antigen, thus directly reflecting the AP capability of MO. The results demonstrated that D10.G4.1 proliferation induced via AP by PMO and splenic adherent cells from hemorrhaged-resuscitated mice was 29% and 24% of control, respectively ($P<0.05$).

The effects of eicosanoids on AP function of MO were also examined. For such studies, PMO were harvested and AP was tested in vitro by incubating various number of MO with 2×10^4 D10.G4.1 cells/well and conalbumin (400 µg/ml) in the presence and absence of different concentrations of prostaglandin E_2 (PGE_2) or thromboxane B_2 (TXB_2). Cultures were incubated for 72 h, pulsed with ^{3}H-thymidine, and harvested. At concentrations of 10 n*M*, 30 n*M* and 100 n*M* of PGE_2, D10.G4.1 proliferation was 38%, 35%, and 20% of control, respectively ($P<0.05$ compared to control). Addition of TXB_2 at the above-mentioned concentrations did not suppress the proliferative responses of D10.G4.1 cells. Thus, PGE_2 but not TXB_2 has a potent immunosuppressive effect on AP of PMO (Stephan et al. 1988 b).

With regard to IL-2 production, the results demonstrated that simple hemorrhage produced a profound depression in splenic IL-2 production (Stephan et al. 1986). This depression was found to be maximal in animals that were killed immediately after hemorrhage without resuscitation but it persisted even on day 3 after hemorrhage despite resuscitation. On day 5 after hemorrhage and resuscitation, IL-2 production was found to be normal.

Another group of control mice and hemorrhaged and resuscitated mice were subjected to sepsis. On day 3 following resucitation or sham operation, the mice were lightly anesthetized with ether and through a 1 cm midline incision, the cecum of each mouse was exposed and ligated below the ileocecal valve permitting intestinal continuity. The cecum was then punctured twice with a 22-gauge needle and returned to the peritoneal cavity and the abdominal incision was closed in layers. Saline (3 ml/100 g body weight) was given subcutaneously at that time. Food and water were allowed ad lib and survival was measured over a period of 6 days. The results indicated that the mortality rate of controls (not subjected to previous hemorrhage) was 58% whereas in the posthemorrhage and resuscitated animals it was 100% (Stephan et al. 1987 a).

We also examined the effects of ATP-$MgCl_2$ as an immunomodulator following hemorrhage. In these studies, the mice were bled to a mean blood pressure of 35 mmHg and maintained at that level for 1 h. One group of mice then received ATP-$MgCl_2$ (0.1 ml volume, 10 µmol each) along with the resuscitation fluid, whereas the second group received an equivalent volume of saline. On day 1 following hemorrhage and resuscitation with and without ATP-$MgCl_2$, the spleens were harvested and IL-2 measured in supernatants of concanavalin A-stimulated splenic cells. The results indicated that the profoundly depressed IL-2 production following hemorrhage (7% of control) was restored to 89% of control in the group of animals which received ATP-$MgCl_2$ following hemorrhage. Thus, ATP-$MgCl_2$ given as an adjunct to the resuscitation fluid in the hemorrhaged animals leads to a marked restoration of IL-2 levels (Stephan et al. 1987 b).

Discussion

The mouse hemorrhage model used in our study is to the best of our knowledge the first experimental model in which controlled hemorrhage was induced in this rodent species. Although excellent surgical skills are required to cannulate the femoral arteries of mice for bleeding and reinfusion of blood volume, this non-lethal and reproducible hemorrhage model offers advantages of investigating in a comprehensive manner the direct effects of hemorrhage (without major tissue trauma) on immunological responses.

The animals used in our studies were C3H/HEJ mice, a murine strain considered to be endotoxin tolerant (Watson and Riblet 1974). This feature was considered important since hemorrhage leading to hypotension renders the gut more permeable to intestinal flora (Mittermayer and Riede 1982). In the endotoxin-non-tolerant mice, the concentration of bacteria and endotoxin in the portal system would be expected to increase, thus making the animals more susceptible to septic complications following hemorrhage. The use of C3H/HEJ mice would therefore permit one to examine the effects of hemorrhage per se without the additional effects of endotoxemia/bacteremia on the immune system. It could be argued that because of this feature, i.e., endotoxin tolerance, the effects observed in these mice may be peculiar to this strain. This argument is not valid, however, since this strain of mice is immunocompetent and does not demonstrate any abnormalities with respect to any other signals that lead to activation of the immune system (Rosenstreich et al. 1978). Thus, it would appear that the utilization of such a mouse strain would be more of an advantage than of a disadvantage for studying specifically the effects of hemorrhage itself. Another major advantage of this model is that it allows the use of well-standardized immunological assays, some of which are available at present only in the murine species. The more comprehensive examination of the complex immunological interaction is thus possible in future studies. In addition, the hemorrhage model used was not severe enough to produce any mortality. Thus, the model used is of clinical relevance since hemorrhage is frequently encountered not only in surgical procedures but also following trauma.

The results demonstrated that profound depression of T-cell blastogenesis in response to mitogenic stimulation with concanavalin A occurred on day 1 following hemorrhage despite adequate resuscitation. The data obtained from mitogen activation assay also indicated that a slow and gradual reversible loss of immunoresponsiveness takes place with the progression of time following hemorrhage and resuscitation. These findings concur with the results seen with the allogeneic mixed lymphocyte reaction and indicate that immunocompetency is adversely affected in the very early phase following hemorrhage despite volume resuscitation. Subsequent improvement of the proliferative responses, however, was seen and by day 9 following resuscitation the responses were normal. Thus, unlike burn injury, in which the earliest immunosuppression was seen at day 3, marked immunosuppression was observed immediately following hemorrhage and even at day 1 following hemorrhage despite adequate resuscitation.

Since the model utilized required the use of anesthesia, heparin and reinfusion of shed blood, it could be argued that the use of ether, heparin, or reinfusion of shed blood rather than hemorrhage per se might be responsible for the observed immunosuppression. Studies have, however, indicated that the use of ether during cannulation was not the cause of the immunosuppression observed following hemorrhage (Stephan et al. 1987a). Furthermore, the results indicated that heparin did not depress lymphocyte function (Stephan et al. 1987a). In addition, no differences in the immunoresponsiveness was observed following hemorrhage irrespective of whether fresh syngeneic blood or the remaining shed blood was administered following hemorrhage (Stephan et al. 1987a, 1988a). Although the studies of Waymack et al. (1986) have shown that whole blood transfusion following thermal injury caused a further impairment in CMI, it is unlikely that it was responsible for the observed immunosuppression following hemorrhage. This was due to the fact that blood was not kept in the syringe for more than 1 h in our studies, whereas it was stored in acid citrate solution at 2 °C for 2 days before transfusion in the above study. Thus, it is possible that the combination of storing the blood in acid citrate solution and the significantly longer storage period might be responsible for the immunosuppression seen in the study of Waymack et al. (1986). In view of the information provided above, it could be concluded that hemorrhage per se rather than ether, heparin, and the transfusion of remaining shed blood was responsible for producing the marked and prolonged immunosuppression following hemorrhage.

Since in most of the studies described above the spleen cells were utilized for measuring the immune responses, it is possible that hemorrhage causes a redistribution of cells such that the results in the spleen may not be representative in other lymphoid organs. Utilizing the fluorescence-activated cell sorter (FACS) technique, the different subpopulations of spleen cells obtained from posthemorrhage and nonhemorrhaged animals were quantitated. The results demonstrated that the splenic population did not undergo a redistribution compared to the control or sham-operated animals (unpublished observations). Thus, it could be concluded that hemorrhage does not lead to mobilization of the spleen cells into the circulation.

The precise mechanisms that lead to the functional impairment of the immune system during and following hemorrhage are not clearly understood. It would be pertinent, however, to discuss the factors that might be responsible for producing immunosuppression following hemorrhage.

Since increased secretion of corticosteroids into the blood stream occurs as a result of hemorrhage (Hume and Nelson 1954), and steroids have been implicated as potent agents that depress T-cell blastogenic transformation when activated with mitogen (Gillis et al. 1979), it is possible that the increased corticosteroid levels during hemorrhage might be responsible for the observed immunosuppression. This possibility, however, seems unlikely for the prolonged immunosuppression seen following hemorrhage since the stimulus for increased production and release of steroids, i.e., low blood flow, should be removed following appropriate resuscitation (Trachte 1983).

Studies have shown that administration of epinephrine in healthy men not only altered the mitogen-induced proliferation capacity of lymphocytes but also produced changes in the ratio of different subsets of lymphocytes (Crary et al. 1983 a, b). This shift in the subset of T-cells is being suggested as the event that leads to the reduction of mitogen responses either when epinephrine is administered or when epinephrine is secreted in large amounts due to stress. It is unlikely, however, that increased catacholamine secretion is responsible for the immunoresponsiveness seen in our study, since a sharp decline in the epinephrine levels occurs rapidly following adequate resuscitation (Beck 1955).

Factors ranging in molecular weight between 10000 and 30000 daltons have been isolated from the serum of traumatized patients and have been shown to suppress mitogen induced lymphocyte proliferation (Wolfe et al. 1981). In our model of hemorrhage, however, the presence or absence of serum factors was not measured, and therefore the possibility that such factors might be responsible for producing immunosuppression following hemorrhage cannot be ruled out. Although the studies of Abraham and Chang (1986) suggest that suppressive serum factors may be present during hemorrhage, it is unlikely that such serum factors are responsible for the immunosuppression seen 3–5 days following hemorrhage. This is due to the fact that the animals were resuscitated adequately following hemorrhage and, thus, the stimulus for the production of such factors should have been eliminated.

Studies have also shown that prostaglandin production and secretion are significantly enhanced by stimuli such as hemorrhage, hypoxia, and ischemia (Lefer 1983). Prostaglandins have been shown to inhibit lymphocyte function by elevating cyclic AMP levels (Smith et al. 1971). Moreover, studies have demonstrated that incubation of glass-adherent splenic T cells with PGE_2 leads to elaboration of a factor that suppresses PHA-induced mitogenesis (Rogers et al. 1980). In view of this, we attempted to determine whether the antigen presenting cell function of MO is altered following hemorrhage. The role of MO as an antigen presenting cell cannot be overemphasized since such a cellular interaction between MO and a T helper cell is a catalytic signal which triggers subsequent secretory and cellular events in response to antigeneic stimulation, thus making a CMI response possible (Unanue 1981). Our results indicate that antigen presentation by MO following hemorrhage is defective despite adequate resuscitation. To determine the potential reasons for this, in vitro experiments were conducted. The results of those studies indicated that PGE_2 down-regulated antigen presentation function of the PMO. This effect was not seen when PGE_2 was replaced by TXB_2. It should also be pointed out that the concentrations of PGE_2 and TXB_2 used in our studies (Stephan et al. 1988 b) are within the physiological range, which varies from about 10^{-11} *M* to as high as 10^{-7} *M* in inflamed tissue sites (Lefer 1983). Thus, our data suggest that PGE_2 at concentrations which are observed during shock and ischemia may depress MO antigen presenting cell function. The defective AP function by MO following hemorrhage could very well be the mechanism which could explain the state of immunosuppression and enhanced susceptibility to sepsis.

Defective antigen presentation function could suggest that antigen-specific activation of the T helper cell is inadequate to promote the production and release of IL-2 which is responsible for the induction of the antigen specific clonal T-cell proliferation. In this regard, PGE_2 has been recently shown to directly suppress IL-2 production by T lymphocytes (Faist et al. 1987). Our results have also shown that IL-2 production by splenocytes following hemorrhage was profoundly depressed despite adequate resuscitation (Stephan et al. 1986).

Since our studies demonstrated depressed immunoresponsiveness following hemorrhage, experiments were conducted to determine whether such animals are more susceptible to sepsis. The results clearly indicated that even 3 days following hemorrhage and resuscitation, a severely compromised host defense system exists due to defective antigen presentation function by MO and depressed proliferation of T lymphocytes, which produces the state of immunosuppression and enhances susceptibility to sepsis. In light of the above-presented results, an hypothesis can be formulated to explain in part the profound immunocompromise and ensuing septic complications in traumatized individuals. Our hypothesis is that massive stimulation of the macrophage in the setting of trauma along with the simultaneous persistent bacterial challenge causes a heightened synthesis of the inhibitory immunomodulator, PGE_2, as well as a decrease in the degradation rate of PGE_2, thus promoting a down-regulatory response of the specific immune system. The consequences of such an event would be the increased susceptibility to sepsis.

With regard to the potential explanation for the generalized effects of pure hemorrhage on immunological alteration, our hypothesis is that even a transient decrease in blood flow during hemorrhage causes a decrease in high-energy phosphate compounds in immunologic organs, which persists for a prolonged period of time despite adequate resuscitation. This may very well be responsible for the significant and prolonged depression of cell-mediated immunity following hemorrhage. In support of this hypothesis are our findings which demonstrated that administration of ATP-$MgCl_2$ following hemorrhage led to marked restoration of IL-2 levels (Stephan et al. 1987b). Whether this is due to provision of energy to the immunologic organs, improvement in blood flow, membrane effects (Chaudry 1983) or mobilization of calcium remains to be determined.

Conclusions

Available evidence indicates that simple hemorrhage (without major tissue trauma) that produces a sustained but nonlethal hypotension profoundly impairs the proliferative responses of T lymphocytes to mitogen and alloantigens, depresses antigen presentation by splenic and peritoneal macrophages, produces a defect in IL-2 generation, and increases the susceptibility to sepsis. In view of this, any additional trauma, i.e., thermal injury or other extensive tissue trauma, would be expected to have an additive effect on immunosuppression when associated with hemorrhage. Therefore, septic complications would be expected to occur more frequently when a combination of hemorrhage and other injuries occur. Administration of ATP-$MgCl_2$ as an adjunct to the resuscitation solution following hemorrhage leads to marked restoration of IL-2 levels. Thus, the increased susceptibility to sepsis following hemorrhage could be decreased by the use of ATP-$MgCl_2$ as an adjunct to the resuscitation fluid.

Acknowledgements. The authors wish to express their thanks to Mrs. Mary Kelly for her skill in typing this manuscript and Mrs. Sharon Waite for editorial assistance. This work was supported by USPHS grants GM37127 and GM39519.

References

Abraham E, Chang Y (1985) The effects of hemorrhage on mitogen-induced lymphocyte proliferation. Circ Shock 15:141

Abraham E, Chang Y (1986) Cellular and humoral bases of hemorrhage-induced depression of lymphocyte function. Crit Care Med 14:81

Alexander JW, Ogle CK, Stinnett JD et al. (1978) A sequential, prospective analysis of immunologic abnormalities and infection following severe thermal injury. Ann Surg 188:809

Alexander JW, Dwight J, Stinnett JD et al. (1979) A comparison of immunologic profiles and their influence of bacteremia in surgical patients with a high risk of infection. Surgery 188:94

Antonacci AC (1986) Immune dysfunction and immunomodulation following trauma. In: Gallis JI, Fauci AS, Davis JM, Shires GT (eds) Advances in host defense mechanisms: host defenses in trauma and surgery, vol 6. Raven, New York, pp 81–109

Baker CC, Opponheimer L, Lewis FR et al. (1980) The epidemiology of trauma death. Am J Surg 140:144

Baker CC, Degutis LC, DeSantis JG et al. (1985) The impact of a trauma service in a University Hospital. Am J Surg 149:453

Baue AE, Chaudry IH (1980) Prevention of multiple systems failure. Surg Clin North Am 60:1167

Beck L, Dontas AS (1955) Vasomotor activity in hemorrhagic shock. Fed Proc 14:318

Bjornson AB, Altemeir WA, Bjornson HS (1978) Host defense against opportunistic micro-organisms following trauma: 1. Studies to determine the association between changes in humoral components of host defense and septicemia in burned patients. Ann Surg 188:93

Chaudry IH (1983) Cellular mechanisms of shock and ischemia and their correction. Am J Physiol 245:R117

Chaudry IH, Kupper TS, Schleck S et al. (1982) Impairment of reticuloendothelial function following thermal injury and its restoration with ATP-$MgCl_2$ administration. Circ Shock 9:297

Christou NV, MacLean L, Meakins JL (1980) Host defense in blunt trauma: interrelationships of kinetics of anergy and depressed neutrophil function: nutritional status and sepsis. J Trauma 20:833

Crary B, Borysenko M, Sutherland DC et al. (1983a) Decrease in mitogen responsiveness of mononuclear cells from peripheral blood after epinephrine administration in humans. J Immunol 130:694

Crary B, Hauser SL, Borysenko M et al. (1983b) Epinephrine-induced changes in the distribution of lymphocyte subsets in peripheral blood of humans. J Immunol 131:1178

Deitch EA, Gelder F, McDonald JC (1982) Prognostic significance of abnormal neutrophil chemotaxis after thermal injury. J Trauma 22:199

Faist E, Kupper TS, Baker CC et al. (1986) Depression of cellular immunity after major injury: its association with post-traumatic complications and its restoration with immunomodulating agents. Arch Surg 121:1000

Faist E, Mewes A, Baker CC et al. (1987) Prostaglandin E_2 dependent suppression of interleukin-2 production in patients with major trauma. J Trauma 28:837

Faist E, Mews A, Strasser T et al. (1988) Alteration of monocyte function following major injury. Arch Surg 123:287

Gillis S, Crabtree GR, Smith KA (1979) Glucocorticoid-induced inhibition of T-cell growth factor production: I. The effect on mitogen-induced lymphocyte proliferation. J Immunol 123:1624

Hume DM, Nelson DH (1954) Adrenal cortical function in surgical shock. Surg Forum 5:568

Keane RM, Birmingham W, Shatney CM et al. (1983a) Prediction of sepsis in the multitraumatic patients by assays of lymphocyte dysfunction. Surg Gynecol Obstet 156:163

Keane RM, Munster AM, Birmingham W et al. (1983b) Suppressor cell activity after major injury: indirect and direct functional assays. J Trauma 22:770

Kupper TS, Green DR (1984) Immunoregulation after thermal injury: sequential appearance of I-J+, LY-1 T suppressor inducer cells and LY-2 T suppressor effector cells following thermal trauma in mice. J Immunol 135:3047

Kupper TS, Green DR, Chaudry IH et al. (1984) A cyclophosphamide-sensitive suppressor T-cell circuit induced by thermal trauma. Surgery 95:699

Kupper TS, Green DR, Durum SK et al. (1985) Defective antigen presentation to a cloned T helper cell by macrophages from burned mice can be restored with interleukin-1. Surgery 98:199

Lefer AM (1983) Role of prostaglandins and thromboxanes in shock. In: Altura BM, Lefer AM, Schumer W (eds) The handbook of shock and trauma, vol 1. Raven, New York, p 355

McIrvine AJ, O'Mahony JB, Saporoschetz I et al. (1982) Depressed immune response in burn patients: use of monoclonal antibodies and functional assays to define the role of suppressor cells. Ann Surg 196:297

Miller SE, Miller LS, Trunkey DD (1982) The immune consequences of trauma. Surg Clin North Am 62:167

Mittermayer C, Riede UN (1982) Human pathology of the gastrointestinal tract in shock, ischemia, and hypoxemia. In: Cowley RA, Trump BE (eds) Pathophysiology of shock, anoxia and ischemia, 1st edn. Williams and Wilkins, Baltimore, pp 301–308

Munster AW (1976) Posttraumatic immunosuppression is due to activation of suppressor T cells. Lancet 1:1329

Ninneman JL, Stockland AE (1984) Participation of prostaglandin E in immunosuppression following thermal injury. J Trauma 24:201

O'Mahony Palder SB, Wood FF, McIrvine A et al. (1984) Depression of cellular immunity after multiple trauma in the absence of sepsis. J Trauma 24:869

Rogers TJ, Nowowiejski I, Webb DR (1980) Partial characterization of a prostaglandin-induced suppressor factor. Cell Immunol 50:82

Rosenstreich DL, Vogel SN, Jacques AR et al. (1978) Macrophage sensitivity to endotoxin: genetic control by a single codominant gene. J Immunol 121:1664

Saba TM (1986) Organ failure with sepsis after trauma or burn: support of the reticuloendothelial host-defense system. In: Sibbald WJ, Sprung CL (eds) Prospectives on sepsis and septic shock. Soc Crit Care Med, California, pp 77–95

Shires GT (1985) Principles and management of hemorrhagic shock: principles of trauma care, 3rd edn. McGraw-Hill, New York, p 3

Smith J, Steiner A, Parker C (1971) Human lymphocyte metabolism: effects of cyclic and noncyclic adenosine monophosphate on stimulation by phytohemagglutinin. J Clin Invest 50:442–448

Stephan RN, Conrad PJ, Janeway CA et al. (1986) Decreased interleukin-2 production following simple hemorrhage. Surg Forum 37:73

Stephan RN, Kupper TS, Geha AS et al. (1987a) Hemorrhage without tissue trauma produces immunosuppression and enhances susceptibility to sepsis. Arch Surg 122:62

Stephan RN, Janeway CA, Dean RE et al. (1987b) Decreased interleukin-2 (IL-2) production following simple hemorrhage and its restoration with ATP-$MgCl_2$ treatment. Magnesium 6:163

Stephan RN, Kisala JM, Dean RE et al. (1988a) Effect of blood transfusion on antigen presentation function and on interleukin-2 generation. Arch Surg 123:235

Stephan RN, Conrad PH, Saizawa M et al. (1988b) Prostaglandin E_2 depresses antigen presenting cell function of peritoneal macrophages. J Surg Res (in press)

Trachte G (1983) Endocrinology of shock. In: Altura BM, Lefer AM, Schumer W (eds) Basic science. Raven, New York, pp 337–354 (Handbook of shock and trauma, vol 1)

Trunkey DD (1982) Overview of trauma. Surg Clin North Am 62:3
Trunkey DD (1983) Trauma. Sci Am 249:28
Unanue ER (1981) Symbiotic relationship between lymphocytes and macrophages. Adv Immunol 31:1
Unanue ER, Beller DI, Lu CT et al. (1984) Antigen presentation: comments on its regulation and mechanism. J Immunol 132:1
Wang BS, Heacock EH, Wu WVO et al. (1980) Generation of suppressor cells in mice after surgical trauma. J Clin Invest 66:200
Watson J, Riblet R (1974) Genetic control of responses to bacterial lipopolysaccharides in mice. J Exp Med 140:1147
Waymack JP, Rapien J, Garnett D et al. (1986) Effect of transfusion on immune function in a traumatized animal model. Arch Surg 121:50
Wolfe JHN, Saporoschetz I, Young AE et al. (1981) Suppressive serum, suppressor lymphocytes and death from burns. Ann Surg 193:513

Blood Transfusions: The Immunologic Sequelae *

J. P. Waymack, G. S. Branfman, and B. A. Pruitt

Prior to the 1970s, it was believed that the administration of blood products to patients resulted in an immunostimulatory effect. This theory was based on two observations. The first was the widely established principle that the administration of incompatible red blood cells generated a strong immunologic reaction which resulted in massive red blood cell lysis (Landsteiner 1900). The second was the demonstration by Medawar that the administration of white blood cells obtained from a specific donor caused an immunization of the recipient that generated a more rapid rejection of skin allografts harvested from the same donor (Medawar 1946). These findings led transplant surgeons to avoid transfusing patients who were awaiting solid organ allografts. This policy continued until the early 1970s when a number of retrospective human studies and experimental animal work demonstrated that pretransplant transfusions decreased the rate and severity of allograft rejection (Halasz et al. 1964; Jenkins and Woodruff 1971; Fabre and Morris 1972; Opelz et al. 1973). As of 1985, there were more than 68 reports documenting that pretransplant transfusions decreased the rate of rejection of transplanted organs (Tiwari 1985).

There have been three hypotheses proposed to explain the beneficial transfusion effect (Waymack and Alexander 1986). The first was a selection hypothesis which stated that those patients more likely to eventually reject a transplant were also more likely to form cytotoxic antibodies in response to the transfusion. With the development of such antibodies, these patients were denied transplantation. The transfusions thus selected out those patients most likely to undergo eventual rejection of the transplanted organ. The second hypothesis was that the transfusions elicited production of an antiidiotypic antibody which protected the donor tissue from the recipient's immune system. Although both these hypotheses may play a role in the beneficial transfusion effect, it has now been demonstrated that the most important component of the transfusion effect is its suppression of the recipient's immune system (Waymack and Alexander 1986).

Once the immunosuppressive effect of transfusions in the transplant population was unequivocally established, a number of retrospective studies were carried out to determine the effect of transfusion on the host response to tumors. There have been 13 such reports evaluating the effect of perioperative transfusions on the rate of tumor growth and metastases in patients undergoing oncologic oper-

* The opinions or assertions contained herein are the private views of the authors and are not to be construed as official or as reflecting the views of the Department of the Army or the Department of Defense.

Immune Consequences of
Trauma, Shock and Sepsis
Eds. Faist/Ninnemann/Green

Table 1. Five-year survival following tumor resection: transfusion versus no transfusion

Investigators	Tumor type/ stage	Number of patients	Five-year survival rate (%)		P value
			Transfused	Not transfused	
Burrows and Tartter (1982)	Colon dukes $B_2C_1C_2$	122	51	84	=0.005
Agarwar and Blumberg (1983)	Colon dukes ABC	197	48	91	<0.005
Foster et al. (1985)	Colon dukes ABC	146	51	68	=0.03
Ota et al. (1984)	Colon dukes ABC	207	72	77	ns
Nathanson et al. (1984)	Colon/rectum all stages	366	43	57	ns
Tartter et al. (1984)	Lung stage I	165	62	75	=0.013
Hyman et al. (1985)	Lung stages I, II	95	27	44	=0.03
Nowack and Ponsky (1984)	Breast stages I–III	81	48	80	=0.03
Tartter et al. (1984)	Breast stages I–III	169	51	65	=0.002
Foster et al. (1984)	Breast stages I–IV	226	80	80	=0.082
Rosenberg et al. (1985)	Extremity sarcoma high grade	156	63	85	=0.004

ations (Waymack and Alexander 1986). Nine of these 13 reports demonstrated decreased long-term survival rates and increased rates of tumor recurrence in those patients receiving perioperative transfusions (Burrows and Tartter 1982; Agarwal and Blumberg 1983; Burrows and Tartter 1983; Tartter et al. 1983; Nowak and Ponsky 1984; Tartter et al. 1984; Foster et al. 1985; Hyman et al. 1985; Rosenberg et al. 1985). The remaining four failed to document any correlation (Foster et al. 1983; Foster et al. 1984; Nathanson et al. 1985; Ota et al. 1985). Table 1 summarizes these reports (excluding those which utilized the same data twice).

The possibility that those patients with more advanced tumors required a greater quantity of the transfusions necessitated the use of animals, which received equal amounts of tumor challenges, to confirm a detrimental transfusion effect. Francis et al. (1981) first reported that allogeneic transfusions increased the rate of tumor growth in rats. More recently, Francis et al. (1987) demonstrated that the detrimental transfusion effect was not seen when using athymic mice. This finding emphasizes the necessity of the presence of an intact immune system in order to elicit the posttransfusion immunosuppressive effect (Foster et al. 1985).

With the demonstration of the beneficial immunosuppressive effect of transfusions in the transplant population and the detrimental effect of such transfusions in oncologic patients, recent investigations have centered on the effect of transfusions on resistance to bacterial infections. Tartter et al. (1986) evaluated the effect of perioperative blood transfusions on the rate of infectious complications in patients undergoing colon cancer surgery. They noted a 7% incidence of infectious complications in patients who did not receive perioperative transfusions. This increased to 25% in patients who were administered blood products during the perioperative period ($P = 0.01$). They also noted that the mean number of transfusions in patients who developed postoperative infections was 2.14 units as compared to 0.82 units in patients who failed to develop such infections ($P = 0.0005$).

To exclude the possibility that the transfusions were necessitated by a more serious overall condition of these patients and that this explained the higher infection rate rather than any immunosuppressive properties of the blood, they examined a number of other variables in their patient population. These variables uniformly failed to show any significant differences between infected and noninfected patients. These included comparisons between infected and noninfected patients with regard to age ($P = 0.78$), sex ($P = 0.95$), degree of tumor differentiation ($P = 0.42$), presence of positive lymph nodes ($P = 0.17$), tumor state ($P = 0.36$), duration of surgery ($P = 0.34$), tumor size ($P = 0.70$), and length of colon specimen ($P = 0.33$). It was also noted that the amount of intraoperative blood loss did not correlate with the development of infections ($P = 0.29$). Tartter et al. (1986) have confirmed that the logical, but startling, conclusion from this data is true, the amount of blood loss does not correlate with the use of perioperative transfusions.

Tartter et al. (1987) also examined the incidence of postoperative infections in patients with Crohn's disease who required surgical intervention. They noted a 26% infection rate in patients who received 2 or more units of blood in the perioperative period as compared to 8% among patients who received 0–1 units of blood ($P = 0.0014$). As in the colon cancer review, evaluation of all other variables failed to demonstrate any significant differences between the groups of patients who developed postoperative infections and those who did not.

Dellinger et al. (1987) prospectively evaluated the risk of developing infections in patients with open fractures of the lower extremities. They noted a 20% infection rate in patients who required perioperative transfusions as compared to 8% in patients not requiring perioperative transfusions ($P < 0.05$).

Graves et al. (unpublished data) reviewed the infection rate for burn patients treated from 1982 to 1986. They documented that in patients with 10%–70% total body surface area burns, the use of blood transfusions was associated with an increased incidence of both invasive burn wound infection and pneumonia.

A multicenter study of patients who had penetrating abdominal trauma found that patients who received transfusions in the perioperative period had a higher infection rate than did those who were not given blood products (Nichols et al. 1984).

It may be argued that human studies cannot exclude the possibility that the more seriously ill patients require a greater quantity of the transfusions and thus the higher incidence of infections were not caused by the transfusions but rather by the patients' overall poorer condition. There have been a number of animal studies which have attempted to answer such criticisms. In one, rats were subjected to a 30% total body surface area scald burn and randomized to receive either allogeneic blood, syngeneic blood, or saline on the day of burn injury (Waymack et al. 1987a). The animals' burn wounds were infected with *Pseudomonas aeruginosa* 24 h postinjury. The survival curves for these animals are shown in Fig. 1. The mean survival times were 26.05 ± 0.73 days for the saline group,

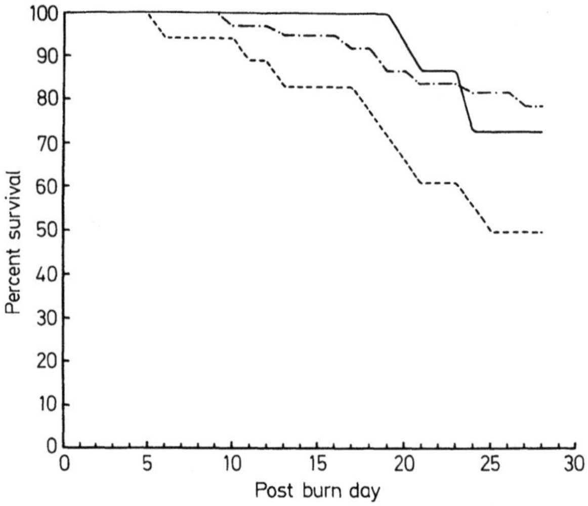

Fig. 1. Survival curves for animals given saline (*dotted line*), syngeneic Lewis blood (*solid line*), or allogeneic ACI blood (*dashed line*) the day of burn injury and then challenged with *Pseudomonas aerguinosa* 24 h later

Table 2. Effect of varying number and volume of transfusions on susceptibility to infectious complications (mean ± standard error)

Group	Mean survival time (days)	Percent survival
Saline control	24.85 ± 0.88	78
Single 0.1-ml transfusion	20.48 ± 1.37	40
Single 1.0-ml transfusion	19.67 ± 0.74	31
Three 1.0-ml transfusions	19.39 ± 1.00	24

26.86 ± 0.68 days for the syngeneic blood group, and 22.72 ± 1.47 days with allogeneic blood ($P < 0.029$).

Since it is well recognized that increasing the number of pretransplant blood transfusions decreases the rate of rejection in an additive manner (Tiwari 1985), Waymack et al. (1987 b) investigated the effect of varying the number and volume of transfusions on the susceptibility to infections. In this study, rats received either saline, a single 0.1-ml allogeneic transfusion, a single 1.0-ml allogeneic transfusion, or three 1.0-ml allogeneic transfusions. The mean survival times and absolute survival rates for these animals are listed in Table 2. Although there was a slight increase in mortality as the number and volume of transfusions increased, these changes did not achieve statistical significance.

Both of the above studies required an immunosuppressive burn injury in addition to the transfusion to demonstrate mortality. More recent work has indicated that the transfusion effect exists even without burn injury. Rats administered allogeneic blood immediately prior to a peritoneal challenge of *Escherichia coli* have been shown to have a significantly diminished mean survival time and absolute survival rate compared to rats which received syngeneic blood or saline (Fig. 2) (Waymack et al. 1987 c).

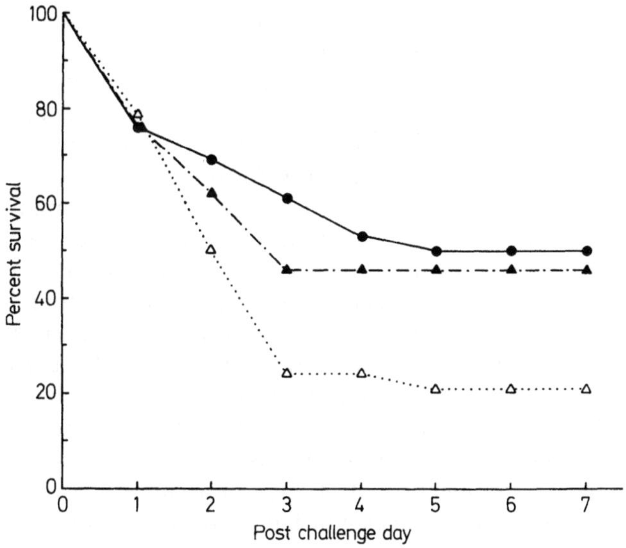

Fig. 2. Survival curves for animals challenged with *Escherichia coli* for the day of administration of saline (●), syngeneic Lewis blood (▲), or allogeneic ACI blood (△)

Investigations into the possible mechanisms by which transfusions increase susceptibility to infectious complications have identified a number of possible causes. Transfusions have been demonstrated in animal models to increase the production of the immunosuppressive arachidonic acid metabolite prostaglandin E (Webb and Osheroff 1976; Waymack et al. 1986a; Waymack et al. 1987d). Blood transfusions have also been shown to impair the normal macrophage/lymphocyte interaction necessary for lymphocyte blastogenic response following exposure to foreign antigens (Waymack et al. 1986b). This impairment can be achieved through the addition of either macrophages obtained from transfused rats or supernatants obtained from the same macrophages. Such macrophages, when infused into nontransfused rats, decreased their ability to resist bacterial infections (Waymack, unpublished data). Macrophages obtained from allogeneically transfused rats have also been shown to have an impaired ability to phagocytize and kill bacteria (Waymack and Yurt, unpublished data). Further evidence of a posttransfusion impairment in macrophage function has been provided by the demonstration that rats which received allogeneic transfusions have a decreased cell-mediated immune response as measured by skin swelling to cutaneous application of hapten dinitrofluorobenzene. Neutrophils did not appear to be adversely affected by allogeneic transfusion in this rat model (Waymack et al. 1986c).

Lymphocyte abnormalities have also been demonstrated in mice following transfusion. Stephen et al. (1988) showed a 70% decrease in interleukin 2 production within three days of transfusion. Multiple transfusions resulted in an additive suppressive effect on its production.

Similar studies on immune function following blood transfusions have been performed in humans who suffer from various anemias. These reports have generated results that are nearly identical to those obtained from experimental animal work. Chronic renal failure patients were documented to have an increased prostaglandin E production (Lenhard et al. 1985) and a decreased cell mediated immune response (Watson et al. 1979) following transfusions. Lymphocytes obtained from transfused patients have been shown to have a decreased blastogenic response compared to those obtained prior to the transfusion (Lenhard et al. 1983). The CD4/CD8 T-lymphocyte ratio has been demonstrated to be diminished in patients who receive transfusions as compared to those with the same blood dyscrasias who do not receive transfusions (Luban et al. 1983; Kaplan et al. 1984). Gascon et al. (1984), in a review of sickle cell anemia patients, found that those who required transfusions had a 50% reduction in their natural killer cell function as compared to those not receiving blood transfusions. Finally, it has been shown that transfusions decrease the serum level of the opsonic protein fibronectin (Synder et al. 1981). Such a decrease in fibronectin may impair phagocytosis of any invading microorganism and thereby increase the susceptibility of the transfusion recipient to the development of infectious complications.

Although studies on the immunologic sequelae of blood transfusion are still in their infancy, the large number of recent reports on the immunosuppressive effect of such transfusions should influence all physicians to consider carefully the necessity for transfusing their patients. When transfusions are essential to maintain adequate hemodynamics and tissue oxygenation, a method for infusing blood without resulting in immunosuppression in the transfusion recipient must be sought. Two possible solutions appear feasible from the preliminary human and animal work.

Since allogeneic transfusions have been repeatedly shown to immunosuppress animals while syngeneic transfusions do not, it appears that exposure of the transfusion recipient to foreign histocompatibility antigens is required to result in posttransfusion immunosuppression. If blood can be administered without exposing the recipient to such foreign antigens, then the blood may be safely administered without compromising immune function in the patient. Frozen washed red blood cells lack such foreign histocompatibility antigens and may, therefore, offer a possible alternative in the anemic, hemodynamically unstable patient. Support for this concept comes from transplantation literature which has documented that frozen washed red blood cells do not result in the beneficial effect generated by whole blood or packed cells (Tiwari 1985). Additional support comes from the finding that the administration of human leucocyte antigen (HLA)-matched blood fails to result in the decreased allograft rejection rate seen with the use of HLA unmatched blood (Albert et al. 1981).

The second possible means of transfusing without immunosuppressing the patient involves the use of autotransfusions. This may be achieved by having the patient donate blood prior to surgery and then transfusing this, the patient's own blood, at the time of surgery. Since the blood cells are the patient's own, there will be no foreign histocompatibility antigens to trigger the posttransfusion immunosuppression.

In conclusion, blood transfusions appear to generate a broad, wide spectrum immunosuppression in the transfusion recipient. This immunosuppression can be used to decrease the rate of allograft rejection in transplant patients. In nontransplant patients, the immunosuppression can result in undesirable sequelae. These include the development of cancer metastases and a higher infection rate. Preliminary investigations into alternate methods of infusing red blood cells without generating an immunosuppressive effect appear promising.

References

Albert ED, Scholz S, Meixner U, Land W (1981) HLA-A, B matching of pretransplant blood transfusion is associated with poor graft survival. Transplant Proc 13:175–177

Agarwal M, Blumberg N (1983) Colon cancer-patients transfused perioperatively have an increased incidence of recurrence (abstract). Transfusion 23:421

Burrows L, Tartter P (1982) Effect of blood transfusions on colonic malignancy recurrence rate (letter). Lancet 2:662

Burrows L, Tartter P (1983) Blood transfusions and colorectal-cancer recurrence – a possible relationship (abstract). Transfusion 23:419

Dellinger EP, Caplan ES, Weaver L, Wertz MJ, Droppert B, Hoyt N, Brumback R, Burgess A, Poka A, Benirschke SR, Lennard ES, Mou MA (1988) Duration of preventive antibiotic administration for open extremity fractures. Arch Surg 12:333–339

Fabre JW, Morris PJ (1972) The effect of donor strain blood pretreatment on renal allograft rejection in rats. Transplantation 14:608–617

Foster RS, Foster JC, Costanza JC (1983) Do blood transfusions have an adverse effect on survival after mastectomy for breast cancer? Proceedings American Society of Clinical Oncology nineteenth annual meeting, abstract C-234, 23 March 1983

Foster RS Jr, Foster JC, Costanza MC (1984) Blood transfusions and survival after surgery for breast cancer. Arch Surg 119:1138–1140

Foster RS Jr, Costanza MC, Foster JC, Wanner MC, Foster CB (1985) Adverse relationship between blood transfusions and survival after colectomy for colon cancer. Cancer 55:1195–1201

Francis DMA, Shenton BK (1981) Blood transfusion and tumor growth: evidence from laboratory animals. Lancet 2:871

Francis DMA, Burren CP, Clunie GJA (1987) Acceleration of B16 melanoma growth in mice after blood transfusion. Surgery 102:485–492

Gascon P, Zoumbos NC, Young NS (1984) Immunologic abnormalities in patients receiving multiple blood transfusions. Ann Intern Med 100:173–177

Halasz NA, Orloff MJ, Hirose F (1964) Increased survival of renal homografts in dogs after injection of graft donor blood. Transplantation 2:453–458

Hyman NH, Foster RS Jr, DeMeules JE, Costanza MC (1985) Blood transfusions and survival after lung cancer resection. Am J Surg 149:502–507

Jenkins AM, Woodruff MFA (1971) The effect of prior administration of donor strain blood or blood constituents on the survival of cardiac allografts in rats. Transplantation 12:57–60

Kaplan J, Sarnaik S, Gitlin J, Lusher J (1984) Diminished helper/suppressor lymphocyte ratios and natural killer activity in recipients for repeated blood transfusions. Blood 64:308–310

Landsteiner K (1900) Zur Kenntnis der antifermentativen, lytischen und agglutinierenden Wirkungen des Blutserums und der Lymphe. Zentralbl Bakterioli I Abt 27:357–360

Lenhard V, Maassen G, Grossewilde H, Wernet P, Opelz G (1983) Effect of blood transfusions on immunoregulatory mononuclear-cells in prospective transplant recipients. Transplant Proc 15:1011–1015

Lenhard V, Gemsa D, Opelz G (1985) Transfusion-induced release of prostaglandin-E_2 and its role in the activation of T-suppressor cells. Transplant Proc 17:2380–2382

Luban NLC, Kelleher JF Jr, Reaman GH (1983) Altered distribution of T-lymphocyte subpopulations in children and adolescents with haemophilia. Lancet 1:503–505

Medawar PB (1946) Relationship between antigens of blood and skin. Nature 157:161–162

Nathanson SD, Tilley BC, Schultz L, Smith RF (1985) Perioperative allogeneic blood transfusions: survival in patients with resected carcinomas of the colon and rectum. Arch Surg 120:734–738
Nichols RL, Smith JW, Klein DB, Trunkey DD, Cooper RH, Adinolfi MF, Mills J (1984) Risk of infection after penetrating abdominal trauma. N Engl J Med 311:1065–1070
Nowak MM, Ponsky JL (1984) Blood transfusion and disease-free survival in carcinoma of the breast. J Surg Oncol 27:124–130
Opelz G, Sengar DP, Mickey MR, Terasaki PI (1973) Effect of blood transfusions on subsequent kidney transplants. Transplant Proc 5:253–259
Ota D, Alvarez L, Lichtiger B, Giacco G, Guinee V (1985) Perioperative blood transfusion in patients with colon carcinoma. Transfusion 25:392–394
Rosenberg SA, Seipp CA, White DE, Wesley R (1985) Perioperative blood transfusions are associated with increased rates of recurrence and decreased survival in patients with high-grade soft-tissue sarcomas of the extremities. J Clin Oncol 3:698–709
Synder EL, Mosher DF, Hezzey A, Gloenwsky G (1981) Effect of blood transfusion on in vivo levels of plasma fibronectin. J Lab Clin Med 98:336–341
Stephen RN, Kisala JM, Dean RE, Geha AS, Chaudry IH (1988) Effect of blood transfusion on antigen presentation function and on interleukin 2 generation. Arch Surg 123:235–240
Tartter P, Papatestas A, Lesnick G, Burrows L, Aufses A Jr (1983) Breast cancer recurrence is associated with perioperative blood transfusion. Proceedings American Society of Clinical Oncology nineteenth annual meeting, abstract C-198, 23 March 1983
Tartter PI, Burrows L, Kirschner P (1984) Perioperative blood transfusion adversely affects prognosis after resection of Stage I (subset NO) non-oat cell lung cancer. J Thorac Cardiovasc Surg 88:659–662
Tartter PI, Quintero S, Barron DM (1986) Perioperative blood transfusion associated with infectious complications after colorectal cancer operations. Am J Surg 152:479–482
Tartter PI, Dreifuss RM, Malon AM, Heimann TM, Aufses AH (1987) Relationship of postoperative septic complications and blood transfusions in patients with Crohn's disease. Am J Surg 155:43–48
Tiwari JL (1985) Review: kidney transplantation and transfusion. In: Teraski PI (ed) Clinical kidney transplants 1985. UCLA Tissue Typing Laboratory, Los Angeles, p 257
Watson MA, Briggs JD, Diamandopoulos A, Hamilton DNH, Dick HM (1979) Endogenous cell-mediated immunity, blood transfusion, and outcome of renal transplantation. Lancet 2:1323–1326
Waymack JP, Alexander JW (1986) Blood transfusions as an immunomodulator – a review. Comp Immunol Microbiol Infect Dis 9:177–183
Waymack JP, Gallon L, Barcelli U, Alexander JW (1986a) Effect of blood transfusions on macrophage function in a burned animal model. Curr Surg 43:305–307
Waymack JP, Balakrishnan K, McNeal N, Gonce S, Miskell P, Warden GD, Alexander JW (1986b) Effect of blood transfusions on macrophage-lymphocyte interaction in an animal model. Ann Surg 204:681–685
Waymack JP, Metz J, Garnett D, Alexander JW (1986c) Effect of transfusion on immune function in a traumatized animal model. Arch Surg 121:50–55
Waymack JP, Robb E, Alexander JW (1987a) Effect of transfusion on immune function in a traumatized animal model. II. Effect on mortality rate following septic challenge. Arch Surg 122:935–939
Waymack JP, Warden GD, Miskell P, Gonce S, Alexander JW (1987b) Effect of varying number and volume of transfusions on mortality rate following septic challenge in an animal model. World J Surg 11:387–391
Waymack JP, Warden GD, Alexander JW, Miskell P, Gonce S (1987c) Effect of blood transfusion and anesthesia on resistance to bacterial peritonitis. J Surg Res 42:528–535
Waymack JP, Gallon L, Barcelli U, Trocki O, Alexander JW (1987d) Effect of transfusions on immune function. III. Alterations in macrophage arachidonic acid metabolism. Arch Surg 122:56–60
Webb DR, Osheroff PL (1976) Antigen stimulation of prostaglandin synthesis and control of immune responses. Proc Natl Acad Sci USA 73:1300

Nutrition and Resistance to Sepsis *

J. W. Alexander

Famine and pestilence have been partners since antiquity. Yet, except for rare glimpses of insight, it has been only in this century that nutritional status has been shown to influence outcome during medical and surgical therapy and only about 2 decades ago that techniques for intravenous hyperalimentation became generally available and specific defects of cellular immunity were found to be associated with malnutrition.

The first prospective controlled study in man that showed better nutrition was associated with outcome in acute traumatic disease was in 1980, in burned children at the Shriners Burns Institute in Cincinnati [1]. In that study, seriously burned children were randomized into two groups, one of whom received a normal diet supplemented by tube feedings of commercially available enteral formulations while the other group received the same diet but also supplemented with whey protein to achieve a protein intake of 22% of calories. Increasing the amount of protein in the diet significantly improved survival by decreasing the number of septic episodes. Serum concentrations of central nutritional proteins such as transferrin were much better in those patients receiving a high-protein diet, and complex protein functions, exemplified by the opsonic index, improved rapidly in patients on a high-protein diet when compared with patients receiving a normal diet.

Translocation, Hyperalimentation, and Enteral Nutrition

The complexities of clinical studies of nutrition following burn injury led to the development of an animal model to study specific nutrients under highly controlled conditions [2]. This model involved placement of a gastrostomy tube in such a way that the tube exited in the intracapular area so that the animals could move freely about their cages while being fed continuously through a swivel apparatus. After a period of stabilization of 7–10 days after placement of the gastrostomy tubes, 30% total body surface full-thickness flame burns were inflicted. Thereafter, the animals were fed with pump-controlled continuous gastrostomy feedings.

As a part of an overall assessment in these studies, it was noted that animals receiving only lactated Ringer's solution by gastrostomy tube developed a loss of approximately 50% of the mucosal mass in the jejunum during the first 24 h. In

* Supported by NIH Grant AI12936 and the Shriners Burns Institute.

Immune Consequences of
Trauma, Shock and Sepsis
Eds. Faist/Ninnemann/Green

contrast, if full-strength enteral feedings of appropriate composition were begun within 2 h after the burn injury, loss of mucosal mass was insignificant. As might be expected, burn injury was associated with a marked increase in plasma cortisol levels drawn 24 h after the burn in animals given only the lactated Ringer's solution by gastrostomy. In contrast, animals receiving full-strength enteral nutrition immediately after burn injury had minimal rise in plasma cortisol. The same observations were true for plasma glucagon. Perhaps of most interest, both serum cortisol and glucagon levels were inversely related to the jejunal mucosal mass for individual animals ($r > 0.8$, $P < 0.001$). In other words, the stress hormonal response of burn injury could be prevented by early enteral feedings which preserved the mucosal mass of the small intestine. This led to the hypothesis that the hypermetabolic response of burn injury was associated with rapid failure of the barrier function of the intestine [3]. More specifically, it seemed rational that with burn injury there was not only a redistribution of fluid to reduce blood flow to the intestine, but also a lack of effect of luminal nutrition on growth of mucosal epithelial cells with acute failure of the intestinal barrier for luminal contents. When bacteria, endotoxin, and other luminal substances enter directly into the intestinal lymphatic and portal venous systems, there is activation of the complement sequence as well as direct activation of macrophages. Macrophages in turn produce large numbers of cytokines including interleukin 1 and tumor necrosis factor (cachetin), as well as thromboxane and prostaglandin E_2 and other biological mediators. These in turn are key elements in production of both the immunosuppressive effect of burn injury and the hypermetabolic response as shown by Roderick, Mannick, and Wilmore and reported elsewhere in this symposium. These cytokines act at least in part through neuromediators which have a secondary effect on the generalized neuroendocrine system.

This hypothesis has been largely validated. Arita et al. [4] have shown that continuous administration of low-dose endotoxin induces hypermetabolism when infused slowly into the portal vein with an osmotic pump. In those studies, the level of endotoxin was directly proportionate to the metabolic rate 3 days after induction of the infusion. Studies in Deitch's lab using *E. coli* [5] and in our laboratory using *Candida albicans* [6] have shown that translocation of viable organisms increased with major burn injury. Using the *C. albicans* model of translocation described by Inoue [6], *C. albicans* appeared to pass directly through the mucosal cells to enter the lamina propria where they are rapidly ingested by macrophages. Viable organisms are then transported directly to the regional lymph nodes, where they are felt to be located primarily in germinal centers and less frequently in the medullary cords. In those studies they were not seen in the thymic dependent paracorticol regions. Inoue et al. [7] have shown further that the regional blood flow to the intestine, particularly the cecum, is increased with enteral feedings following burn injury. Furthermore, translocation of *C. albicans*, which has an approximate 70-fold increase following burn injury, can be reduced by a factor of 7 even with a single bolus feeding 12 h after burn [8].

The importance of translocation following injury has been further emphasized by studies of Sori et al. [9], who showed that mortality was related directly to the degree of translocation of isotope-labeled bacteria in the intestine of animals subjected to hemorrhagic shock.

To further evaluate the importance of early enteral feedings in burn patients, we have partially analyzed an ongoing study [10]. Seriously burned patients have been randomized to receive enteral feedings beginning within 12 h of their burn injury or to have delayed enteral feedings for 72 h. In the patients fed early, a nasoenteral tube as well as a nasogastric tube was introduced. Feedings were given through the nasoenteral tube while aspiration of the nasogastric tube was accomplished. The treated patients had a total body surface area averaging 37.6% total/21.8% third degree, whereas the controls had a total body surface area of 42.7%/15.3% third degree. Six episodes of infection occurred in treated patients versus 12 in the controls. Four episodes of diarrhea occurred in the treated patients versus eight in the controls. Resting energy expenditure (Kcal/kg per day) was 35.7 in treated patients compared with 43.4 in controls. None of these differences were significant. However, IgG levels, serum plasma, serum albumin, total serum protein, and nitrogen balance were all significantly higher during the 1st week in the patients receiving early feeding compared with controls. Additional animal models have supported the concept that enteral feeding is superior to parenteral feeding.

Kudsk et al. [11] demonstrated that animals fed intravenously have greater susceptibility to bacterial infection than animals fed enterally. Using nutritional and metabolic parameters, Saito et al. [12] showed superiority of intragastric feedings versus intravenous feedings in the burned guinea pig model. Finally, Alverdy et al. [13] showed that total parenteral nutrition promoted bacterial translocation from the intestine using a noninjured rat model.

Together, these clinical and laboratory studies provide clear indication that the intestine is a central organ in hypermetabolism and in the septic state. Most importantly, it is clear that changes in the intestinal barrier function including prevention of translocation occurs within hours of injury and can be modulated by early administration of enteral nutrition following injury.

Effect of Dietary Composition on Outcome

In a series of studies using the animal model described above, individual components of the diet were examined to determine the optimal amounts for support of immunological and nutritional outcome variables following burn injury. More specifically, the following were evaluated: total energy, total amount of protein as a percentage of energy, carbohydrate/fat ratio, type of lipid, amount of branched chain amino acids, and arginine content. It was found that a diet optimal for support of burned guinea pigs contained 20% of energy in the form of a high-quality protein (whey), 2% of energy as arginine, and 15% of nonprotein energy as lipid, one-half of which was from fish oil, which is relatively rich in omega 3 fatty acids including eicosapentaenoic acid and docosahexaenoic acid. The addition of carnitine, branched-chain amino acids, or medium-chain triglycerides had no beneficial effect. Using the data from the animal studies, a modular tube feeding was designed for use in seriously burned patients which also had histidine and cysteine added, each in a concentration of 0.5% energy. The modular tube feeding was initially given to a small group of patients in a noncontrolled study, which suggested that infection, hospital stay, and the incidence of diarrhea could be reduced. A subsequent prospective, randomized study was instituted in which the modular tube feeding was compared with the diet with which we have previously had the most success (Osmolite with Promix added to increase the protein concentration to 22%), and also Traumacal, a commercially available product. Preliminary results of this study have been reported by Gottschlich et al. [14]. Demographic characteristics of the three groups were similar. However, the patients receiving the modular tube feeding had a reduction in the length of hospital stay (0.82 days/percentage burn compared with 1.26 and 1.15 days in the groups receiving Osmolite-Promix, or Traumacal). Wound infections were also significantly reduced in the patients receiving the modular tube feedings.

These studies in burn patients strongly suggest that dietary composition influences outcome variables. Particularly important in these studies has been the observation that normal amounts of dietary lipid may have harmful effects which are related, at least in part, to activation of the arachidonic acid pathway and the generation of prostaglandins, leukotrienes, and thromboxanes. Substitution of lipids high in omega 6 fatty acids with lipids rich in omega 3 fatty acids has a beneficial effect, at least in part by limiting the amount of prostaglandin E_2 and thromboxane produced.

Nutrition in Established Sepsis

Virtually all of the models of experimental peritonitis which have been previously described have resulted in either death or recovery of the animal within a short period. Injection of bacteria singly or in mixtures, or with adjuvants, usually causes death within 24–48 h. Mixtures of bacteria, fecal pellets, insertion of bacteria in capsules or entrapped in fibrin clots, or cecal ligation and puncture characteristically cause death within 1–5 days, a time clearly insufficient for nutritional intervention. Because of this, a new model was developed which involves insertion of an osmotic pump filled with bacteria into the peritoneal cavity [15]. By placing a long length of tubing to the outlet of the pump, the delivery of bacteria can be delayed for approximately 36–48 h after implantation of the pump. This model results in a peritonitis, usually with abscess, which causes death of approximately 50% of the animals by 2 weeks depending on the bacterial mix and inoculation. After preliminary trials, animals were allowed to feed freely for 3 days before pump-controlled gastrostomy feedings were administered. In previous studies, using similar-sized burned guinea pigs, feeding 175 Kcal/kg per day of a balanced diet resulted in maintenance of weight after the 3rd day whereas 200 Kcal/kg per day was well tolerated and associated with a slight weight gain. Freely feeding nonburned guinea pigs spontaneously ingest approximately 125 Kcal/kg per day and gain weight. Four groups of animals were studied initially receiving 175, 150, 125, or 100 Kcal/kg per day. The animals receiving 150 and 175 Kcal/kg per day maintained their body weight whereas the ones receiving 125 or 100 Kcal/kg per day lost weight. However, the group that lost the most weight had the best survival and all animals receiving 150 Kcal/kg per day or more died. Additional studies in animals receiving 125 Kcal/kg per day showed no difference in the survival of animals caused by varying the amount of lipid from 0% to 50% of nonprotein calories, a marked contrast from previous studies in burned animals. From these studies using a model of prolonged acute peritonitis, it is apparent that overfeeding may be harmful and, in fact, slight underfeeding may have an advantage. Use of the intestinal tract for feeding is highly desirable and may be accomplished even in the face of extensive peritonitis. In sepsis, lipids may not be all that bad and, from other studies, excess arginine may be helpful [16].

Summary

There is clear evidence in both experimental animals and man that dietary intervention may play a major role in outcome from acute injury and/or infection. However, the dietary composition should be tailored for the specific disease. Optimal enteral diets for burn injury and severe trauma have been partially developed, but optimal diets for septic individuals remain a matter of speculation. The optimal diet for burn patients requires increased calories to meet metabolic demands, increased protein (greater than 20% of total calories using a high-quality protein), enrichment with arginine (2% of energy), enrichment with cysteine and histidine (0.5% each), reduction in lipid calories to approximately 15% of nonprotein energy, and a change in lipid composition to include the omega 3 fatty acids. In contrast, the optimal diet for septic subjects should be hypocaloric rather than hypercaloric and the optimal compositions are yet to be determined and will probably be different for different types of infection.

It is also clear that the intestines play a major role in consequences of the injury process. Following a major thermal injury, the intestinal mucosal mass will atrophy rapidly (within hours) and lose its barrier function against the translocation of intestinal products including bacteria. The sudden surge of endotoxin into the portal venous and mesenteric lymphatic circulations trigger the activation of macrophages and the catabolic and hypermetabolic processes. These events can be attenuated by early dietary intervention.

References

1. Alexander JW, MacMillan BG, Stinnett JD, Ogle CK, Bozian RC, Fischer JE, Oakes JB, Morris MJ, Krummel R (1980) Beneficial effects of aggressive protein feeding in severely burned children. Ann Surg 192:505–517
2. Dominioni L, Stinnett JD, Fang CH, Trocki O, Berlatzky Y, Kaufman T, Alexander JW (1984) Gastrostomy feeding in normal and hypermetabolic burned guinea pigs: a model for the study of enteral diets. J Burn Care Rehabil 5:100–105
3. Mochizuki H, Trocki O, Dominioni L, Brackett KA, Joffe SN, Alexander JW (1984) Mechanism of prevention of postburn hypermetabolism and catabolism by early enteral feeding. Ann Surg 200:297–310
4. Arita H, Ogle CK, Alexander JW (1988) Continuous administration of low-dose endotoxin induces hypermetabolism in guinea pigs. 1st international congress on the immune consequences of trauma, shock and sepsis. Mechanisms and therapeutic approaches. Munich, Germany, 3–5 March, 1988
5. Maejima K, Deitch E, Berg R (1984) Promotion by burn stress of the translocation of bacteria from the gastrointestinal tracts of mice. Arch Surg 119:166–172

6. Inoue S, Wirman JA, Alexander JW, Trocki O, Cardell RR *Candida albicans* translocation across the gut mucosa following burn injury. J Surg Res (in press)
7. Inoue S, Luke S, Alexander JW, Trocki O, Silverstein EB Preservation of gut blood flow by early enteral feeding in burned guinea pigs. (Submitted for publication)
8. Inoue S, Epstein M, Alexander JW, Trocki O, Gura P Prevention of yeast translocation across the gut by a single enteral feeding after burn injury. (Submitted for publication)
9. Sori AJ, Rush BF Jr, Lysz TW, Smith S, Machiedo GW (1988) The gut as source of sepsis after hemorrhagic shock. Am J Surg 155:187–191
10. Jenkins M, Gottschlich M, Waymack JP, Alexander JW, Warden GD (1988) An evaluation of the effect of immediate enteral feeding on the hypermetabolic response following severe burn injury. 20th annual meeting of the American Burn Association. Seattle, WA, 23–28 March, 1988
11. Kudsk KA, Stone JM, Carpenter G, Sheldon GF (1983) Enteral and parenteral feeding influences mortality after hemoglobin – *E. coli* peritonitis in normal rats. J Trauma 23:605–609
12. Saito H, Trocki O, Alexander JW, Kopcha R, Heyd T, Joffe SN (1987) The effect of route of nutrient administration on the nutritional state, catabolic hormone secretion, and gut mucosal integrity after burn injury. JPEN 11:1–7
13. Alverdy JC, Aoys E, Moss GS (1988) Total parenteral nutrition promotes bacterial translocation from the gut. 49th annual meeting of the Society of University Surgeons. San Antonio, TX, 11–13 February, 1988
14. Gottschlich MM, Jenkins M, Carey M, Warden GD, Alexander JW (1988) Differential effects of three enteral regimens on tube feeding tolerance, body composition and patient outcome. Abstract presented 20th annual meeting of the American Burn Association. Seattle, WA, 23–26 March, 1988
15. Alexander JW, Gonce SJ, Peck MD A new experimental model for studying the effect of nutrition on peritonitis. The adverse effect of overfeeding. (Submitted for publication)
16. Barbul A (1986) Arginine: biochemistry, physiology, and therapeutic implications. JPEN 10:227–238

The Gut-Origin Septic States

J. R. Border

Normal Physiology

The gut contains sufficient bacteria and toxins to kill the host millions of times over. In normal life these toxic entities are confined to the gut by processes dependent upon food ingestion, defecation, the interactions of the gut associated lymphoid tissue and the systemic immune system, and the function of various valves such as the glottis and gastroesophageal junction. Food ingestion stimulates salivary gland secretion, stomach digestion, biliary tract secretions, replication of enterocytes, mucous secretion, and growth of commensal bacteria. Secretory IgA is delivered to the lumen of the gut by the salivary gland, biliary tract secretions and in mucous. Secretory IgA binds to bacteria and thus prevents binding of the bacteria to the enterocyte in preparation for penetration. The gut mucosa wall is continually renewed by a process of cell and mucous shedding which also aids in preventing bacterial binding and penetration. Finally, commensal bacteria bind to the enterocytes where they consume available nutrients, prevent pathogenic bacteria binding, and release metabolites toxic to pathogenic bacteria. It is the growth of commensal bacteria that is the primary factor that prevents growth of pathogenic bacteria in the gut.

In the upper gut, stomach digestion is the major bacteriocidal mechanism that kills the bacteria continually supplied from the environment and the oropharynx to maintain the stomach and proximal small bowel largely sterile. Biliary tract secretion of bile salts is the major in vivo detoxifier of endotoxin. This has major importance in preventing endotoxin penetration of the gut mucosa. In the colon the commensal bacteria are largely obligatory anaerobes. These bacteria even if they penetrate the colonic mucosa cannot survive in the systemic body. The metabolism of the obligatory anaerobes consumes residual nutrient and releases short-chain fatty acids. These are both toxic to pathogenic bacteria and provide nutrients that support cell replication in the colonic mucosa and thus aid in maintaining the integrity of the colonic mucosa.

The enterocytes are highly polar cells which are best supported metabolically from the lumen of the gut to maintain the gut mucosa as a barrier to entry of bacteria and endotoxin. From the vascular side the enterocytes are heavily dependent upon ketone bodies and glutamine as energetic fuels. In starvation the gut is both emptied of its contents of bacteria and endotoxin and well supplied with enterocyte fuel from ketone bodies. Thus, although severe atrophy of the gut mucosa rapidly occurs, no gut-origin septic state evolves.

Immune Consequences of
Trauma, Shock and Sepsis
Eds. Faist/Ninnemann/Green

Pathophysiology

In blunt multiple trauma (Hospital Trauma Index – Injury Severity Score >18, e.g., fractured femur and ruptured spleen) conservative fracture management involving femur traction routinely leads, if prolonged more than 48 h, to a pulmonary failure septic state. This is directly proportional in duration to the number of days of femur traction and is associated in days 3 to 10–14 with an increasing magnitude of septic organ failures. Positive blood cultures begin on days 8–10 and thereafter increase in number per day on the ventilator. Continued femoral traction leads to a considerable increase in multiple-system organ failure and late septic deaths. These observations are uniformly reported in every report that examines this problem [1–10].

Figure 1 shows the alveolar arterial oxygen tension difference and positive end-expiratory pressure for two groups of patients. These patients were initially equally injured by 20 different criteria and differed only in the fact that group I had immediate internal fixation of their fractures so that they could be sitting up at 36 h while group II had an average of 10 days of femoral traction. It is to be noted that the group in femoral traction has a much higher alveolar arterial oxygen tension difference, a higher positive end-expiratory pressure, and if anything, is extubated physiologically earlier than group I. This difference mandates continued tracheal intubation in the group in femoral traction. Table 1 shows the Pearson cross-correlations of 10 criteria of the pulmonary failure septic state to the initial Injury Severity Score and to the days of femoral traction. It is immedi-

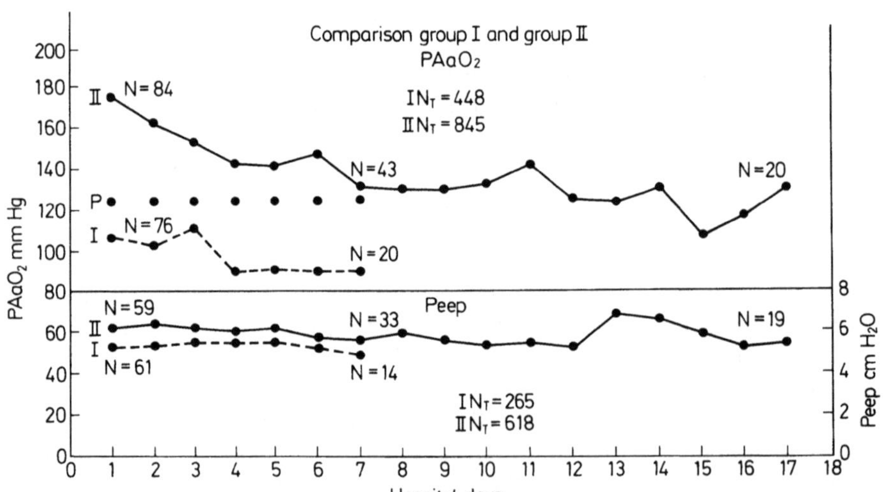

Fig. 1. A comparison of the group mean daily values for groups I and II for PAa O_2 and positive end expiratory pressure (PEEP). Group I (*dashed line*) has the present criteria for weaning of a PAa O_2 of 80–100 mmHg, and 5 cm H_2O of PEEP by day 3 and is appropriately weaned. Group II (*solid line*) is weaned at day 10 when the PAa O_2 is 130 mmHg, and the PEEP is about 5 cm. The difference in the pulmonary problems between group I and group II is also reflected in their NTs for PAa O_2 of 448 and 845, and for PEEP of 265 and 618. ●, $P \leqq 0.001$

Table 1. Pearson cross correlations of hospital trauma index injury severity score (HTI-ISS) and days of femoral traction to several measures of the pulmonary failure septic state together with the asscociated *P* value and *n* number (N)

	HTI ISS	Days of femur traction	Acute care days	Ven-tilator days	ICU days	Number of arterial gases	Number of elevated white counts	Febrile days (101F)	Blood cultures taken	Total number of cultures taken	Bili-rubins >1.5 mg/ppml	Number of anti-biotics utilized
HTI-ISS	1.000	−0.1290	0.0235	−0.0099	0.1130	−0.0190	0.1359	−0.0654	−0.2050	−0.1381	0.1381	0.0461
P values	0.000	0.348	0.863	0.943	0.407	0.894	0.337	0.638	0.137	0.324	0.357	0.743
n	–	55	56	56	56	52	52	54	54	53	51	53
Days of femur traction	−0.1290	1.000	0.7310	0.6257	0.5996	0.5688	0.6684	0.6469	0.7592	0.7040	0.2883	0.3604
P values	0.348	0.000	0.001	0.001	0.001	0.001	0.001	0.001	0.001	0.001	0.042	0.009
n	55	–	55	55	55	51	51	53	53	52	50	52

Note that three are no significant *P* values for any measure of the pulmonary failure septic state to the initial HTI-ISS. In contrast every measure of the pulmonary failure septic state has a significant to highly significant *P* value for the cross correlation with days of femoral traction. These data strongly suggest that it is not the magnitude of the original injury that determines the magnitude and duration of the pulmonary failure septic state but rather it is our treatment of the original injury with femoral shaft traction that determines the magnitude and duration of the pulmonary failure septic state. These data are entirely compatible with the concept of the gut-origin septic states.

Table 2. Comparison of positive blood cultures per patient in groups I, II, and III[a]

Group	Number of positive blood cultures/patients[b]	Number of patients with positive blood cultures[b]
I	0.05	1/20
II	0.50	8/20
III	3.7	6/9

[a] These data show the numbers of positive blood cultures per patient and the number of patients with positive blood cultures in groups I, II, and III. Groups I and II were equally injured in terms of 20 different emergency room and operating room measurements with any bias being toward group I being more injured (12 vs. 9 chest injuries). Groups I and II differ only in that group I had immediate internal fixation of fractures and was sitting up at 36 h while group II had an average of 10 days of femoral traction. Group III was clearly less injured than groups I and II (HTI-ISS = 36 vs. 29) but was immediately extubated (all had to be reintubated) and was left on average in 30 days of femoral traction.
[b] Note that the number of positive blood cultures expressed as per patient or as number of patients increases in direct proportion to the number of days of femoral traction and has no relation to HTI-ISS as in Table 1. Group III had the only two patients who nearly died a late septic death from multiple systems organ failure.

ately apparent that there are no significant Pearson cross correlations to the magnitude of the Injury Severity Score, while every cross correlation to the days of femoral traction is significant or highly significant. We have also found no significant cross correlations for the initial bicarbonate or the first 48 h of fluid volume. Table 2 shows the average number of positive blood cultures per patient and the number of patients with positive blood cultures. Both increase from group I to group II to group III. Group III was the least injured group initially, but were immediately extubated (all had to be reintubated) and were left on average for 30 days in femoral traction.

Figure 2 shows the alveolar arterial oxygen tension difference and positive end-expiratory pressure for group III relative to group I. It is again apparent that femoral traction is associated with a considerable increase in alveolar arterial oxygen tension difference, positive end-expiratory pressure, and that group III is extubated physiologically earlier than group I. It is to be noted that group III had the only two patients who nearly died of multiple-system organ failure. It is of some interest that immediate internal fixation of fractures not only drastically reduced the duration and magnitude of the pulmonary failure septic state but also drastically reduced the number of fracture complications [10].

All of these data show very clearly that it is not the magnitude of the original injury as judged by the Injury Severity Score that determines the magnitude and duration of the pulmonary failure septic state (or number of late septic deaths), but that it is our therapy of the original injury that determines the magnitude and duration of the pulmonary failure septic state. Femoral traction is tightly associated in the multiple trauma patients with the enforced supine position and an increased magnitude of pulmonary failure that requires continued tracheal intubation. This leads to use of drugs to maintain the endotracheal tube that reduce consciousness.

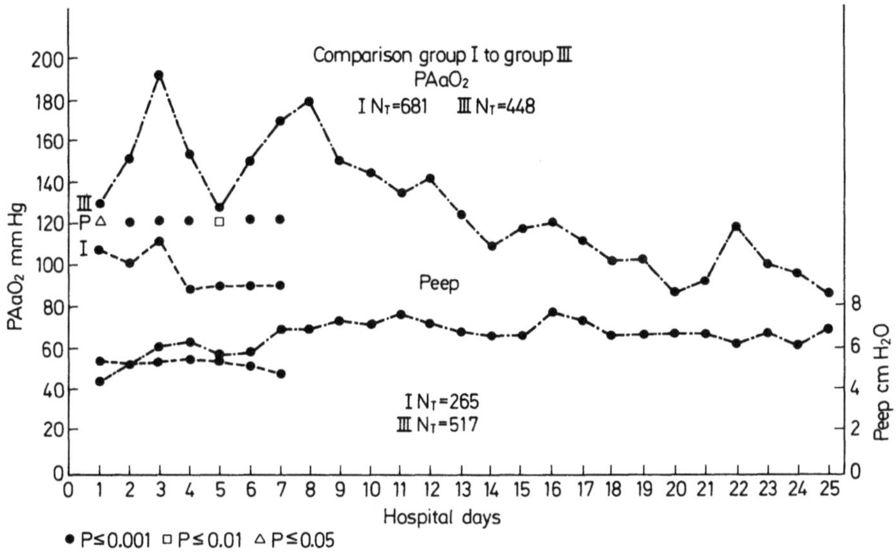

Fig. 2. A comparison of the group mean daily observations for PAa O_2 and PEEP for groups I (*dashed line*) and III (*broken line*). Group III attains a PAa O_2 of 80–100 mmHg on days 19–20 and is actually weaned on day 21. The PEEP at this time is 6 cm H_2O. There are significant differences in PAa O_2 for the 7 days in which comparisons are possible to group I but no significant difference in PEEP. ●, $P \leqq 0.001$; □, $P \leqq 0.01$; △, $P \leqq 0.05$

These events together largely prevent oral food intake while the enforced supine position also greatly impedes defecation. The oral endotracheal tube also allows the mouth to dry out so that salivary gland secretions do not wash out the oropharynx, prevents the normal expulsion of the tracheal mucosa blanket with its contained bacteria, and provides access of oropharyngeal bacteria to the pulmonary airways. In addition, because the intubated patient becomes more septic he has his stomach alkalinized to prevent stress ulcers and receives broad-spectrum antibiotics for suspected infection. Finally, the metabolic response to the septic state largely shuts off hepatic ketogenesis and thus shuts off a vital vascular fuel supply to the enterocyte.

This effect is compounded by the fact that the amino acids given intravenously do not contain glutamine. Glutamine under these conditions is produced by muscle catabolism of valine. These patients rapidly develop muscle protein malnutrition that impedes conversion of valine to glutamine. One sign of an impending septic death is rising plasma valine and falling plasma glutamine [11].

The essential point is that our management of the original injury and its consequences impedes in almost every way the factors which normally confine the gut bacteria and toxins to the gut and the factors which prevent growth of pathogenic (largely aerobic) bacteria in the gut. In addition the antibiotics used are used in an almost ideal way to support growth of pathogenic antibiotic-resistant bacteria in the gut.

Pathophysiology: Hypothesis

We will hypothesize that the septic states observed in blunt multiple trauma are predominantly gut-origin septic states due to gut mucosa malnutrition which allows at 48–96 h entry of gut endotoxin and at 8–10 days entry of gut endotoxin and bacteria [12, 13]. The entry of these materials then activates the hepatic macrophage which releases cytokines to produce the septic state, immunosuppressive products to suppress all T cell-dependent immunity, and tissue destructive elements which damage the lung to increase the magnitude of the pulmonary failure. It is to be noted that the wound macrophage releases the same materials but has a large variety of processes which largely confine them to the wound while the hepatic macrophage lives in a system designed to deliver hepatocyte products to the blood stream. It is probably equally good at delivering macrophage products [14, 15].

Pathophysiology: Revised with New Hypothesis

To investigate this hypothesis, we will construct a septic severity score (SSS) based upon standard deviational units of change in the septic direction for the 16 measurements commonly made every day in the intensive care unit (ICU). These are the electrolytes, blood gases, inspired oxygen, positive end-expiratory pressure, leukocytes, temperature (highest of the day), bilirubin, creatinine, blood glucose, and platelets. This creates a totally objective measure which works exactly the way the clinician works in evaluating the magnitude of the septic process. Normal man has an SSS of zero, patients discharged from the ICU have an SSS of 34 ($n=62$), and patients who die of sepsis have an SSS of >100. We will examine the correlations of SSS in 2.4 megabytes data covering 66 patients and 1649 patient days. These patients have an average initial Injury Severity Score of 40, age of 29, 14 diagnoses, and 12 procedures. This study is retrospective with all of the caveats that implies. These patients are divided into five groups based upon weeks in the ICU and a sixth group that died of sepsis. These groups have initial equal characteristics statistically as judged by ANOVA statistics and differ only in terms of time in the ICU on the ventilator, or death [14].

Overall, Pearson cross correlations quickly reveal that an increased SSS is tightly associated with an increased number of days on the ventilator ($r=+0.52$), an increased number of positive cultures ($r=+0.32$), and increased nasogastric suction volume ($r=+0.41$) (all $n=1626$; $P<0.001$). In addition, an increased number of antibiotics per day is associated with an increased SSS ($r=+0.38$), increased ventilator days ($r=+0.26$), and increased total positive cultures ($r=+0.15$) (all $n=1615$; $P<0.001$). Only an increased enteral protein intake is tightly associated with a reduced SSS ($r=-0.38$), reduced ventilator days ($r=-0.48$), reduced total positive cultures ($r=-0.18$) (all $n=1636$ and $P<0.001$). The fundamental dichotomy of an increasing SSS with increasing days on the ventilator and a decresing SSS with increasing enteral protein holds for all individual components of the SSS and not just the total SSS ($r=-0.38$ to -0.10 for enteral protein while $r=+0.70$ to $+0.19$ for ventilator days, all $n=1475$, $P<0.001$) [14].

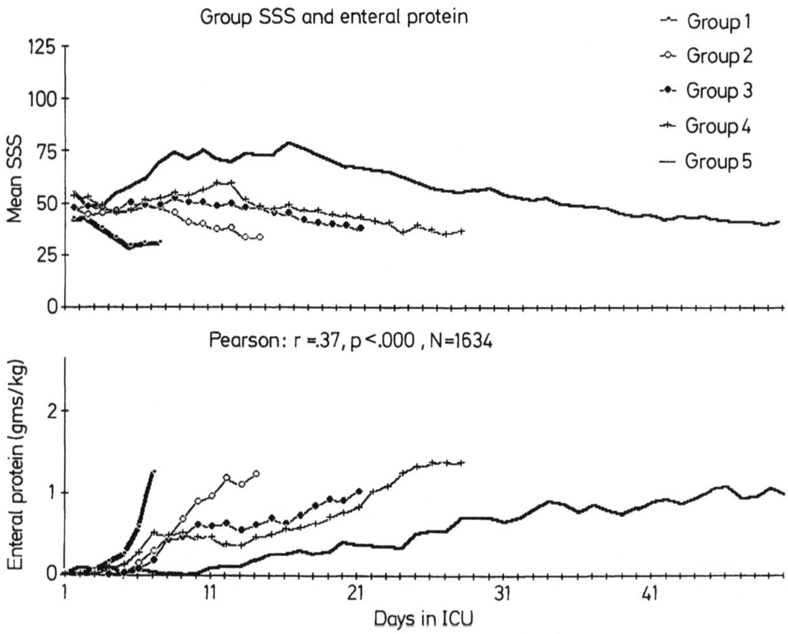

Fig. 3. A comparison of SSS by group daily mean to enteral protein (EnP) by group daily mean. This data base has a constant N per group achieved with a mean data fill between the time of earliest ventilator weaning in a given group to the time when one half the patients had been discharged from the ICU. The relationship of a rising EnP to a falling SSS for each group is obvious and confirms the Pearson correlations

Thus all overall correlations strongly support the concept that an increased number of ventilator days (and its associated use of broad spectrum antibiotics and stomach alkalinization) is associated with an increased magnitude of SSS (septic organ failures) and increased bacteriological evidence of sepsis while only increased enteral protein is associated with a reduction in SSS and reduced bacteriologic evidence of sepsis. An increased number of antibiotics does not reduce the magnitude of the septic state and, if anything, is associated with an increased magnitude of the septic state and increased number of positive cultures [14].

Figure 3 shows the SSS for the individual groups of patients who survived and the associated enteral protein intake. It is to be noted in each group that as enteral protein intake rises SSS falls. It should further be noted that initially there is a period of 48–72 h when SSS is stable or falls and that then SSS rises until 8–12 days. After 8–12 days, SSS is largely stable until enteral protein intake rises. Group 1 has immediate total surgical care, is sitting up in 24–48 h, and with this therapy has a prompt drop in SSS and rise in enteral protein. We hypothesize that at 48–72 h endotoxin activates the hepatic macrophage to produce the increase in SSS. We know that at 8–11 days the number of positive blood cultures drastically increases and hypothesize that at this time the hepatic macrophage is activated by both endotoxin and bacteria from the gut [14].

The question must be raised as to whether increased enteral protein produced the reduction in SSS or occurs because of the reduction of SSS. Figure 4 shows

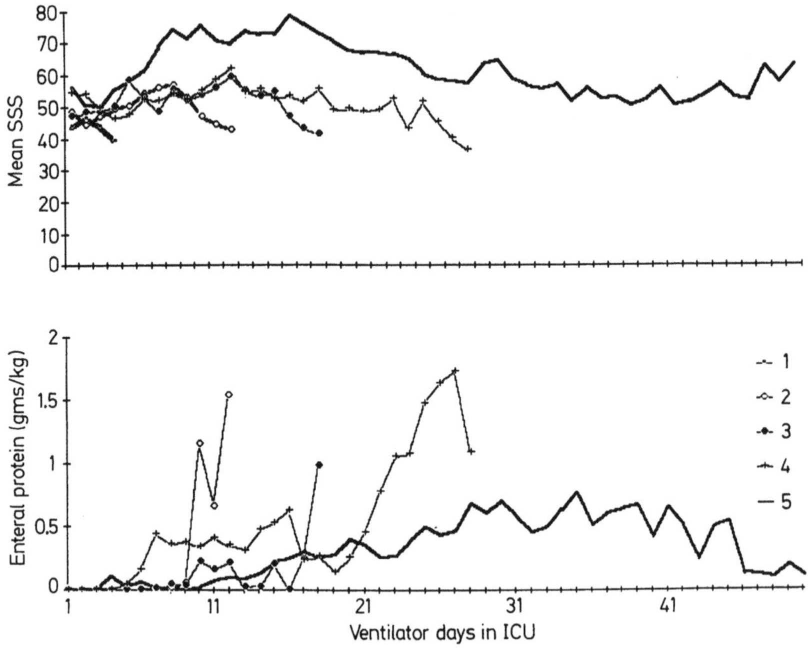

Fig. 4. A comparison by group of SSS and enteral protein (EnP) daily mean values for those patients still on the ventilator. This produces a variable *n* as the patients are weaned but has no mean data fill. SSS in each group after the initial 10 days is stable and falls abruptly in groups 2–4 as EnP rises rapidly. This occurs when they are gotten out of bed and sitting up while on the ventilator. Group 1 is sitting up out of bed at 2–3 days and the patients eat after coming off the ventilator. Group 5 has the expected reciprocal relationship between SSS and EnP but does not have the rapid rise in EnP that groups 2–4 have

the relationship that exists in patients still on the ventilator and thus truly shows the effects of forced feeding. It is to be noted that the relationship of SSS and enteral protein is the same as in Fig. 3. This tends to confirm the basic hypothesis. A second way of asking the question is to examine the SSS of those patients who received no enteral protein. This effect is shown in Fig. 5 for the first 20 days. It is apparent that those who received no enteral protein but received almost twice as much total protein intake became progressively more septic relative to the control group that received 0.61 g of protein enterally per kilogram per day. We began with the question of femoral traction and protein intake. Figure 6 shows that the patients who were in femoral traction 20 or more days had only 0.18 g enteral protein intake per day and became progressively more septic relative to those who had internal fixation who had 0.55 mg enteral protein. This comparison is clouded by the reduced total protein intake of patients in femoral traction [14].

All of the proceding evaluations of the data have involved the variation of an intensive variable over days. An alternative evaluation using extensive variables with one variable per patient is shown in Fig. 7. This plot shows the number of patients in the ICU for each day postinjury. It is apparent that we can rather accurately predict this line (adj. $R^2=0.85$, $F=104$, $P<0.000$) using the variables number of delayed operations (DORS), day of rising enteral protein to 0.3 g/kg

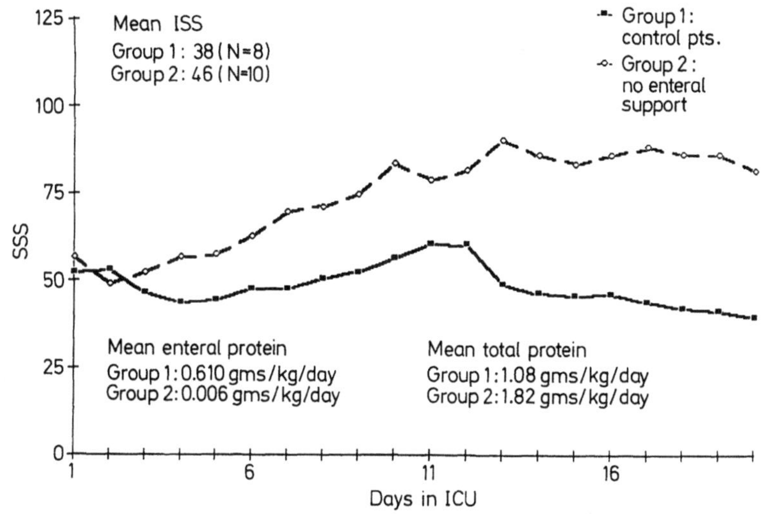

Fig. 5. A comparison of the associations of zero enteral protein (EnP) or 0.61 g of EnP with SSS on a group daily mean basis. The group with zero EnP has a progressively rising SSS, whereas the group with 0.61 g of EnP has a stable to falling SSS over the 21 days of observations. The group with zero EnP receives much more total protein (1.82 *vs.* 1.08 g). There is no mean data fill in this comparison. ANOVA: $F=90.4, P<0.00$

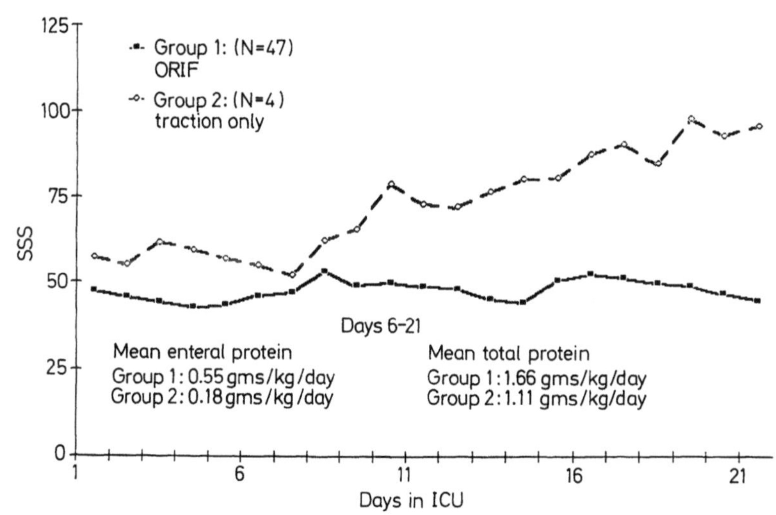

Fig. 6. A comparison of the associations of femoral fracture internal fixation or femur traction over 21 days with the group daily mean SSS. The group with femur traction has a progressively increasing SSS over the 21-day period relative to the stable or falling SSS of those with internal fixation. There is no mean data fill in this comparison. ANOVA: $F=179.9$, $P<0.000$

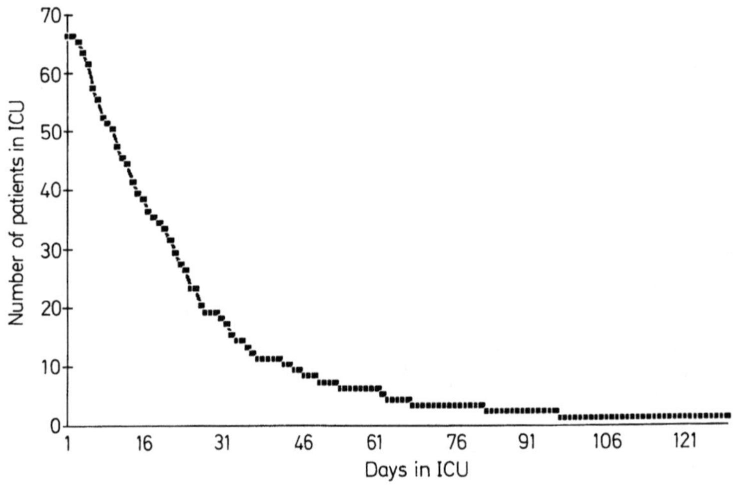

Fig. 7. A plot of ICU days and number of patients in the ICU each day shows a logarithmically decreasing curve. Total ICU days is best predicted with the independent variables: number of delayed operations (*DORS*), day of rising enteral protein (*DREnP*), and total positive cultures (*TPC*) (adj. $R^2=0.84$, $F=104$, $df=3/59$). The variable of greatest importance is *DORS* and the next greatest is *DREnP*. *TPC* is highly correlated with both of these variables but does contain some new information. Total ICU days=0.65 TPC+0.52 DREnP+2.78 DORS

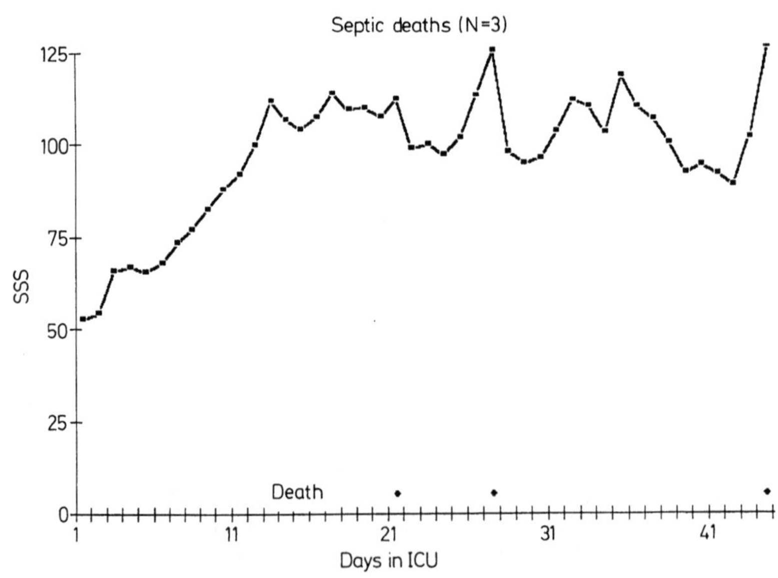

Fig. 8. This shows the behavior of SSS in the three patients who died with zero EnP. The hospital days of their deaths are noted at the bottom. Death (·) is associated with an SSS between 100 and 125 and occurs earliest in the patient who received the least exogenous protein. Septic deaths=3; mean enteral protein=0; mean total protein=2.03 g/kg/day

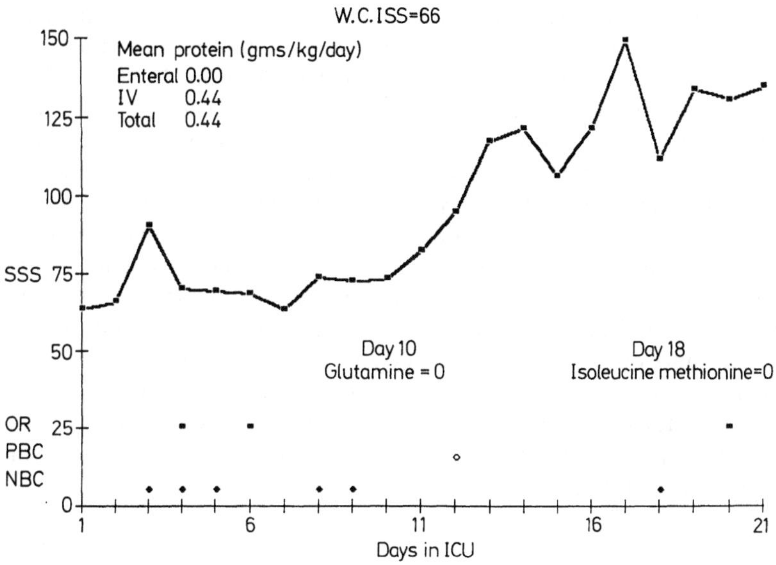

Fig. 9. The association of SSS in a patient who died of sepsis with zero enteral protein (EnP) and very small total protein intake with splanchnic extraction. We have reported on this patient in great detail metabolically [16, 17]. We therefore thought we should construct a SSS to compare with these metabolic measurements. SSS rises abruptly as glutamine extraction goes to zero on day 10 (see text for discussion) and then continues to rise as isoleucine and methionine extraction go to zero at day 17. These falling splanchnic extractions of glutamine and isoleucine are based on very low plasma concentrations produced by changes in muscle metabolism. OR, operation; NBC, negative blood culture; PBC, positive blood culture. ISS = 66; mean protein (g/kg/day): enteral = 0; IV = 0.44; total = 0.44

(DRENP), and total positive cultures (TPC). These variables are listed in order of statistical importance. It is of considerable interest that the two major variables (DORS and DRENP) are clearly and totally under the surgeon's control. This again supports the basic contention that these are gut-origin septic states which result not from the original injury, but from the surgeon's management of the original injury [14].

Figure 8 shows the SSS of three of the patients who died of sepsis. It is to be noted that they died with an SSS above 100 after about 21 days and typically have zero enteral protein. They also have massive use of broad-spectrum antibiotics, persistent stomach alkalinization, and on average 2 g total protein per kilogram. Figure 9 shows one patient we reported on metabolically in great detail in 1981. It is to be noted that on day 10 that gut plus liver extraction of glutamine goes to zero and the patient rapidly becomes more septic with increased SSS. On day 17 the splanchnic extraction of both isoleucine and methiomine went to zero as the patient had a continued increase in SSS and then died of sepsis on day 22. This patient had one positive blood culture (*Staphylococcus epidermidis*) and clearly had grossly inadequate total protein intake as well as no enteral protein [14].

Died of sepsis has typically been taken to mean died of bacterial infection. Our patients who died of sepsis had an average of two positive blood cultures out of an average of 16 blood cultures taken. These patients have the same number of positive cultures as the patients who survived who were on the ventilator the same length of time. In fact, the patients who were on the ventilator longest, all of whom survived, had far more bacteriologic evidence of infection. One must wonder if died of sepsis has far more relation to entry of gut endotoxin then entry of gut bacteria. We were unable to show any beneficial effect of added antibiotics in terms of reducing the magnitude of SSS or clearing bacteria from the blood stream. In addition, the overall correlations of number of antibiotics per day suggest that antibiotics do not benefit these patients and may make them worse. This is entirely consistent with the antibiotics killing the commensal bacteria and thus supporting growth of pathogenic antibiotic-resistant bacteria in the gut. These then enter the immunocomprised systemic body to produce pneumonia, wound infections, urinary tract infections, sinusitis, parotitis, bacteremias, and probably intraperitoneal infectious and abscesses. The immunosuppressed state is produced both directly by endotoxin from the gut and by the effect this endotoxin has on the hepatic macrophage [14].

Discussion

Our data are retrospective and therefore allow only the firm conclusion that enteral protein intake and the septic state are tightly associated as shown. The prospective studies of severely burned children and adults by Alexander et al. and Antonacci et al. show clearly that increased enteral protein intake is associated tightly with reduced mortality rates and reduced evidence of the septic state. These are discussed by Alexander in this volume. The work of Deitch (also in this volume) clearly shows that under a variety of conditions that bacteria can translocate from the gut into the systemic body and that this is greatly supported by endotoxin. This year has seen a great expansion in the surgical literature on the gut-origin septic states with many papers showing bacterial overgrowth in the alkalinized stomach [16], reduced secretory IgA secretion with parenteral nutrition relative to enteral nutrition [17], increased gut bacterial translocation with parenteral nutrition relative to enteral [18], that hemorrhagic shock produced bacterial translocation and that this is blocked by blocking oxygen free radicals [19], that endotoxin in healthy man increases gut permeability as does infection in burned patients [20, 21], that antibodies against endotoxin protect against death from sepsis [22], and that added intravenous glutamine and epidermal growth factor enhance gut mucosal cellularity and thickness [23]. Mochiguki et al. previously showed that enteral protein feeding within 24 h in burned guinea pigs increased gut mucosal thickness and largely shut off the hypermetabolic response [24]. Alexander and associates have shown that portal vein infusion of endotoxin at a low rate elicits the hypermetabolic response [25].

There is, therefore, a rapidly evolving literature which supports the concept of the gut-origin septic states from any points of view. Crucial to that literature is the concept of gut endotoxin entering the systemic body to activate the hepatic macrophage. One must wonder if a large portion of the immune suppression that follows severe trauma is an effect of endotoxin both directly and via its effect on the hepatic macrophage. In any event, the need for improved support of the gut mucosa as a barrier is evident.

References

1. Riska EB, Von Bonsdorff H, Hakkinen S, Jaroma H, Kiviluoto O, Paavilainen T (1976) Prevention of fat embolism by early internal fixation of fractures in patients with multiple injuries. Injury 6:110–116
2. Riska E, Von Bonsdorff H, Hakkinen S (1977) Primary operative fixation of long bone fractures in patients with multiple injuries. J Trauma 17:111–121
3. Wolff G, Dittman M, Ruedi T, Allgöwer M (1978) Koordination von Chirurgie und Intensivmedizin zur Vermeidung der posttraumatischen respiratorischen Insuffizienz. Unfallheilkunde 81:425–442
4. Goris R, Gimbrere J, Van Niekerk J, Schoots F, Booy L (1982) Early osteosynthesis and prophylactic mechanical ventilation in the multiple trauma patient. J Trauma 22:895–903
5. Meek R, Vivoda E, Crichton A (1981) A comparison of mortality in patients with multiple injuries according to the method of fracture treatment. J Bone Joint Surg [Br] (63 b):465
6. Meek R, Vivoda E, Pirani S (1986) Comparison of mortality of patients with multiple injuries according to type of fracture treatment: a retrospective age and injury matched series. Injury 17:2–4
7. Johnson KD, Cadami A, Seibert G (1985) Incidence of adult respiratory distress syndrome in patients with multiple musculoskeletal injuries. J Trauma 25:375–385
8. Bone L, Johnson K, Weigett J (1989) Prospective randomized study of early versus delayed femoral fracture stabilization. J Bone Joint Surg
9. Lozman J, Deno C, Feusetel P, Hewell J, Stratton H, Sedraush N, Detton R, Fortune J, Shah D (1986) Pulmonary and cardiovascular consequences of immediate fixation or conservative management of long bone fractures. Arch Surg 121:992–1000
10. Seibel R, LaDuca J, Hassett J, Babikian G, Mills B, Border D, Border J (1985) Blunt multiple trauma (ISS 36), femur traction, and the pulmonary failure septic state. Ann Surg 202:283–295
11. Border JR (1982) Trauma and sepsis. In: Worth MH (ed) Principles and practice of trauma care. Williams and Wilkins, Baltimore, pp 330–388
12. Alexander JW, Macmillan BG, Stinnet JD, Ogle G, Bozian R, Fischer JE, Oakes J, Morris M, Krummnel R (1980) Beneficial effects of aggressive protein feeding in severely burned children. Ann Surg 192:505–518
13. Antonacci A, Cowles S, Reaves L (1984) The role of nutrition in immunologic function. Infect Surg 3:590–597
14. Border J, Hassett J, LaDuca J, Seibel R, Steinberg S, Mills B, Losi P, Border D (1987) The gut origin of septic states in blunt multiple trauma (ISS = 40) in the I.C.U. Ann Surg 206:427–448
15. Border J (1988) Hypothesis: Sepsis, multiple systems organ failure, and the macrophage. Arch Surg 123:285–287
16. Marshall J, Meakins J, Christou N (1988) Small bowel bacterial overgrowth and systemic immunosuppression in a rat model of intra-abdominal sepsis. Program Society University Surgeons, San Antonio, 11–13 Feb, 1988, p 62
17. Alverdy J, Sang Chi H, Sheldon G (1985) The effect of parenteral nutrition on gastrointestinal immunity: the importance of enteral stimulation. Ann Surg 202:681–685
18. Alverdy J, Aoyes E, Moss G (1988) Total parenteral nutrition promotes bacterial translocation from the gut. Program Society University Surgeons, San Antonio, 11–13 Feb, 1988, p 23
19. Deitch E, Bridges W, Baker J, Jing W, Berg R, Granger N (1988) Hemorrhagic shock induced bacterial translocation is reduced by blocking xanthine oxidase activity. Program Society University Surgeons, San Antonio, 11–13 Feb, 1988, p 24

20. O'Dwyer S, Michie H, Zeigler T, Reohaug A, Smith R, Wilmore D (1988) A single dose of endotoxin increases intestinal permeability in man. Program Surgical Infection Society, San Francisco, 5–6 May, 1988
21. Zeigler T, O'Dwyer S, Demling R, Smith R, Wilmore D (1988) Increased intestinal permeability associated with infection in burn patients. Program Surgical Infection Society, San Francisco, 5–6 May, 1988
22. Dunn D, Priest B, Condie R (1988) Protective effect of polyclonal and monoclonal antibodies directed against endotoxin during experimental sepsis. Program Surgical Infection Society, San Francisco, 5–6 May, 1988
23. Jacobs D, Evans G, Smith R, Wilmore D (1988) Combined effect of glutamine and epidermal growth factor (EGF) on G.I. mucosal cellularity. Program Society University Surgeons, San Antonio, 11–13 Feb, 1988, p 51
24. Mochiguki H, Trocki O, Dominioni L, Brackett K, Jaffe S, Alexander J (1984) Mechanism of prevention of postburn hypermetabolism and catabolism by early enteral feeding. Ann Surg 200:297–310
25. Arita H, Agle C, Alexander J (1988) Continuous administration of low dose endotoxin through the portal vein induces hypometabolism in guinea pigs. Program Surgical Infection Society, San Francisco, 5–6 May, 1988

The Influence of Anesthetic Agents on the Immune Response: A Crucial Factor in Immune Suppression?

P. Schmucker and C. Hammer

The immunological status, subsequent to surgery, plays a crucial part in the recovery of the patient. It is now entirely clear that immunological parameters are influenced by a multitude of factors induced by trauma or surgery. Neural and humoral factors are influenced by traumatic events and surgical operations resulting in the liberation of mediators. So far, in the event of trauma the situation is clear, but it is impossible to undertake surgical procedures without some type of anesthesia or analgesia. However, the anesthesia itself could exert an immunodepressive or immunostimulative influence or anesthesia might modify the surgical effects on the immunological state of the patient. The effect of anesthesia itself could again give rise to alterations in neurohumoral mechanisms, secondarily influencing immunologic parameters, or quite simply influence the immunological state by some direct action of the anesthetics on immunocompetent cells.

In 1983, Ledingham reported increased mortality in trauma patients treated in his intensive care unit. He attributed the increase in mortality to the use of etomidate infusion for sedation of patients as an alternative to opiate and benzodiazepine injections used prior to the establishment of etomidate infusion. The overall increase was from 25% with opiates and benzodiazepines to 69% with etomidate. Mortality was particularly increased in patients with a high trauma score [1].

It has been suggested that this is because serum cortisol levels are decreased for several hours due to inhibition of cortisol biosynthesis after even a single injection of etomidate, but not with thiopentone [2]. From a superficial point of view, one might assume that there should be improved immune function after etomidate, since cortisol does exert a suppressive effect on cellular immunity. However, increased serum cortisol levels are obviously necessary after trauma or surgical procedures.

The decrease in serum cortisol levels gives rise to a number of secondary effects. Therefore, adrenocorticotropic hormone (ACTH) levels increase significantly after injection of etomidate due to the decrease in plasma cortisol concentrations [2]. This demonstrates that anesthetics can in fact influence humoral factors which may in turn influence immunological function. It must also be remembered that there is an ACTH receptor located in human mononuclear leukocytes, and that both B cells and T cells can be modified functionally by ACTH. ACTH suppresses antibody production by an unknown mechanism [3, 4]. Moreover, ACTH is one part of a peptide hormone precursor from which it is enzymatically separated. The other part of this peptide, which is released by the same reaction, is beta-endorphin which inhibits human leukocyte proliferation and enhances natural killer cell activity [3].

Immune Consequences of
Trauma, Shock and Sepsis
Eds. Faist/Ninnemann/Green

Recent papers by von Haefen [5] and Crozier [6] demonstrate the influence of an anesthetic procedure both on the lytic activity of natural killer cells and on the number of natural killer cells. There is for example a decrease in the number of natural killer cells preoperatively, as determined by the Leu-7 antibody, as well as 6 and 20 h postoperatively following induction of anesthesia by injection of etomidate. After etomidate injection, there is a marked decrease in the number of natural killer cells but not after midozalam injection [6].

It seems clear so far that anesthesia and analgesia influence immunological parameters via modulation of neural and humoral factors. However, the true mechanisms of this reaction seem as yet to be somewhat unclear. Quite apart from these subtle mechanisms, cytostatic effects of a number of anesthetics have been demonstrated.

As early as 1968, Fink demonstrated that several volatile anesthetics slowed the multiplication rate of mouse heteroploid cells [7]. In 1969, Bruce demonstrated a prolongation of DNA synthesis in rat small intestine cells caused by halothane [8]. During the same period of time, the lymphocytes of patients after surgical operations were demonstrated as being less reactive to stimulation by phytohemagglutinin (PHA) [9]. This was attributed by the authors both to anesthetic action and alterations secondary to the surgical trauma. In 1972, Bruce proved that halothane in vitro directly inhibits lymphocyte proliferation induced by PHA [10]. This effect was later shown to be independent of intracellular levels of cyclic AMP and is therefore probably a more nonspecific effect and not directly dependent on interference with receptors influencing the intracellular level of this second messenger [11].

Not only volatile anesthetics were demonstrated as exerting an effect on immunological parameters. In a paper by Neuwelt published in 1982, inhibition of mitogen-induced lymphocyte proliferation in vitro was shown. This inhibition is dependent on concentration and the same concentration of other barbiturates exerts a different inhibition [12]. Moreover, Puppo demonstrated an effect of the barbiturate phenobarbital in vivo, i.e., following oral uptake of this drug. Following a single oral dose, the lymphocytes of volunteers showed reduced response to mitogens [13].

Apparently, volatile and intravenous anesthetics have an immunosuppressive effect which has been shown in vitro, i.e., by the effect of anesthetics on previously prepared lymphocytes, and, as in the last example from Puppo, also in vivo, i.e., on lymphocytes prepared from patients or volunteers who had ingested the drug prior to the lymphocyte preparation. Most of the studies deal with the effects of anesthetics on lymphocyte proliferation induced by mitogens. The reason is that this is a parameter which can be measured relatively easily and which gives, to a certain degree, information regarding cellular immunocompetence.

In order to elaborate on the theories and the studies already discussed, approximately three years ago I carried out investigations in cooperation with the Institute of Surgical Research, University of Munich.

In vitro studies were carried out during the first stage of our investigations. Peripheral blood lymphocytes of volunteers were incubated together with various intravenous anesthetics with and without halothane. Peripheral blood lymphocytes were prepared in the usual way by centrifugation over a Ficoll-Isopaque gradient. After preparation the lymphocytes were kept in culture with and without optimal concentrations of phytohemagglutinin (PHA), pokeweed mitogen (PWM), and concanavalin A (ConA), as well as with the addition of different concentrations of thiopentone, methohexitone, etomidate, and ketamine, and with and without halothane at a concentration of 2%. As a measure of the degree of transformation of the inserted lymphocytes into lymphoblasts, DNA synthesis was measured by incorporation of tritium-labelled methylthymidine. The incorporated radioactivity was determined by means of a liquid scintillation counter. The differences between the counts of the stimulated cultures and those of the controls without mitogens are given.

The influence of increase in concentration of the i.v. anesthetics on the responsiveness to stimulation by ConA is shown in Fig. 1. There is a suppressive influence of thiopentone and to a smaller degree also of methohexitone. Etomidate exhibits an influence only at concentrations far above clinical serum levels. In contrast to these anesthetics, ketamin seems to have no influence at all. The influence of the anesthetics on the cells stimulated by PHA is less pronounced, as it was in the cells stimulated by PWM.

Since thiopentone showed the most pronounced influence on lymphocyte transformation, this anesthetic was investigated more thoroughly. In Fig. 2 the influence on cells stimulated by PHA is shown. It becomes clear that PHA-stimulated cells are suppressed only by concentrations far higher than the ConA-stimulated cells. This becomes even more obvious in cells stimulated by PWM (Fig. 3). On account of this, we concluded that T cells are more subject to the influence of thiopentone than B cells. There is also a suppression of the mixed lymphocyte reaction by thiopentone at rather high concentrations (Fig. 4).

In order to evaluate the influence of the time of action of thiopentone, thiopentone was added to aliquots of the same lymphocyte preparation 24, 48, 72, and 96 h before termination of the culture by freezing of the cells. In Fig. 5 the stimulation rates are shown as a percentage of those of aliquots from the same lymphocyte preparations cultured entirely without addition of thiopentone. It becomes clear that the suppressive influence of thiopentone on mitogen-induced lymphocyte proliferation is not only dependent on concentration but also on the time of action.

In another series of experiments we investigated the influence of halothane on mitogen-induced lymphocyte proliferation. Figure 6 demonstrates the influence of halothane, 2% for 96 h, combined with thiopental, 32 μg/ml for 96 h. Please note that the stimulation rates are given as a percentage of those of anesthetic-free control cultures. As could be expected the combination of the two agents leads in a synergistic manner to a suppression of lymphocyte transformation again especially pronounced in cells stimulated by ConA. In contrast, halothane alone leads to a reduced transformation rate only after stimulation with ConA, even at as high a concentration as 2% for as long as 96 h.

We can now question the clinical significance of these findings. There is marked suppression of lymphocyte transformation by thiopental which is statistically significant for concentrations of 16 μg/ml and more and for a period of action of 24 h or more. In this connection it should be noted that thiopental serum levels during thiopental-induced anesthesia amount to approximately 16 μg/ml

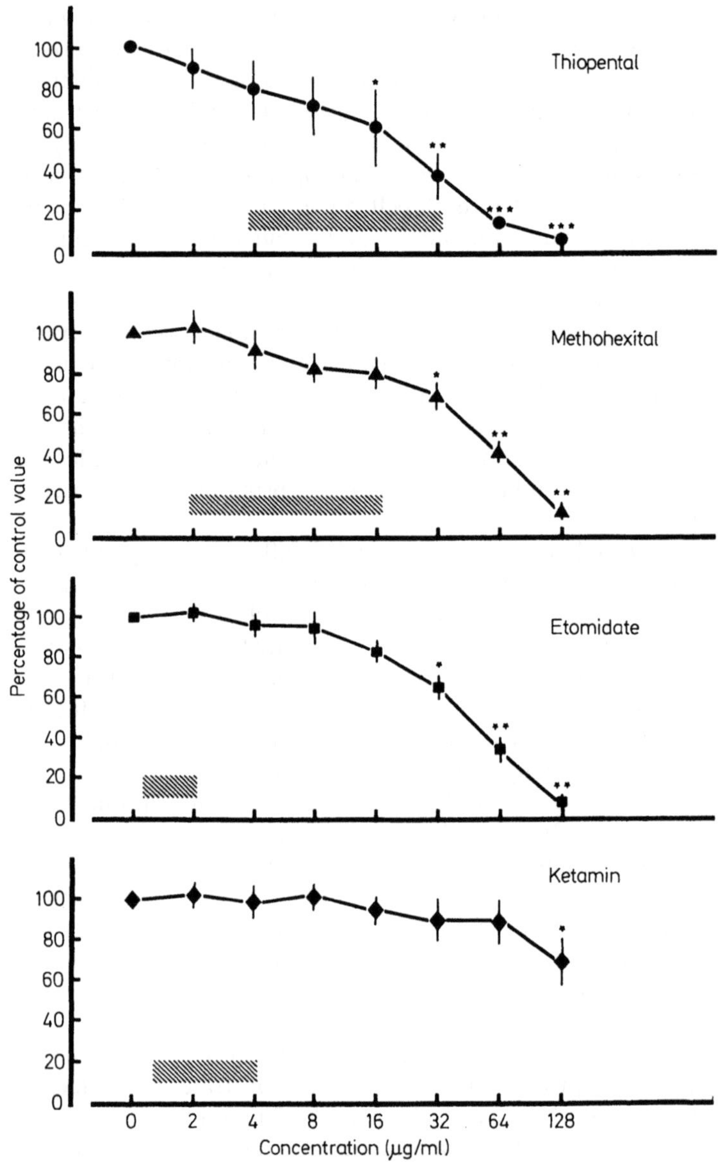

Fig. 1. The influence of intravenously applied anesthetics thiopental ($n=12$), methohexital ($n=8$), etomidate ($n=6$) and ketamine ($n=6$) on the lymphocyte proliferation induced by stimulation with ConA. Depicted are the stimulation rates (cpm) of cultures following the addition of anesthetics, as percentage of the control cultures without addition of narcotics, which were equal to 100% for each set of experiments. Statistics were performed based on the original values before transformation into percentage (Wilcoxon test for paired data). In the case of cultures with addition of narcotics, mean values and standard error of means are given. The *abscissa* shows the concentration of anesthetics; the *dotted bars* near to the respective base lines symbolize the serum concentrations of the respective anesthetics, which can be measured during anesthesia. The numbers (n) give the number of the respective lymphocyte donors. *$P<0.05$; **$P<0.01$; ***$P<0.001$

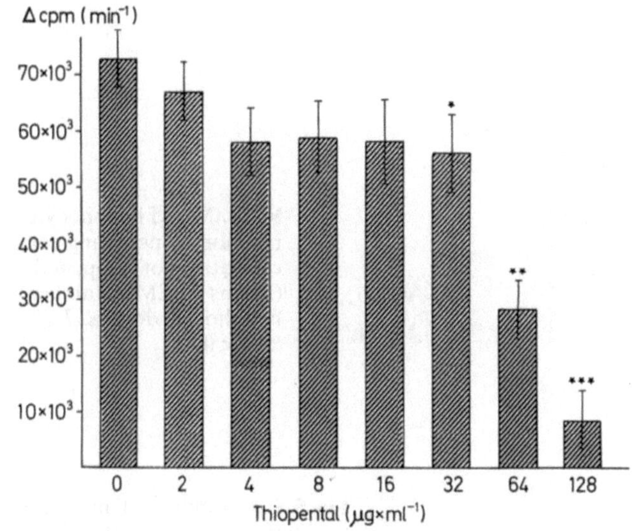

Fig. 2. Transformation of lymphocytes after stimulation by PHA with increasing concentrations of thiopental (means ± SEM). Number of lymphocyte donors, 12. *$P<0.05$; **$P<0.01$; ***$P<0.001$

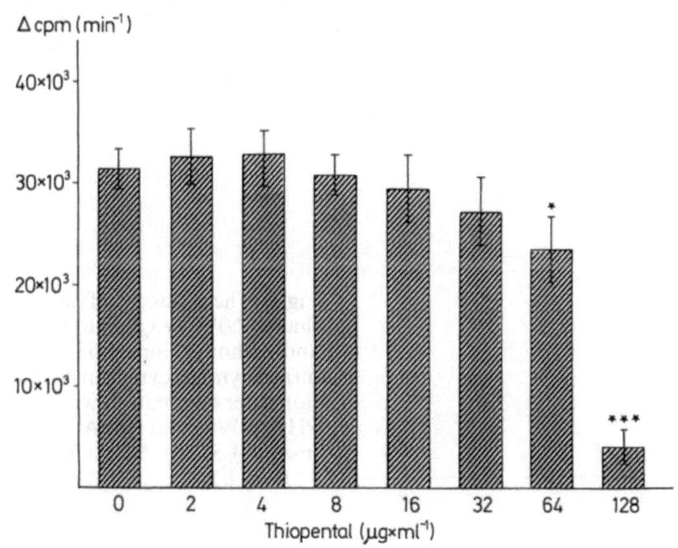

Fig. 3. The influence of thiopental on the PWM induced lymphocyte proliferation (means ± SEM). Number of lymphocyte donors, 12. *$P<0.05$; ***$P<0.01$

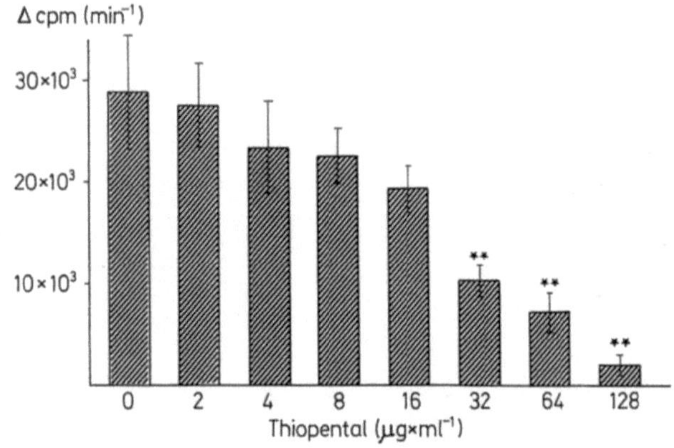

Fig. 4. Mixed lymphocyte reaction in increasing concentrations of thiopental (means ± SEM). Number of lymphocyte donors, 7. $^{**}P<0.01$

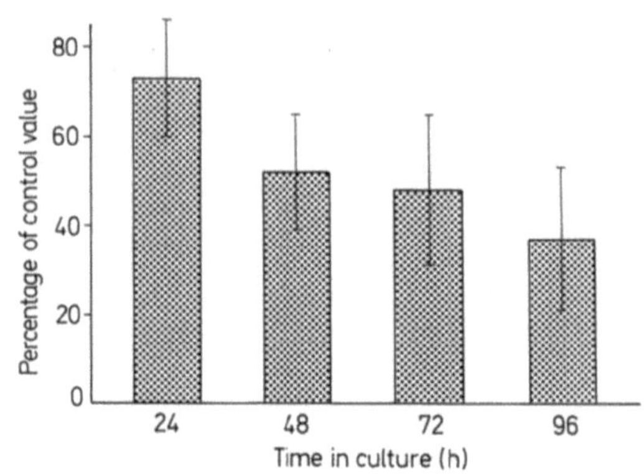

Fig. 5. ConA induced lymphocyte proliferation in thiopental (32 μg/ml) added at different periods of time before termination of the culture. The *columns* on the left symbolize the cultures with a short action for thiopental, the *columns* on the right the cultures with a long action for thiopental (means ± SEM). Number of lymphocyte donors, 6

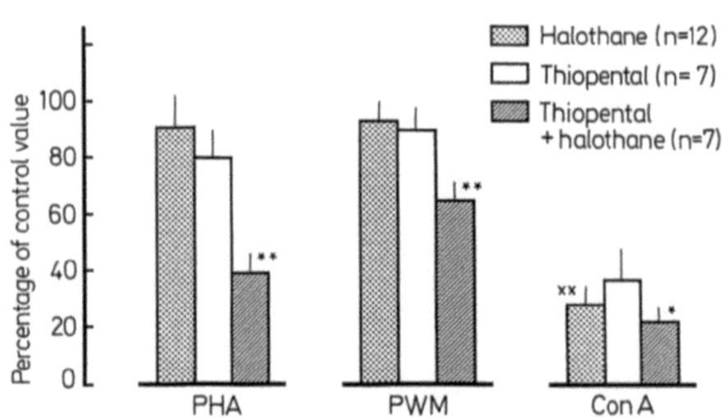

Fig. 6. The influence of halothane (2.0% by volume) with and without thiopental (32 μg/ml) on lymphocyte transformation after stimulation with PHA, PWM and ConA (means ± SEM). $^{*}P<0.05$; $^{**}P<0.01$

during the induction phase and range between 2 and 8 μg/ml in the further course of anesthesia. In the case of high dosage thiopental therapy, as used, e.g., in patients with severe head injury, thiopental serum levels between 30–60 μg/ml are found. With halothane, even at a concentration as high 2% by volume and for as long as 96 h, we could demonstrate in vitro only a moderate suppressive effect, statistically significant only in cells stimulated by ConA. But is this clinically significant?

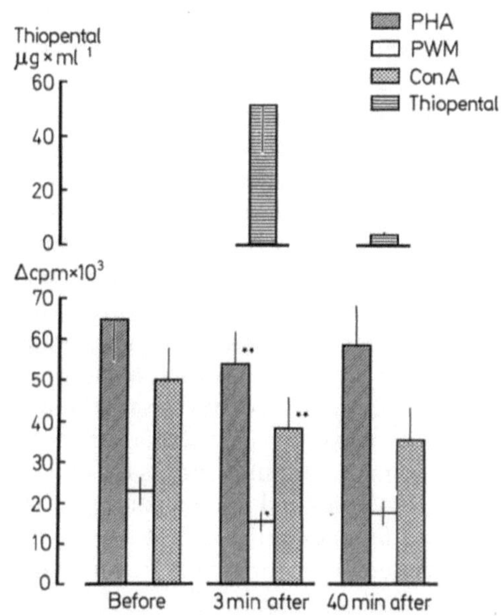

Fig. 7. Mitogen-induced lymphocyte proliferation before and 3 or 40 min after intravenous injection of thiopental. The *upper columns* represent gas chromatography measurements of thiopental serum concentrations; the *bars* on the *lower part* of the illustration represent transformation into lymphoblasts measured as [^{3}H]thymidine incorporated. The lymphocytes were prepared from patients before as well as 3 and 40 min after induction of anesthesia by injection of thiopental 5 mg/body weight (means ± SEM). Numbers of lymphocyte donors, 8. *$P<0.05$; **$P<0.01$; n.s., not significant

The next study was performed to find an answer to this question and to discover whether inhibition of mitogen-induced lymphocyte proliferation can be demonstrated subsequent to intravenous injection of thiopental. Eight male patients were examined who had to undergo coronary artery bypass operations for coronary heart disease. After taking a blood sample for extraction of control lymphocytes, anesthesia was induced by injection of thiopental at a dose of 5 mg/kg body weight. Following the induction of anesthesia, the patient was ventilated via a mask with pure oxygen and 3 min after injection of thiopental a second blood sample was taken. Subsequently the patient was relaxed and intubated and ventilated with pure oxygen to which halothane at an inspiratory concentration of 0.3%–0.8% by volume was added. During this period all the necessary preoperative measures were undertaken. Forty minutes after induction of anesthesia – but still prior to making the first skin incision – the third blood sample was drawn. The results are shown in Fig. 7.

A moderate but statistically significant reduction in the stimulation rates with all mitogens 3 min after induction of anesthesia is clearly demonstrated. These reduced rates of stimulation coincide with a comparatively high thiopental serum level of approximately 60 μg/ml. However, 40 min subsequent to induction of anesthesia and following an additional inhalation of halothane, the stimulation rates with all three mitogens are moderately reduced compared to control values. Statistically, however, this reduction was not significant.

So, taking into account the present results, the conclusion is that the reactivity of lymphocytes to mitogens is reduced by thiopental, both in vitro and in vivo. In vivo, however, i.e., after injection of thiopental in patients, this effect is short-lived and corresponds only to high levels of thiopental.

The question of whether anesthetic agents are a crucial factor in immunosuppression can only be answered to the following extent. On the one hand, the results of the aforementioned study seem to be rather reassuring, since they appear to demonstrate that the anesthesiologist is not apparently responsible for immunosuppression during surgical operations. On the other hand, only a small number of the substances utilized in the course of normal anesthesia were tested, and only one test was used to measure the cellular immunocompetence, on account of the fact that this particular test is easy to perform. However, as is by now entirely clear, the immune system is immensely complicated, and so it would be nonsense to draw conclusions regarding the whole system on account of the results of a few tests. However, in my opinion, from these simple results the conclusion can be drawn that anesthetics are only anesthetics and not cytostatics. If immunological parameters are in fact influenced by anesthetics or anesthesia, this seems to be much more the result of a complicated interaction with the regulation system than simply a cytostatic action on immunocompetent cells.

References

1. Ledingham IM, Watt I (1983) Influence of sedation on mortality in critically ill multiple trauma patients. Lancet 1:1270
2. Allolio B, Stuttmann R, Leonhard U, Fischer H, Winkelmann W (1984) Adrenocortical suppression by a single induction dose of etomidate. Klin Wochenschr 62:1014–1017
3. Plaut M (1987) Lymphocyte hormone receptors. Annu Rev Immunol 5:621–669
4. Smith EM, Brosnan P, Meyer WJ, Blalock JE (1987) An ACTH receptor on human mononuclear leukocytes. Relation to adrenal ACTH-receptor activity. N Engl J Med 317:1266–1269
5. von Haefen B, Zenner HP (1987) Zum Einfluß verschiedener Anästhesieverfahren auf die Natürliche-Killer-Zell-Aktivität. Anaesthesist 36: Zentral Europäischer Anaesthesiekongreß, ZAK 87 München, p. 412
6. Crozier TA, Beck D, Schuff-Werner P, Kettler D (1987) Veränderte Expression lymphozytärer Oberflächenmarker nach Gabe von Etomidat, Midazolam oder Methohexital. Anaesthesist 36:692–695
7. Fink RB, Kenny GE (1968) Metabolic effects of volatile anaesthetics in cell culture. Anesthesiology 29:505–516
8. Bruce DL, Harold HH (1969) The effect of halothane on the cell cycle in rat small intestine. Anesthesiology 30:401–405
9. Park SK, Brody JJ, Wallace HA, Blakmore WS (1971) Immunosuppressive effect of surgery. Lancet 53:108
10. Bruce DL (1972) Halothane inhibition of phytohemagglutinin-induced transformation of lymphocytes. Anesthesiology 36:201–205
11. Bruce DL (1976) Halothane action on lymphocytes does not involve cyclic AMP. Anesthesiology 44:151–154
12. Neuwelt EA, Kikuchi K, Hill SA, Lipsky P, Frenkel E (1982) Barbiturate inhibition of lymphocyte function. J Neurosurg 54:254
13. Puppo F, Adami GF, Corsini G, Zavarise GM, Zattoni J (1980) Effect of single oral dose of phenobarbitone on lymphocyte blastogenesis response in man. Br J Anaesth 5:1205–1207

Comparison of the Effects of General Endotracheal and Epidural Anesthesia on the Immune Functions *

M. Udovic-Sirola, B. Radosevic-Stasic, L. Ribaric, and D. Rukavina

Introduction

It has been known for a long time that anesthetics and operation might provoke changes in the immune response [1, 2]. The observed immunodepression is usually related to the direct toxic effects of some anesthetics on various cells involved in immune reaction [3–5] and to the transitory neuroendocrine changes, provoked by the action of anesthesia or by the activation of the hypothalamohypophyseal adrenal axis by the concomitant operative stress [6, 7]. Since the incidence of postoperative septic complications correlates to the extent of immunodepression, it is very important to choose those anesthetic methods that are less harmful for the immune system, especially in some risk groups of patients (elderly patients, preoperative immunodeficiency, presence of tumor or similar).

One of the favored methods in this sense could be the use of epidural anesthesia, in which the side effects of surgical stress are probably less expressed owing to the neurogenic blockade of the adrenal gland. Data showing the lower increase of endocrine-metabolic response to trauma [8], prevention of postoperative lymphopenia and granulocytosis [9] and the lower impairment of polymorphonuclear neutrophil chemotaxis after epidural than after general anesthesia [10] support this hypothesis. In this study we compared the effects of general endotracheal and epidural anesthesia on the number of lymphocyte subpopulations in peripheral blood and their functional reactivity. We tried to obtain additional information from the analysis of serum, by the determination of its rosette-forming inhibitory properties.

Methods

The research series comprised 64 patients (male and female) of different ages (20–60 years), who were admitted for elective surgical operations in the clinical hospital center. Twenty-seven underwent general endotracheal anesthesia with combined halothane or combined neurolept anesthesia (group A), while 37 underwent epidural anesthesia (group B). Classification of surgical trauma in group A was the following: cholecystectomy, mastectomy, vertebrosynthesis, sigmoidectomy, and ureterotomy; and in group B – osteosynthesis, prostatectomy, embolectomy, and herniorhaphy.

* Supported by grant 2.05.01.04.04. from the Republic of Croatia Research Fund, Zagreb.

Immune Consequences of
Trauma, Shock and Sepsis
Eds. Faist/Ninnemann/Green

In both groups patients with congenital or acquired immunodeficiency and those receiving medication affecting immune response were avoided. Combined halothane anesthesia was induced with thiopentone and pancuronium bromide and then maintained with 0.5%–1% halothane and 70% nitrous oxyde in oxygen, while neurolept analgesia was induced by dehydrobenzperidol and phentanyl. Epidural anesthesia (Th_6-L_3) was performed with 0.5% Marcaine and 2% Xilocaine. Samples of peripheral blood were obtained 24 h before and 24 h after the operation. Lymphocyte subpopulations were monitored immediately after that by the determination of rosette-forming cells (RFCs). Active and avid T-RFCs were determined by our modification of standard methods [11]. Avid cells were considered lymphocytes with ten or more sheep red blood cells (SRBCs). M-RFCs were determined with murine and H-RFCs with human erythrocytes. The functional reactivity of lymphocytes was analyzed by the slight modification of the method of Hartman et al. (1971) [12]. As stimulators of cultured lymphocytes phytohemagglutinin (PHA), concanavalin (ConA), and pokeweed mitogen (PWM) were used. The results were expressed as absolute values of counts per minute of [^{3}H]thymidine incorporated in the culture (cpm) and as transformation index, calculated as the ratio of stimulated and unstimulated cultures.

Sera, separated from the samples of blood collected 24 h before, during, and 24 h after the anesthesia and operation were frozen until use. The existence of immunosuppressive factors in them was then evaluated by the analysis of the number of total E rosettes, formed with lymphocytes of a healthy person in the presence of this serum in comparison with the number of E rosettes formed in the presence of control, AB serum. The deviations from normal values (100%) were then expressed as the index of inhibition.

Statistical analysis was performed by Student's *t*-test.

Results

The effects of general endotracheal and epidural anesthesia in operated patients on the number of RFCs are shown in Fig. 1.

Twenty-four hours after the operation, E rosettes (active, avid, and total) as well as EAC and M rosettes were found to be significantly lower in relation to their preoperative values in patients given general endotracheal anesthesia (group A) than in those operated on under epidural anesthesia (group B). Similar signs of immunosuppression in group A were found in tests of blastic transformation of lymphocytes with polyclonal mitogens (Fig. 2).

In contrast to decreased transformation response to all examined mitogens in group A, responsiveness of lymphocytes to nonspecific antigens in group B was postoperatively unchanged (for PHA and PWM) or even increased (for ConA). In both groups, however, the spontaneous transformation of lymphocytes postoperatively was found to be lower than preoperatively. The analysis of serum revealed that in both groups of patients are present some factors capable of inhibiting the formation of E rosettes of lymphocytes from normal persons with SRBCs (Fig. 3).

Some inhibitory activity was found even in preoperative samples of blood.

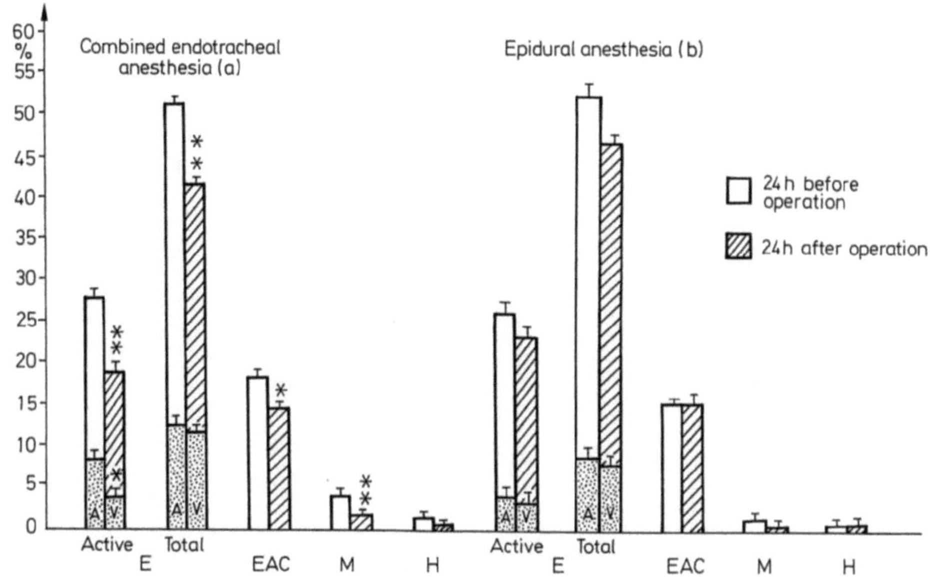

Fig. 1. Effects of combined endotracheal (group A) and epidural anesthesia (group B) on the rosette-forming tests. Values are means ±SEM. Inside the columns of E rosettes, the level of avid rosettes (AV) is shown. *$P<0.05$; **$P<0.01$

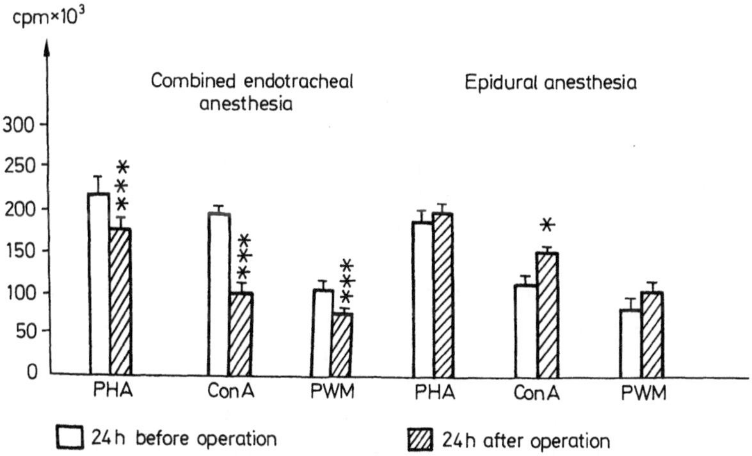

Fig. 2. Effects of combined endotracheal and epidural anesthesia on lymphocyte transformation assays to polyclonal mitogen. Values are means of total number of counts per minute (cpm) ±SEM. *$P<0.05$; ***$P<0.001$

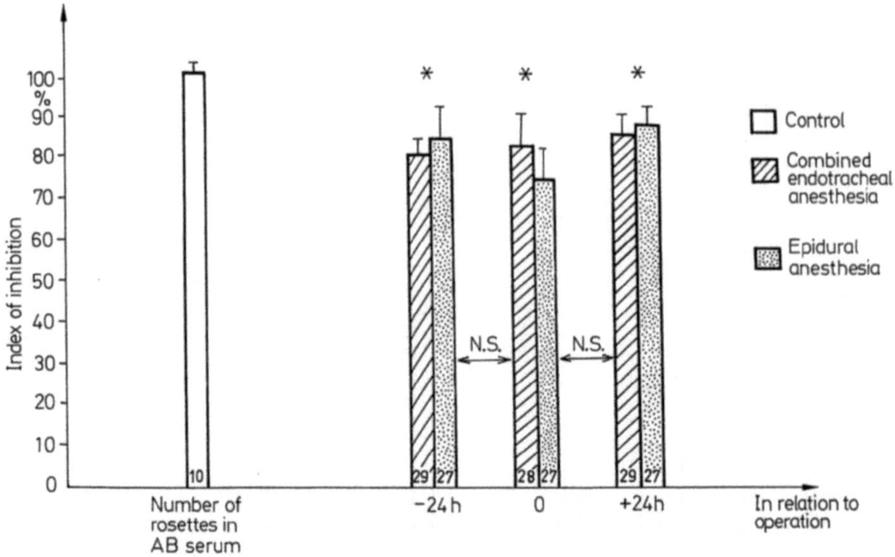

Fig. 3. Rosette inhibitory properties of serum obtained from patients operated on under combined endotracheal or epidural anesthesia. Number of rosettes formed between the lymphocyte from a healthy person in the presence of AB serum is shown as the 100% value. In the columns the number of examined sera is presented. $*P<0.01$ in relation to the control group

Discussion

The data point to the higher incidence of immune suppression in patients operated on under general endotracheal anesthesia in comparison to those operated on under epidural anesthesia. The number of both T- (E rosettes) and B-lymphocytes (EAC rosettes) were found to be decreased only in group A, as well as functional reactivity to these nonspecific mitogens that stimulate mostly T- (PHA and ConA) or B-lymphocytes (PWM).

One possible explanation of the observed difference between these two types of anesthesia is a connection between the immunosuppression and the effects of halothane or neurolept analgesia alone. It is known that halothane anesthesia leads to the depression of both nonspecific [13, 14] and specific immune functions [15, 4, 16]. This is partly the consequence of its toxic effects on several cellular organelles [5] and impairment of mitosis [3]. Besides these direct effects, in vivo application of halothane and neurolept anesthesia leads to the development of transient neuroendocrine changes that might also affect the immune response. Among them it seems that particularly important are those affecting the dopaminergic, serotonergic, and autonomic nervous system because recently published evidence points to immunomodulatory activities not only of many hormones [17] but also of numerous peptides [18] connected with the action of these pathways. Activation of the serotonergic system usually leads to an inhibition of immune response with realization of the effects via the hypothalamo-hypophyseal-adrenal axis, while activation of the dopaminergic system leads to the stimulation of immune response [19]. A direct relationship also exists between the sympathetic nervous system and lymphocytes and other cells of the immune microenvironment. Activation of α-adrenergic receptors usually augments, while stimulation of β-adrenergic receptor inhibits, the lymphocyte proliferation [20]. Since it is known that halothane and drugs used in neurolept analgesia affect almost all of the mentioned structures, it is obvious that greater immunodepression observed in group A than in group B, in our investigation, is probably provoked by the action of general endotracheal anesthesia alone. It must, however, be emphasized that surgical stress in patients operated on under general endotracheal anesthesia is usually greater than in patients operated on under epidural anesthesia. In the latter the operations are simpler and shorter, except that the blockade of splanchnic efferent impulses to the adrenal medulla exists, which reduces sympathetic nervous system activity. Experimental evidence showing that stress suppresses immunity in proportion to the intensity of the stressor and to the degree of operative trauma [6] supports this hypothesis, as well as the findings showing that adrenocortical and hyperglycemic responses to surgery might be blocked by the use of epidural anesthesia [8]. It is therefore often concluded that in patients operated on under general endotracheal anesthesia surgical stress has a principal role for the induction of immunosuppression. In most cases in the plasma of these patients the levels of cortisol and adrenalin were found to be increased more than after epidural anesthesia. This obviously could also explain the finding of the decreased number of E, EAC, and M rosettes and inhibition of blastic transformation in our study after operations performed in general endotracheal anesthesia. From our data, however, it does not seem that differences between the effects of general endotracheal and epidural anesthesia are provoked by the different amount of some inhibitory substance in the blood because a factor that inhibits the formation of rosettes between the normal lymphocytes and SRBCs was present postoperatively, not only in group A with immunodepression, but also in group B, without the signs of impairment of immune functions. Moreover, in both groups of patients, some inhibitory activity was present in serum, even 24 h before the operation, suggesting that emotional stress may also play a role in its formation. Similar stress-behavior influences on the immune system are well documented [21].

The lack of correlation between the rosette inhibitory properties of serum and degree of immunosuppression, of course, does not mean that humoral changes are not involved in the development of observed changes. The possibility exists that susceptibility of lymphocytes to, and recovery from, the action of inhibitory substance, present in the serum, is different in group A than in group B, because halothane and/or greater surgical stress do not affect the same lymphocyte subpopulation as that after epidural anesthesia. Stressful situations usually induce a marked redistribution of cell-possessing suppressor or helper functions [19]. So, adrenalin injected in human volunteers may cause a transient increase of T-suppressor cells, a decrease of circulating T-helper cells, and a decrease of mitogen-induced blastic lymphocyte transformation [22]. It is likely that similar changes were expressed more in group A than in group B in our investigation.

Regardless of the exact mechanism of the induction of immunosuppression after general endotracheal anesthesia, our data suggest that impairment of surgical stress by neurogenic blockade of the adrenal gland with epidural anesthesia may prevent the development of postoperative inhibition of immune function. As a consequence, protection of the patient from the induction of septic and other complications connected with the impairment of the immune system might be assumed to occur simultaneously with the prevention of other endocrine-metabolic changes, provoked by stress response to surgery, such as development of catabolic state, increased oxygen consumption, and increased incidence of postoperative thromboembolism [8, 23].

It seems therefore that in suitable situations regional anesthesia may have some advantages in comparison to endotracheal anesthesia.

Acknowledgment. The excellent technical assistance of Mrs. Marija Kastela and Mrs. Neda Kruzic is gratefully acknowledged.

References

1. Walton B (1979) Effects of anaesthesia and surgery on immune system. Br J Anaesth 51:37–43
2. Watkins J (1980) Immunological problems in anaesthesia. Br J Hosp Med 23:583–590
3. Bruce DL, Koepke JA (1966) Changes in granulopoiesis in the rat associated with prolonged halothane anesthesia. Anesthesiology 27:811–816
4. Bruce DL (1972) Halothane inhibition of PHA-induced transformation of lymphocytes. Anesthesiology 36:201–205
5. Kusyk CJ, Hsu TC (1976) Mitotic anomalies induced by three inhalation halogenated anesthetics. Environ Res 12:366–370
6. Berenbaum MC, Fluck PA, Hurst NP (1973) Depression of lymphocyte response after surgical trauma. Br J Exp 54:597–607
7. Ryhanen P (1977) Effects of anaesthesia and operative surgery on the immune response of patients of different ages. Ann Clin Res 9:7–75
8. Brandt MR, Fernande A, Mordhors R et al. (1978) Epidural analgesia improves postoperative nitrogen balance. Br Med J 1:1106–1108
9. Rem J, Brandt MR, Kehlet H (1980) Prevention of postoperative lymphopenia and granulocytosis by epidural analgesia. Lancet 1:283–295
10. Stanley TH, Hill GE, Hill HR (1978) The influence of spinal and epidural anesthesia on neutrophil chemotaxis in man. Anesth Analg 57:567–571
11. Rukavina D (1983) A modified test of active T lymphocytes and its clinical significance. Period Biol 85:243–245
12. Hartman RJ, Segall M, Bach ML et al. (1971) Histocompatibility matching. VI. Miniaturization of the mixed leucocyte culture test: a preliminary report. Transplantation 11:268–274
13. Bruce DL (1966) Effect of halothane anesthesia on extravascular mobilisation of neutrophils. J Cell Physiol 68:81–83
14. Moudgil GC, Allan RB, Russell RJ et al. (1977) Inhibition by anaesthetic agents of human leucocyte locomotion towards chemical attractants. Br J Anesth 49:97–105
15. Humphrei LJ, Wingard DW, Lang R (1969) The effect of surgery and anesthesia on the immunologic responsiveness of the rat. Surgery 65:946–951
16. Lewis RE, Cruse JM, Hayelwood J (1980) Halothane-induced suppression of cell-mediated immunity in normal and tumor-bearing C3Hf/He mice. Anesth Analg 59:666–671

17. Pierpaoli W, Fabris N, Sorkin E (1970) Development hormones and immunological maturation. In: Wolstenholme GEW, Knight J (eds) Hormones and the immune response. Churchill, London, pp 126–143 (Ciba Foundation Study Group no 36)
18. Morley JE, Kay NE, Solomon GF et al. (1987) Neuropeptides: conductors of the immune orchestra. Life Sci 41:527–544
19. Devoino L, Idova G, Alperina E et al. (1986) Distribution of immunocompetent cells underlying psychoneuroimmunomodulation. Ann NY Acad Sci 496:292–300
20. Hall NR, Goldstein AL (1981) Neurotransmitters and the immune system. In: Ader R (ed) Psychoneuroimmunology. Academic, New York, pp 521–543
21. Ader R, Grota LJ, Cohen N (1986) Conditioning phenomena and immune function. Ann NY Acad Sci 496:532–544
22. Crary B, Borysenko M, Sutherland DC et al. (1983) Decrease in mitogen responsiveness of mononuclear cells from peripheral blood after epinephrine administration in humans. J Immunol 130:604–697
23. Thornburn J, Louden JR, Vallance R (1980) Spinal and general anaesthesia in total hip replacement: frequency of deep vein thrombosia. Br J Anaesth 52:1117–1121

Effect of Splenectomy Upon the Antibody Response to Pneumococcal Immunization

M. A. Malangoni and J. C. Peyton

Introduction

Splenectomized man is at increased risk for overwhelming infection due to encapsulated bacteria, in particular *Streptococcus pneumoniae*. Studies in man and animals have linked the virulence of *S. pneumoniae* to the presence of a thick polysaccharide capsule that surrounds the cell. This capsular polysaccharide is type specific and is the basis for the current multivalent pneumococcal vaccine used to protect against infection due to *S. pneumoniae* following splenectomy.

The spleen acts as a reticuloendothelial filter of bacteria and particulates from the bloodstream and also is an important source of antibody production. Splenectomy may impair bacterial clearance as well as diminish the ability to manufacture antibody in response to a bacterial challenge, even after immunization has occurred. Indeed, immunization after splenectomy improves survival from a pneumococcal challenge yet this restoration is not complete [1].

This study investigates the primary and secondary antibody responses both to pneumococcal whole cell or protein vaccine and to capsular polysaccharide and examines the effect of splenectomy upon the production of antibody.

Methods

Adult Sprague-Dawley rats were immunized 3 weeks following sham laparotomy or splenectomy. Initial immunization was with either 0.2 μg type 3 pneumococcal capsular polysaccharide or with 10^5 heat-formalin-killed whole cells (*S. pneumoniae*, type 3, American Type Culture Collection #6303). These doses were chosen since prior study has shown that they elicit optimal antibody responses in this model. Twenty-one days later, all rats were reimmunized with 0.2 μg type 3 pneumococcal polysaccharide. Blood was withdrawn intermittently throughout the experiment for determination of total, IgM, and IgG antibody as determined by enzyme-linked immunosorbent assay (ELISA).

The ELISA was a modification of the microassay described by Voller et al. [2] with polysaccharide antigen coating as described by Kalin and Lindberg [3]. In brief, low protein-binding 96-well microtiter plates were coated with 1 μg type 3 pneumococcal polysaccharide in barbital buffer, pH 8.6, and incubated at room temperature overnight. After washing with phosphate-buffered saline (PBS, pH 7.3), with 0.1% Tween 20 (T), serum diluted 1 : 150 in PBS-T was added, incubated for 2 h, and washed with PBS-T × 3. Alkaline phosphatase-conjugated

Immune Consequences of
Trauma, Shock and Sepsis
Eds. Faist/Ninnemann/Green

goat anti-rat immunoglobulin (Ig) was added to detect total Ig or specific IgM or IgG pneumococcal antibody (anti-Ig, Sigma Chemical, St. Louis, MO; anti-IgM, Cappel Biochemical, Malvern, PA; anti-IgG, Rockland, Inc, Gilbertsville, PA). Following 45 min incubation the reaction was stopped by adding 0.1 *N* NaOH and the plates read at 410 nm. All samples were done in duplicate and mean values were expressed in units of optical density (OD).

Statistical comparisons were done using Student's *t*-test for unpaired values.

Results

Total Ig rose following immunization to a maximum at day 5 after both primary and secondary vaccinations. Splenectomy did not alter the time to peak response. The primary IgM antibody peaked on day 5 and was reduced significantly by splenectomy (1.5 OD vs. 0.08 OD, $P<0.05$). The initial IgG response peaked on day 12 and was greatest following polysaccharide vaccination in sham-operated rats ($P<0.05$ vs. others). Secondary immunization accentuated the IgM response in all animals; however, IgM levels remained lower in splenectomized rats than in the sham-operated animals (0.28 vs. 0.57 OD, $P<0.05$). While polysaccharide vaccine resulted in greater IgG production after primary immunization compared with the whole cell vaccine, the levels of IgM and IgG were similar in both groups following secondary immunization. Splenectomy impaired the anamnestic response to both vaccine types.

Discussion

Following splenectomy, pneumococcal challenge is characterized by persistent bacteremia and an increased mortality. This excessive mortality following splenectomy is likely due to loss of the splenic reticuloendothelial mass, which is an important site for clearance of unopsonized bacteria. Immunization improves survival in this setting by stimulating antibody production, which results in an increased clearance of opsonized bacteria by the hepatic Kupffer's cells.

While protein antigens characteristically induce an anamnestic or immunologic memory response, vaccination with carbohydrate antigens such as pneumococcal polysaccharide may not elicit such a response. This difference is likely due to the manner in which the antigens are processed in the spleen. Protein antigens are preferentially routed through the red pulp to the germinal centers, where large numbers of antibody-producing cells reside [4]. On the contrary, carbohydrate antigens such as pneumococcal polysaccharide are routed to the splenic white pulp, where less antibody-producing cells are available.

The antibody response to pneumococcal vaccination illustrates two important points. First, an optimal antibody response to a carbohydrate antigen such as pneumococcal capsular polysaccharide occurs within a very narrow dose of antigen [5]. Larger doses of capsular polysaccharide actually impair the antibody response, a phenomenon known as "immunologic paralysis" [6]. Second, the anamnestic response to capsular polysaccharide may be limited unless this carbohydrate is coupled with a particulate such as sheep red blood cells or is given in the form of a whole cell vaccine, which is a protein antigen. Failure of IgG production on subsequent bacterial challenge may be associated with a lack of protection against pneumococcal infection. In contrast, prior exposure to the whole cell vaccine leads to an appropriate anamnestic response even when using only pneumococcal capsular polysaccharide.

Besides acting as a reticuloendothelial filter for the bloodstream, the spleen also has an important role in the production of antibody. In this model splenectomy significantly impaired the antibody response to immunization with both whole cell and polysaccharide capsular pneumococcal vaccine. Despite differences in antibody production following primary immunization, both vaccine types provided similar levels of antibody following secondary immunization, suggesting that the immunogen chosen is not critical in these circumstances. In the absence of the spleen, the reduced primary and secondary antibody responses may augment other deficits in pneumococcal clearance that are either preexistent or induced by splenectomy and these synergistic deficits may explain the increased mortality observed in this model.

Summary

The primary and anamnestic antibody responses of Sprague-Dawley rats immunized with either pneumococcal polysaccharide or whole cell vaccine were assessed. Splenectomy led to a significant impairment of primary and secondary antibody responses. The spleen is essential for antibody production following immunization, and production of antibody upon reimmunization with pneumococcal polysaccharide occurs only in animals with intact spleens.

References

1. Dawes LG, Malangoni MA, Speigel CA, Schiffman G (1985) Response to immunization after partial and total splenectomy. J Surg Res 39:53–58
2. Voller A, Bidwell DE, Bartlett A (1979) The enzyme-linked immunosorbent assay (ELISA): a guide with abstracts of microplate applications. Zoological Soc London, London, pp 23–40
3. Kalin M, Lindberg AA (1985) Antibody responses against the type-specific capsular polysaccharide in pneumococcal pneumonia measured by enzyme-linked immunosorbent assay. Scand J Infect Dis 17:25–32
4. Lockwood CM (1983) Immunological functions of the spleen. Clin Haematol 12:449–465
5. Coonrod JD, Rylko-Bauer B (1976) Antigenicity of type-specific pneumococcal polysaccharides in rats. Infect Immun 13:1554–1558
6. Jones JM, Amsbaugh DF, Prescott B (1976) Kinetics of the antibody response to type III pneumococcal polysaccharide. II Factors influencing the serum antibody levels after immunization with an optimally immunogenic dose of antigen. J Immunol 116:52–64

Summary

References

Surgical Aspects of AIDS

D. A. August and H. Rice

Trauma, shock, and sepsis are accompanied by profound immunosuppression. This immunosuppression is evidenced by abnormalities in cellular immunity, humoral immunity, macrophage function, and neutrophil function [1, 2]. The resultant immunodeficiency is not merely of academic interest, but rather expresses itself in the form of increased susceptibility of severely injured patients to infections caused not only by organisms usually considered pathogenic, but also by so-called nonpathogenic microbes. A major difficulty encountered in studying this immunosuppression in vivo is the multiplicity of factors causing it. It is often impossible to sort out the interrelating effects of trauma, sepsis, surgery, and anesthesia on the patient's immune system. An additional confounding issue is often the emergent appearance of clinical problems in severely injured patients. The rapidity with which clinical events occur usually makes it impossible to establish a baseline with which subsequent measurements may be prospectively compared.

The immunologic abnormalities observed in patients with the acquired immunodeficiency syndrome (AIDS) in many ways mirror those seen in severely injured patients. Among the major immunologic derangements measured in AIDS patients are a decreased T-helper: T-suppressor cell ratio, decreased proliferative responses to soluble antigens, impaired delayed-type hypersensitivity reactivity, decreased humoral response to specific immunization, decreased proliferative responses to T-cell mitogens, decreased interleukin-2 production, decreased natural killer cell activity, and impaired macrophage and neutrophil chemotaxis [3]. All of these abnormalities have been reported in human or animal model investigations of severely injured and septic patients [1, 2]. Although the severity and consequences of the immunologic abnormalities associated with AIDS are by no means homogeneous, they evolve with a much slower time course than similar deficiencies in the severely injured patient. This permits better prospective investigation of the clinical consequences of the immunodeficiency.

AIDS also offers a unique opportunity to understand the specific consequences of surgery in a host with a well-characterized immunodeficient state. As this state in some ways mimics the immunodeficiency observed in the severely injured patient, an understanding of the immune consequences of surgery in AIDS patients may offer insight into the consequences of surgery in severely injured patients. Additionally, many surgical procedures in AIDS patients are less urgent than those in severely injured patients and may occur in situations not clouded by acute sepsis and tissue destruction. Thus, these procedures in some ways offer an "experiment of nature," permitting insight into the consequences of surgery in an immunodeficient host in the absence of many of the confounding variables inherent in trauma and sepsis settings.

Immune Consequences of
Trauma, Shock and Sepsis
Eds. Faist/Ninnemann/Green

There have been few reports addressing broad surgical issues in AIDS patients. The natural history of surgical disease in AIDS patients, the indications for diagnostic and therapeutic operations, and the outcomes of these procedures is poorly characterized. At Yale we have reviewed the surgical treatment of AIDS patients during the period January 1981 through September 1987 to answer questions regarding clinical patterns of presentation, indications for surgery, efficacy of surgical intervention, and operative morbidity and mortality.

During this period, 63 surgical procedures were performed in 48 patients. Diagnostic open lung biopsy was the most common procedure undertaken, and was diagnostic in 91% of cases. Frequent findings were pneumocystitis carinii, *Mycobacterium avium*-intracellular, and cytomegalovirus pneumonias. Open brain biopsy was also commonly performed and was diagnostic in more than 80% of cases. Toxoplasmosis and lymphoma were the most frequent findings. Operative complications with both of these procedures were limited to two instances of ventilator dependence.

Eleven procedures were performed to establish venous access in nine patients. Three transcutaneous venous access devices (Hickman catheter-type devices) were inserted. Two became infected within 14 days, and the third at 6 months. All infections involve staphylococcal organisms. Only one of the totally implantable devices became infected. Although the organisms causing these episodes of catheter sepsis were those typically seen, it is possible that the synergy of the AIDS immunodeficiency coupled with the break in the skin barrier necessitated by a transcutaneous venous access device contributed to the high incidence of infection seen with the Hickman-type devices.

Of interest are the AIDS patients who underwent laparotomy. There were 9 such patients in whom 11 procedures were performed. The only complication occurred in a patient who underwent liver biopsy and biopsy of a portal lymph node. Ascites developed postoperatively that necessitated closure of an ascitic leak and ultimately a peritoneovenous shunt. Despite such intraoperative findings as a bleeding candidal gastric ulcer, *Candida* cholecystitis, hepatic MAI, and retroperitoneal MAI, there were no infectious complications.

In this entire series, there were no complicating opportunistic infections. Despite the severe impairment of these patients' immune systems, they tolerated surgery quite well, experiencing only complications routinely seen in ill patients requiring operative intervention. Preoperative and postoperative assessment of serum albumin, white blood count cell, and total lymphocyte count did not reveal any differences at the two time points, nor did they allow prediction of those patients who would experience complications. We are currently undertaking a prospective study to investigate the specific effect of surgery on a battery of immune parameters in AIDS patients. Thirty-three of 48 patients survived to leave the hospital; none of the in-hospital deaths were surgery related.

This experience, which is in agreement with a number of other reported series [4, 5], suggests that surgery in AIDS patients is an appropriate therapeutic modality. Although the indications for diagnostic procedures (e.g., lung biopsy, brain biopsy, lymph node biopsy) differ from those in the general population, therapeutic procedures may be considered independent of the underlying immunodeficiency. The low incidence of postoperative infectious complications and the absence of complicating opportunistic infections is somewhat surprising. This correlates with surgical experience in profoundly neutropenic patients, but these patients do not suffer from the myriad of immune deficiencies that AIDS patients do. This may, however, suggest that the immunosuppression associated with surgery is not of great clinical significance in the setting of an underlying immunodeficient state. This supports the generally shared belief that surgery, as it debrides devitalized tissue, drains walled-off infections, stabilizes fractures, and provides access for nutritional support, remains the most important modality in the treatment of the severely injured patient.

References

1. Baker CC (1986) Immune mechanisms and host resistance in the trauma patient. Yale J Biol Med 59:387–393
2. Abraham E (1985) Immunologic mechanisms underlying sepsis in the critically ill surgical patient. Surg Clin North Am 65(4):991–1003
3. Seligmann M, Pinching AJ, Rosen FS et al. (1987) Immunology of human immunodeficiency virus infection and the acquired immunodeficiency syndrome. Ann Intern Med 107:234–242
4. David JM, Mouradian J, Fernandez RD et al. (1984) Acquired immune deficiency syndrome. A surgical perspective. Arch Surg 119:90–95
5. Robinson G, Wilson SE, Williams RA (1987) Surgery in patients with acquired immunodeficiency syndrome. Arch Surg 122:170–175

Section 7

Restoration of Impaired Immune Response: In Vitro Models and Clinical Trials

Immunomodulation and the Surgeon

J. L. Meakins and D. Franco

The infectious complications of surgical illness and trauma continue to have a major impact upon morbidity and mortality. Advances in trauma care and a clearer understanding of the physiology of surgery and surgical illness have reduced many formerly common complications such as renal and respiratory failure. These improvements have reduced the incidence of early mortal illness and injury, but have been costly in terms of late complications such as multiple system organ failure and the septic syndrome. Control of infection and infectious complications therefore remains an important objective. The determinants of infection as a biological framework applicable to all surgery will be presented together with the evidence that the surgeon, operatively and otherwise, can have a meaningful influence on the ability of the surgical patient to resist both colonization and infection locally and systemically. Manipulation of these responses, immunomodulation (Meakins et al. 1979; Polk 1984; Alexander et al. 1987), has been promising so far, but disappointing in its clinical application. The search for a single magic bullet – levamisole, muramyl dipeptide, BCG, fibronectin, steroids, prostaglandin inhibitors, glucan – has not been fruitful. This chapter will consider quality of care as the immunomodulator. Surgeons will be shown to have an important influence upon host factors which contribute to the reduction of infection and its impact upon morbidity and mortality.

Determinants of Infection

The development of an infection is a dynamic process involving many factors; these can be classified into three kinds of determinants: (1) the microorganism(s) producing the infection, (2) the environment in which it takes place, the local defenses, and (3) the host–defense mechanisms, the systemic responses to bacteria established in tissue, the immune system. Normally there is continuous interaction among these factors, in that there are frequent breaks in mucosal and cutaneous barriers which, despite having organisms present, do not become infected. In addition, the commensal flora prevent pathogenic organisms from invading, and those that do invade are dispersed by local (environmental) and systemic responses. There is a dynamic balance between the determinants.

Immune Consequences of
Trauma, Shock and Sepsis
Eds. Faist/Ninnemann/Green

If all of the interwoven factors could be identified and weighted, an equation would result:

$$\begin{aligned} P\ (\text{infection}) = K &+ A\ (\text{bacteria}) \\ &+ B\ (\text{environment:local factors}) \\ &+ C\ (\text{host defense mechanisms:systemic factors}). \end{aligned}$$

The schematic approach is presented to introduce the concept of sepsis as a process in which the surgeon can influence each determinant (Meakins 1988). All surgeons have been faced with the patient who appeared to have a negligible injury or a successful operation, but who rapidly dissolved in pus. Any one of the three determinants might be responsible: an extraordinarily virulent organism, a local, minor technical error, or abnormal resistance to infection with an inability to contain even the slightest microbiologic contamination, or more likely a combination of small abnormalities of two, or even three, determinants.

The Surgical Patient: An Altered Host

Acquired immunodeficiency is a very fashionable area of study when caused by a virus. It should, however, be noted that many more patients have acquired defects of host resistance and secondary infections as a result of surgical disease, surgery itself, its complications, and all aspects of trauma with major health care implications for disease, disability, and death (Meakins et al. 1980, 1981). Two questions come to mind: Who has these abnormalities, and do they really matter? This text answers the first question. The next is more problematic. Can anything be done about abnormal host–defense mechanisms? There are several patient populations with grossly altered host defenses from whom surgeons have learned a great deal about the control of infection. These are patients with thermal injury, recipients of organ transplants and trauma elective surgical, and surgical intensive care patients. The following touches on some of these, but does not review in any detail the acquired abnormalities identified in surgical patients. The preceding chapters in this book will have reviewed these in detail. Rather it will address some areas which have led to change in therapeutic behaviors and/or to improvements in care and will show that abnormalities in host defense really do matter.

Thermal Injury

The burn patient is well known to have an increased risk of infection (Deitch 1988). With the shock phase controlled, sepsis has become the principal hazard of thermal injury. The burn presents an obvious example of an altered environment permitting infection – the wound providing a warm, wet, nutritient-rich environment in which bacteria flourish. The importance of systemic host factors and their study evolved concurrently with topical therapy and at an increased pace as patients still died of sepsis. Almost every component of host resistance to infection is affected by burns (Deitch 1988).

Thermal injury incorporating 30% of body surface or more has become the prototype of acquired derangement of host defenses which because of the magnitude and breadth of the abnormalities has become a common laboratory model (Tchervenkov et al. 1986). The profound immunosuppressive effect of thermal injury and attendant catabolism is largely responsible for the high incidence of and mortality from sepsis. All abnormalities are resolved when the burn wound has healed. The determinants of infection in thermal injury are decreased host defenses in the presence of an abnormal environment – the burn wound – and account for the high probability of infection.

Age and Chronic Health Status

Advancing age is associated with a decline in strength and changes in physiological function which decreases linearly with age. Immune function is no exception (Christou 1988). These changes affect all aspects of the immune response and both specific and nonspecific effector mechanisms. The simplest measure of altered immune function is skin testing. Anergy increases with age and is associated with increased septic complications. The altered physiology of the elderly makes it more difficult for them to respond to stress (Knaus et al. 1985). The Apache II (acute physiology and chronic health evaluation) system is a measure of chronic health status and physiological variables which together with age make a reliable score for predicting outcome in serious illness. Host defenses are abnormal. Infection rates are high.

Surgery and Trauma

Both surgery and trauma can influence most aspects of the immune response (Meakins 1981). The principal concept is that the degree of injury, whether from a motor vehicle accident or from controlled surgical trauma, is directly (Slade et al. 1975) related to the magnitude in the postinjury abnormalities of host resistance (Christou et al. 1980, 1982; Meakins et al. 1978).

Previous health status and age of the patient are significant variables which will affect the expression of host–defense abnormalities following surgery and trauma. With increasing age, less injury is required to produce anergy (Meakins 1978). While studied within the context of fractured hips and multiple trauma with high injury severity scores, the natural extension to surgery as trauma demonstrates that the magnitude of an operation is directly proportional to the postoperative changes in the reaction skin testing and neutrophil function (Christou et al. 1982).

The two critical variables seem to be the state of host resistance (age, immunosuppression, chronic disease) at the time of trauma (burn, fall, operation) and its magnitude as measured by blood loss, shock, tissue injury and dissection, number of broken bones, etc.

Infection

Infection itself, whether viral, fungal, or bacterial, is immunosuppressive. The control of an infectious process can eliminate the cycle of stimulant and mediator which leads to immunosuppression. There are innumerable clinical examples, but two will suffice: the loss of tuberculin skin responses in miliary tuberculous or following measles and the increased incidence of pneumonia following epidemic flu.

The Surgeon: An Immunomodulator

The surgeon is too often thought of as a technician with little involvement in the pre- and postoperative management decisions which may play a role in outcome. This is particularly apparent when anesthetists decide who is fit for operation, thereby distancing the surgeon from important modulating decisions with respect both to how to prepare the patient and when to operate. It must be recognized that surgeons can influence the determinants of infection (Meakins 1988) and results of surgery (Fielding et al. 1978; Franco et al. 1989). In the following discussion we would like to demonstrate how good surgical care influences outcome with respect to modulation of the host's response to bacteria, i.e., the surgeon as an immunomodulator.

The anergic patient, known to have an increased incidence of infection, is represented in Fig. 1. Our goal is to decrease susceptibility to infection, allowing the patient to cope with a larger inoculum of bacteria, while having the same or lower incidence of infection.

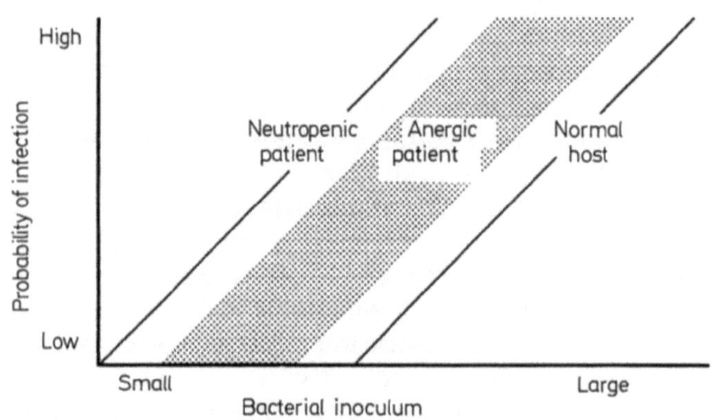

Fig. 1. The relationship between the inoculum (high or low) and the incidence of infection (high or low) is presented as a function of the patient–host resistance to infection. The normal host and the neutropenic patient represent the extremes. The anergic patient who does have an increased risk of infection lies between them. Surgical care objectives are to move the patient representation to the right, which would show tolerance of more bacteria with the same or fewer infections

Specific Clinical Situations

The following clinical problems provide examples of how the total approach to the patient influences host responses.

Shock

The wide range of effects shock has upon the patient are well known. There are generalized ischemic effects which influence specific organ systems such as acute tubular necrosis, peripheral ischemia, stroke, myocardial infarction, intestinal ischemia with ulcers, to name but a few. There is clear evidence that specific resistance to infection is altered at the time of shock (Miles et al. 1957) and for up to 5 days afterwards (Livingstone and Malangoni 1989). In both time frames there is an inoculum effect, that is, infection rates are markedly altered by numbers of bacteria. Animals in shock require far fewer organisms to generate infection when compared to normal animals (Livingstone and Malangoni 1989). These results would be expected in the short term because altered perfusion decreases the inflammatory response and resistance to infection at the time of contamination (Miles 1980; Livingstone and Malangoni 1988; Nichols et al. 1984). Of great significance is that for up to 5 days after shock, the resistance to infection is reduced. This can only be mediated through a significantly altered systemic immune response as all local perfusion defects will have long been corrected. The implications for care are clear. Bleeding and trauma, the basic causes of shock, are surgical diseases. Resuscitation, speed, and efficacy are critical to reducing the late systemic effects of shock. Prevention and control of hemorrhage in the operating room is crucial both for early and late effects. Once shock has occurred, the patient must be considered immunocompromised.

Burns and Other Wounds

Burns are the prototype injury in humans and animals which is used to demonstrate the wide influence of trauma upon the immune response (Deitch 1988; Tchervenkov et al. 1986). In recent years there have been a number of areas in which specific approaches to therapy have radically altered outcome. Topical agents facilitated management by suppressing bacterial growth, at the cost of delaying separation of eschar and prolonging the period of immune suppression secondary to the wound. The next obvious step was early excision of the burn wound and coverage with autografts or a mixture of auto- and allograft skin. With excision and coverage of the burn wound, *the stimulus,* although multifactorial and multidimensional, for the generation of mediators and the array of humoral messengers which downregulate and render the immune response less effective is removed. The wound is closed, and with closure the patient is converted from a hypermetabolic, immunocompromised patient to one requiring reconstruction.

The control of the shock phase of the burn injury is well understood and a standard part of therapy (see above). Better understanding of the catabolic and hypermetabolic aspects of thermal injury has led to nutritional support with either specific nutrients (see Alexander, this volume) or routes of therapy (see Border, this volume) to provide the fuel and building blocks permitting early ex-

Table 1. Host defense mechanisms and severity of diseases in ten patients with Crohn's disease

	Normal	Abnormal
Severity of disease (CDAI)	63.7±23.1	341.2±33.0
Skin test		
Normal	10	–
Relative anergic	–	7
Anergic	–	3
Neutrophil chemotaxis	126.6± 2.3	103.7± 3.2
Neutrophil delivery into skin windows $\times 10^6$		
6 h	11.4± 2.0	0.5± 0.2
12 h	144.4±23.1	25.2±12.5

CDAI, Crohn's disease activity index.

cision and grafting and control of the negative response to trauma and dead tissue.

These concepts of burn wound management have their roots in the management of other wounds where "nettoyage et débridement" and rapid closure are the cornerstones of management. The implications for the patient are that they resist bacterial contamination better, not only in the wound, but also elsewhere.

Crohn's Disease

Crohn's disease has been postulated to be a result rather than the cause of abnormal host defenses. Superina et al. (1980) have shown (Table 1) that control of the disease with associated reduction of the Crohn's disease activity index (CDAI) to resonable levels is closely correlated with an improvement in skin tests, neutrophil chemotaxis, and polymorphonuclear neutrophil (PMN) delivery into skin windows over Rebuck-like abrasions (Superina et al. 1980). This approach to preoperative preparation, quality of care, and control of inflammation has recently (Hill et al. 1988) been linked to significant improvements in operative outcome. Controlling the disease controls its expression, one factor of which is immunosuppression.

Intra-abdominal Infection

As part of a study on immunomodulators in anergic surgical patients (Meakins et al. 1979), we examined the impact on immune function of surgery to resolve specific lesions and to drain intra-abdominal abscesses (Tables 2, 3). It is apparent that reactions to skin tests improved promptly following surgical correction of the inciting lesion. In particular, drainage of pus can be seen to resolve anergy. Surgery can clearly be as effective as an antibiotic or an immune modulator.

In persistent peritonitis (Maddeus and Simmons 1987; Walsh et al. 1989) not only are the bacteria different (Rotstein et al. 1986), but the host response is abnormal. The failure of nonspecific responses can be followed closely in an infected peritoneum where there is loose watery pus and complete failure of localization

Table 2. Definitive therapy and recovery of skin-test responses

Operation	Patients	Days A/RA → N
Biliary tract surgery	11	5.7
Resection of colon cancer	8	6.6
Relief of bowel obstruction	5	8.2
Control of hemorrhage	5	5.8
Miscellaneous	3	5

Table 3. Drainage of postoperative, postpancreatitis intraperitoneal abscesses and skin tests

Patients	Drainage procedures	Skin tests
7	1	$A/RA \xrightarrow{5.4} RA/N$
2	2/3	$A \xrightarrow{6} N$
2	2/3 unsuccessful	$A \longrightarrow A$[a]

[a] Both died of sepsis.
A, anergy; RA, relative anergy; N, normal skin test response.

or fibrin formation. In addition, the granulation in the wound is unhealthy, has a pallid, ragged look, and shows no evidence of healing. During the period required to control the infection and remove necrotic material, supportive care, in particular nutrition, is mandatory to fuel the patient's hypermetabolism. With control of infection (supportive care, dressings and drainage, nutrition, antibiotics), there is a sudden dramatic change in the apearance of the wound's granulation tissue and the development of fibrous adhesions in the peritoneum. The change to pink healthy granulation covering the wound signals the beginning of the healing process and the end of the hypermetabolic, septic syndrome period.

Cirrhosis and Ascites

The presence of ascites uncontrolled by salt restriction, bed rest, and diuretics is invariably associated with a serious state of malnutrition and altered immune competence (Franco et al. 1983). If ascites cannot be controlled, prognosis is dismal. Peritoneovenous shunting, when performed in a meticulous manner (Meakins et al. 1988; Smadja and Franco 1985), permits cirrhotic patients to recover their normal body composition (Blendis et al. 1986) and immunocompetence via a number of mechanisms (Franco et al. 1983). The shunt must be placed with zero mortality and low morbidity to be justifiable. The act, however, allows immunomodulation since the control of ascites is associated with recovery of appetite, sense of health, and other imponderables leading to some recovery of liver function.

Surgery

Surgeons are very sensitive about the quality of surgery and generally assume excellence. While this seems correct, it has become apparent that postoperative infection rates vary between patient groups and between surgeons.

Wound Infection

Wound infection following elective surgery provides a fine example of the interplay between the determinants of infection and the surgeon's role in its prevention. During preoperative care the surgeon can best equip his patient to resist infection by improving host variables and diminishing potential bacterial contamination. In the operating room, bacteria can be controlled; the operation can be performed perfectly, leaving a wound best able to resist infection. For example, a patient with 12 h of fecal peritonitis should not have the wound closed primarily. Infection rates are 50%–70% and have important sequelae. Cruse (1987) and Olson et al. (1984) have shown that keeping individual surgeons informed of their wound infection rates keeps them low. The quality of hemostasis has been shown by Polk and Lopes-Mayor (1969) to be crucial to the number of bacteria required to infect a wound. Poor hemostasis reduces by 2–3 log (10000 to 10–100) the number of bacteria required for a 20% wound infection rate. There are variables under the surgeon's control which have impact on the host determinants of infection (Meakins 1988).

Operative Site Infection

Those factors which influence wound infection will also influence the results of major surgery. However, rather than a simple wound infection, the resulting infection or complication will be more serious and mortality may increase. The principles of gentle tissue handling, atraumatic anatomic dissection, careful hemostasis, preservation of blood supply, and anastomoses without tension will improve results. In addition, modern anesthesia and monitoring techniques have eliminated the demand for speed which was once a measure of skill. The surgeon's reputation no longer needs to be linked to the length of the procedure; results count. There is enormous variation in infectious morbidity after hepatic resection (Pachter et al. 1983; Schwartz 1983; Franco 1989). Subphrenic abscesses remain common, yet it is possible to do resectional surgery of the liver with very low (1%) mortality and infection rates (Franco 1989). Therefore excellence of surgical technique and the preservation of local and systemic host responses by gentle, nontraumatic surgery has a major role as a potential immunomodulator.

Testing an immunomodulator under circumstances as described by Fielding et al. (1978), where in a multicenter trial differences in anastomotic leak rates and mortality in patients who have undergone colorectal surgery have been demonstrated to be surgeon related, would not lead to comprehensible results. Maintenance of local and systemic host defenses and control of bacteria – functions of surgical technique – should make results from all centers equivalent. It would then be possible to study a biological response. In addition, the skilled operating surgeon, by remembering the germ theory of disease, keeps bacterial inoculation to a minimum so that the concept of the inoculum effect works to the patient's benefit.

Unintended Effects of Therapy

Pharmacological regimens have many effects, some of them unintended. These unintended effects can, in precarious situations, create complications. The use of cimetidine or antacids for the prevention of stress ulcer and hemorrhagic gastritis is very common in surgical intensive care units. The unintended effect is an overgrowth of bacteria and a gastric reservoir of organisms with loss of acidity which is responsible for many, if not most, nosocomial bacterial pneumonias (Driks et al. 1987; Dumoulin et al. 1982; Marshall et al. 1988). In addition, there is now evidence that bacteria in the proximal gut may be associated with multiple organ failure and its associated infectious complications (Marshall et al. 1988). Some incidental data from Driks et al. (1987) indicate that in patients with an abnormal gastric acid barrier, there is improvement not only in infection rates, but also in noninfectious respiratory morbidity and death, suggesting that the stimulus to end-organ failure is controllable.

The problem of steroids and septic shock has been resolved (Bone et al. 1987; Hinshaw et al. 1987). Steroids do not improve the outcome in septic shock or the septic syndrome, despite animal models, and appear to substantially increase mortality rates from secondary infection, but not its incidence. This can only be the result of an altered host defense. The infection rates are the same, but the compromised patient is less able to resist the same number of bacteria (Bone et al. 1987), showing the significance of the interplay between the determinants.

The Surgeon, Infection, and the Determinants of Infection

Since primitive time the drainage of infected material has been known to have salutary effects on a patient's health. An abscess necessitates naturally surgical intervention. It is now evident that the surgeon's role may be more biological. Drainage reduces bacterial numbers to a level manageable by the host. Fever drops, as does hypermetabolism, because the stimulus for the immune cells to generate mediators (interleukin-2, tumor necrosis factor etc.) for both the responses, fever and hypermetabolism, and the immune suppression (Table 2) have been removed. Nettoyage et débridement of the area manages the local environment, restoring its capacity to resist contamination. Immune function returns to normal. The improved host factors prevent reinfection. Surgery may be an antimicrobial.

Summary

Immunomodulation is fashionable (Nohr and Meakins 1985). There has been a search for the magic bullet (Meakins et al. 1979; Polk 1986; Alexander et al. 1987) similar to Ehrlich's to resolve our patients' immunosuppression. To date it has been unsuccessful. Before studies of immunomodulators can be properly done in humans, all other variables of care must be standardized and maximized. Surgeons have the opportunity to dominate the determinants of infection to prevent or control infectious complications. There are two aspects to this role, the first is the quality of care in pre- and postoperative management to reduce and control factors leading to altered immunity, and in the operating room where technical excellence controls bacteria and preserves host resistance locally and systemically. The second is that surgery now, in addition to demanding surgical perfection, requires an understanding of the biological implications of disease, its manifestations, and how our behavior can control that biology. Within the biological framework introduced initially, the surgeon is an immunomodulator.

References

Alexander JW, Babcock GF, Waymack JP (1987) Immunotherapeutic approaches to the prevention and treatment of infection in the surgical patient. In: Howard RJ, Simmons RL (eds) Surgical infectious diseases. Appleton and Lange, Norwalk, Chap 17

Blendis LM, Harrison JE, Russel DM et al. (1987) Effects of peritoneovenous shunting on body composition. Gastroenterology 90:127–134

Bone RC, Fisher CJ, Clemmer TP et al. (1987) A controlled trial of high-dose methylprednisolone in the treatment of severe sepsis and septic shock. N Engl J Med 317:653–658

Christou NV (1988) Immune function and the aged surgical patient. In: Meakins JL, McClaran JC (eds) The surgical care of the elderly. Yearbook Chicago, Chap 11

Christou NV, McLean APH, Meakins JL (1980) Host defence in blunt trauma: interrelationships of kinetics of anergy and depressed neutrophil function, nutritional status and sepsis. J Trauma 20:833–841

Christou NV, Superina RA, Broadhead M, Meakins JL (1982) Postoperative depression of host resistance: determinants and effect of peripheral protein sparing therapy. Surgery 92:786–792

Cruse PJE (1987) Wound infections: epidemiology and clinical characteristics. In: Howard RJ, Simmons RL (eds) Surgical infectious diseases. Appleton and Lange, Norwalk

Deitch EA (1988) Infection in the compromised host. Surg Clin North Am 68:181–198

Driks MR, Craven DE, Celli BR et al. (1987) Nosocomial pneumonia in intubated patients given sucralfate as compared with antacids or histamine type 2 blockers: the role of gastric colonisation. N Engl J Med 317:1376–1382

Du Moulin GC, Paterson DG, Hedley-Whyte J, Lisbon A (1982) Aspiration of gastric bacteria in antacid-treated patients: a frequent cause of postoperative colonisation of the airway. Lancet I:242–245

Fielding LP, Stewart-Brown S, Dudley Haf (1978) Surgeon related variables and the clinical trial. Lancet II:778–779

Franco D, Charra M, Jeambrun P et al. (1983) Nutrition and immunity after peritoneovenous drainage of ascites in cirrhotic patients. Am J Surg 146:652–657

Franco D, Smadja C, Meakins JL et al. (1989) The operative risk of elective hepatic resection for liver tumours: results of a series of one hundred consecutive hepatectomies in cirrhotic and noncirrhotic patients. Arch Surg (Submitted)

Hill GL, Bouchier RG, Whitney GB (1988) Surgical and metabolic management of patients with external fistulas of the small intestine associated with Crohn's disease. World J Surg 12:191–197

Hinshaw LB, Peduzzi P, Young E et al. (1987) Effect of high-dose glucocorticoid therapy on mortality in patients with clinical signs of sepsis. N Engl J Med 317:659–665

Knaus WA, Draper EA, Wagner DP, Zimmerman JE (1985) Apache II. A severity of disease classification system. Crit Care Med 13:818–829

Livingstone DH, Malangoni MA (1989) An experimental study of susceptibility to infection after hemorrhagic shock. Surg Gynecol Obstet (In press)
Maddeus M, Simmons RL (1987) Leave the abdomen open for peritonitis: yes, no, maybe? Adv Surg 21:1–18
Marshall JC, Christou NV, Horn R, Meakins JL (1988) The microbiology of multiple organ failure: the proximal GI tract as an occult reservoir of pathogens. Arch Surg (In press)
Meakins JL (1981) Clinical importance of host resistance to infection in surgical patients. Adv Surg 15:225–255
Meakins JL (1988) Guidelines for the prevention of wound infection. In: Wilmore DD, Brennan M, Harken A, Holcroft J, Meakins JL (eds) The care of the surgical patient. Scientific American, New York, Chap 6
Meakins JL, McLean APH, Kelly R, Pietsch JB, Bubenik O, Maclean LD (1978) Delayed hypersensitivity response and neutrophil chemotaxis: effect of trauma. J Trauma 18:240–247
Meakins JL, Christou NV, Shizgal HM, Maclean LD (1979) Therapeutic approaches to anergy in surgical patients: surgery and levamisole. Ann Surg 190:285–296
Meakins JL, Wicklund B, Forse RA, McLean APH (1980) The surgical intensive care unit: current concepts in infection. Surg Clin North Am 60:117–132
Meakins JL, Hillaire S, Vons C, Smadja C, Franco D (1988) Perioperative antibiotics (2 doses) control early but not late infectious complications of peritoneovenous shunts (PVS). Surg Res Commun 3:51:45
Miles AA (1980) The inflammatory response in relation to local infections. Surg Clin North Am 60:93–105
Miles AA, Miles EM, Burke J (1957) The value and duration of defense reactions of the skin to the primary lodgement of bacteria. Br J Exp Pathol 38:79–96
Nichols RL, Smith JW, Klein DB et al. (1954) Risk of infection after penetrating abdominal trauma. N Engl J Med 311:1065
Nohr CW, Meakins JL (1985) Biologic response modifiers. In: Meakins JL (ed) Surgical infection in critical care medicine. Churchill Livingstone, Edinburgh, Chap 16
Olsen M, Connor M, Schwartz ML (1984) Surgical wound infections: a 5-year prospective study of 20,193 wounds at the Minneapolis VA Medical Center. Ann Surg 199:253–265
Pachter JL, Spencer FC, Hofstetter SR et al. (1983) Experience with finger fracture technique to achieve intra-hepatic hemostasis in 75 patients with severe injuries of the liver. Ann Surg 197:771–778
Polk HC Jr (1984) Enhancement of host defenses against infection. Search for the Holy Grail? Surgery 99:1
Polk HC Jr, Lopez-Mayor JF (1969) Postoperative wound infection: a prospective study of determinant factors and prevention. Surgery 66:97–103
Rotstein OD, Pruett TL, Simmons RL (1986) Microbiologic features and treatment of persistent peritonitis in patients in the intensive care unit. Can J Surg 29:247–250
Slade MS, Simmons RL, Yunis EJ, Greenberg LJ (1975) Immunodepression after major surgery in normal patients. Surgery 78:363
Smadja C, Franco D (1985) The LeVeen shunt in the elective treatment of intractable ascites in cirrhosis. A prospective study on 140 patients. Ann Surg 201:488–493
Superina RA, Christou NV, Meakins JL (1980) Failure of neutrophil delivery into skin windows in anergic surgical patients. Surg Forum 31:68–70
Tchervenkov JI, Diano E, Meakins JL, Christou NV (1986) Susceptibility to bacterial sepsis: accurate measurement by delayed-type hypersensitivity skin test score. Arch Surg 121:37–40
Walsh G, Chaisson P, Hedderich G, Wexler MJ, Meakins JL (1989) The open abdomen: marlex mesh and zipper, a method of managing intraperitoneal infection. Surg Clin North Am (In press)

Immune Consequences of the Acute Stress Response and Sepsis

A. C. Antonacci

Introduction

Of the numerous types of injuries possible, burn injuries rank among the most devastating, affecting all organ systems, and severely challenging every adaptive survival mechanism known. Ultimately, an organism that successfully adapts to the consequences of its injury will survive, and those that do not, will not. In the past, I have stressed that the degree to which we understand the "adaptive response to injury" will determine the limits of our success in the treatment of the disease processes involved. I will reiterate that concept once again.

In his now famous treatise of 1897, *Adaptation in pathological processes,* Doctor William Welch discussed the dynamic physiologic and evolutionary mechanisms at work in an organism's adaptive response to various life-treatening pathologic processes. In his paper, Doctor Welch aptly suggested:

... that the adaptability of this mechanism to bring about useful adjustments has been in large part determined by the factors of organic evolution, but that in only relatively few cases can we suppose these evolutionary factors to have intervened in behalf of morbid states. For the most part, the agencies employed are such as exist primarily for physiologic uses, and while these may be all that are required to secure a good pathologic adjustment, often they have no special *fitness for this purpose ...*

In any discussion of the adaptive responses to the pathologic processes induced by trauma, the alterations observed in host defense mechanisms are among the most important to the survival of the organism in the morbid state. Whether a good pathologic adjustment is secured depends, in large part, on a successful "series" of pathologic adjustments to the recurrent threats of immune deficiency and septic infection. However, these threats often arise as the final "coup de grace" in an organism's frequently unsuccessful struggle to adapt to the complex phenomenon of trauma. As such, trauma must be viewed as a dynamic insult, extending and increasing in complexity well beyond the initial encounter with the host as a series of interactions among adaptive responses, the pathophysiologic sequelae of adaptation, and the introduction of new influences. Indeed, host defense must not be viewed as an isolated entity, but rather as an integral element of the clinical didactic, sensitive to the effects of organ system change and capable of exerting its own beneficial and deleterious effects on other organ systems. Successful immunologic adaptation, therefore, is more accurately determined by how significantly immunologic homeostatic balance is affected by the complex phenomenology of trauma, i.e., the immunologic effects of (a) the acute stress (ad-

Immune Consequences of
Trauma, Shock and Sepsis
Eds. Faist/Ninnemann/Green

renocortical response), (b) neuroendocrine influences, (c) nutritional deficiency, (d) the infection itself, or (e) medical intervention, and others.

The role of the physician and scientist in this adaptive process is that of a modulatory force active in maintaining a comfortable homeostatic range within which the organism itself may initiate the physiologic adjustments necessary to survival and recuperation. Without this modulatory influence, survival would be impossible since, as Doctor Welch wrote, "the agencies employed ... often have no special fitness for this purpose." Success in these efforts is evidenced by advances in fluid resuscitation and treatment of the acute cardiopulmonary effects of shock, modern blood banking, anesthesia and improvements in surgical technique, an increasing awareness of the importance of nutritional support, the development of antibiotics, the principles of wound care, and other factors. Failure in these efforts is evidenced by an increase in septicemia-related deaths at approximately 5%/year, with a persistent 50% mortality rate associated with polymicrobial and fungal infection [1].

It is the purpose of this presentation to examine immune dysfunction following burn trauma as related to the acute stress response and sepsis. Through an understanding of their potential synergies, we may gain some insight into the clinical challenges posed by the injury as a whole.

Experimental Models

During the course of the past 7 years, our laboratory has recognized what we believe to be critical differences in the adaptive response to burn injury between the rodent and human species (Table 1). Simply put, rats tolerate a 50% full-thickness thermal injury quite well following one time fluid resuscitation and demon-

Table 1. The adaptive response to a 50% third-degree burn in rat and man

	Rat	Man
Mortality	Low (<5%–10%)	High (about 50% or greater)
Wound healing	Sheds eschar	Requires grafting
Sepsis	Low spontaneous rate	High spontaneous rate
Weight loss	<10%	>10%–15%

Table 2. Important functional differences between rat and man

	Rat	Man
Corticoid levels	24–48 h	Spike 24–48 h; 3–4 week elevation
Effect of septic inoculum	High mortality with time postburn	High mortality all time points
Immune parameters	Transitory changes responses in some tissues	Pan depression for significant time postburn
Metabolic stresses	Well tolerated	Poorly tolerated

strate little significant morbidity and low mortality rates, whereas humans suffer both significant morbidity and mortality. Some of the more important functional differences are outlined in Table 2.

The most apparent difference rests in a chronic elevation of corticosteroids in humans with only an acute increase observed in rats. It was hypothesized that this differential adrenocortical response to burn injury was related to the markedly different clinical course of the two species as manifest by the distinct differences in immune function, metabolic sequelae, and the effects of septic inoculi.

Human Data

Cortisol Levels Following Thermal Injury in Man

Thermally injured patients ($n=31$) have significantly elevated free (10-fold) and total (2-fold) cortisol levels compared to normal controls ($n=50$) [2]. Mean concentrations of free cortisol for thermally injured patients were always above the 95th percentile for the normal control samples while mean concentrations of total cortisol dipped within the normal range at postburn days (PBD) 7 and 14. Cortisol binding globulin capacity (CBGC) was decreased relative to normals in the 48-h period following burn, but by PBD 7 all patients had mean levels of CBGC within the normal range. Plasma albumin was uniformly decreased throughout. These data confirm that burn injury results in an exaggerated adrenocortical response with an increase in biologically active free cortisol to 2–10 times normal levels.

Changes in Lymphocyte Subpopulations Following Thermal Injury in Man

Within 24–48 h of severe thermal injury, CD4+ helper/inducer T cells decline significantly with little or no change in CD8+ suppressor/cytotoxic cells [3, 4]. These changes are reversible with recovery. In addition, the decrease in CD4+ cells can be totally accounted for by a concomitant decrease in the suppressor-inducer subset of CD4 as defined by two-color fluorescence flow cytometry with CD4 and CD45 receptor antibodies. Percentages of T cells in the helper-effector subset of CD4, as assessed by staining with CD4 and Leu8 antibodies, were not significantly affected.

In addition, it has been demonstrated by Damle et al. [5] and Morimoto et al. [6] that T cells which proliferate in the autologous mixed lymphocyte response (AMLR) belong to the CD4/CD45 receptor subset. Interestingly, burn patients demonstrate markedly defective proliferation in AMLR which correlates with the observed decrease in the percentage of the CD4 subset. Also, studies by Ilfeld et al. [7] demonstrate that pathophysiological concentrations of corticosteroids significantly depress the response of normal T cells in AMLR suggesting that corticosteroids may have specific functional effects on the CD4+ subset as well.

Effect of Continuous Pathophysiological Infusions of Hydrocortisone on Peripheral Blood Phenotype in Normal Controls

In the present study, the relationship between increased corticosteroids and immunologic changes following thermal injury was elucidated further by administration of a constant infusion of hydrocortisone to normal human subjects at a rate designed to produce steady state plasma concentrations which mimic those observed after burn [8, 9]. Hydrocortisone rose to 49 µg/100 ml during infusion, similar to the mean of 47.5 µg/100 ml for burn patients. Infusion subjects showed significant lymphopenia, monocytopenia, and granulocytosis. Additionally, there were significant decreases in percentages of T3, T4 and T11 lymphocytes; no significant changes in percentages of T8 or HLA-DR; and an increase in percentages of Leu7+ cells. These changes in lymphocyte subsets mimicked those of burn patients. The number of T3, T4 and T11 cells significantly decreased during hydrocortisone infusion while numbers of T8, HLA-DR and Leu7 lymphocytes did not change. Burn patients showed decreased numbers of T3 and T4 cells, but this T3/T4 lymphopenia was not as great as during hydrocortisone infusion.

These data support the hypothesis that elevation of plasma hydrocortisone is responsible for the lymphocyte phenotype changes that occur in the early postburn period.

Rat Data

Corticosterone Alterations Following Thermal Injury in the Rat

Thermal injury-induced endocrinologic changes may contribute to post burn defects in metabolism, fluid/electrolyte balance and immune function. To further investigate burn injury–endocrine hormone relationships, total corticosterone, corticosterone binding globulin capacity, free corticosterone and albumin were measured in the serum of rats at 0.5, 1, 2, 6, 12 and 24 days following 50% total body surface area scald burns [7]. Results were compared to normal control rats as well as sham-injured animals studied at 0.5 and 2 days postsham. Total corticosterone is significantly elevated at 0.5 and 1 day postburn, but promptly returned to normal by day 2. Due mostly to a 75% decrease in corticosterone binding globulin

Table 3. Hormone/protein responses in burn injury

Hormone/protein	Control	Day postburn					
		0.5	1	2	6	12	24
Total B (ng/ml)	96	263*	350*	112	36	55	8
Free B (ng/ml)	3	71*	114*	54*	1	3	
CBGC (ng bound/ml)	408	206*	239*	75*	322*	317*	22
Albumin (g/dl)	3.1	2.2*	2.1*	2.2*	2.3*	2.6*	2

Values are means, $n = 5$ at each time point.
* $P<0.01$ vs. control by analysis of variance and Dunnett's test; B, corticosterone.

capacity, free corticosterone was still elevated 20-fold on postburn day 2, but decreased to normal by day 6. Finally, serum albumin concentrations were uniformly decreased by approximately 30% throughout the 24 day study period. The rats in this study, despite 50% total body surface area burns, showed no infectious complications or mortality. This suggests that rapid resolution of the endocrine response to injury is beneficial to ultimate outcome (Table 3).

Effects of Chronically Elevated Plasma Corticosterone Levels on Body Weight and Composition Following Thermal Injury in the Rat

The present study sought to evaluate basic nutritional/metabolic effects of corticosteroids following thermal injury. Lewis rats ($n = 16$) were anesthetized and administered a 40% total body surface area scald burn immediately followed by subcutaneous implantation of corticosterone (B) pellets designed to maintain plasma B at chronically elevated, pathophysiological levels. Control animals ($n = 16$) were similarly injured but underwent the implantation procedure without pellet insertion. Controls were pair-fed to rats receiving pellets. At various times postburn, body weight and plasma B were evaluated. Animals were sacrificed on postburn day 24 for gravimetric analysis of body composition (Tables 4 and 5).

Following pellet implantation, a significant chronic elevation in plasma B was achieved throughout the course of the study. Weight loss was significantly greater in the experimental group at all time points postburn. Body composition analysis demonstrated a significant decrease in both lean tissue and body water in the animals implanted with pellets as compared to controls while body fat was significantly higher.

Table 4. Plasma corticosterone level and body weight following burn

	Pre-study	Day postburn			
		2 days	5 days	11 days	20 days
Plasma B (−pellet) (ng/ml)	12	71	42	68	40
Plasma B (+pellet) (ng/ml)	8	243*	125*	164*	262*
Body weight (−pellet) (g)	353	347	337	338	324
Body weight (+pellet) (g)	348	330*	308*	288*	274*

Values are means, $n = 16$.
* $P < 0.01$ vs. control animals by two-way analysis of variance and Newman-Keuls test.
B, corticosterone.

Table 5. Body composition – postburn day 24

	Total weight	Lean tissue	Water	Fat
−pellet ($n = 3$) (g)	344.4	86.3	248.3	9.8
+pellet ($n = 4$) (g)	275.4*	65.6*	179.4*	30.4*

* $P < 0.01$ vs. control animals by t-test.

These data suggest that chronic elevations of plasma corticosterone in thermally injured rats are associated with an exacerbation of metabolic derangements. Further, these results support a hypothesis that a persistent adrenal response following burn injury in humans may contribute to a clinically unstable course.

Maintenance of Pathophysiologic Elevations of Plasma Corticosterone Promotes Postburn Mortality in *Pseudomonas* Infected Rats

As stated above, burn patients sustaining severe or nonsurvivable thermal injury demonstrate chronic elevations of plasma corticosteroids while burned rats manifest only acute increases in adrenal steroids. Since thermally injured rats show minimal or no mortality, it was hypothesized that this differential adrenocortical response may be related to the interspecies variation in postburn mortality.

This study examined the effects of chronic plasma corticosterone elevations, maintained within a pathophysiologic rather than a pharmacologic range, on postburn mortality in *Pseudomonas*-infected rats. Male Lewis rats ($n = 21$) were anesthesized and administered a 40% total body surface area scald burn immediately followed by the subcutaneous implantation of corticosterone pellets which maintain plasma corticosterone levels at approximately 150–250 ng/ml. Control animals ($n = 18$) were similarly injured but underwent the implantation procedure without pellet insertion and were pair-fed to rats receiving pellets. On the fourth day postburn, dorsal burn wounds were superficially inoculated with either 10^2, 10^4, 10^6, or 10^8 colony-forming units (CFU) of *Pseudomonas aeruginosa* (Table 6).

No significant differences in mortality were noted between experimental and control animals with inoculations less than 10^6 CFU. Overall mortality was significantly affected by pellet implantation in the 10^6-inoculum group. Temporal changes in mortality were seen in the 10^8 group with a diminished postinoculation survival time in pelleted animals but ultimate mortality was not affected. Plasma corticosterone maintained at pathophysiologic levels in postburn rats increased overall mortality following inoculation with 10^6 CFU of *Pseudomonas aeruginosa*. Pathophysiologic corticosterone levels diminished survival time with a larger (10^8 CFU) inoculum. These data suggest that chronic elevations of plasma corticosteroids observed in burn patients may in part be responsible for the difference in postburn mortality that exists between man and rat.

Table 6. Rat dorsal burn wounds infected with *P. aeruginosa:* percentage cumulative mortality

	Days postinoculation					
	2	6	10	14	18	22
10^8 CFU (−pellet) ($n = 5$)	0	0	0	0	0	100
10^8 CFU (+pellet) ($n = 5$)	0	0	40	60*	100**	100
10^6 CFU (−pellet) ($n = 4$)	0	0	0	0	25	25
10^6 CFU (−pellet) ($n = 5$)	0	40	40	40	40	80*

* $P < 0.05$; ** $P < 0.001$ vs. control (−pellet) animals by testing of proportions.

Sepsis

A meaningful study of sepsis in a clinical setting is fraught with difficulties primarily because of the numerous clinical variables at work at the same time. Therefore, we chose to study the immunologic and endocrinologic effects of a single intravenous bolus injection of purified lipopolysaccharide (LPS) in normal human volunteers. The following complex study was performed in collaboration with Stephen Lowry and coworkers, and represents preliminary data obtained from four normal volunteers who were admitted to the Clinical Research Center at The New York Hospital, Cornell Medical Center. The experimental design consisted of baseline immune and endocrine studies followed by a single intravenous bolus injection of LPS. Phenotypic and endocrinologic data were obtained every 5 min during the first hour following injection and hourly thereafter for 6 h. A postinfusion study point of 24 h was the last sample taken. Baseline immunologic data were obtained utilizing mononuclear cell drawn prior to infusion. Each patient's baseline immunologic profile served as control. Patients were screened for normal immunologic function 2 weeks prior to study.

Monocyte T-cell Interaction Cultures

Monocyte T-cell interaction cultures' responses used purified T cells as responders and irradiated monocytes as mitogen presenting cells. T cells from baseline and 4 h after LPS infusion were cultured as the responder cell and monocytes from either baseline or 4 h after LPS infusion were the mitogen presenting cells or effector cells. Monocytes were cultured for 4 h at 37 °C with and without an optimal dose of PHA (0.1 μg/ml), washed three times, and irradiated with 3000 rads from a ^{137}Cs source. The mitogen-free suspension of monocytes (both baseline and 4 h after post-LPS infusion) were then added to responder T cells from either baseline or 4 h after LPS infusioin in round-bottomed microtiter plates at a cell density of 100000 T cells/well and 25000 monocytes/well in a total volume of 200 μl. Cultures were performed in quadruplicate for 72 h and incubated at 37 °C in a humidified atmosphere of 5% CO^2 and air. Cells were pulsed with 1 μCi [^{3}H]thymidine (New England Nuclear Corporation, Boston, Mass.) for 8 h prior to harvest with an automatic cell harvester (Flow Laboratories). [^{3}H]Thymidine incorporation was measured in a liquid scintillation counter and expressed as net counts per minute (c.p.m.). Simultaneous monoclonal antibody labelling and flow cytometric analysis was performed. Schematically, the experimental design of the above experiment is depicted below:

$$\text{Monocytes*} \longrightarrow + \text{PHA} \xrightarrow[\text{wash}]{\text{4 h culture}} + \text{T cells} \longrightarrow \text{Final culture}$$

Monocytes* – irradiated or treated with mitomycin C; isolated from time zero and 4 h after LPS infusion. T cells – isolated from time zero and 4 h after LPS infusion were the responders.

It is important to realize that this system represents a mitogen-free final culture and can be utilized to assess both primary T-cell and monocyte alterations as a function of LPS infusion. When T cells isolated from either time zero or 4 h after LPS infusion are presented mitogen by monocytes isolated prior to LPS infusion, proliferative capacity is normal. However, when T cells isolated from either time zero or 4 h after LPS infusion are presented mitogen by monocytes isolated 4 h following LPS infusion, proliferative capacity is dramatically and consistently reduced between 50%–80%. These data suggest that the immunosuppressive effect of LPS can be seen as early as 4 h following infusion (although the phenotypic data that follows suggests that phenotypic effects are generated as early as 15 min following infusion) and are mediated via the macrophage with T-cell function remaining normal at this time point. Activation of suppressor macrophage pathways is a possible explanation. However, macrophage supernatants and three-way mitogen presentation studies demonstrate a lack of adequate macrophage mitogen presentation.

Simultaneous Phenotype and Cortisol Analysis Following LPS Infusion

Monoclonal antibody phenotyping by flow cytometry was performed together with simultaneous sampling for cortisol levels following LPS infusion. As early as 15 min following infusion of LPS, a 40% depletion of lymphocytes bearing the OKT3, OKT4 and OKT8 markers was observed from the peripheral blood. A further decrease to the 60%–80% level is observed 1 h after infusion as suggested by the change in slope of the decline. The early phase 1 decline in lymphocytes does not correlate to the elevation in cortisol which begins 1 h after LPS infusion, peaks and achieves pathophysiologic levels between 2–4 h post LPS infusion.

Effect of In Vitro Hydrocortisone on Monocyte and T-cell Function

It has been shown that LPS infusion is associated with a significant increase in plasma cortisol levels. Since cortisol can mediate profound immune effects and in order to clarify the precise cellular effects of both LPS and cortisol in this assay system, we performed the following in vitro experiment. Using an assay system similar to the proliferation assay described above, we assessed the effect of varying doses of hydrocortisone [10^{-7} *M* physiological, 10^{-6} *M* pathophysiological (burns), and 10^{-5} *M* pharmacological levels) on monocyte capacity to present PHA and the T-cell response to such a stimulus. The final assay system was mitogen free and either monocytes or T cells or both were pretreated with varying doses of hydrocortisone.

The data suggest that the effect of hydrocortisone is mediated via the T cell and that hydrocortisone pretreatment of monocytes exposed to PHA does not affect proliferative responses. However, treatment of T cells with hydrocortisone demonstrates a monotonic decrease in proliferation with increasing dose of hydrocortisone. Treatment of both monocytes and T cells with hydrocortisone recapitulates the treatment of T cells alone. Interestingly, when monocytes are treated with physiological doses of hydrocortisone (10^{-7} *M*), whether or not T cells are exposed to hydrocortisone, enhancement is observed. These data confirm that a facultative effect of hydrocortisone on T-cell proliferation at physiologic levels is exerted via the monocyte and the T cell, and a suppressive effect is exerted at pathophysiologic and pharmacologic levels via the T cell alone.

Summary

Data suggest that both adrenocortical stress responses and infection (LPS exposure) alter immunologic function via more than one mechanism. These effects involve significant changes in lymphocyte phenotype, in part accounted for by cortisol, which may be characterized by a decrease in suppressor-inducer cells from the circulating pool. Cortisol's direct effects on immunologic functions are mediated via the T cell and probably involve decreased capacity for the production of IL-2. LPS, however, has both immunologic and endocrine effects. Its immediate effects on lymphopenia are not well understood, but LPS administration does increase cortisol levels one hour after infusion. Primary immunologic effects of LPS are mediated via the macrophage and are characterized by a defect in mitogen presentation and does not represent active suppression.

References

1. Kiani D, Quinn E, Burch KH (1979) The increasing importance of polymicrobial bacteremia. JAMA 242:1044–1047
2. Calvano SE, Chiao J, Reaves LE, Antonacci AC, Shires GT (1984) Changes in free and total levels of plasma cortisol and thyroxine following thermal injury in man. J Burn Care Rehabil 5:143–151
3. Antonacci AC, Reaves LE, Calvano SE, Amand R, deRiesthal HF, Shires GT (1984) Flow cytometric analysis of lymphocyte subpopulations following thermal injury in man. Surg Gynecol Obstet 159:1–8
4. Calvano SE, deRiesthal HF, Marano A, Antonacci AC (1988) The decrease in peripheral blood CD4+ T cells following thermal injury in humans can be accounted for by a concomitant decrease in suppressorinducer CD4+ T cells as assessed using anti-CD45R. Clin Immunol Immunopathol (In press)
5. Damie NK, Mohagheghpour N, Engleman EG (1984) Soluble antigen-primed inducer T cells activate antigen-specific suppressor T cells in the absence of antigen-pulsed accessory cells. J Immunol 134:1508–1515
6. Morimoto C, Letvin NL, Boyd AW, Hagan M, Brown HM, Kornacki MM, Schlossman SF (1985) The isolation and characterization of the human helperinducer T cell subset. J Immunol 134:3762–3769
7. Ilfeld DN, Krakauer RS, Blaese RM (1977) Suppression of the human autologous mixed lymphocyte reaction by physiologic concentrations of hydrocortisone. J Immunol 119:428–434
8. Calvano SE, Albert JD, Organ BC, Tracey KJ, Lowry SF, Antonacci AC (1986) Hydrocortisone but not epinephrine infusion in normal subjects mimics burn injury with respect to changes in lymphocyte subset percentages. Surg Forum 37:95–98
9. Calvano SC, Albert JD, Legaspi A, Organ BC, Tracey KT, Lowry SF, Shires GT, Antonacci AC (1987) Comparison of numerical and phenotypic leukocyte changes during constant hydrocortisone infusion in normal subjects with those in thermally injured patients at 24–48 h following burn: hydrocortisone infusion mimics thermal injury with respect to changes in lymphocyte subset percentages. Surg Gynecol Obstet 164:415–422

Immunomodulation in Animal Models of Injury

J. F. Hansbrough and M. A. Gadd

Introduction

Burn injury and multisystem trauma have been shown to produce multiple aberrations in the various host-defense systems. The clinical and experimental impressions of many investigators and surgeons have indicated that the immunologic sequelae following burn injury are more severe than those following nonburn trauma.

For the last five years our laboratory has investigated immunologic alterations after controlled injury in mice and rats. We have concentrated our work on these animals for several reasons. Firstly, precise types of injury have been described in these animals, including burn injury, musculoskeletal and abdominal trauma. The effects of these types of injury on subsequent immunologic changes can then be studied in the absence of associated factors, such as blood transfusions, further surgery, anesthetics, infections, and drugs, all of which may have separate effects on immunity. Secondly, large numbers of animals can be conveniently studied, and inbred populations of animals are readily available. This facilitates the use of experiments in which cell populations are to be combined, or in which large numbers of animals are desirable to optimize statistical evaluation of experiments.

In this discussion we will present some of our data regarding T-cell activation and maturation and neutrophil functions in small-animal models of burn and nonburn trauma.

T-Cell Activation Processes After Injury

Although several tests for T-cell functions have been used to study postinjury immune suppression, limitations in the applicability, reproducibility, and ease of use of most such tests are hindrances to their use. Two of the most commonly used assays are the measurement of incorporation of radioactive DNA precursors following mitogen stimulation of lymphocytes, or following mixed lymphocyte culture. These tests are commonly termed "functional tests" of lymphocyte activity. However, these assays have been shown to have wide variability and their clinical usefulness may be limited in many situations. Furthermore, lymphocyte culture conditions may result in stimulation and proliferation of many cell populations, including suppressor cells as well as helper cells; isotope incorporation by proliferating suppressor cells might thus lead to a "positive" interpretation for the

Immune Consequences of
Trauma, Shock and Sepsis
Eds. Faist/Ninnemann/Green

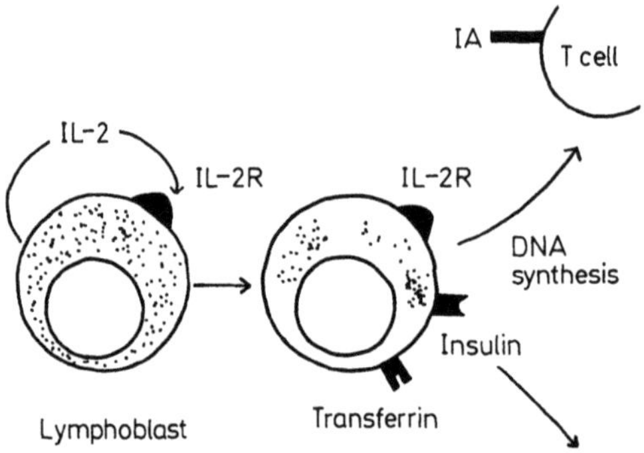

Fig. 1. T-lymphocyte activation after mitogen stimulation involves expression of early surface antigens (IL-2, transferrin and insulin receptors); Ia antigen (HLA-DR in humans) occurs during or after S phase

test when in fact suppressive activity is dominating. Indeed, purified Lyt-2^+ cells, in the presence of accessory cells, proliferate readily upon concanavalin A (Con-A) stimulation, express IL-2 receptors, and produce IL-2 [1]. In addition, DNA synthesis may not parallel other indicators of blast transformation; Cotner et al. [2] demonstrated that blast transformation may result in the appearance of several surface "activation antigens" well before DNA synthesis. Identification of the exact steps in T-cell activation which are affected by injury might be expected to yield valuable information, particularly regarding the study of potentially immune-modulating therapies.

We therefore utilized a potentially more useful type of lymphocyte stimulation test to study immunity in injured mice. In addition to measuring incorporation of isotopically labeled precursors into DNA, we followed the expression of lymphocyte surface antigens during the culture period using monoclonal antibodies and two-color flow cytometry. Stimulation and proliferation of small, resting T lymphocytes have been shown to be accompanied by the appearance of new surface antigens, which have been termed T cell activation antigens; these include the transferrin receptor [3], the insulin receptor [4], Ia or HLA-DR [5], and "Tac" or IL-2 receptor [6]. In addition, cell surface coexpression of both "helper" and "suppressor" major histocompatibility (MHC) antigens has been shown to be an early step in T-cell blastogenesis [7]. In normal cells there is a definite pattern of surface antigen expression; IL-2, transferrin and insulin receptors are expressed early after mitogen stimulation, for example, while Ia (HLA-DR in humans) is expressed much later, either during or after S phase (Fig. 1) [2].

We have studied the lectin-induced expression of surface markers on murine lymphocytes following controlled injury (musculoskeletal trauma, 25% body surface area burn injury, simple laparotomy and laparotomy–partial hepatectomy). Representative results after burn and musculoskeletal trauma are seen in Fig. 2. Similar studies after laparotomy and partial hepatectomy in the mouse showed that these types of trauma produced minimal defects in lymphocyte activation processes. Clearly, the block in lymphocyte surface receptor expression is much more evident after burn injury than after nonburn trauma.

In further experiments, we have shown that the addition of prostaglandin E_2 (PGE_2) to normal splenocytes during culture and mitogen stimulation results in a block in surface antigen expression similar to that seen after burn injury, and

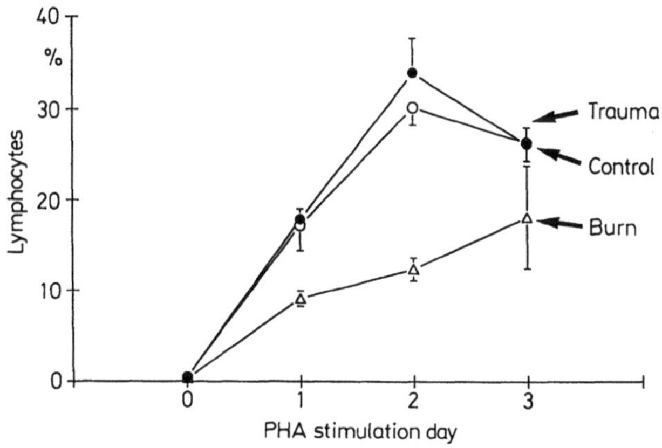

Fig. 2. Typical block in surface receptor expression on day 10 after murine burn injury, evidenced by marked depression of "helper" antigen (L3T4) coexpressed with IL-2 receptor. These defects were minimal after musculoskeletal injury (shown here), or after laparotomy or laparotomy/partial hepatectomy in the mouse

that indomethacin can partially restore surface antigen expression after burn injury. However, complete restoration of surface antigen expression is seen only in cells from indomethacin-treated animals which are also cultured in the presence of indomethacin. This indicates the PGE_2 blockade by cyclooxygenase inhibitors, while immune enhancing in vivo in our earlier work [8, 9], is rapidly reversible when cells are taken from the animal. Finally, we have been disappointed to find that early excision of burned tissue in the mouse model does not prevent the multiple blocks in receptor expression.

These results suggest that characterization of lymphocyte surface antigen expression after culture and stimulation may be a useful indicator of postinjury T-cell dysfunction, and that the block in T-cell blastogenesis following severe injury occurs very early in the activation process. Finally, the experiments indicate that T-cell dysfunction is much more severe after burn injury than after musculoskeletal trauma.

Neutrophil Phagocytosis and Opsonic Defects

We modified a phagocytic assay similar to one which has been used by others [10]. Briefly, selected microorganisms were heat killed and then labeled with fluorescein isothyocyanate (FITC). Leukocytes (5×10^5) were then incubated in suspension with FITC microorganisms at a ratio of 5 bacteria to 1 leukocyte, or 2 yeast to 1 leukocyte in 6.25% serum. The standard serum concentration for incubation was 10%. The suspension was incubated at 37 °C with shaking (160 revolutions/min) for 90 min. At the end of the incubation period EDTA solution was added to stop phagocytosis. Prior to analysis by flow cytometry, 200 µl of 0.1% trypan blue was added to the suspension to quench extracellular, adherent organisms. Cells were analyzed within 15 min of addition of trypan blue to avoid intra-

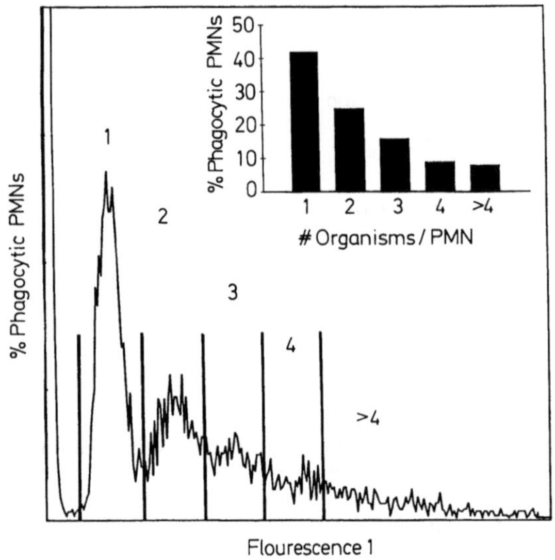

Fig. 3. Typical fluorescence histogram displaying neutrophil phagocytosis of fluorescein labeled organisms. The percentage of neutrophils ingesting various numbers of organisms can be easily calculated, and these values are displayed in the *inset*

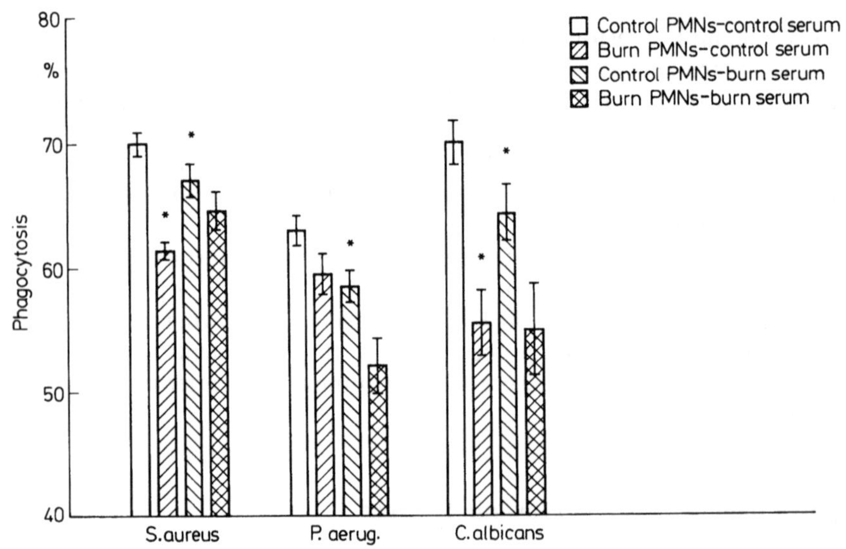

Fig. 4. Phagocytosis of various fluorescein labeled organisms by murine peritoneal neutrophils (PMNs) on day 5 after burn injury, displaying both neutrophil and serum defects. $^{*}P<0.05$

cellular penetration of the dye. Cell suspensions were analyzed on a Becton Dickinson FAC Star flow cytometer. Neutrophils were selected by gating for forward and side scatter to eliminate mononuclear cells from analysis, and the percentage of fluorescent cells was determined. Computer analysis of fluorescence histograms demonstrates the percentages of phagocytic cells containing 1, 2, 3, 4, and

>4 organisms per cell (Fig. 3). Data were calculated from the following equations:

$$\% \text{ phagocytic neutrophils (PMNs)} = \frac{\text{No. fluorescent neutrophils}}{\text{Total no. neutrophils}} \times 100$$

$$\% \text{ (PMNs engulfing} \varkappa \text{organisms} \frac{\text{No. PMNs engulfing} \times \text{organisms}}{\text{No. fluorescent neutrophils}} \times 100$$

where $\varkappa = 1, 2, 3, 4$ and >4.

Typical results in burned animals are shown in Fig. 4. We noted neutrophil phagocytic defects and serum opsonic defects after burn injury, but only with certain organisms. These data contrast with phagocytic data obtained by others using labeled, inert beads, which failed to shown phagocytic defects after injury. We feel that the use of particular organisms for the phagocytosis evaluation provides for a more clinically meaningful assay than the use of labeled, inert beads. In addition, the addition of the quenching agent trypan blue to eliminate fluorescence by adherent but noningested particles is a valuable feature of the assay. Phagocytic defects were much less severe after musculoskeletal trauma.

Measurement of Neutrophil Oxidative Burst After Injury

The microbicidal and cytotoxic activity of neutrophils begins with reduction of NADPH to superoxide which rapidly converts to H_2O_2. The peroxidase enzyme system then acts on H_2O_2 to produce hydroxyl radicals. Hydroxyl radicals and H_2O_2 have been implicated as primary mediators of microbial killing [11].

We used a flow-cytometric assay [12] which measures the generation of intracellular hydrogen peroxide after appropriate stimulation of neutrophils. Control or burn PMNs, 10^6/ml, are preincubated with 10% control or burn serum for 15 min at 37 °C. After the initial incubation, 10 μM 2′7′dichlorofluorescin diacetate (DCFH-DA) is added to the PMN suspension and incubated for 15 min at 37 °C with shaking. Fluorescence of the cells is measured following the second incubation by flow cytometry and designated as zero time. The suspension is then stimulated with 100 ng/ml phorbol myristate acetate (PMA) for 15 min at 37 °C with shaking and reanalyzed by cytometry to detect the percentage change in fluorescence at 15 and 60 min. The flow cytometer isolates PMNs by forward (size) and side (granularity) scatter characteristics, thus making complete manual cell separation unneccessary. Fluorescent emission at 827 nm is recorded with the use of photomultiplier gain settings to ensure that approximately 75% or more of the fluorescence at zero time remained between channels 0 and 110 (250 channel capacity). Fluorescence histograms are compared using the Kolmogorov-Smirnov test to compare fluorescence histograms [13].

Typical fluorescence histograms are shown in Fig. 5, and overall results using burned mice are shown in Fig. 6. On postburn day 1, control and burn neutrophils produced equal amounts of H_2O_2 as measured by the change in percent positive fluorescent cells after stimulation with PMA. The presence of day 1 burn serum did not alter the capacity of normal neutrophils to produce H_2O_2.

Burn neutrophils demonstrated a significant defect in their ability to produce H_2O_2 compared to control neutrophils on postburn day 5. Similarly, the addition of postburn day 5 serum to control neutrophils significantly reduced control neutrophils' production of H_2O_2. Burn serum in the presence of burn neutrophils did not appear to have an additional inhibitory effect on burn neutrophil H_2O_2 production on day 5.

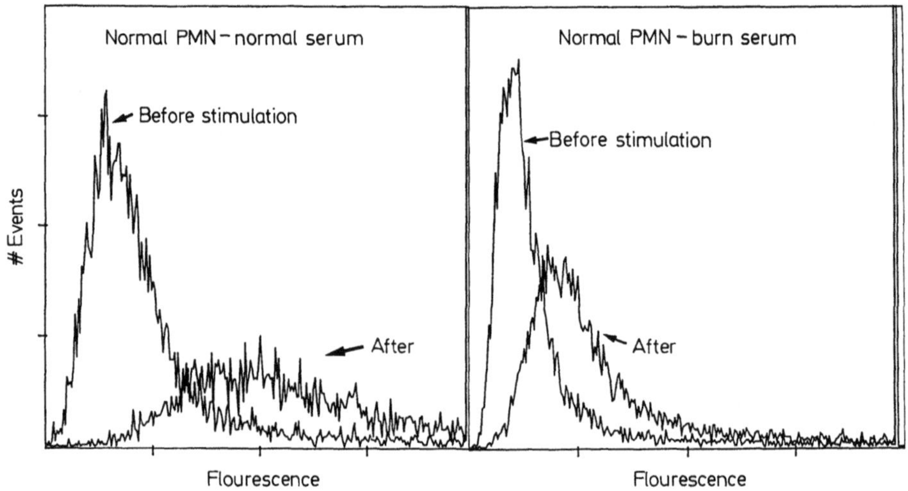

Fig. 5. The neutrophil PMA-stimulated oxidative burst can be measured using a dye which reacts with intracellular H_2O_2, thereby becoming fluorescent

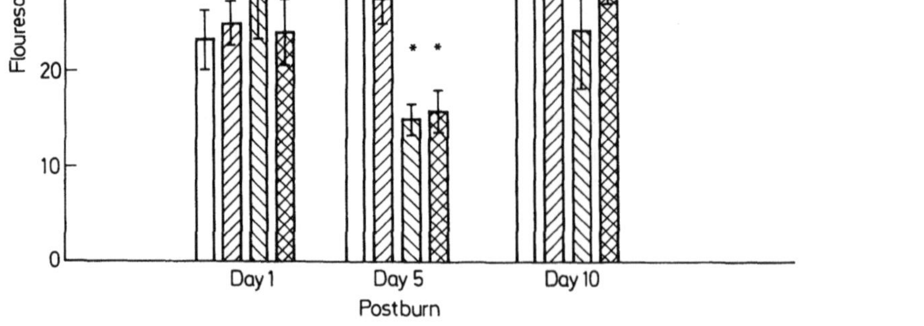

Fig. 6. Multiple defects in the neutrophil oxidative burst are seen after burn injury, including serum suppressive effects.* $P<0.05$

On postburn day 10, burn neutrophil H_2O_2 production remained significantly depressed compared to controls. The presence of burn serum in the assays with control or burn neutrophils slightly enhanced H_2O_2 production compared to the same assay in control serum.

The previous data indicate the number of fluorescent-positive cells in each group. Using Kolmogorov-Smirnov statistical analysis, the distribution pattern of fluorescence between histograms can be compared, so that one can determine whether the *amount* of H_2O_2 within each active cell is the same. Derived critical values are compared against standard critical values which are a function of the confidence level and number of samples listed in Table 1 of Young's paper [13]. The mean $D/s(n)$ for control PMNs with control serum compared to control PMNs with day 5 burn serum was 2.3 ± 0.8. The $D/s(n)$ for control PMNs with control serum compared to burn PMNs with control serum was 5.5 ± 1.5. Both critical values demonstrate a significant difference between the groups at a 95% confidence level. This indicates a qualitative defect in the stimulated oxidative burst of burn neutrophils, reflecting their inability to generate normal amounts of H_2O_2 within each active cell. Defects in the neutrophil oxidative burst were less evident in mice after musculoskeletal injury.

We are now measuring the stimulated oxidative burst in neutrophils after various potential immunomodulating therapies. We have been disappointed to find that immediate excision of burned tissue, with wound closure, did not prevent the subsequent development of neutrophil defects in oxidative metabolism. This again indicates a unique and overwhelming immune suppressive phenomenon which occurs almost simultaneously with burn injury.

Nutritional Effects on Immunity

Numerous investigators have shown the effects of malnutrition on the immune response. Figure 7 reflects data from our laboratory on immune functions in rats after 8 weeks of severe protein depletion. Lymphocyte proliferation, neutrophil

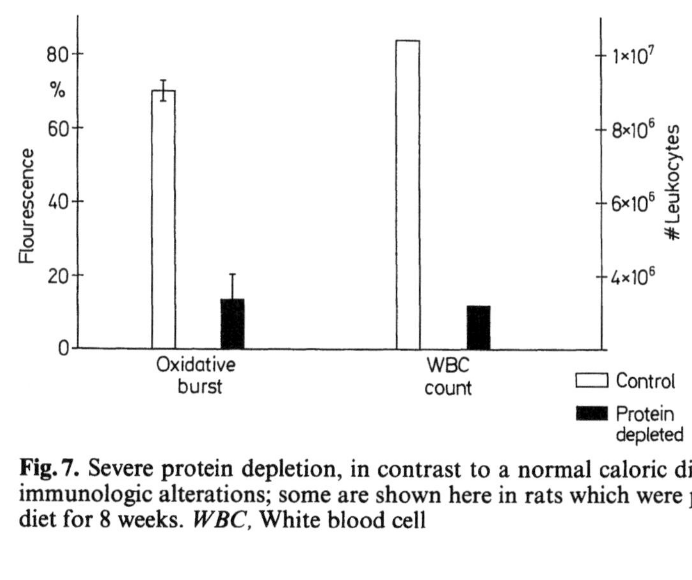

Fig. 7. Severe protein depletion, in contrast to a normal caloric diet, produces numerous immunologic alterations; some are shown here in rats which were placed on a 2% protein diet for 8 weeks. *WBC*, White blood cell

numbers and neutrophil oxidative burst activity were severely depressed. Clearly, successful immune modulation must include the maintenance of a high-quality dietary regimen in the injured patient.

References

1. Kern DE, Lachmann LB, Greenberg PD (1987) Lyt-2^+ cells. Requirements for concanavalin A-induced proliferation and interleukin 2 production. J Immunol 139:2880–2887
2. Cotner T, Williams JM, Christenson L et al. (1983) Simultaneous flow cytometric analysis of human T cell activation. Antigen expression and DNA content. J Exp Med 157:461–472
3. Trowbridge IS, Omary MB (1981) Human cell surface glycoprotein related to cell proliferation is the receptor for transferrin. Proc Natl Acad Sci USA 78:3039–3043
4. Helderman JH, Strom TB (1979) Role of protein and RNa synthesis in the development of insulin binding sites on activated thymus-derived lymphocytes. J Biol Chem 254:7203–7207
5. Evans RL, Faldetta J, Humphreys RE et al. (1978) Peripheral human T cells sensitized in mixed leukocyte culture synthesize and express Ia-like antigens. J Exp Med 148:1440–1445
6. Uchiyama T, Broder S, Waldman TA (1981) A monoclonal antibody (anti-Tac) reactive with activated and functionally mature human T cells. J Immunol 126:1393–1397
7. Blue M-L, Daley JF, Levine H, Schlossman SF (1985) Coexpression of T4 and T8 on peripheral blood T cells demonstrated by two-color fluorescence flow cytometry. J Immunol 134:2281–2286
8. Zapata-Sirvent RL, Hansbrough JF, Bartle EJ (1986) Prevention of posttraumatic alterations in splenic lymphocyte subpopulations in mice by immunomodulating drugs. Arch Surg 121:116–122
9. Zapata-Sirvent RL, Hansbrough JF et al. (1986) Postburn immunosuppression in an animal model. IV. Improved resistance to septic challenge with immunomodulating drugs. Surgery 99:53–59
10. Bjerknes R, Bassoe C-F (1984) Phagocyte C3-mediated attachment and internalization: flow cytometric studies using a fluorescence quenching technique. Blut 49:315–323
11. Babior BM (1978) Oxygen-dependent microbial killing by phagocytes. I and II. N Engl J Med 298:659–665; 721–726
12. Keston AS, Brandt R (1965) The fluorometric analysis of ultramicro-quantities of H_2O_2. Anal Biochem 11:1–5
13. Young IT (1977) Proof without prejudice: use of the Kolmogorov-Smirnov test for the analysis of histograms from flow systems and other sources. J Histochem Cytochem 25:935–941

Use of Plasma Exchange in Thermally Injured Patients

G. D. Warden

Introduction

Major thermal injuries produce pathophysiologic changes in the external and internal systems of the body, the initial life-threatening alterations occurring in the internal environment. Numerous reports, beginning with the cross-circulation studies of Baxter and Shires [1] in 1968, suggest that serum from thermally injured patients has "factors" that alter cellular function. Although these factors remain to be identified, it is obvious from studies on cellular function that placing dysfunctional cells (usually leukocytes of lymphocytes) into a normal environment such as donor whole blood or fresh frozen plasma generally returns the particular function to normal [2–5].

With the development of in vivo blood cell separators, isolation and removal of specific blood components for therapeutic purposes has become a practical possibility. Since in this technique a volume of removed plasma must be replaced, plasma exchange is probably a better term than plasmapheresis for this procedure. Removal of plasma followed by the return of cellular components to the blood was first described in 1913 by Abell et al. to relieve uremia in dogs following bilateral nephrectomy [6]. During the twentieth century, whole blood exchange revolutionized the management of hemolytic disease of the newborn.

Table 1. Medical conditions using plasma exchange

Antibody-mediated disease	Goodpasture's syndrome (anti-GBM AB) Myasthenia gravis (anti-AchR AB) Herpes gestationis Idiopathic thrombocytopenic purpura Hypogammaglobulinemia Rhesus isoimmunization
Immune-complex disease	Rapidly progressive nephritis (including polyarteritis nodosa and Wegener's granulomatosis) Systemic lupus erythematosus Tumors Some cutaneous vasculitis
Diseases of excess plasma factors	Paraproteinemias Homozygous familiar hypercholesterolemia
Miscellaneous	Renal transplantation Raynaud's disease Thrombotic thrombocytopenic purpura Drug overdose

Immune Consequences of
Trauma, Shock and Sepsis
Eds. Faist/Ninnemann/Green

Ten years have elapsed since the introduction of in vivo blood cell separators into clinical medicine. These machines were initially developed for the collection of granulocytes and platelets from normal donors; however, their availability in general hospitals has led to therapeutic use in a wide range of medical conditions (Table 1). Plasma exchange has a role in the management of many immunoproliferative and autoimmune disorders [7]. The success of plasma exchange in correcting these disorders has provided direct evidence for the involvement of circulating mediators.

These concepts have led to the use of plasma exchange in thermally injured patients in an attempt to remove circulating toxic factors, replenish injury-triggered host deficiencies, correct cellular defects, and control unchecked altered immunoregulation.

Methods

Plasma Exchange Protocol

The plasma exchange procedure involved performing plasmapheresis in adult patients and simultaneously replacing milliliter for milliliter 1.5 times the patient's calculated blood volume with type-specific fresh frozen plasma (FFP) [8, 9]. The blood volume for adult males was estimated to equal approximately 7% of the total body weight in kilograms. Fluid resuscitation with Ringer's lactate solution was continued throughout the course of plasma exchange, and was modified according to urine output as outlined above.

The plasma exchange procedure was accomplished using either the IBM Model 2997 continuous blood cell separator (IBM Systems, Endicott, NY) or the Haemonetics Model 30 discontinuous blood cell processor (Haemonetics, Natick, MA). The continuous cell separator has been used almost exclusively since 1981 because it is particularly well suited for patients with elevated hematocrits and hyperviscosity (i.e., hemoconcentration during burn shock). This machine separates whole blood into major components (erythrocytes, platelet-rich plasma, platelet-poor plasma, and leukocytes) with the advantage over discontinuous cell separators of requiring virtually no initial volume from the patient to prime the device (100 ml normal saline is utilized). A double vascular access technique was employed. Blood was removed through a 12- or 14-gauge femoral venous catheter (Intracath, Deseret, Sandy, UT) and directed into the centrifuge. The platelet-poor plasma fraction was removed and collected in sterile bags for research purposes. The remaining fractions were recombined with FFP and returned to the patient through a 16-gauge femoral or central venous catheter.

Exchange transfusions were performed in children less than 5 years of age using whole blood and platelets in an isovolemic fashion. Again, the volume of exchanged fluid was calculated to be 1.5 times the circulating blood volume as defined above. Blood was removed from the patient through a femoral arterial catheter in increments of 30–50 ml with the simultaneous infusion of an equal volume of cross-matched whole blood through a femoral or central venous catheter. Six to eight pooled platelet packs were administered at the end of the procedure to replenish the anticipated platelet deficit. Throughout both plasma exchange and exchange transfusion procedures, intake and output data were carefully balanced to ensure that the procedures were isovolemic.

Mixed Lymphocyte Cultures

Previous reports have documented the reliability of the one-way mixed lymphocyte reaction (MLR) as an in vitro monitor of serum immunosuppressive activity [10–13].

A one-way mixed lymphocyte culture was used as the standard assay for immunologic activity of burn serum specimens. The assay used normal human lymphocytes from two unrelated adult donors. Fifty-milliliter donations of heparinized blood were diluted, one part 6% dextran 70 in saline to five parts whole blood, and allowed to sediment at 37 °C for 1 h. The leukocyte-rich plasma was then drawn off, and the cells were passed through an RPMI 1640 primed column, constructed by packing a 50-ml syringe barrel with 2.0 g sterile cotton. After 15 min, nonadherent cells were eluted with three volumes of RPMI 1640. Finally, the leukocytes were washed twice and counted. This method consistently yielded more than 95% lymphocytes with greater than 95% viability. Lymphocytic yield was approximately 5×10^5 to 7×10^5 cells/ml blood. Approximately 75% were erythrocyte rosette-forming cells, as determined by the method of Jondal et al. [14].

Triplicate mixed lymphocyte cultures were established in the wells of 96-well tissue culture plates with each well containing 2×10^5 responder lymphocytes and 2×10^5 allogeneic stimulator lymphocytes in a total of 200 µl RPMI 1640. Stimulator cells were pretreated with 50 mg/liter mitomycin C for 30 min at 37 °C, then washed three times to remove any remaining mitomycin C. Wells were supplemented to contain 10% normal human or burned patient serum. Cultures were maintained at 37 °C for 144 h under 5% carbon dioxide, then pulsed by the addition of 1.0 µCi/well of methyl tritiated thymidine. After an additional 18-h incubation, cultures were harvested.

Counting was accomplished by using a scintillation cocktail, plastic vials, and a scintillation counter. Radioisotope incorporation was determined as quench-corrected disintegrations per minute (DPM). Suppressive activity was calculated as follows: % Suppression = 1-[(DPMe-unstimulated DPMc)/(stimulated DPMc-unstimulated DPMc)] × 100, where e indicates experimental, and c, control. Each assay was performed at least twice, with the data representing reproducible effects.

Plasma-Exchange Therapy During Burn Shock

Although burn shock almost invariably accompanies major thermal injury, it is rarely refractory to fluid resuscitation. Baxter has stated that 95% of children and 80%–90% of adults will achieve resuscitation after burns with fluid volumes predicted by the Parkland formula [15]. This formula is the most liberal of those commonly employed to guide resuscitation in the treatment of burn shock, and many patients are resuscitated successfully with substantially smaller volumes of fluid [16]. However, in selected patients, failures of burn shock resuscitation still occur despite administration of massive volumes of fluid. Such patients are characterized by either extreme age and exceptionally extensive tissue trauma or major electrical injuries, major inhalation injury, delay in initiating adequate fluid resuscitation, or underlying disease which limits metabolic and cardiovascular reserve [17]. In these patients, refractory burn shock and resuscitation failure remain major causes of early mortality despite advances in emergency care and transport, resuscitation regimens, and physiologic stabilization.

The use of plasma exchange was evaluated in a group of patients with major thermal injuries who failed to respond to conventional fluid volumes during resuscitation from burn shock [9].

During a 3-year period, 22 patients underwent plasma exchange during burn shock resuscitation [9]. The mean age was 22.7 years (range 1–60 years). The mean total body surface area (TBSA) burn was 47.9% (range 25.5%–100%) with a mean full-thickness TBSA injury of 31.9% (range 3.5%–88%). The patient group consisted of 14 adults (all male) and 8 children (5 male, 3 female). The etiology of tissue injury was flame burns in 16 patients and electrical injuries in 3. Twelve patients suffered concomitant inhalation injuries, as documented by ^{133}Xe perfusion scan [10]. Significant preexisting medical conditions were present in five patients.

In 17 patients, the indications for plasma exchange were ongoing fluid requirements exceeding twice those predicted by Parkland formula guidelines despite conversion to hypertonic lactated saline resuscitation fluid [39]. In an additional five patients, plasma exchange was performed for massive myoglobinuria in addition to resuscitation failure. Patients failing to respond to fluid resuscitation also demonstrated persistent lactic acidemia, depressed mental status, and arterial hypotension. In most patients, the diagnosis of resuscitation failure could not be made for at least 12 h postburn during which time the patients often required fluid volumes in excess of those predicted by the entire 24-h Parkland calculation. The decision to perform plasma exchange was not made until the above criteria were satisfied. The procedure was often instituted as a last resort in an attempt to salvage the patient from irreversible burn shock. Plasma exchange was performed only once in this group of patients.

The response to plasma exchange is outlined in Table 2 [9]. The mean delay in initiating adequate fluid resuscitation was 3.0 h. Plasma exchange was performed at a mean time of 17.0 h postburn. The plasma exchange procedure required a mean 4.3 h to complete, while exchange transfusions required 1.0 h. Sixteen patients underwent plasma exchange and exchange transfusions were performed in six patients. A therapeutic response was documented in 21 of the 22 patients. This response was characterized by a sharp decrease in fluid requirements from a mean of 260% above the predicted hourly volume by the resuscitation formula to within calculated requirements at a mean time of 2.3 h following plasma exchange. Rapid clearing of pigment was seen in five patients with myoglobinuria. Only one patient, with a 100% total body surface area (TBSA) burn (88% full-thickness injury), failed to respond to plasma exchange and ex-

Table 2. Results of plasma exchange therapy during burn shock

Mean delay in initiating resuscitation	3.0 h (range 0.5–12 h)
Mean time postburn of plasma exchange	17.0 h (range 7–48 h)
Mean duation of:	
Plasma exchange	4.3 h (range 1–7 h)
Exchange transfusion	1.0 h
Procedure performed:	
Plasma exchange	16 patients
Exchange transfusion	6 patients
Therapeutic response to plasma exchange	21/22 (95.4%)
Percentage resuscitation volume above calculated requirements at time of plasma exchange	260% (range 100%–500%)
Mean time to return to calculated volume requirements following plasma exchange	2.3 h (range 0–8 h)
Clearing of myoglobinuria	5/5 (100%)
Mortality (three early, three late: one to resuscitation failure)	4.5% during burn shock
Complications (major)	27.3% overall (in-hospital)
	None

Table 3. Plasma exchange therapy during burn shock. Resuscitation characteristics

Total resuscitation received:		
Mean duration	27.3	h (range 14–52)
Mean fluid volume	6.77	ml/kg/% burn (range 1.3–15 mg/kg/% burn)
Mean sodium load	1.24	mEq Na/kg/% burn (range 0.4–2.7 mEq/kg/% burn)
Effect of plasma exchange on resuscitation volume:		
Pre	0.39	0.04 ml/kg/% burn/h
Post	0.17	0.02 ml/kg/% burn/h*
Effect of plasma exchange on urine output:		
Pre	1.04	0.13 ml/kg/h
Post	3.26	0.71 ml/kg/h*

* $P<0.001$.

pired at 18 h postburn. The overall in-hospital mortality for the patient group was 27.3%. Three early deaths occurred within 5 days of injury (one each due to irreversible burn shock, cerebral hemorrhage, or respiratory failure), while three late deaths (at 22, 41, and 55 days postburn) were attributed to sepsis. No major complications were associated with the plasma exchange procedure.

The patient group achieved resuscitation at a mean time of 27.3 h postburn (Table 3) [9]. The mean resuscitation volume was 6.77 ml/kg/% burn with a sodium load of 1.24 mEq Na/kg/% burn. Plasma exchange resulted in a dramatic and statistically significant decrease in resuscitation volume and increase in urine output when comparing group means pre- and post-plasma exchange. Figure 1 illustrates the effect of plasma exchange on resuscitation volume [9]. Immediately before plasma exchange, the mean volume of resuscitation fluid necessary to

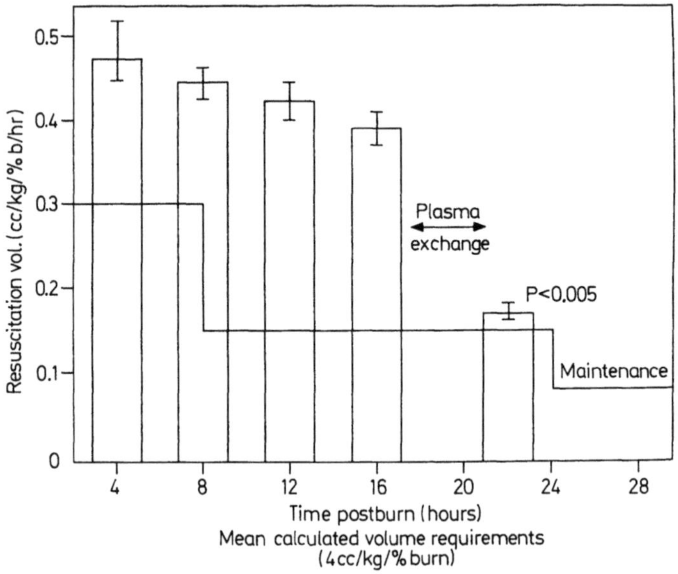

Fig. 1. Effect of plasma exchange on resuscitation volume. The mean ±SEM resuscitation volume for the entire patient group ($N = 22$) is depicted on the *ordinate* in ml/kg/% burn/h versus time postburn in hours on the *abscissa*. Plasma exchange was performed at a mean time postburn of 17 h, required approximately 4 h to complete, and resulted in a statistically significant decrease in fluid requirements approaching the volume predicted by the resuscitation formula. (J Trauma 23:947, 1983)

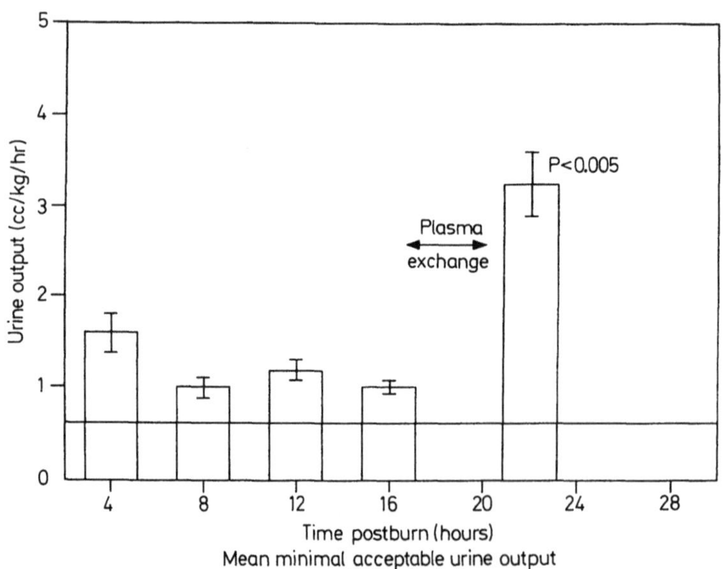

Fig. 2. Effect of plasma exchange on urine output. The mean ±SEM urine output is depicted on the *ordinate* in ml/kg/h versus time postburn in hours on the *abscissa*. Plasma exchange resulted in a brisk diuresis despite a marked reduction in fluid administration following the procedure. This change is statistically significant. (J Trauma 23:947, 1983)

maintain a minimum acceptable urine output was 260% of the level predicted by the Parkland formula based upon burn size and body weight in kilograms. However, plasma exchange permitted a sharp decrease in fluid resuscitation volume within 2 h after the procedure was completed. Similarly, Fig. 2 illustrates the effect of plasma exchange on urine output [9]. Immediately before plasma exchange, urine output was adequate only because of the massive volume infusions being administered at this time. Plasma exchange resulted in a brisk diuresis despite a marked decrease in fluid volume administration. Plasma exchange resulted in a statistically significant decrease in serum lactate levels within 2–4 h. A significant increase in serum bicarbonate, pH, and base excess levels was seen immediately post-plasma exchange as metabolic acidosis resolved. No significant effect was observed on serum sodium concentration. However, a significant increase occurred in serum albumin levels. The colloid content of the replacement fluid (FFP) was measured and compared with the mean total protein and albumin content of burn plasma removed by plasmapheresis. Plasma exchange resulted in a mean net gain in colloid of 131 g total protein and 80 g albumin to the patient.

Discussion

An expanding body of evidence supports the concept that the etiology of burn shock may be secondary to a number of alterations in the internal environment of the organism [19–22]. Baxter et al. in 1966 demonstrated in cross-perfusion studies from burned to unburned dogs a decrease in cardiac output in the unburned animals, suggesting that there were circulating factors in the burn serum responsible for burn shock [1]. A number of other studies have addressed the issue of a circulating "myocardial depressant factor" or "shock toxin" responsible for the characteristic dysfunction of myocardial contractility observed in burn shock both in experimental animals and in man [21, 23].

A variety of circulating serum factors have been implicated in the pathophysiology of burn shock, including the release and consumption of many mediators of the inflammatory response which lead to increased vascular permeability and cellular membrane dysfunction [24–27]. These substances include vasoactive amines, products of platelet and complement activation, products of arachidonic acid metabolism, kinin polypeptides, endotoxin, metabolic hormones, fibronectin, and other substances:

1. Vasocative amines – histamine, serotonin
2. Products of platelet activation – thromboxanes
3. Products of complement activation – C_{3a}, C_{5a} (anaphylatoxins)
4. Products of arachidonic acid metabolism – prostaglandins, leukotrienes
5. Kinin polypeptides, coagulation/fibrinolytic proteins
6. Exogenous substances – endotoxin
7. Metabolic hormones – catecholamines, cortisol
8. Other – neutrophil products, denatured protein, serum proteins, fibronectin

In addition to the activation and release of the postulated toxic effect on substances, thermal injury is associated with the consumption of a number of serum components, including fibronectin, complement components, platelets, and other inflammatory mediators [26, 28–31].

It is clear from the discussion that an altered internal environment exists following major thermal injury. Plasma exchange may provide a potential alternative in burn shock resuscitation by returning the altered internal milieu toward normal. Whether the mechanism of action of plasma exchange involves a removal of circulating toxic factors, a replenishment of specific deficiencies, or a combination of the two remains to be determined. Although the plasma exchange procedure resulted in a positive albumin balance, the net gain in albumin of only 80 g/plasma exchange procedure suggests that the positive effect of plasma exchange is not due merely to colloid replacement.

Effect of Plasma Exchange on Postburn Lymphocyte Suppression

Since the early 1950s, convincing clinical and experimental evidence has documented the acquired immunodepression that occurs within 24 h following major thermal injury [32, 33]. This immunodepression results in enhanced susceptibility to infection, in which active suppression of host defense mechanisms plays a critical role. Despite advances in general medical and surgical treatment modalities, infection remains a significant problem in treating thermally injured patients, with 75%–85% of deaths at most burn centers due to sepsis [33, 34].

It is clear from numerous studies that the internal milieu in burned patients contains circulating factors toxic to cellular function and presumably responsible for immunosuppression after burn injury [34–37].

Excisional therapy has gained wide acceptance in the management of thermal injuries. These procedures are associated with rapid and voluminous blood loss [38]. The similarity between plasma exchange and the rapid blood loss and replacement that accompany excisional therapy prompted the evaluation of the immunomodulatory potential of plasma exchange and excisional therapy on postburn lymphocyte function [41, 42].

Plasma Exchange

Twenty-one adult patients underwent plasma exchange during their postburn recover [42]. The mean age was 33.5 years. The mean TBSA burn was 52.6%, with a mean full-thickness TBSA injury of 32.6%. Twelve patients sustained inhalation injuries as documented by ^{133}Xe perfusion scan [18]. Significant preexisting medical conditions were present in six patients (31.6%), including substance abuse in three patients, chronic obstructive pulmonary disease in two patients, and one patient with iatrogenic Cushing's syndrome after bilateral adrenalectomy.

Plasma exchange therapy was used in five clinical settings including: (1) failure to respond to conventional fluid resuscitation during burn shock, (2) the presence of massive myoglobinuria after electrical injury, (3) adult respiratory distress syndrome, (4) metabolic exhaustion or "presepsis," and (5) documented sepsis. These indications for plasma exchange essentially defined patient groups that represented a complication of or inability to respond appropriately to conventional burn treatment regimens.

The criteria for initiating plasma exchange in patients treated for failure to resuscitate is described in the previous section.

Adult respiratory distress syndrome, or respiratory failure, was defined as arterial hypoxemia, tachypnea, increased shunt fraction, and bilateral diffuse pulmonary infiltrates in the absence of infection, true inhalation injury, or elevated pulmonary capillary wedge pressures.

The syndrome of metabolic exhaustion, or "presepsis," is a clinical condition that generally occurs 7 days after burn injury and is manifested by poor wound healing, intolerance of caloric support, mild loss of capillary integrity, and mild metabolic acidosis, all in the absence of documented infection [40].

The category of documented sepsis included patients with positive blood cultures or with positive burn wound biopsy specimens growing greater than 10^5 organisms/cm^3 or showing evidence of tissue invasion by bacteria.

Plasma exchange was performed only once in the resuscitation failure and myoglobinuria groups. However, two patients in the resuscitation failure group underwent an additional plasma exchange procedure on the second postburn day for recurrent "capillary leak." Another patient received daily plasma exchanges for the first 3 days after burn injury because of persistent myoglobinuria after a large electrical injury. Patients who met the criteria for respiratory failure, metabolic exhaustion, or sepsis underwent plasma exchange at 24-h intervals for three consecutive days unless marked clinical improvement obviated further therapy after the first or second procedure.

Fifty-four plasma exchange procedures were performed in 21 patients, with 12 patients undergoing multiple plasma exchange procedures. The mean volume of plasma exchanged was 5079 ml (range 2100–7500 ml), with the procedure requiring a mean duration of 4.3 h (range 2–7 h) to complete. No major complications were associated with the plasma exchange procedures. Nine septic episodes were documented in six of the patients (28.6%), five of whom underwent plasma exchange before developing clinical sepsis. The overall mortality rate for the patient group was 28.6%, with two early deaths attributed to irreversible burn shock and four late deaths caused by sepsis.

The effect of plasma exchange on postburn lymphocyte suppression, as measured by the mixed lymphocyte reaction for each of the treatment groups, demonstrated a statistically significant decrease in suppressive activity in each of the patient groups after plasma exchange (Table 4) [42]. The decrease in suppressive activity was greater than 50% in all but the sepsis group. The suppressive activity of burn plasma removed by plasma exchange was 50% or greater in all groups. The duration of the plasma exchange-induced reduction in serum suppressive activity varied according to the indications for and the timing of plasma exchange. However, the improvement in mixed lymphocyte reactivity in most instances appeared to be more than just a transient effect, as return of suppressive activity to pre-plasma-exchange levels often required several days.

Plasma exchange therapy in patients who failed to resuscitate from burn shock resulted in a dramatic reversal of fluid requirements accompanied by a brisk diuresis, resolution of lactic acidosis, and restoration of capillary integrity as described previously. Serum suppressive activity appeared very quickly after thermal injury, often within 12 h in each of these patients, and plasma exchange

Table 4. Effect of plasma exchange on mixed lymphocyte reaction

	Failure to resuscitate	Massive myoglobinuria	Respiratory failure	Metabolic exhaustion	Documented sepsis
Patients (no.)	10	3	4	6	5
Plasma exchange procedures (no.)	12	5	10	12	15
Mean time postburn of plasma exchange	15.7 h (7–30)	30.6 h (10.66)	4 days (1–7)	11.75 days (4–20)	24.7 days (4–52)
% TBSA burn (mean)	56.4 (35–100)	39.3 (29–53)	46.4 (29–84)	60.5 (38–84)	64.4 (38–84)
Before mixed lymphocyte reaction (% suppression)	77.7 5.5	51.6 15.1	68.6 8.2	57.9 12.1	56.9 5.1
After mixed lymphocyte reaction (% suppression)	36.9 6.7*	20.0 11.6*	15.8 4.6*	29.0 6.3*	32.8 3.8*
Duration of mixed lymphocyte reaction	4.6 (1–21)	2.0 (1–3)	13.2 (2–24)	7.2 (4–16)	1.7 (0–10)

* $P<0.05$

reduced immunosuppression in all instances. Only two of these patients subsequently developed septic complications during postburn convalescence, with one late death.

Plasma exchange after major electrical injury resulted in not only lowered resuscitation volumes but also marked clearing of myoglobinuria without supervening renal compromise. Of the three patients in this treatment group, one patient died of irreversible burn shock. The remaining two patients recovered without incident.

The four patients who underwent plasma exchange for respiratory failure, or adult respiratory distress syndrome, demonstrated a dramatic improvement in their respiratory status characterized by a decrease in pulmonary artery pressure, a marked improvement in oxygenation, and radiographic clearing of pulmonary infiltrates within 30 h. The dramatic clinical response was paralleled by a 74% reduction in serum suppressive activity that lasted nearly 2 weeks. One of these patients developed late sepsis that resulted in ultimate death.

Patients who underwent plasma exchange for metabolic exhaustion or "presepsis" demonstrated marked clinical improvement with reversal of target-organ damage and restoration of lymphocyte function. All six of the patients in this category demonstrated decreased fluid requirements, increased urine output, and resolution of lactic acidosis after plasma exchange. The mortality rate of these patients was 33.3%, with the two deaths caused by the subsequent development of sepsis. The septic episodes occurred at 11 and 40 days after resolution of metabolic exhaustion. However, plasma exchange was effective in restoring lymphocyte function. The mean duration of mixed lymphocyte reaction improvement was 7.2 days.

Table 5. Effect of plasma exchange on mixed lymphocyte reaction in sepsis

	Group means (±SEM)		
	First plasma exchange	Second plasma exchange	Third plasma exchange
Before mixed lymphocyte reaction (% suppression)	47.8±2.3	47.0±6.5	53.6± 9.4
After mixed lymphocyte reaction (% suppression)	27.0±3.9*	32.6±2.2[a]	28.0±10.6*
Duration of mixed lymphocyte reaction improvement	24 h	24 h	5.5 days (range 4–10)

* $P<0.05$.
[a] Not significant ($P=0.10$).

In the five patients who underwent plasma exchange therapy for documented sepsis, there was only transient (mean 1.7 days) improvement in lymphocyte function. However, the results of the plasma exchange procedures performed at 24-h intervals for three consecutive days demonstrated that the initial plasma exchange produced a significant reduction in suppressive activity that was of short duration lasting only 24 h (Table 5) [42]. The second plasma exchange resulted in a decrease in suppressive activity; however, this decrease was not significant. The final plasma exchange procedure resulted in a significant improvement in lymphocyte reactivity of 51.2%. This beneficial effect lasted a mean of 5.5 days. These patients also demonstrated a transient improvement in metabolic and cardiovascular parameters. Four patients eventually died of sepsis at a mean time of 7 days (range 1–18 days) after exchange and 34.1 days after burn injury.

Excision and Grafting

Thirty adult patients underwent excisional therapy [42]. The patients had a mean age of 31.9 years. The mean TBSA burn was 42.8%, with a mean full-thickness injury of 24.1%. Inhalation injury was documented in 15 patients (50%) by ^{133}Xe perfusion scan.

Initial excision and autografting of burns was performed as soon as the patient had stabilized after fluid resuscitation. The excision and grafting procedure was a two-stage technique that required a layered excision of eschar followed by an overnight stabilization period for restoration of normal body temperature and blood volume [38]. Excised wounds were covered with bulky gauze dressings that were kept moist by soaking the dressing through irrigating catheters every 4 h.

On the day after excision, patients were returned to the operating room for autograft coverage of the excised burns. Freshly applied autografts were dressed with fine mesh gauze and covered with bulky dressings and irrigating catheters. Patients were returned to the burn unit where attention was given to temperature control and blood volume replacement.

Table 6. Plasma exchange versus excisional therapy on mixed lymphocyte reaction

	Plasma exchange		Excisional therapy	
Before mixed lymphocyte reaction (% suppression)	62.7	3.4	42.2	3.3
After mixed lymphocyte reaction (% suppression)	28.3	2.9*	29.1	2.9*
Volume exchanged (% blood volume)	150		64.1	
Duration of procedure (HR)	4.2		3.0	

* $P<0.05$.

Blood loss was calculated separately for each excision and grafting procedure and then totaled. Blood for hematocrit tests was drawn before and after operation and 24 h after each procedure. The intraoperative and postoperative transfusion records of each patient were noted. Blood loss was calculated on the assumption of an average blood volume of 7% [38].

Seventy-eight excision and grafting (E/G) procedures were performed in 30 patients, with 25 patients undergoing multiple E/G procedures. The initial E/G procedure was performed at a mean time of 7.5 days after burn injury (range 3–13 days). The mean burn size excised and skin grafted at each procedure was 7.5% TBSA (range 0.8%–22% TBSA) or 2372 cm^2 (range 320–5000 cm^2). In this group of patients there were six septic episodes documented in four patients. The overall mortality rate for the patient group was 6.7%, with the two deaths caused by late sepsis.

The main blood transfusion requirement per E/G procedure was 3355 ± 235 ml (range 0–8150 ml). The mean percentage of circulating blood volume required per E/G procedure was $64.1\% \pm 4.5\%$. The mean volume of blood transfusion required per percent burn excised and grafted was 462.7 ± 32.4 ml or 1.4 ± 0.1 ml/cm^2.

The effect of E/G on postburn lymphocyte suppression demonstrated a statistically significant decrease in suppressive activity after excisional therapy. The mean percentages decrease in suppressive activity was 24.2%, returning the mixed lymphocyte reaction suppression to only 29.1% by 24 h after the procedure (Table 6) [42]. The mean duration of reversal of suppressive activity after excisional therapy was 5.0 days (range 2–14 days). The mean admitting suppression of normal lymphocyte function was 73.1% and in the surviving patients (93.3%) the mean mixed lymphocyte reaction suppression was 18.0% at the time of discharge on mean postburn day 47.7.

Discussion

There is extensive evidence that lymphocyte responses in patients with major thermal injuries are severely impaired, and normal lymphocyte function is compromised when placed in culture in the presence of burn sera [34, 36, 43]. Evidence has implicated both exogenous (bacterial endotoxin, various medications) and endogenous (prostaglandins, thromboxanes, vasoactive amines, products of complement activation, metabolic hormones) factors in the systemic circulation as possible causes of postburn immunodepression [19, 44, 45]. The presence of immunosuppressive substances in burn sera appears to precede the dysfunction of patient lymphocytes. Since it appears that multiple circulating lymphocyte-suppressive mediators are present and of importance during the clinical course of burn management, plasma exchange may have a unique advantage in its potential to correct the multiple causes of impaired lymphocyte function in burn patients.

Although plasma exchange reversed lymphocyte suppression during sepsis, clinical efficacy of this modality could not be clearly demonstrated since four of these five patients eventually died of sepsis. These results suggest that immunologic restoration of the patients was ineffective in reversing the inexorable progression of vital tissue and organ damage [46]. However, the syndrome of metabolic exhaustion, or "presepsis," may represent a point in time when immunorestorative therapy is still of benefit in the prevention of invasive infection.

There is convincing evidence that surgical trauma and/or anesthesia results in altered immunocompetence [47–49]. Riddle and Berenbaum [50] demonstrated postoperative lymphocyte suppression using phytohemagglutinin stimulation of blastogenesis. Jubert et al. [47] reported decreased lymphocyte blastogenesis after operation. They correlated lymphocyte suppression with length of operation and the particular anesthetic agent administered. All anesthetic agents were associated with some degree of immunosuppression. However, lymphocyte suppression also occurs during operations with spinal anesthesia [48].

The effect of blood transfusions on lymphocyte suppression remains controversial. In surgical patients (Jubert et al. [47]), as welldas patients with uremia (Fehrman et al. [51] and Giacchino et al. [52]), it was demonstrated that decreased lymphocyte function is associated with transfusion therapy. However, Hunt and Trotter [53] reported that the reduction in lymphocyte transformation seen after operation was partly reversed by blood transfusions during operation. In the present study, excisional therapy was associated with large blood losses and replacement was associated with a significant decrease in lymphocyte suppressive activity. The mean blood transfusion requirement per excisional procedure was 64.1% of the calculated circulating blood volume of an adult. The decrease in lymphocyte suppression associated with excision therapy returned the serum suppressive activity to a level that was similar to that obtained with plasma exchange – postplasma exchange 28.3% versus post-E/G 29.1% (Table 7) [42]. In 1982, Gray et al. [54] reported less burn wound sepsis and serious wound contamination with excisional therapy as compared with conservative wound management. In addition, in a guinea pig burn model, thymic DNA synthesis returned to normal by day 6 in the animals that were excised but remained depressed in the unexcised group [55]. In contrast, Fried and Munster [56] demonstrated no improvement in T-cell function with early excision. However, the wounds were not immediately closed with skin grafts or primary closure, as performed in the previous study.

The beneficial effect of excisional therapy with large volume blood replacement on lymphocyte suppression may be due to multiple factors. Possibilities include removal of circulating suppressive factors, replacement of injury-triggered host deficiencies, or removal of toxins contained within the burn wound. The return to pre-excisional suppression levels in approximately 5 days in burn patients whose wounds cannot be closed in a single excisional procedure suggests that the beneficial effect of excisional therapy may be due to removal of circulating factors or replacement of host deficiencies. Although the reasons for the beneficial effect of excisional therapy remain to be elucidated, it is clear that excisional procedures do not produce more lymphocyte dysfunction, as has been demonstrated in other varieties of surgical trauma.

Summary

Since it appears that multiple circulating mediators are present and of importance during the clinical course of burn treatment, plasma exchange may have a unique advantage in its potential to correct the multiple causes of both burn shock and altered immunological function following thermal injury. The studies performed to date have demonstrated that plasma exchange can be performed safely in critically ill thermally injured patients.

Plasma exchange has a beneficial effect in restoring lymphocyte immunocompetence in a group of thermally injured patients not responding to conventional therapy; however, the effect in reducing the risk of infection remains to be determined. Excisional therapy with large blood volume replacement also has a beneficial effect in restoring lymphocyte immunosuppression and may partially account for the decrease in septic episodes reported in burn centers using excisional therapy.

Plasma exchange facilitates resuscitation from burn shock in a select group of patients who do not respond to conventional volume therapy by arresting ongoing burn shock through an as yet undefined mechanism, resulting in a dramatic reversal of fluid requirements, a brisk diuresis, a resolution of lactic acidosis, and restoration of capillary integrity.

Although this report is preliminary and involves a heterogeneous patient population without adequate controls, the return toward normal of various clinical parameters is encouraging. As a research tool, plasma exchange has great potential; however, it must be emphasized that plasma exchange has not been established as a tool for the treatment of routine burns and many questions remain to be answered before plasma exchange becomes an established adjunct to the management of the thermally injured patient.

References

1. Baxter CR, Shires GT (1968) Physiological response to crystalloid resuscitation of severe burns. Ann NY Acad Sci 150:874
2. Miller CL, Baker CC (1979) Changes in lymphocyte activity after thermal injury: the role of suppressor cells. J Clin Invest 63:202–210
3. Warden GD, Mason AD, Pruitt BA Jr (1975) Evaluation of leukocyte chemotaxis in vitro in thermally injured patients. J Clin Invest 54:1001
4. Edgar MA, Heck E, Okita R et al. (1979) Defective superoxide production in PMN leukocytes from burned patients. Proceedings of the annual meeting of the American Burn Association, New Orleans, March 16
5. Meakins JL, McLean AP, Kelly R et al. (1978) Delayed hypersensitivity and neutrophil chemotaxis: effect of trauma. J Trauma 18:240

6. Orosez JJ (1981) A short history of bloodletting. Artif Organs 5:226
7. Isbister JP, Biggs JC, Penny R (1978) Experience with large volume plasmapheresis in malignant paraproteinaemia and immune disorders. NZ Med J 8:154
8. Warden GD, Saffle JR, Kravitz M (1982) A two-stage technique for excision and grafting of burn wounds. J Trauma 22:98–103
9. Warden GD, Stratta RJ, Saffle JR, Kravitz M, Ninnemann JL (1983) Plasma exchange therapy in patients failing to resuscitate from burn shock. J Trauma 23:945–951
10. Ninnemann JL (1981)Suppression of lymphocyte response following thermal injury. In: Ninnemann JL (ed) The immune consequences of thermal injury. Williams and Wilkins, Baltimore, pp 66–89
11. Baker CC, Miller CL, Trunkey DD (1979) Predicting fatal sepsis in burn patients. J Trauma 19:641–648
12. Sakai H, Daniels JC, Beathard GA et al. (1974) Mixed lymphocyte culture reaction in patients with acute thermal burns. J Trauma 14:53–57
13. Keane RM, Birmingham W, Shatney CM et al. (1983) Prediction of sepsis in the multitraumatic patient by assays of lymphocyte responsiveness. Surg Gynecol Obstet 156:163–167
14. Jondal M, Hohn G, Wigzell H (1972) Surface markers on human T and B lymphocytes: I. A large population of lymphocytes forming nonimmune rosette with sheep red blood cells. J Exp Med 136:207–215
15. Baxter CR (1978) Problems and complications of burn shock resuscitation. Surg Clin North Am 58:1313
16. Pruitt BA Jr (1978) Fluid and electrolyte replacement in the burned patient. Surg Clin North Am 58:1291
17. Pruitt BA Jr (1978) Advances in fluid therapy and the early care of the burn patient. World J Surg 2:139
18. Moylan JA, Wilmore DW, Mouton DE et al. (1972) Early diagnosis of inhalation injury using ^{133}xenon lung scan. Ann Surg 176:477
19. Baxter CR, Cook WA, Shires GT (1966) Serum myocardial depressant factor of burn shock. Surg Forum 17:1
20. Kremer B, Allgower M, Graf M et al. (1981) The present status of research in burn toxins. Intens Care Med 7:77
21. Raffa J, Trunkey DD (1978) Myocardial depression in acute thermal injury. J Trauma 18:90
22. Rosenthal SR (1972) Purified burn toxin and its competition. Surgery 71:527
23. Fozzard HA (1961) Myocardial injury in burn shock. Ann Surg 154:113
24. Alexander JW, McClellan MA, Ogle CK et al. (1976) Consumptive opsoninopathy: possible pathogenesis in lethal and opportunistic infections. Ann Surg 184:674
25. Bjornson AB, Altemeier WA, Bjornson HS (1977) Changes in humoral components of host defense following burn trauma. Ann Surg 186:88
26. Ninnemann JL (ed) (1983) Traumatic injury: infection and other immunologic sequelae. University Park Press, Baltimore
27. Warden GD, Ninnemann JL (1981) The immune consequences of thermal injury: an overview. In: Ninnemann JL (ed) The immune consequences of thermal injury. Williams and Wilkins, Baltimore, pp 1–20
28. Daniels JC, Larson DL, Abston S et al. (1974) Serum protein profiles in thermal burns. J Trauma 14:137
29. Alexander JW, Ogle CK, Stinnett JD et al. (1978) A sequential prospective analysis of immunologic abnormalities and infection following major thermal injury. Ann Surg 188:809
30. Lanser ME, Saba TM, Scovill WA (1980) Opsonic glycoprotein (plasma fibronectin) levels after burn injury. Ann Surg 192:776
31. Ninnemann JL (1982) Immunologic defenses against infection: alterations following thermal injuries. J Burn Care Rehabil 3:355
32. Warden GD, Ninnemann JL (1981) The immune consequences of thermal injury: an overview. In: Ninnemann JL (ed) The immune consequences of thermal injury. Williams and Wilins, Baltimore, pp 1–21

33. Polk HC (1979) Consensus summary on infection. J Trauma 19:894–896
34. Ninnemann JL (1983) Immune depression in burn and trauma patients: the role of circulating suppressors. In: Ninnemann JL (ed) Traumatic injury: infection and other immunologic sequelae. University Park Press, Baltimore, pp 33–57
35. Hakim AA (1977) An immunosuppressive factor from serum of thermally traumatized patients. J Trauma 17:908–919
36. Ninnemann JL, Condie JT, Davis SE et al. (1982) Isolation of immunosuppressive serum components following thermal injury. J Trauma 22:837–844
37. Constantian MB, Menzoian JO, Nimberg RB et al. (1975) Suppression of T cell function by a peptide fraction in the serum of traumatized patients. Clin Res 23:410A
38. Warden GD, Saffle JR, Kravitz M (1982) A two-stage technique for excision and grafting following thermal injury. J Trauma 22:98–103
39. Moylan JA, Reckler JM, Mason AD Jr (1973) Resuscitation with hypertonic lactate saline in thermal injury. Am J Surg 125:580
40. Warden GD, Saffle JR, Kenfield K, Kravitz (1983) The use of plasma exchange in thermally injured patients not responding to conventional burn management. J Burn Care Rehabil 4:264–270
41. Ninnemann JL, Stratta RJ, Warden GD, Saffle JR, Weber ME (1984) The effect of plasma exchange on lymphocyte suppression after burn. Arch Surg 119:33–38
42. Warden GD, Ninnemann JL, Stratta RJ, Saffle JR (1984) The effect of exchange therapy on postburn lymphocyte suppression. Surgery 96:321–329
43. Ninnemann JL, Fisher JC, Wachtel TL (1979) Thermal injury associated immunosuppression: occurrence and in vitro blocking effect of convalescent serum. J Immunol 122:1736–1741
44. Alexander JW, McClelland MA, Ogle CK et al. (1976) Consumption opsoninopathy: possible pathogenesis in lethal and opportunistic infections. Ann Surg 184:672
45. Bjornson AB, Altemeier WA, Bjornson HS (1977) Changes in humoral components of host defense following burn trauma. Ann Surg 186:88
46. Levinson SA, Hume DM (1972) Effect of exchange transfusion with fresh whole blood on refractory septic shock. Am Surg 38:49
47. Jubert AV, Lee ET, Hersh EM, McBride CM (1973) Effect of surgery, anesthesia and intraoperative blood loss on immunocompetence. J Surg Res 15:399–403
48. Kent JR, Geist S (1975) Lymphocyte transformation during operations with spinal anesthesia. Anesthesiology 42:505–508
49. Roth JA, Golub SH, Lukingnan RA, Brazier J, Morton D (1981) Cell-mediated immunity is depressed following cardiopulmonary bypass. Ann Thorac Surg 31:350–356
50. Riddle PR, Berenbaum MC (1967) Postoperative depression of the lymphocyte response to phytohemagglutinin. Lancet I:746
51. Fehrman I, Ringden O, Moeller E, Lundgren G, Groth CG (1981) Is cell-mediated immunity in the uremic patient affected by blood transfusion. Transplant Proc 13:164–166
52. Giacchino F, Belardi P, Coppo R et al. (1981) Effects of blood transfusion on cellular immunity. Proc Eur Dial Transplant Assoc 18:465–468
53. Hunt PS, Trotter S (1976) Lymphocyte response after surgery and blood transfusion. J Surg Res 21:57–61
54. Gray DT, Pine RW, Harnar TJ, Marvin JA, Engrav LH, Heimbach DM (1982) Early surgical excision versus conventional therapy in patients with 2% to 40% burns: a comparative study. Am J Surg 144:76–80
55. Echinard CE, Sajdel-Sulkowska E, Burke PA, Burke JF (1982) The beneficial effect of early excision on clinical response and thymic activity after burn injury. J Trauma 22:560–565
56. Fried DA, Munster AW (1975) Does immunosuppression by thermal injury depend on the continued presence of the burn wound? J Trauma 15:486–495

In Vivo Infusion of a Single Dose of Endotoxin in Healthy Humans Causes In Vitro Alterations of Both T-Cell and Adherent Cell Functions *

M. L. Rodrick, H. R. Michie, N. M. Moss, J. T. Grbic, A. Revhaug, S. T. O'Dwyer, D. B. Gough, D. Dubravec, J. McK. Manson, D. W. Wilmore, and J. A. Mannick

Introduction

Following severe traumatic or thermal injury significant suppression of the immune response has been demonstrated [1–4]. It has been proposed that the primary inducers of this alteration may be bacterial endotoxins [5].

When postinjury infection is due to gram-negative bacterial infection, exposure of the host to high levels of endotoxin is inevitable. In the noninfected patient, alterations in the gastrointestinal mucosal barrier may allow intestinal endotoxins to enter the circulation. This response has been associated with burn injury [6, 7] and endotoxin [8].

Although changes in humoral immunity following endotoxin administration in healthy humans have been studied [9], there is virtually no information concerning T-cell or monocyte-mediated immune function. In order to study the effects of endotoxin without the influence of injury and therapy we monitored cellular immune function before and following administration of a reference endotoxin from *Escherichia coli* and during separate saline control periods in paired studies in healthy male subjects.

Materials and Methods

Subjects

The volunteers were 20 normal males (mean age 33 years, range 26–39 years), who were healthy as determined by history, physical examination, hematology, blood chemistry, and exercise electrocardiogram. They were admitted 4 days prior to the study to the Clinical Research Center of the Brigham & Women's Hospital, Boston, MA for acclimatization and evaluation. Written informed consent was obtained from each subject and approved by the Committee for the Protection of Human Subjects from Research Risks of Brigham & Women's Hospital.

* Supported by NIH Grant # 2R01 GM35633-03A1, Trauma Center Grant P50 GM 36428-02, the Brigham Surgical Group Foundation, and Clinical Research Center NIH Grant # R01-RR 02635-05.

Immune Consequences of
Trauma, Shock and Sepsis
Eds. Faist/Ninnemann/Green

Infusions

Volunteers were given an intravenous bolus infusion via an antecubital vein catheter of either endotoxin, 20 IU/kg body weight (4 ng/kg), or the equivalent volume of 0.9% saline. Endotoxin was UJS standard endotoxin (RSE), Lot EC-5 [10], derived from *E. coli*, 10000 endotoxin units/vial, reconstituted with pyrogen-free water. In additional investigations, volunteers received 800 mg ibuprofen (Upjohn, Kalamazoo, MI) by mouth at time −90 min and again at 0 h before either saline or endotoxin infusion as above.

Blood Samples

Immediately prior to infusion (0 h), 30 ml heparinized blood was obtained and samples were again taken 4 h after infusion, and 24 h after infusion in study 1 and 3 ($n=7$). Samples were taken at 0, 1, and 4 h postinfusion of either saline or endotoxin in study 2 ($n=6$).

Peripheral blood mononuclear cells (PBMCs) were obtained by Ficoll-Hypaque separation, washed three times at 4 °C in minimal essential medium (MEM) containing 1% penicillin/streptomycin/fungizone (10000 units / 10000 μg / 25 μg/ml), HEPES and 2 m*M* glutamine and taken up in media as above with addition of 5% heat-inactivated (56 °C, 30 min) fetal bovine serum (FCS) (MEM-FCS). All media and additives were obtained from Grand Island Biological Co., New York. The cells were always found to be more than 95% viable by trypan blue. The cells were counted on the basis of mononuclear cells excluding all polymorphonuclear cells from the count using a nuclear stain. To control for interassay variability, PBMCs from two normal laboratory volunteers were studied on each day.

Mitogenic Response of Lymphocytes

1×10^5 PBMCs/200 μl in MEM-FCS as above were incubated with an optimally stimulating dose of 6.0 μg/ml phytohemagglutinin (PHA) for 48 h at 37 °C, followed by an 18-h pulse with 1 μCi tritiated thymidine (^{3}HTdr) 6 Ci/mmol (New England Nuclear, Boston, MA). Uptake of ^{3}HTdr was determined using an LKB liquid scintillation counter (Gaithersburg, MD) and the assay performed in triplicate. In experiments to test the effect of indomethacin, it was added to cultures at 1 μg/ml final concentration. IL-1 (Genzyme, Boston, MA) and recombinant human IL-2 (Amgen, Thousand Oaks, CA) were added at 1, 10, and 100 units/ml culture (Genzyme, Boston, MA).

Generation and Assay of IL-2

Interleukin 2 was generated by culturing PBMCs at 1×10^5 cells/well in 200 μl volume for 24 h in MEM-FCS with or without 2.5 μg PHA. Supernatants were collected and stored at −20 °C. Assay was as previously described [4] using the

IL-2-dependent cell line (CTLL-2). All supernatants were assayed two times in different assays.

Generation and Assay of IL-1

Peripheral blood mononuclear cells (200 µl cells at 5×10^6/ml) in MEM-FCS were allowed to adhere to flat-bottomed plastic microtiter plates for 1 h at 37 °C, 5% CO_2, and 95% air. Nonadherent cells were removed by washing three times in RPMI-1640 medium containing antibiotics, 1-glutamine, and 10 m*M* HEPES buffer as above without FCS, and the adherent cells were cultured as above for 24 h in 200 µl of the same medium in the presence of 1.0 µg/ml lipopolysaccharide [lipopolysaccharide (LPS): *Escherichia coli* 055:B5, Sigma Chemical Co., St. Louis, MO]. Supernatant solutions were pooled from three to four wells, frozen, and assayed for IL-1 as previously described [4] using the C3H/HeJ mouse thymocyte costimulator assay. Supernatants were also tested for IL-1 beta using a radioimmunoassay (Cistron Biotechnology, Pine Brook, NJ).

Measurement of T-Lymphocyte Subsets Using Monoclonal Antibodies

A quantity of 5×10^5 PBMCs in 100 µl was stained with monoclonal antibodies following manufacturer's instructions (Ortho Diagnostics, Raritan, NJ). The number of cells that stained with the antibodies OKT3, OKT4, and OKT8 which label the total T-cell, cluster designation (CD) (CD3), helper/inducer (CD4), and cytotoxic/suppressor (CD8) cell populations, respectively, was assayed using fluorescence-activated flow cytometry, by the Hematology Laboratory of Brigham and Women's Hospital.

Statistics

Statistical analysis of the data was performed using Student's paired *t*-test or, for nonparametric data, the Mann-Whitney U-test. Data processing and statistical analysis was performed using a VAX 11/780 computer (Digital Equipment Corporation, Maynard, MA) and a standard software package (Minitab, State University of Pennsylvania, 1982).

Results

Clinical Response

These results have been reported in detail elsewhere [11]. Briefly, following administration of endotoxin, subjects experienced a flu-like syndrome with elevation of body temperature, chills, increased heart rate, headache, and myalgia. Symptoms were maximal at about 4 h postinfusion of endotoxin. Plasma levels of cortisol, ACTH, epinephrine, and C-reactive protein were all elevated during this same period. No clinical response occurred following saline infusion.

Effect of Endotoxin on White Blood Cell Count and Mononuclear Cells Harvested

Total white blood cell (WBC) counts were significantly increased 4 h post endotoxin infusion, but were normal by 24 h. Maximum WBC count was at 6 h post endotoxin infusion [11]. The increase was due to granulocytes.

The number of PBMCs harvested from equivalent volumes of blood after these time points was significantly reduced 4 h after endotoxin infusion, although at that period there was a significant increase in total white blood cell count. In study 2 (Table 1) it was found that this decrease was not statistically significantly different from controls until the 4-h sample.

Effect on T-Cell Mitogen Response

A significantly decreased response to PHA occurred 4 h following endotoxin infusion and a decrease was observed at this time in the response of PBMCs of seven out of seven volunteers (Table 1). This shift in response was not found following saline infusion or in normal laboratory volunteers. In study 2 no significant decrease in response to PHA was seen at 1 h post endotoxin infusion (data not shown).

Table 1. Effect of in vivo endotoxin on PBMCs, PHA response, and IL-1 and IL-2 production

	Time post infusion	Infusion: Saline	Infusion: Endotoxin
PBMCs[a]	0	4.1±0.5[b]	4.3 ±0.9
	1	4.8±0.7	3.64±0.04
	4	4.5±0.7	1.5 ±0.3*
	24	3.5±0.6	4.1 ±0.9
PHA (cpm)[c]	0	101476±15629	99037±19675
	1	126800±25335	91842±23735
	4	104134±15364	44236±13987*
	24	115511±15364	143186±22614
IL-2 (units)	0	1.3±0.4	1.0 ±0.2
	1	1.5±0.4	0.51 ±0.2
	4	1.8±0.3	0.19 ±0.1*
	24	1.3±0.4	1.8 ±0.6
IL-1 (units)	0	1.6±0.9	2.2 ±1.1
	1	2.4±0.7	0.03 ±0.03*
	4	1.5±0.4	0.002±0.0005*
	24	1.6±0.2	4.6 ±1.37

* Significantly different from saline infusion, $P = < 0.02$.
[a] Peripheral blood mononuclear cells harvested ($\times 10^{-6}$) from 30 ml whole blood.
[b] All values expressed as mean ± standard error (SEM).
[c] cpm, mean counts per minute.

Effect on Production of IL-2

A marked decrease was observed in the production of IL-2 4 h following endotoxin infusion in study 1.

In study 2 IL-2 production by PBMCs from some of the volunteers was decreased from normal or saline infusion values by 1 h post endotoxin infusion but the difference was not significant. All were significantly decreased by 4 h ($P<0.01$). No significant effect was seen following saline infusion or in normal controls sampled at the same time.

Effect on IL-1 Production

At 4 h after endotoxin infusion (study 1) in most cases there was a marked decrease in IL-1 production by adherent cells to undetectable levels (0.001 units/ml). This decrease was followed in three out of seven volunteers by a marked increase over normal (7.57, 8.99, and 8.69 units) but the other four volunteers' adherent cells produced normal amounts of IL-1 (1.51, 2.02, 1.79, and 1.44 units/ml) so overall the results after 24 h were not significantly different from saline or normal control values ($P>0.05$). Thcsc supernatants when assayed by the RIA for IL-1 beta contained less than detectable IL-1B (<250 pg/ml). This assay has been shown [12] to be able to detect IL-1B in supernatants of human mononuclear cells stimulated by endotoxin. In study 2, unlike the case of IL-2, IL-1 production by adherent cells was markedly diminished at 1 h after endotoxin infusion in all volunteers (Table 1). No IL-1 (<0.001 units/ml) could be detected in supernatants of unstimulated adherent cells at any time.

T-Cell Phenotypes

Peripheral blood mononuclear cells were stained with monoclonal antibodies to total T (CD3), T-helper (CD4), and T-suppressor/cytotoxic (CD8) markers of T cells, and the percentage of positively stained cells in the lymphocyte gate counted. The results in studies 1 and 2 (Table 2) showed that there was no significant change in the numbers of cells bearing these markers, at any time tested, following saline or endotoxin infusion.

Effect of Addition of IL-2, IL-1, or Indomethacin to Endotoxin-Induced Suppressed PHA Response

Three doses of IL-2 or IL-1 were added to cultures of PBMCs from volunteers post endotoxin or saline infusion. A representative experiment is shown in Table 3. At 4 h post endotoxin infusion when the PHA response had been found to be suppressed, addition of either 10 (not shown) or 100 units of IL-2/ml culture restored the response to near pre-infusion levels. Addition of IL-1, conversely, did not cause restoration of the response at any dose (Table 3). Since we have previously reported that endotoxin infusion causes volunteers' PBMCs to be more

Table 2. Effect of endotoxin or saline infusion on T-cell phenotypes

Infusion	Hours post infusion	CD3[a]	CD4	CD8
Saline	0	51.3 ± 5.9	36.8 ± 3.2	16.9 ± 1.6
Endotoxin	0	52.6 ± 11.1	39.8 ± 6.8	17.6 ± 5.4
		NS[b]	NS	NS
Saline	1	55.8 ± 2.7	39.3 ± 2.7	16.3 ± 1.2
Endotoxin	1	55.5 ± 12.3	41.0 ± 9.5	12.3 ± 2.7
		NS	NS	NS
Saline	4[c]	52.6 ± 3.3	38.1 ± 2.9	17.1 ± 2.0
Endotoxin	4[c]	65.0 ± 6.2	40.6 ± 6.2	13.5 ± 6.2
		NS	NS	NS
Saline	24	60.1 ± 5.9	42.4 ± 2.8	19.9 ± 6.1
Endotoxin	24	57.2 ± 8.9	46.1 ± 6.6	15.1 ± 5.2
		NS	NS	NS

[a] Percentage of cells in PBMC-bearing phenotypic markers for CD3, CD4, and CD8 (OKT3, OKT4, OKT8 positive defining total, helper, and suppressor/cytotoxic T cells respectively), mean ± SEM.
[b] Data from studies 1 and 2 combined.
[c] Not significantly different from saline controls at the same time period.

Table 3. Effect of addition of IL-1 or IL-2 or indomethacin to PHA response of PBMCs 4 h following saline or endotoxin infusion

Infusion	Response to PHA (cpm)			
	0	IL-1	IL-2	Indo
Saline	152432[a]	159484	164879	165548
Endotoxin	10383	13613	133923*	27288*

[a] Expressed as mean of triplicate cultures. SEM was always $<10\%$.
* Statistically significantly different from 0 addition, $P<0.01$.

sensitive to the suppressive effects of PGE2 [13], we also sought to restore the response to PHA by the addition of indomethacin to the culture to block de novo activation of the cyclooxygenase pathway. This resulted in a restoration toward normal and in fact doubled the response, but was not as effective as the addition of IL-2 (Table 3).

Effect of Therapy with Ibuprofen In Vivo on Effects of Endotoxin

Pretreatment of volunteers with ibuprofen as described in "Methods" essentially abolished all symptoms and attenuated fever and normal responses [11]. The effect of this therapy on in vitro production of cells obtained 4 h after endotoxin infusion is seen in Table 4. IL-2 production was restored to 70% of the preinfusion response. However, IL-1 production was essentially unchanged. There was

Table 4. Effect or ibuprofen therapy on endotoxin effect on interleukin production

	% of pre-endotoxin infusion level	
	IL-2	IL-1
Saline	10.8	9.1
Endotoxin + ibuprofen	70.2[a]	17.7

[a] Significantly different from endotoxin alone, $P = <0.0001$.

no significant suppression of the PHA response when endotoxin was administered to ibuprofen-treated subjects (not shown).

Discussion

These results suggest that endotoxin alone can induce effects on two major cell types of the immune response, the T-cell and the monocyte, as well as on two important immunoregulatory molecules produced by them, IL-2 and IL-1. Some of these effects depend on activation of the cyclooxygenase pathway as they can be inhibited both in vitro and in vivo by drugs which inhibit that pathway.

The finding that the PHA response of PBMCs from volunteers 4 h after receiving endotoxin can be returned to near normal by addition of IL-2 and partially by indomethacin in vitro and not by IL-1 suggests that the suppression is due not to a lack of IL-1 production, but to a lack of IL-2 production, which may be due to inhibition by a product of the cyclooxygenase pathway such as PGE2. This is further suggested by the fact that there was no change in the percentages of T cells or ratios of helper to suppressor/cytotoxic T cells in the PBMCs following endotoxin infusion.

The effect of endotoxin on IL-1 production was not anticipated as LPS is known to stimulate IL-1 production in vitro, and, in fact, was used in these studies to stimulate production by adherent PBMCs in vitro. No stimulation of IL-1 was found without LPS addition. There are several possible explanations for this that are currently being investigated. The monocytes could have produced a large amount of IL-1 in vivo and were been unable to respond again in vitro. This is unlikely because no evidence of increased IL-1 was found in the serum of individuals at any time post endotoxin infusion (Michie H. et al., submitted for publication). Secondly, the monocytes could have been rendered "tolerant" to the second stimulation with the same LPS. Thirdly, since it has been shown that the mononuclear cells leave the circulation for some time after endotoxin infusion, the cells returning at 4 h may be less mature. We have found that the monocytes in differentials of PBMCs isolated 4 h post endotoxin infusion have the appearance of "activated" cells (ruffled edges and increased spreading) [14] and therefore may be at a stage of maturation where they cannot produce IL-1.

The suppression of IL-1 production following endotoxin was not prevented by ibuprofen. In contrast, IL-2 production 4 h following endotoxin was much greater in subjects pretreated with ibuprofen than in the nonpretreated group (1.1 ± 0.4 and 0.2 ± 0.1 units respectively). These data suggest that products of the cyclooxygenase pathway are responsible for the suppression of IL-2 but not IL-1. Alternatively, such low concentrations of products of the cyclooxygenase pathway may suppress IL-1 production that the dose of ibuprofen used in the present study was insufficient to attenuate this response.

These effects of endotoxin on regulation of the immune response were the result of a single bolus infusion. The effects of continuous infusion or several separate infusions are not known. Humans are the most susceptible of all species to the effects of endotoxin, but they do develop a tolerance to the febrile effects of endotoxin after several injections [15]. However, the WBC response is not subject to this tolerizing effect. Whether this would be the same for immune changes is not known and is a subject for further investigation. The effects we have observed on the immune response caused by endotoxin alone may have significant importance in the immunosuppression observed in burn and trauma patients which leads to morbidity and often mortality in spite of antibiotics and other therapeutic protocols.

Summary

We have studied the effects of a small bolus intravenous infusion of endotoxin in normal male volunteers admitted to our Clinical Research Center. The first group of seven were studied before and 4 h and 24 h after infusion of normal saline or saline plus 4 ng/kg endotoxin. Peripheral blood mononuclear cells (PBMCs) obtained at these times showed marked decreases in response to T-cell mitogens and production of interleukin 2 (IL-2), and adherent PBMCs (A) exhibited markedly decreased production of interleukin 1 (IL-1) 4 h postinfusion, returning to normal or supranormal values at 24 h post endotoxin infusion, when compared with saline infusions in the volunteers or with normal laboratory controls studied at the same time. A second study of six volunteers showed that the decrease in IL-1 production occurred as early as 1 h post endotoxin infusion, but the decrease in IL-2 production was more variable (three out of six decreased at 1 h, six out of six at 4 h). In vitro addition of ibuprofen to PBMC cultures responding to T-cell mitogens reduced the suppression observed after in vivo endotoxin, and in vivo administration of ibuprofen prior to endotoxin infusion caused a significant decrease in the suppression of IL-2 production, but had no effect on the suppression of IL-1 production by A cells, 4 h post endotoxin infusion. These results indicate that the immunosuppressive effects of in vivo endotoxin on in vitro immune responses of T cells and adherent cells do not occur through a common pathway.

Acknowledgments. The authors are very grateful for the excellent technical assistance of Ms. Inna Saporochetz, Ms. Kathryn Collins, and Ms. Andrea Jordan and for the excellent assistance of Ms. Ann Braswell in the preparation of this manuscript. We are also indebted to the nursing staff of the Clinical Research Center of Brigham & Women's Hospital.

References

1. Miller CL, Claudy BJ (1979) Suppressor T-cell activity induced as a result of thermal injury. Cell Immunol 44:201–208
2. Antonacci AC, Calvano SE, Reaves LE, Prajapati A, Bockman R, Welte K, Mertelsmann R, Gupta S, Good RA, Shires GT (1984) Autologous and allogeneic mixed-lymphocyte responses following thermal injury in man: the immunomodulatory effects of interleukin 1, interleukin 2, and a prostaglandin inhibitor WY-18251. Clin Immunol Immunopathol 30:304–320
3. Wood JJ, Rodrick ML, O'Mahony JB, Mannick JA (1984) Inadequate interleukin 2 production: a fundamental immunological deficiency in patients with major burns. Ann Surg 200:311–320
4. Rodrick ML, Wood JJ, O'Mahony JB, Davis CF, Grbic JT, Demling RH, Moss NA, Saporoschetz I, Jordan A, D'Eon P (1986) Mechanisms of immunosuppression associated with severe nonthermal traumatic injuries in man: production of interleukin 1 and 2. J Clin Immunol 6:310–318
5. Winchurch RA, Munster AM (1983) The involvement of bacterial lipopolysaccharides in trauma-induced immune depression. In: Ninneman JL (ed) Traumatic injury, infection and other immunologic sequelae. University Park Press, Baltimore, pp 103–117
6. Maejima K, Deitch EA, Berg R (1984) Promotion by burn stress of the translocation of bacteria from the gastrointestinal tracts of mice. Arch Surg 119:166–172
7. Zeigler TR, O'Dwyer ST, Demling RH, Smith RJ, Wilmore DW Increased intestinal permeability associated with infection in burn patients. Arch Surg (in press)
8. O'Dwyer ST, Michie HR, Zeigler TR,Revhaug A, Smith RJ, Wilmore DW A single dose of endotoxin increases intestinal permeability in healthy humans. Arch Surg (in press)
9. Morrison DC, Ryan JL (1979) Bacterial endotoxins and host immune responses. Adv Immunol 28:293–350
10. Hochstein JD, Mills DF, Outschoorn AS, Rastogi SC (1983) The processing and collaborative assay of a reference endotoxin. J Biol Stand 11:251–260
11. Revhaug A, Michie HR, McK Manson I, Watters JM, Dinarello CA, Wolff SM, Wilmore DW (1988) Inhibition of cyclo-oxygenase attenuates the metabolic response to endotoxin in humans. Arch Surg 123:162–170
12. Lisi PJ, Chu C-W, Koch GA, Endres S, Lonnemann G, Dinarello CA (1987) Development and use of a radioimmunoassay for human interleukin-1B. Lymphokine Res 6:229–244
13. Grbic JT, Rodrick ML, Gough DB, Moss NM, Revhaug A, Michie HR, O'Dwyer ST, Wilmore DW, Mannick JA (1987) Endotoxin causes increased sensitivity of lymphocytes to inhibitory effects of prostaglandin E2. Surg Forum 38:91–93
14. Morland B, Kaplan G (1977) Macrophage activation in vivo and in vitro. Exp Cell Res 108:279–288
15. Greisman SE, Hornick RB (1973) Mechanisms of endotoxin tolerance with special reference to man. In: Wolff SM, Kass EH (eds) Bacterial lipopolysaccharides. University of Chicago Press, Chicago, pp 257–268

Treatment of Burn Patients with Polymyxin B: Effects on Lymphokine Regulation *

R. A. Winchurch, G-X. Xiao, A. M. Munster, W. H. Adler, C. White, and B. Bender

Endotoxins are among the most potent agents known to affect mammalian metabolism. The body's responses to bacterial endotoxins were recognized as early as the 1920s by such notables as Sanarelli [1], Shwartzman [2], and Hanger [3]. In 1924 Sanarelli observed that animals injected with a small, sublethal dose of *Vibrio cholerae* died when subsequently exposed to a nonlethal dose of colon bacilli. Soon afterward Shwartzman described this phenomenon in detail and characterized the reaction which still bears his name; namely, the ability of substances produced by gram-negative bacteria to induce a temporary, nonspecific sensitivity which results in local or systemic hemorrhagic necrosis upon subsequent challenge. In the 60 odd years since these early reports much has been written about the biological effects of endotoxins. Within this compendium the greatest bulk of the literature concerns the effects of endotoxins on host resistance. This devotion to the study of endotoxins is not at all surprising since all mammalian species carry a large and potentially fatal burden of endotoxins derived from the gram-negative flora of the gut. In the normal, young adult animal this burden does not appear to affect the host adversely provided that the mechanisms for containment and detoxification are intact. When the ability to contain endotoxins is compromised, as might occur in the aged [4], or when detoxification fails as in the case of liver malfunction [5], the systemic exposure to endotoxins can produce dramatic changes in the host defense posture.

Traumatic Injury and Endotoxins

The notion that endotoxins were involved in the pathogenesis following burns and trauma was first advanced by Fine and his colleagues 16 years ago [6, 7]. Using a crude limulus assay, Fine observed increases in circulating limulus-activating substances after injury. These increases were not always associated with gram-negative sepsis and the origin of the putative endotoxin remained obscure. Fine proposed that the gut was the source of the endotoxin but was unable to demonstrate conclusively that these endotoxins were of endogenous origin. The fact that endotoxin increases were not clearly associated with infectious sequelae led many investigators to discount Fine's observations and to conclude that the limulus test was of limited diagnostic usefulness [8, 9].

---

* Supported in part by NIH grant GM 26235 and funding from Whittaker, M.A. Bioproducts, Inc.

Immune Consequences of
Trauma, Shock and Sepsis
Eds. Faist/Ninnemann/Green

Our laboratories attempted to reproduce Fine's experiments in 1980. These studies were prompted by the observation that many of the immunological consequences of thermal injury resembled the immune depression generated in response to purposeful endotoxin exposure. Our studies centered around three basic questions: (1) Are there significant increases in endotoxins in the burn patient? (2) If so can these increases be reduced to "normal" levels? (3) What, if any, are the immunological consequences of endotoxin therapy? We reasoned that if the immunological consequences of burn injury were related to endotoxin exposure then the treatment of endotoxemia should prevent or minimize the burn-induced immunodepression. Successful implementation of such therapy favoring the restoration of the host's immunological defenses would open an important avenue in the management of infection in the burn patient. More importantly, success in these endeavors would constitute a significant step in understanding the immunopathology of burn injury.

In our initial studies we encountered the same problems of plasma inhibitors and the lack of quantitation that had plagued the earlier investigators. The development of a commercial, quantitative assay in the early 1980s [10] enabled us to measure accurately the levels of endotoxin in plasma samples and to compensate for the presence of inhibitors. Using this assay we initiated a long-term study of endotoxemia in populations of burn patients. Our results showed that there were indeed increases in circulating endotoxins in burn patients [11]. These increases were correlated with the extent of injury, as shown in Fig. 1, and generally increased to maximum levels at about 3–5 days after injury (Fig. 2). On the strength of these observations we concluded that Fine's hypothesis was correct and that burn injury was associated with increased endotoxin exposure.

Armed with definitive data showing the association of burn injury with increased endotoxin levels we addressed the question of whether the endotoxin levels in burn patients could be reduced to "normal" levels. Our initial experiments were conducted in laboratory mice using the antibiotic polymyxin B. Polymixin B had been shown to neutralize the toxic and immunologic effects of endotoxin by combining stoichiometrically with the lipid A portion of all endotoxins [12, 13]. Initially, we tested polymyxin B in mice subjected to burn injury and

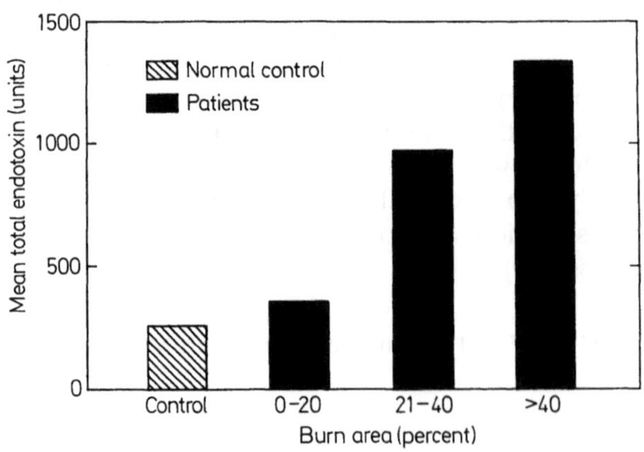

Fig. 1. Mean total endotoxin levels for all patients according to the extent of burn area. The relationship between burn area and the endotoxin levels is significant at $P = < 0.01$

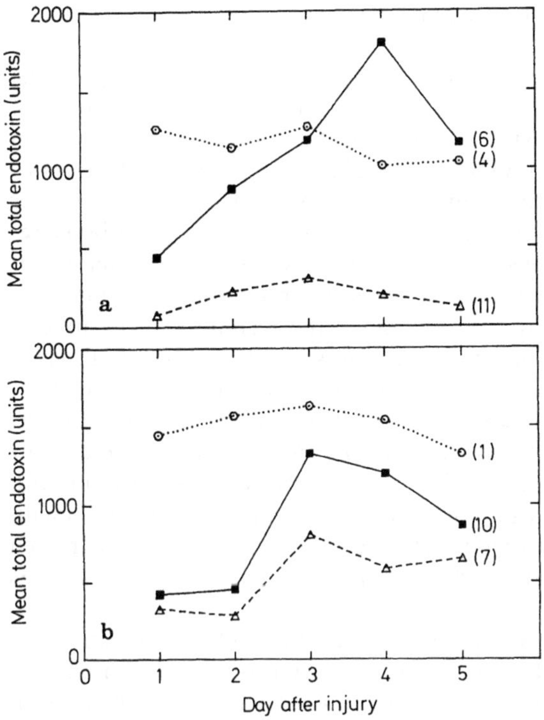

Fig. 2 a, b. Sequential measurement of endotoxin levels in burn patients. Each point represents the mean total endotoxin level for each group per day of assay. The number of patients per group are shown in parentheses. **a** All patients less than 40 years old; **b** all patients over 40 years old; △—△, burn area <20%, ■—■, burn area between 21% and 40%; ○—○, burn area over 40%

Table 1. Protocol for polymyxin B administration

Day	Dosage (U/kg/day)
1	3000
2	4000
3	5500
4	5500
5	4000
6	3000

Administered i.v. in two divided daily doses.

found that the drug did indeed restore antibody production [14]. This restoration occurred despite the fact that the drug was immunosuppressive in normal animals. The immunorestorative effects in the thermally injured mouse were proportional to the extent of burn-induced immunodepression. This suggested that polymyxin B neutralized immunosuppressive factor(s) released in response to injury, i.e., endotoxins [15]. The potential immunosuppression associated with the drug indicated that the dosage of the drug should not be excessive and that the levels of drug administered therapeutically should reflect the expected increases in endotoxin. A protocol of therapy was established for use in man based on the general profile of endotoxin increase observed over the first several days after injury (Table 1).

Effects of Endotoxin Therapy in Burn Patients

Polymyxin B was effective in reducing the endotoxin burden in burn patients. Typical results are illustrated in Fig. 3. However, the most important question remained to be answered. If endotoxins were responsible for immune dysfunction in the burn patient then polymyxin B therapy should concomitantly reduce endotoxin levels and improve the immunological posture of the burn patient. In our pilot experiments in mice we showed that polymyxin B restored antibody responses. In the patient studies we elected to study parameters of cell-mediated immunity since CMI is the most consistently depressed parameter of immunity following thermal injury in man. First we examined the responses of peripheral blood lymphocytes from control and treated patients to selected bacterial, viral, and fungal antigens [16]. In each patient the responses soon after injury were compared with the responses after a 2-week interval of therapy. The presumption was that if the therapy was effective the patients in the treated group would show greater improvement than the controls. The data showed that responses in both populations were depressed early after injury. Treatment with polymyxin B facilitated the improvement in responses such that the cells of patients from the treated group responded significantly better when compared with untreated controls (Table 2).

In a separate study we also examined the natural killer (NK) cell activity in patients treated with polymyxin B [17]. Thermal injury produces a dramatic inhibition of NK activity [18]. Burn injury impairs NK activity very early after injury. Our data also showed that this activity declined further over a 2-week period of observation. Stein et al. reported that burn patients' NK cells were unrespon-

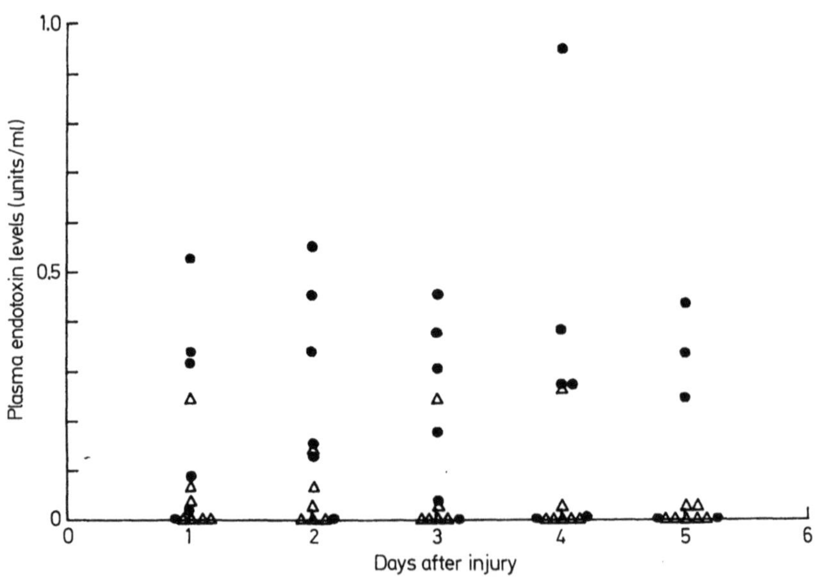

Fig. 3. Sequential measurement of endotoxin concentration (units/ml) in blood plasma from (●) control ($n=6$) and (○) polymyxin B treated patients ($n=7$)

Table 2. Net change in burn patients' in vitro responses to recall antigens 2 weeks post-admission

Antigen	Control patients mean cpm/culture (SEM)	Polymyxin B patients mean cpm/culture (SEM)
SKSD	+ 112 (527)	+ 2568 (287)
PPD	− 510 (1064)	+ 780 (589)
Mumps	+ 456 (684)	+ 3573 (1364)
Candida	+ 7 (3851)	+11490 (4309)
Mixed lymphocyte cultures	+2921 (1581)	2658 (1279)

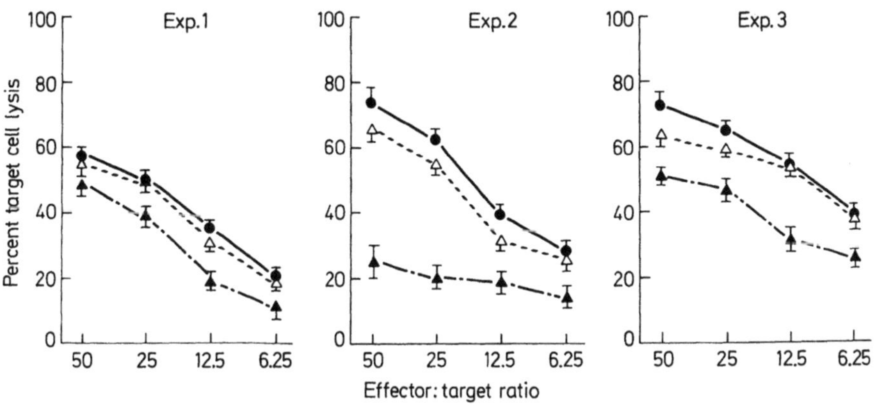

Fig. 4. Effects of burn sera on normal NK activity. Experiments a, b, and c. Sera from burn patients were tested for effects on NK activity before (▲) and after (△) passage over polymyxin B-Sepharose 4B affinity columns. NK activity in the presence of normal serum (●).

sive to lymphokine interferon [19]. Our data showed a similar unresponsiveness to Il-2 [17]. Treatment of patients with polymyxin B had no apparent effect on initial depression of NK activity and did not restore Il-2 responsiveness in these cells. However, polymyxin B did prevent a further decline in NK activity.

The depression of NK activity in the burn patient appeared to be associated with circulating serum factor(s) (Fig. 4). If normal cells were treated with burn serum their NK activity was also depressed. The passage of burn serum over affinity columns of Sepharose-coupled polymyxin B removed the NK-inhibiting factors, suggesting the endotoxins were either directly or indirectly responsible for producing the inhibition of NK activity.

Mechanisms Underlying Immunodepression in the Burn Patient

The cumulative evidence gathered thus far indicates that bacterial endotoxins are responsible for at least some of the immune abnormalities in the burn victim. The precise mechanism(s) by which endotoxin elicits its effects are unknown. Endo-

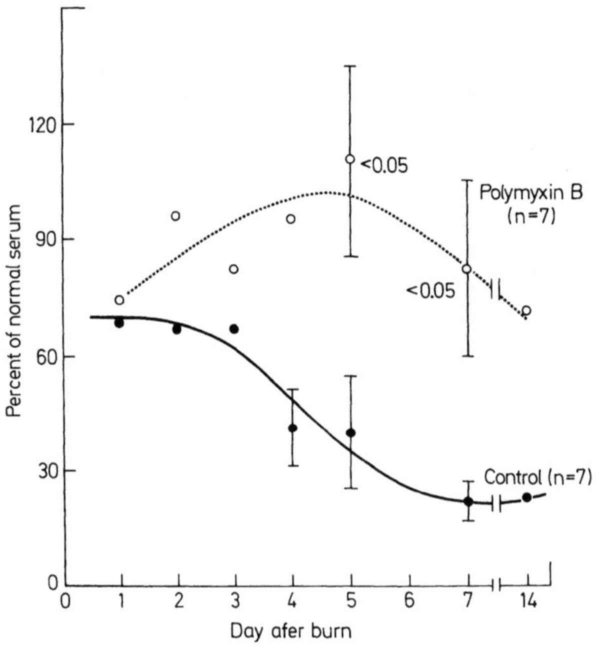

Fig. 5. The effects of burn sera on Il-2-dependent proliferative responses. Serum from either control (●——●) or polymyxin B treated patients (○---○) were added to CTLL-2 cells to a final concentration of 1.25%. Fifty units/ml Il-2 was added and the proliferation determined after 24 h. Results are expressed as the percentage of proliferation in the presence of pooled normal serum

toxin may affect the cells of the immune system directly, but it is more likely that endotoxins induce the production of other factors which, in turn, downregulate various components of the immune system. Ample evidence has been presented showing the inhibitory activity of peptides and proteins such as SAP [20, 21]. Prostaglandins and leukotrienes have also been implicated in burn-induced immunodepression [22] and these factors are known to be generated in response to endotoxins.

The failure of T-cell functions and, in particular, the crippling of T-helper cells is a prominent observation among the perturbations of immune homeostasis that accompany acute thermal injury. As yet, the reasons for the depression of helper T-cell activity are not fully understood. However, recent observations highlight a basic defect in the repertoire of T-cell activities. This is the depression in the production of lymphokines essential for T-cell function and the inability of T cells from burn patients to respond to lymphokines. Theodorczyk-Injeyan and her colleagues as well as Wood et al. have demonstrated the depressed production of Il-2 in the burn patient and have shown that the addition of exogenous Il-2 to burn patients' cells produces only minimal effects [23–25].

Thus aberrant lymphokine regulation appears to be the central defect in the immune profile of the burn patient. Theoretically, it might be possible to compensate for this defect by administering the essential lymphokines therapeutically. However, it is unlikely that the cells will respond to supplemental lymphokines. There are two reasons why burn cells do not respond to lymphokines. First, as mentioned above, burn serum contains factor(s) which impair immune responsiveness. Apparently, this impairment is due, at least in part, to the ability of burn sera to inhibit the responses of T cells to lymphokines. This impairment was ob-

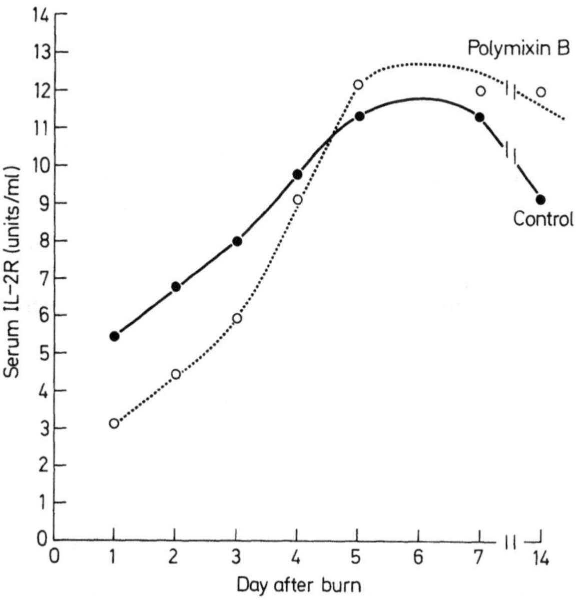

Fig. 6. Il-2R levels in burn serum. Serum taken sequentially from either control (●—●) or polymyxin B treated patients (○---○) was analyzed for soluble cell-free Il-2R as described in "Methods." Results are expressed as units/ml

served by Roderick et al. [26] and has been studied in our laboratories. Our data showed that concentrations of burn serum as low as 1.25% inhibit the responses of Il-2-dependent T cells (Fig. 5). This inhibition was the result of exposure to endotoxin because treatment of patients with polymyxin B abrogated the ability of serum to inhibit Il-2 responses. However, the factors in serum were not endotoxins since heating of burn serum to 56 °C abolished the Il-2-inhibiting properties. Thus, the failure of T cells to respond to lymphokines is at least partially due to inhibitory factors generated in response to endotoxin exposure. Inhibitors may contribute to the blockade of Il-2 responses in burn T cells, but current evidence suggests that there is an inherent defect in the cells themselves. Analyses of burn sera reveal that these sera contain abnormally high levels of soluble, cell-free Il-2 receptors (IL-2R) (Fig. 6). Early after injury the levels of Il-2R in burn sera are near normal but increase dramatically over a period of days so that by 6–7 days after injury these levels are four- to fivefold over normal. The Il-2R in burn sera do not bind additional Il-2 and the inhibitory properties of burn sera on Il-2 responses are not due to competitive inhibition by these receptors. It is of some interest that increased shedding of soluble Il-2R is a characteristic of other immunodepressed conditions including organ transplant patients and AIDS victims. The treatment of burn patients with polymyxin B does not appear to affect the generation of soluble IL-2R. These increases may not be related to endotoxin exposure.

Summary

Many of the immune aberrations in the burn victim are related to increased exposure to endotoxins and, as such, are amenable to modes of therapy such as polymyxin B. Parmount among these immune abnormalities is the inability to respond to lymphokines. This lack of responsivenes is due, in part, to a blockage of lymphokine responses, chiefly Il-2 responses, by serum factors generated in response to endotoxin exposure. However, burn patients' cells are deficient in surface Il-2R and show increased shedding of Il-2R in the serum. These increases may not be the result of endotoxin exposure and may not be amenable to conventional modes of therapy.

References

1. Sanarelli G (1924) Experimental cholera. Ann de L'Inst Pasteur 38:11
2. Shwartzman G (1928) Studies on *Bacillus typhosa* toxic substances. J Exp Med 48:247
3. Hanger FM (1956) In: Boyd WC (ed) Fundamentals of immunology. Interscience, New York, p 457
4. Winchurch RA, Birmingham W, Hilberg C, Munster A (1982) Effects of endotoxin on immunity in aging mice. Cell Immunol 67:384
5. Trejo RA, Di Luzio NR (1971) Impaired detoxification as a mechanism of lead acetate-induced hypersensitivity to endotoxin. Proc Soc Exp Biol Med 136:889
6. Cardis DT, Reinhold RB, Woodruff PWH, Fine J (1972) Endotoxaemia in man. Lancet I:1381
7. Cuevas P, Shiyama M, Koizumi S, Woodruff R, Kaufman A, Fine J (1974) Role of endotoxaemia of intestinal origin in early death form large burns. Surg Gynecol Obstet 138:725
8. Stumacher RJ, Kovnat MJ, McCabe WR (1973) Limitations of the usefulness of the limulus assay for endotoxin. N Engl J Med 288:1261
9. Elin RJ, Robinson RA, Levine AS, Wolff SM (1975) Lack of clinical usefulness of the limulus test in the diagnosis of endotoxemia. N Engl J Med 293:521
10. Thomas LLM, Sturk A, Kahle LH, ten Cate JW (1981) Quantitative endotoxin determination in blood with a chromogenic substrate. Clin Chim Acta 116:63
11. Winchurch RA, Thupari JN, Munster AM (1987) Endotoxin in burn patients: levels of circulating endotoxins are related to burn size. Surgery 102:808
12. Butler T, Smith E, Hammarstrom L, Moller G (1977) Polymyxins as inhibitors of polyclonal B cell activators in murine lymphocyte cultures. Infect Immun 16:449
13. Jacobs DM, Morrison DC (1977) Inhibition of the mitogenic response to lipopolysaccharide (LPS) in mouse spleen cells by polymyxin B. J Immunol 118:21
14. Chiccone TG, Munster AM, Birmingham W, Winchurch RA (1983) Successful immunomodulation in burned animals and human beings with homeopathic doses of polymyxin B. J Burn Care Rehabil 4:153
15. Winchurch RA, Munster AM (1983) The involvement of bacterial lipopolysaccharides in trauma-induced immune depression. In: Ninnemann J (ed) Traumatic injury: infection and other immunologic sequelae. University Park, Baltimore, p 103
16. Munster AM, Winchurch RA, Thupari JN, Ernst CB (1986) Reversal of postburn immunosuppression with low-dose polymyxin B. J Trauma 26:995
17. Bender BS, Winchurch RA, Thupari JN, Proust JJ, Adler WH, Munster AM (1988) Depressed natural killer cell function in thermally injured adults: successful in vivo and in vitro immunomodulation and the role of endotoxin. Clin Exp Immunol 71:120
18. Antonacci AC, Gupta S, Good RA, Shires GT, Fernandes G (1983) Natural killer and antibody-dependent cytotoxicity following thermal injury in humans. Curr Surg 40:20

19. Stein MD, Gamble DN, Klimpel KD, Herndon DH, Klimpel GR (1984) Natural killer cell defects resulting from thermal injury. Cell Immunol 86:551
20. Wolfe JHN, Saporoschetz AB, Young AE, O'Connor NE, Mannick JA (1981) Suppressive serum, suppressor lymphocytes and deaths from burns. Ann Surg 193:513
21. Ozkan AN, Ninnemann JL (1985) Suppression of in vitro lymphocyte and neutrophil responses by a low molecular weight suppressor active peptide from burn-patient sera. J Clin Immunol 5:172
22. Ninnemann JL, Stockland AE (1984) Participation of prostaglandin E in immunosuppression following thermal injury. J Trauma 24:201
23. Teodorczyk-Injeyan JA, Sparkes BG, Mills GB, Falk RE, Peters WJ (1987) Impaired expression of interleukin-2 receptor (Il-2R) in the immunosuppressed burn patient: reversal by exogeneous Il-2. J Trauma 27:180
24. Teodorczyk-Injeyan JA, Sparkes BG, Mills GB, Peters WJ, Falk RE (1986) Impairment of T cell activation in burn patients: a possible mechanism of thermal injury-induced immunosuppression. Clin Exp Immunol 65:570
25. Roderick ML, Wood JJ, O'Mahony JB, Davis CF, Grbic JT, Demling RH, Mouse MM, Saporoschetz I, Jordan A, D'Eon P, Mannick JA (1986) Mechanisms of immunosuppression associated with severe nonthermal traumatic injuries in man: production of interleukin 1 and 2. J Clin Immunol 6:310
26. Roderick ML, Saporoschetz I, Wood J, Davis CF, Mannick JA (1986) Serum suppression of interleukin 2 (Il-2) production and IL-2 action in thermal injury. Surg Forum 36:98

Mechanisms of Neutralization of Endotoxin by Monoclonal IgG Antibodies to Lipopolysaccharide

T. Sagawa, Y. Abe, S. Kimura, Y. Hitsumoto, and S. Utsumi

Introduction

Endotoxemia is a serious and cumbersome illness, especially for immunocompromised patients who are susceptible to drug-resistant enteric bacteria. In an attempt to explore immunoprophylactic measures applicable to humans, protective efficacies of antibodies to lipopolysaccharide (LPS) have been extensively studied. Thus antibodies to heterologous R core (Braude et al. 1977; Davis et al. 1978; Marks et al. 1982; Ziegler et al.1982) as well as those to homologous O polysaccharides (Freedman 1959; Dunn et al. 1985) are now believed to be able, at least to some extent, to prevent animals and humans from developing endotoxemia. However, it is not yet clear how antibodies to O and R resions located at different spacings from lipid A can equally neutralize the toxic activities of LPS, whereas antibodies to the toxic lipid A moiety itself often fail to do so. In this study, we have prepared mouse monoclonal antibodies (mAbs) of the IgG class to these three regions of LPS and compared their effects on the toxic activities of LPS in vivo and in vitro to look into the mechanism for neutralization by these antibodies.

Materials and Methods

Monoclonal Antibodies

Lipopolysaccharides from *S. minnesota* and O-defective *E. coli* J5 and a synthetic lipid A of *E. coli* type (Dai-ichi Chemical Corp.) coupled to Keyhole Limpet hemocyanin (Galanos et al. 1971) were used as immunogens. Balb/c mice were primed with each immunogen in Freund's complete adjuvant and boosted weekly with soluble immunogen until serum IgG antibody appeared. Hybridomas were prepared by the polyethylene glycol method (Oi and Herzenberg 1980) with Sp2/O-Ag14 cells as fusion partner, and cell lines producing antibodies specific for O saccharide of *S. minnesota* (IgG3 type), R core of J5 (IgG1), and lipid A (IgG3), respectively, were established. Monoclonal antibodies were purified from culture or peritoneal fluids by using protein A-Cellulofine columns (Seikagaku Kogyo LTD).

Immune Consequences of
Trauma, Shock and Sepsis
Eds. Faist/Ninnemann/Green

Effects of mAbs on LPS Activities

Lipopolysaccharide from *S. minnesota* (Boivin fraction) was used throughout this study, since this, after being treated at pH 9.6, could bind nearly equal amounts of anti-O, anti-R, and anti-lipid A mAbs in ELISA. For the protectivity to endotoxin shock, C57Bl/6 mice (5–7 weeks old) given a prophylactic dose of each mAb (100 μg, i.v.) or saline were challenged 2 h later with D-galactosamine (2.6 mmol/kg, i.p.) and LPS (10 ng, i.v.) and mortality within 24 h was scored. For the antipyrogenic effect, rabbits were given mAbs (500 μg, i.v.) 2 h prior to LPS (0.8 μg/kg, i.v.) and rectal temperature was followed at intervals. Unimmunized rabbits gave a biphasic fever response with peaks at 60 and 180 min, respectively. Tumor necrosis factor (TNF) production by bacille Calmette-Guérin (BCG)-activated macrophages (10^6/ml) in response to various concentrations of LPS (1 ng–10 μg/ml)in the presence or absence of mAbs (10 μg/ml) was assayed at intervals by the lytic activity to actinomycin D-treated L929 cells using the crystal violet method (Aggarwell 1985). Effects of mAbs on LPS-induced IL-1 and PGE_2 productions were examined in a similar manner, but resident unactivated peritoneal macrophages were used. IL-1 was assayed by the thymocyte proliferation method (Mizel et al. 1978) and PGE_2 by RIA (NEN Research Products).

Analysis of Immune Complexes

The size distribution of LPS antibody complexes was analyzed with ^{125}I-labeled mAbs by sedimentation in 9%–41% sucrose density gradient at 30000 rpm for 16 h.

Results

Prophylactic administration of homologous anti-O and heterologous anti-R mAbs reduced mortality of endotoxin shock in galactosamine-sensitized mice by 20 LD_{50} of LPS to 27.3% and 37.5%, respectively, and abrogated the second fever onset in rabbits completely (data not shown), consistent with previous reports (Freedman 1959; Radvany 1966). The anti-lipid A mAb used in this study was practically ineffective in both systems.

Parallel to the protective potentials of these antibodies were their effects on the TNF-inducing activity of LPS in vitro. Thus 10 μg anti-O and anti-R mAbs reduced the activity of 10 μg LPS to 1% or less, whereas the same amount of antilipid A could not neutralize 1 μg or higher amounts of LPS (Fig. 1). On the contrary, both anti-O and anti-R mAbs enhanced the IL-1 production in 2 h culture at least twofold (data not shown). The IL-1 production in vivo too was enhanced by the two mAbs.

The effects of these mAbs on PGE_2 production were quite singular. Although the range of LPS doses tested (1 ng–10 μg/ml) induced barely detectable PGE_2 production in the macrophage culture within ½ h, the anti-R mAb greatly enhanced the early PGE_2 production (Fig. 2a). However, when amounts of PGE_2

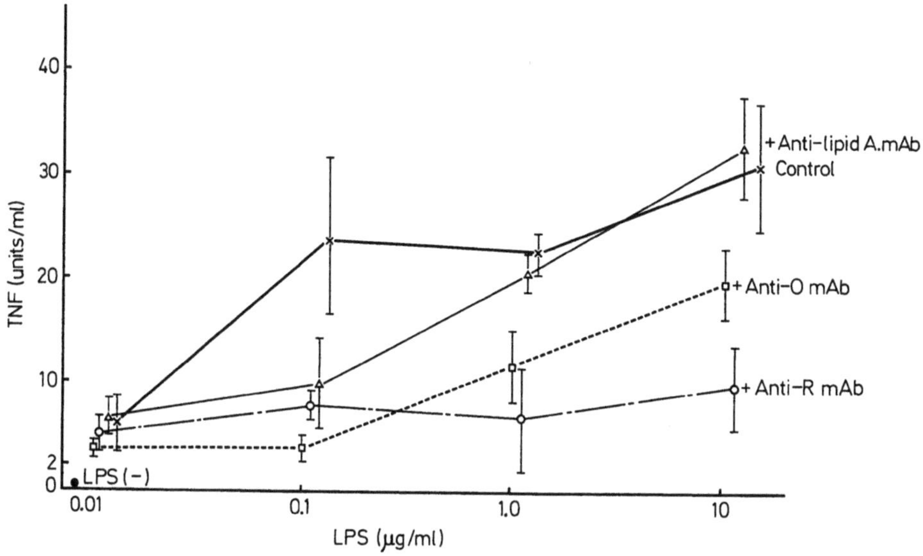

Fig. 1. Effects of anti-LPS mAbs on LPS-induced TNF production by BCG-activated macrophages. Data represent amounts (units) of TNF produced during 2-h-culture in the presence of LPS with or without mAbs ($n = 4$). *Vertical bars* indicate standard deviation

in 2-h cultures were compared, suppression by the anti-O mAb was evident (Fig. 2b). Again the effect of anti-lipid A was obscure.

Each of these monoclonal antibodies to different regions of LPS showed characteristic behavior in their complex formation with LPS. Figure 3 shows sedimentation patterns of these mAbs with or without LPS. The bulk of anti-O mAb was associated with complexes larger than 19S, except for unbound antibody in the 7S region (Fig. 3a). Anti-R mAb formed only small and homogeneous complexes of approximately 9S (Fig. 3b). This can hardly be ascribed to small complexes due to excess antigen as usually seen with protein antigens, since the *S. minnesota* LPS, like other LPSs, formed large micelles of 20–40S in the physiological solvents. Although self-aggregation of the IgG3 anti-lipid A mAb obscured the sedimentation pattern of its complexes, it was still obvious that only a small portion of this antibody was associated with LPS, and the complexes formed were on average smaller than those with anti-O but definitely larger than complexes with anti-R (Fig. 3c).

Discussion

We tentatively interpret the results obtained according to a hypothetical model as illustrated in Fig. 4. In solution, LPS is presumed to be in a transition between the micellic and smaller oligomeric forms and the equilibrium may well be biased to the former under physiological conditions. We postulate that the TNF- and PGE_2-inducing activities of LPS are largely ascribed to the micellic and oligo-

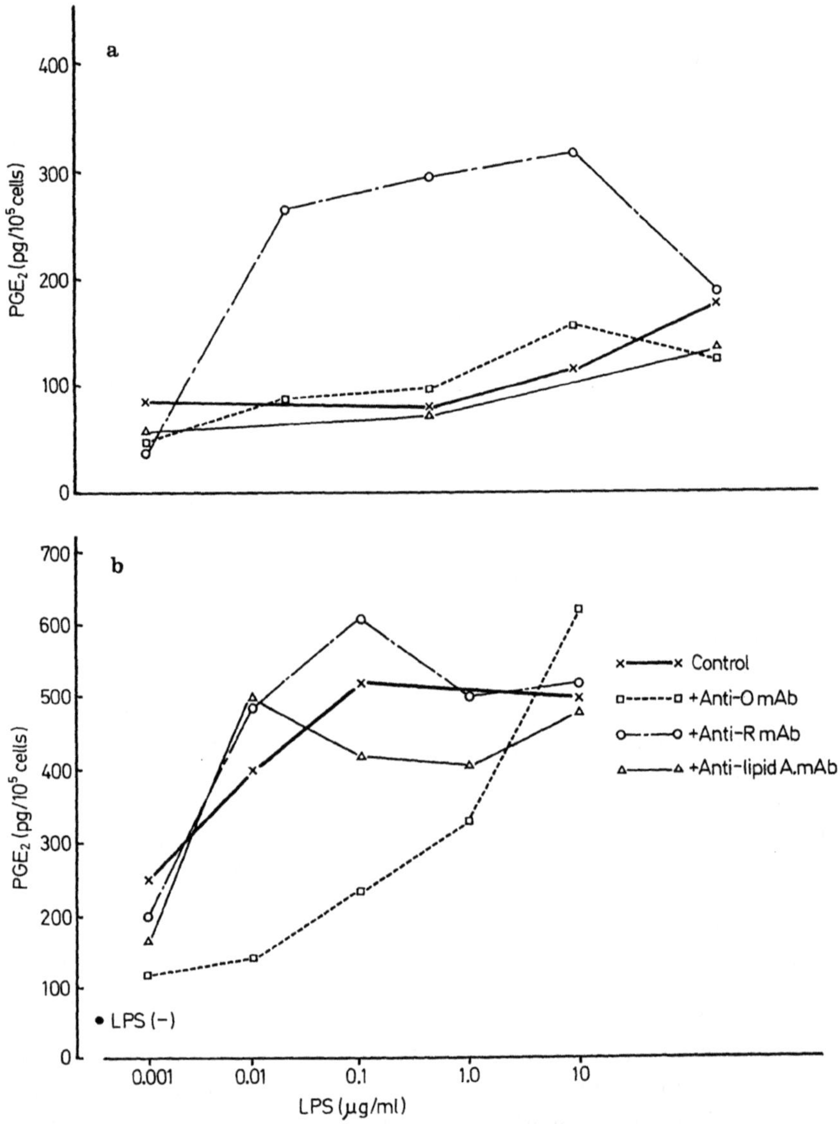

Fig. 2 a, b. Effects of anti-LPS mAbs on the LPS induced PGE_2 production by peritoneal resident macrophages. Data represent PGE_2 activities **a** in 0.5-h culture and **b** in 2-h culture in the presence of various amounts of LPS with or without anti-LPS mAbs

meric forms, respectively. Though antibodies to O and R moieties of LPS suppress the TNF-inducing activity of LPS equally well, they probably do so through entirely different mechanisms. The binding of anti-O antibody molecules to the outermost surface of LPS micelles will not disrupt the micellic structure but will either block the LPS activity or facilitate the Fc receptor-mediated ingestion of the micelles by phagocytes. On the other hand, antibody binding to the region

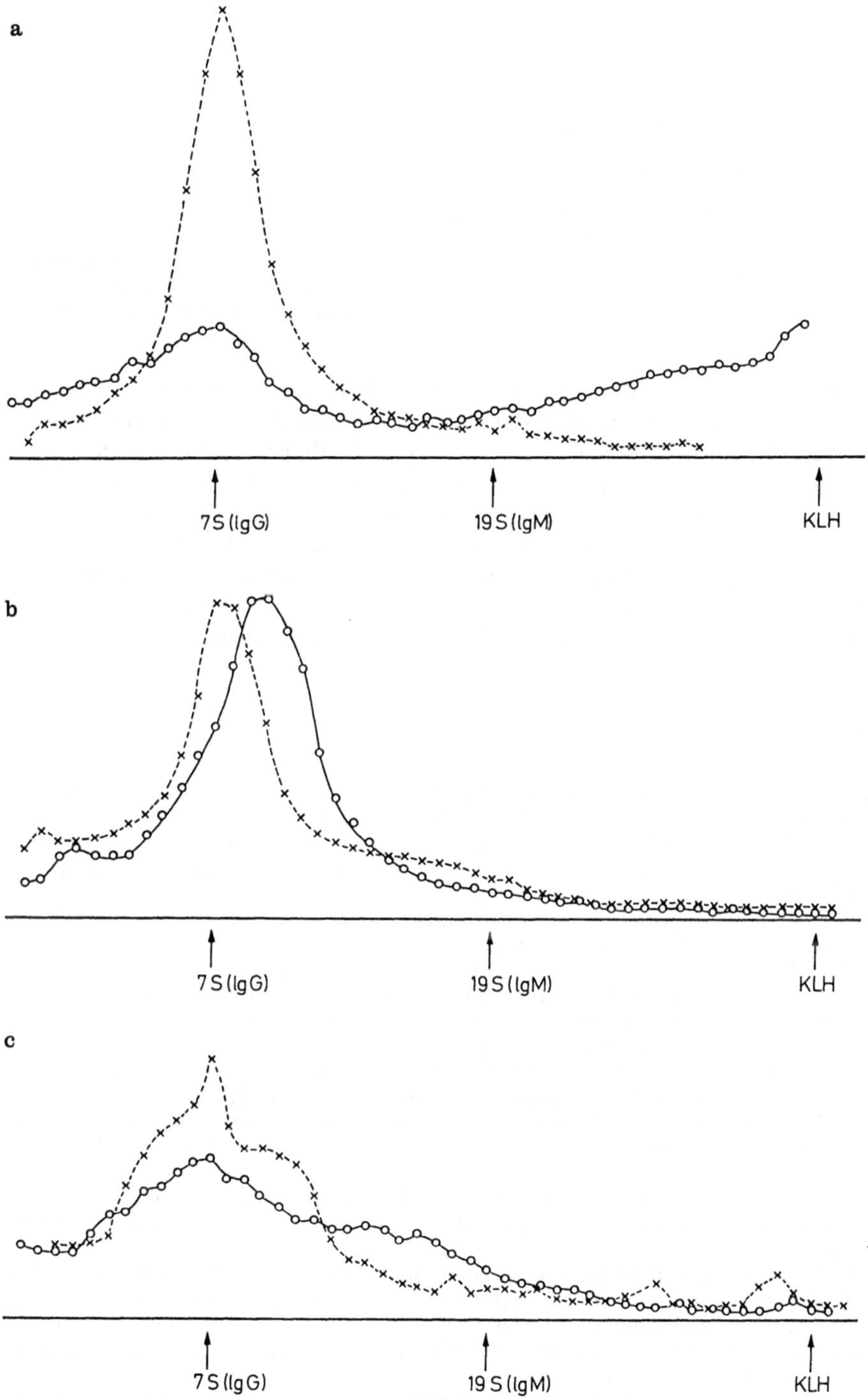

Fig. 3. Sucrose density gradient sedimentation patterns of ^{125}I-labeled **a** anti-O mAb, **b** anti-R mAb, and **c** anti-lipid A mAb with (o---o) or without (X---X) LPS

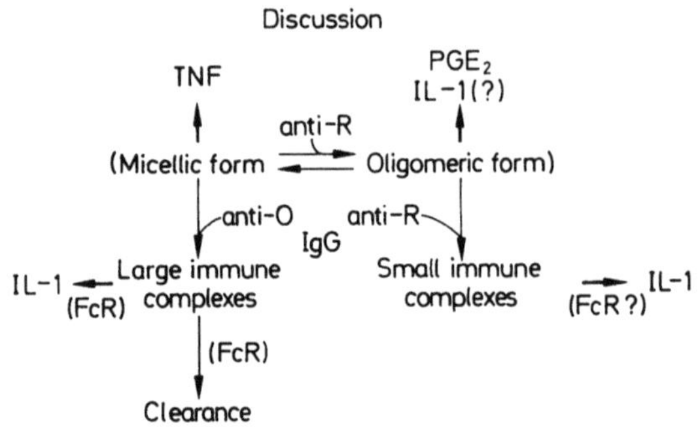

Fig. 4. A hypothetical model of the mechanism for endotoxin neutralization by anti-LPS antibodies

more proximate to the lipid A moiety would interfere with the hydrophobic association between LPS molecules and hence disrupt the micellic structure, resulting in reduction in the TNF-inducing activity and enhancement of the PGE_2-inducing activity of LPS. Antibody would hardly be accessible to the core region of a compact micelle. Whether such hypothetical modes of LPS-antibody interactions are applicable to all classes or subclasses of immunoglobulin is not clear. However, it may be worthwhile mentioning that monoclonal anti-TNF antibodies of all IgG subclasses were found to be protective to endotoxin shock due to TNF-LPS with efficacies indistinguishable from each other.

References

Aggarwell BB, Kohr WJ, Harkins RN (1985) Human tumor necrosis factor. Production, purification and characterization. J Biol Chem 260:2345–2354

Braude AI, Douglas H, Ziegler EJ (1977) Antibody to cell wall glycolipid of gram-negative bacteria: induction of immunity to bacteremia and endotoxemia. J Infect Dis S136:S167–173

Davis CE, Ziegler EJ, Arnold KF (1978) Neutralization of meningococcal endotoxin by antibody to core glycolipid. J Exp Med 147:57–67

Dunn DL, Bogard WC, Cerra FB (1985) Enhanced survival during murine gram-negative bacterial sepsis by use of a murine monoclonal antibody. Arch Surg 120:50–53

Freedman HH (1959) Passive transfer of protection against lethality of homologous and heterologous endotoxins. Proc Soc Exp Biol Med 102:504–506

Galanos C, Lüderitz O, Westphal O (1971) Preparation and properties of antisera against the lipid A component of bacterial lipopolysaccharides. Eur J Biochem 24:110–122

Marks MI, Ziegler EJ, Braude AI (1982) Induction of immunity against lethal *Haemophilus influenzae* type b infection by *Escherichia coli* core lipopolysaccharide. J Clin Invest 69:742–749

Mizel SB, Oppenheim JJ, Rosenstreich DL (1978) Characterization of lymphocyte activating factor (LAF) produced by a macrophage cell line. P388D1. J Immunol 120:1497–1503

Oi VT, Herzenberg LA (1980) Immunoglobulin-producing hybrid cell lines. In: Mishell BB (ed) Selected methods in cellular immunology. Freeman, San Francisco, pp 351–372

Radvany R, Neale NL, Novotny A (1966) Relation of structure to function in bacterial O-antigens. VI. Neutralization of endotoxic O antigens by homologous O-antibody. Ann NY Acad Sci 133:763–786

Ziegler EJ, Douglas H, Blaude AI (1982) Treatment of gram-negative bacteremia and shock with human antiserum to a mutant *Escherichia coli*. N Engl J Med 307:1225–1230

Investigations to Demonstrate the Antibacterial and Antitoxic Efficacy of an IgM-Enriched Intravenous Immunoglobulin Preparation

W. Stephan

Introduction

There are two primary objectives in the development of drugs: demonstration of efficacy and tolerance. Both efficacy and tolerance are optimal in antibodies from human plasma since in contrast to numerous synthetic drugs antibodies are highly specific. Owing to their molecular structure, they react specifically with viruses, bacteria, and toxins. In addition, they activate via the Fc part immunobiological activities in the body. In terms of tolerance, antibody products are autologous natural substances. Correspondingly, the rate of side effects is exceedingly low (in accordance with our statistics, less than one per thousand).

Immunobiological Functions of Antibodies

Immunoglobulins M and G differ markedly in their physical and biological properties. IgM is present in the serum in an eight to ten times lower concentration than IgG [1–3]. Moreover, the half-life of the smaller IgG molecule is four times greater than that of the large IgM molecule [4]. If the concentration of IgM in serum is so much less than that of IgG, the question arises as to the significance of immunoglobulin M for host defense function.

A preeminent property of IgM is its capacity to produce pronounced activation of complement. If the IgM molecule binds to surface antigen structures of a bacterium, the entire molecule undergoes a change in conformation, which leads to a concentration of the Fc moieties [5] (Fig. 1). In this way, the classical complement activation is started. At the end of this reaction pathway, a protein complex arises from the complement component C5b to C9, which leads to irrevers-

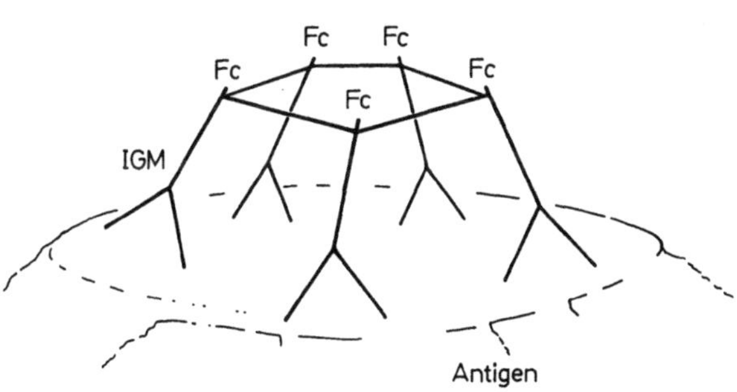

Fig. 1. Concentration of Fc moieties

Immune Consequences of
Trauma, Shock and Sepsis
Eds. Faist/Ninnemann/Green

ible damage of the bacterial membrane. In statistical terms, roughly one thousand times more IgG molecules are required to damage the cell than IgM molecules.

The potency of IgM antibodies in agglutination of large and complex structures, e.g., salmonellae, is ten times greater than that of IgG. In the same system, the killing of bacteria by IgM is more effective, since it activates 100–400 times more complement than IgG. In the opsonization of bacteria, IgM proves to be more than 1000 times more active than IgG [6, 7]. The IgM antibody thus plays a special role as a drug.

Intravenous IgM

Immunoglobin M antibodies are stabilized in human plasma by a variety of proteins. During the purification of IgM from human plasma, albumin and other proteins are removed by fractionation. As a consequence of the removal of stabilizing proteins insoluble IgM aggregates are formed. It was found that IgM is stabilized by IgG and IgA, so that the problem of aggregating immunoglobulins can be prevented when the IgG, IgM, and IgA complex is isolated. Treatment with β-propiolactone reduces the anticomplementary activity to obtain optimal i.v. tolerance [8]. In addition, β-propiolactone inactivates viruses [9].

Efficacy of Intravenous IgM

The efficacy of a drug is of particular interest. The efficacy of blood products can be demonstrated in various ways. The immunoglobulin concentrations and antibody activity can be tested in vitro and in vivo. In vitro parameters for the IgM preparation Pentaglobin are summarized in Table 1. The purity of the immunoglobulins is about 99%. The anticomplementary activity is so low that its intravenous tolerability is as good as for i.v. IgG preparations.

It can be expected that the antibody titers against bacteria in an IgM preparation are higher than those of pure IgG preparations. This is of particular importance in septicemia. The antibody titers of Pentaglobin against bacterial antigens are summarized in Table 2.

This preparation contains not only antibodies against *Escherichia coli, Pseudomonas,* or *Klebsiella* but also antibodies against gram-positive organisms: *Staphylococcus aureus, Enterococcus, Streptococcus viridans,* and *Streptococcus pyo-*

Table 1. Composition of Pentaglobin (mean values of ten lots)

	IgG (mg/100 ml)	IgA (mg/100 ml)	IgM (mg/100 ml)
Mean value	3887	575	647
±SD	164	22	71
Range	3750–4060	568–600	613–730

Nephelometric determination; margin of error ±10%.

Table 2. Reciprocal antibody titers against bacterial antigens in Pentaglobin (mean values of ten lots)

Antigens	Median titer
Escherichia coli	640
Pseudomonas aeruginosa	1280
Klebsiella pneumoniae	1280
Staphylococcus aureus	320
Streptococcus faecalis	160
Streptococcus pyogenws	160
Streptococcus viridans	160

Passive hemagglutination test. Margin of error; ± 1 titer step.

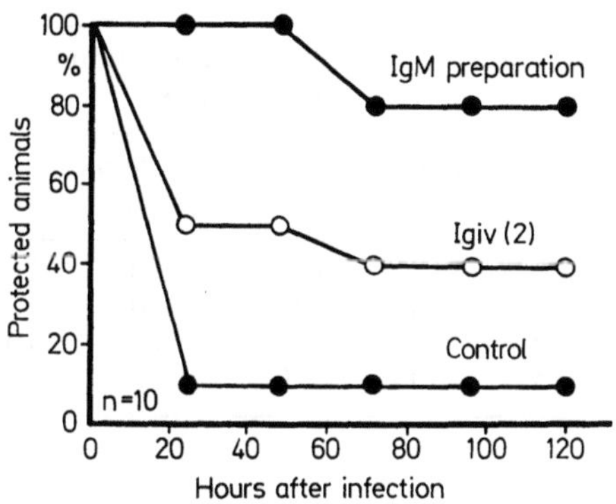

Fig. 2. Infection of mice with *Pseudomonas*. ●, treated with Pentaglobin; ○, treated with Intraglobin

genes. Antibodies against gram-positive organisms are hardly detectable in immunoglobulin preparations of the conventional i.v. IgG type.

Immunoglobulin preparations should have antibodies against the surface antigens of bacteria and they should be capable of neutralizing the bacterial toxins. In contrast to the very variable lipopolysaccharide structures which characterize the serotype of the bacterium, the structural element lipid A is common to all gram-negative bacteria. Lipid A is considered to be responsible for pathological effects which play a major role in septicemia. Antibodies against lipid A have been demonstrated in Pentaglobin [10].

Let us consider now the in vivo efficacy of the immunoglobulin preparations. For our investigations [10], we have used a mouse model which is very similar to the test system with which the Federal Office for Sera and Vaccines, Frankfurt/Main, tests the efficacy of tetanus immunoglobulins. In our tests system, mice were infected with *Pseudomonas* and then treated with either Pentaglobin or Intraglobin (0.5 ml, 5% solution). The results are shown in Fig. 2. Mice were infected with 10^7 *Pseudomonas* infectious units and both products were applied intravenously at the same dosage directly after infection. Compared with controls, the survival rate of the immunoglobulin-protected mice was significantly higher. Eighty percent of the Pentaglobin- and 40% of the Intraglobin-protected mice survived the infection. Because of the above-mentioned differences between the

Table 3. Immunoglobulin-antibiotic synergism in Endoxan-treated mice

Infection	Treatment	Survival (%) 4 days after infection
Pseudomonas aeruginosa	Pentaglobin (P)	40
	Cefsulodin (C)	20
	P+C	70
	Control	10
Staphylococcus aureus	Pentaglobin	20
	Ampicillin (A)	60
	P+A	90
	Control	20

Table 4. Immunoglobulin preparations, composition, and activity

Pre-para-tion	Method	Number of batches investi-gated	Immunoglobulin content %			Reciprocal antibody titers (PHA)		
			IgG	IgA	IgM	*E. coli*	*Ps aeru-ginosa*	*St. aureus*
1	IgM-enriched[a]	4	75.1	10.3	14.6	640	1280	320
2	β-Propiolacton[b]	4	97.0	2.9	0.1	80	160	10
3	pH 4/pepsin	4	97.9	2.0	0.1	80	160	≦10
4	PEG/HES	2	>99.5	<0.5	<0.1	80	160	10

[a] Biotest, Pentaglobin.
[b] Biotest, Intraglobin.

IgM and IgG molecule, we have predicted the superiority of the IgM preparation, which was then documented by these experimental results.

The interaction of antibodies and antibiotics (Table 3) is important. Mice were infected with *Pseudomonas aeruginosa* and directly afterwards they were treated with cefsulodin, the IgM preparation, or a combination of both products. It is seen that cefsulodin is almost ineffective under the experimental conditions chosen; the IgM preparation still provides a protective effect of 40% at a suboptimal dosage (0.1 ml, 5% solution). If both preparations are used together, 70% protection is obtained, so that antibody preparations of the IgM type and antibiotics supplement each other very well. These results do not suggest that antibiotics should be replaced by IgM immunoglobulins, but suggest that the two substances potentiate each other and should be used together. In a gram-positive infection with *Staphylococcus aureus,* the effect of ampicillin and IgM was tested. Under the experimental conditions chosen, the IgM preparation alone has practically no efficacy (0.1 ml, 5% solution), and ampicillin has an efficacy of 60%. If the two preparations are administered simultaneously, the efficacy of the IgM preparation is potentiated. This is also again an indication that antibody preparations do not replace antibiotic therapy but support each other.

The observations made so far apply to animal experiments carried out with bacteria. The efficacy of IgM immunoglobulins in the neutralization of bacterial

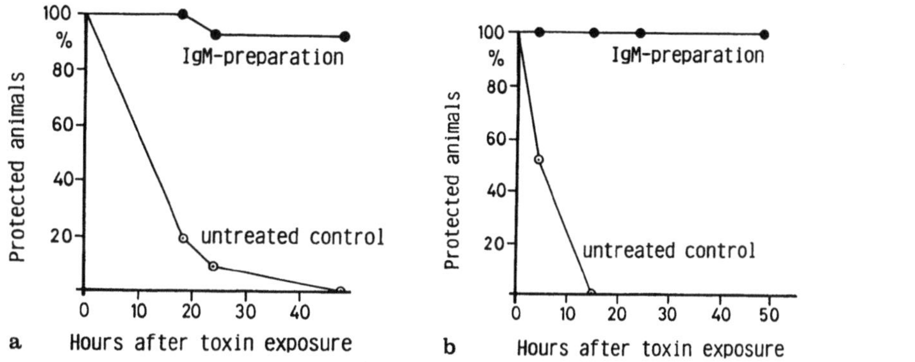

Fig. 3 a, b. Neutralization by Pentaglobin of toxin-containing supernatants of **a** *Pseudomonas aeruginosa* and **b** *Staphylococcus aureus*

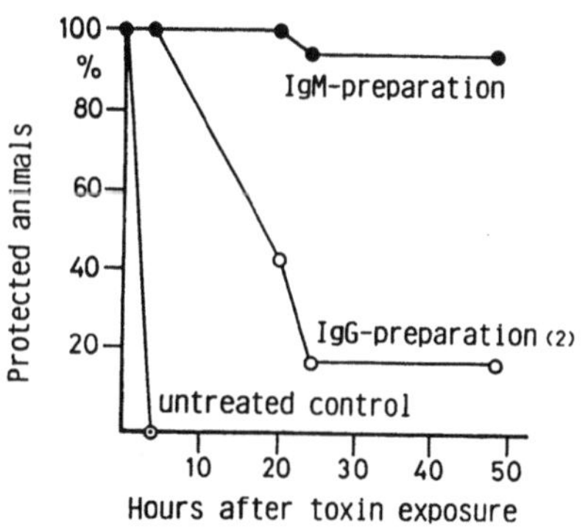

Fig. 4. In vivo toxin neutralization by products 1 (●) and 2 (○) against supernatants of *Pseudomonas aeruginosa*

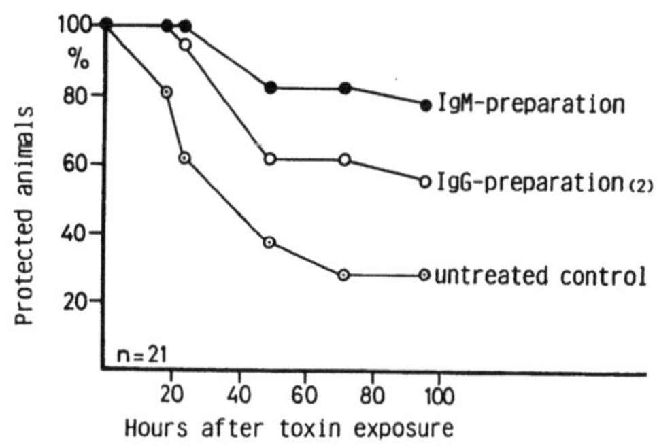

Fig. 5. In vivo toxin neutralization by products 1 (●) and 2 (○) against supernatants of *Staphylococcus aureus*

toxins was studied as follows [11]: 0.05 ml of the germ-free supernatant of the overnight culture of the respective bacterium was applied intraperitoneally for infection. Immunoglobulin (1; Table 4) was administered i.p. as a 5% solution 30 min after infection (0.5 ml/animal).

Figure 3 a, b shows the effect of the toxin-containing culture supernatants of *Pseudomonas aeruginosa* and *Staphylococcus aureus* and their neutralization by Pentaglobin. In both cases, the administration of IgM-enriched immunoglobulin brings about a significant reduction of lethality due to the toxin.

Figures 4 and 5 show the results of comparative investigations on in vivo toxin neutralization by products 1 and 2 (Table 4) against supernatants of *Pseudomonas aeruginosa* and a toxic shock syndrome toxin (TSST)-producing strain of *Staphylococcus aureus*. In both cases, preparation 1 has a significantly higher protection rate than preparation 2.

The toxin-neutralizing activity of Pentaglobin was investigated in comparison to conventional IgG preparations (2, 3 and 4) in the hemolysis inhibition test with

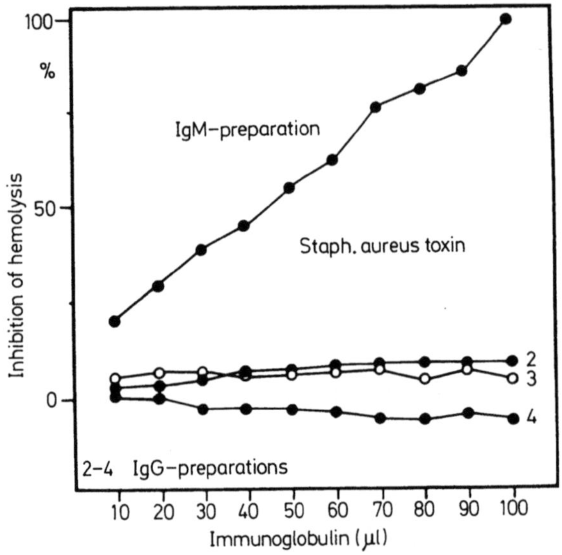

Fig. 6. Toxin-neutralizing capacity of Pentoglobin and conventional IgG preparations in the hemolysis inhibition test

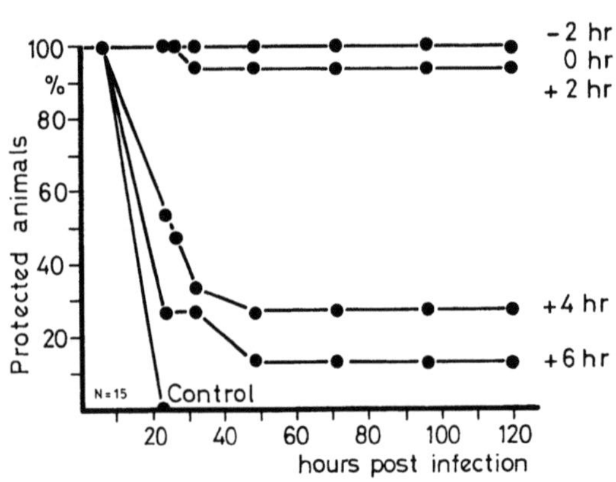

Fig. 7. Time-dependent efficacy of Pentoglobin in *Pseudomonas aeruginosa* infected mice

the toxin-containing supernatant of *Staphylococcus aureus* Smith 3 used as an example (Fig. 6). Inhibition of the toxin-induced hemolysis was only inhibited by preparation 1. Increasing amounts of IgG preparations 2, 3, and 4 had no effect.

Recently, we have carried out experiments in which the time between infection with *Pseudomonas aeruginosa* and antibody administration was prolonged (Fig. 7). In an experimental series, the IgM preparation was administered 2 h before infection, at the time of infection, and 2 h afterwards. Practically no difference in activity was observed. It is interesting that even with an application 4 h after infection an effect was still seen, and that this effect was still apparent (even in a very moderate form) after 6 h. These times should not directly be extrapolated to clinical situations. However, the results indicate that not only prophylaxis of septicemia with antibodies of the IgM type, but also therapy, is possible, especially due to the antitoxic effect.

References

1. Humphrey JH, White RG (1972) Lehrbuch der Immunologie. Thieme, Stuttgart
2. Riesen W (1980) Struktur und biologische Eigenschaften von Immunglobulinen und γ-Globulin-Präparaten. Schweiz Med Wochenschr 110:74
3. Opferkuch W (1985) Immunoglobulin M – physiologische Mechanismen und Wirkungsweise. In: Ungeheuer E, Heinrich D (eds) Bakterien, Endotoxine, Sepsis – Immunglobulin M. Springer, Berlin Heidelberg New York
4. Morell A, Skvaril F (1980) Struktur und biologische Eigenschaften von Immunglobulinen und γ-Globulin-Präparaten. Schweiz Med Wochenschr 110:80
5. Huber R (1982) Spacial structure of the immunoglobulin molecule. Eur Surg Res 14:447
6. Cohen S, Porter RR (1964) Structure and biological activity of immunoglobulins. Adv Immunol 4:287
7. Porter RR (1966) A discussion on the chemistry and biology of immunoglobulins. Proc R Soc Lond [Biol] 166:113
8. Stephan W (1983) Intravenous IgM by means of treatment of Cohn fraction III with β-propiolactone. In: Curling JM (ed) Pharmacia fine chemicals. Uppsala, p 153 (Budapest 1982)
9. Stephan W, Dichtelmüller H (1983) β-Propiolacton als sterilisierendes Agens bei der Herstellung eines intravenösen Immunglobulin-Präparates. Arzneimittelforschung 33(II)9:1230
10. Stephan W, Dichtelmüller H, Schedel I (1985) Eigenschaften und Wirksamkeit eines humanen IgM-Präparates für die intravenöse Anwendung. Arzneimittelforschung 35(I)6:933
11. Dichtelmüller H, Stephan W (1987) Untersuchung zur Wirksamkeit von IgM i.v. Immunglobulinen gegen bakterielle Infektionen und zur Neutralisation bakterieller Toxine. Arzneimittelforschung 37(II)11:1273

Therapy of Secondary T-Cell Immunodeficiencies with Biological Substances and Drugs

J. W. Hadden

Introduction

The immunodeficiencies of trauma and burns have various levels of complexity and it is difficult to treat them as a single common entity (Davis and Shires 1986). They seem to have in common an acute phase reaction which, to a significant degree, is glucocorticoid mediated. This acute phase reaction is associated with lymphopenia and leukocytosis. Depending on the circumstances, a number of mediators are released including cycloxygenase products (thromboxanes and prostaglandins) lipoxygenase products (eicosanoids and leukotrienes), histamine and other mast cell, granulocyte and platelet products, and complement derived products. As the acute phase resolves, the situation may become further complicated by blood and serum losses, fluid and electrolyte imbalances, protein/caloric and nutrient deficiencies, and the many consequences of sepsis. All in all, not a simple metabolic or immunologic circumstance.

In these cascading events, a number of factors impair one or another form of body defense and deficits of granulocyte, macrophage and lymphocyte function have been described. For the purposes of this discussion I would like to focus on the T cell-related defects and to discuss the prospects for bolstering T-cell immunity in the prevention and management of infections which result from these defects.

The T cell-related defects associated with trauma and burns have been well summarized by Antonacci (1986) who has had many years of experience in this area. He has emphasized the early lymphopenia associated with interleukin 2 (IL2) deficiency and depressed mitogen and mixed leukocyte culture responsiveness. The causes of this lymphopenia are not absolutely clear. Steroid-mediated redistribution of T cells, principally T4 cells, is clearly a significant factor. Loss of T cells (lymph node depletion and thymus involution) has also been emphasized, particularly in the studies of steroid-sensitive murine species. Even T-cell and macrophage-mediated suppressor cell mechanisms have been invoked. He has focused on the controversy as to whether the situation should be defined in terms of immunodeficiency versus immunosuppression and has summarized the evidence which supports both views. Finally, he has granted that surely a balanced view includes both sides of the controversy. On these points, we agree fully.

On looking at the T-cell disturbances in trauma and burns and in pondering about the most appropriate means for attacking the problem immunopharmacologically, I find two approaches logical. The first is geared toward contrasup-

Immune Consequences of
Trauma, Shock and Sepsis
Eds. Faist/Ninnemann/Green

pression and the second toward immunorestoration. Many of the mediators associated with both specific and nonspecific immune suppression have been demonstrated to impinge on the prostaglandin/cyclic AMP pathway (see Hadden 1987c for review) and it has been postulated that agents which interfere with these mechanisms may counter the immunosuppressive influences. Agents which either block prostaglandin and cyclic AMP production (e.g., indomethacin) or promote the cyclic GMP system (thymopentin, levamisole, IL2, and cimetidine) have been useful both in vivo and in vitro in reversing burn-induced immune dysfunction (see Calvano 1986 for review). Much can be said in favor of this type of immunopharmacology as a basis for developing therapeutic approaches; however, brevity dictates that I focus, for the purposes of this discussion, on the second approach of immunorestoration. I do so with the recognition that the agents and actions I will discuss also apply to the reversal of immunosuppressive influences. I will review some aspects of the molecular components which regulate the T-cell system and discuss what the therapeutic prospects are for regulating the system with biologicals and drugs in the treatment of secondary T-cell deficiencies in burns and trauma.

The T-cell population is made up of two main components. The major population (approximately 5×10^{10}–5×10^{11}) circulates in blood, percolates through the body's tissues, and circulates through lymphatics back into the blood. The second major population of approximately the same size resides in defined areas of lymph nodes (deep cortex and paracortical area), of spleen (periarteriolar region of the white pulp), and of Peyer's patches and tonsils. The system is populated from the thymus during late fetal life and early childhood and, once populated, can expand in reaction to specific antigenic challenge. Normally, the system is a balanced and effective one capable of meeting a large variety of challenges quickly and efficiently and, once resolved, retains resistance and memory for decades thereafter.

Defects of the T-cell system associated with burns, trauma and irradiation are generally, but not invariably, associated with decreased number of circulating T cells. In addition, T cells which are present may be dysfunctional or nonfunctional due to intrinsic or extrinsic causes (e.g., suppressor factors). An appropriate immunorestorative strategy then is one which seeks to promote the development and/or function of these cells.

So far, clinical treatment *specifically* designed to correct T-cell deficiencies has been restricted to the following (see Hadden 1987a, b for reviews):

1. Fetal thymus transplantation in certain patients with severe combined immunodeficiency disease (SCID)
2. Thymic hormone therapy in primary immunodeficiency, particularly DiGeorge syndrome and SCID with B cells
3. Thymic hormones and transfer factor treatment in collected acquired T-cell deficiencies
4. Levamisole and thymosin treatment of cancer patients
5. A variety of substances (isoprinosine, azimexon, imreg, thymosin, thymopoietin, thymulin and IL2 in acquired immunodeficiency syndrome (AIDS) and the AIDS-related complex

All of these treatments are presently considered experimental in the United States. All have shown some degree of efficacy and it is reasonable to expect that as our clinical efforts, both diagnostically and therapeutically, become more precise these treatments will ultimately become accepted in clinical practice. The following discussion will focus briefly on the preclinical immunopharmacologies of the biologicals and drugs which are likely candidates for future clinical use in the correction of T-cell deficiencies associated with trauma and burns.

Thymic Hormones

A number of substances have been extracted from the thymus gland and termed thymic hormones (see Goldstein 1984). These substances are thought to be extracted from the hormone-producing cells of the thymus, the thymic epithelial cells. Unfortunately, the entire thymus has been used in their preparation so that in the partially purified preparations (like thymosin fraction V and thymostimulin TP-1) lymphocyte and epithelial constituents must be present in addition to thymic hormones (Table 1).

Three thymic hormone preparations have been purified to homogeneity and synthesized either by chemical synthesis or genetic engineering. These are: thymopoietin, thymosin alpha 1, and thymulin (previously FTS). All of these thymic hormones have been shown to modulate prothymocyte and thymocyte function in one or another assay; however, few direct comparisons have been made to allow a proper assessment of differences in their actions. By way of general statement it can be said that several different substances show activity and can be considered to meet the criteria of a thymic hormone. Their capacity to modulate thymocyte development is consistent with events which are known to occur in the thymus and in the periphery in the presence of a thymus; however, none of these preparations are sufficiently potent to restore cell mediated immunity in the absence of a thymus or when the defect is well established and severe.

Table 1. Thymic hormone characterization

	Source	Molecular weight (daltons) (isolectric point)	Sequenced	Demonstrated epithelial origin	In vitro induction of markers	Active on CMI in vivo
Thymosin fraction V	Bovine thymus	>34 peptides	–	+	+	+
			–	ND	+	+
Thymostimulin (TP-1)	Bovine thymus	Multiple	–	ND	+	+
Thymosin alpha 1	Bovine thymus	3107	+	+	+	+
Thymopoietin	Bovine thymus	5662	+	+	+	+
Thymulin (FTS)	Pig serum	$857 + Zn^{++}$	+	+	+	+

ND, Not determined; CMI, cell-mediated immunity.

Interleukins 1 and 2

IL2 is a product of mature T cells and immature large granular lymphocytes (probably pre-T cells). The production of IL2 by mature T cells results from the action of a monocyte/macrophage product called interleukin 1 (IL1). IL2 acts to allow antigen-primed mature T cells (triggered to synthesize RNA and protein) to enter DNA synthesis and to replicate clonally. It was previously thought that only mature T cells respond to IL1 to make IL2; however, immature T cells have recently been described to have IL2 cell receptors (Raulet 1985). Their possible roles in T-cell development will be discussed later in this chapter.

Transfer Factor/Dialyzed Leukocyte Extract

A variety of small dializable factors has been extracted from T cells and given various names. All have been described to modulate nonspecifically T cell mediated immunity. Transfer factor has been ascribed specificity in that it can transfer sensitivity from a nonsensitized to a sensitized donor. It is important to note, for purposes that will become apparent, that while the structure of transfer factor has not been elucidated, it is thought to contain inosine as part of its structure. If one accepts both the specific and the nonspecific aspects of the transfer factor phenomena, the logical postulate is that lymphocytes when killed or perhaps following antigen challenge release transfer factor. It then circulates in the blood and acts on immature or precommitted cells to make them responsive to the particular antigen and acts nonspecifically to prime generally the T-cell system to be more active. How these postulated events occur is not clear.

Thymomimetic Drugs

The two main classes of compounds having thymomimetic action (see Hadden 1985) are represented by levamisole and isoprinosine (Table 2). They act directly or indirectly via induced factors to promote the differentiation of prothymocytes and to modulate mature T-cell receptors and functions. Each class is also represented by structurally similar compounds which, insofar as have been examined, share similar immunopharmacologies. Representatives of both classes of agents augment cell-mediated immune responses as measured both in vitro and in vivo.

Not all of the activities of the two compounds can be termed thymomimetic. Additional features of levamisole's in vitro actions which are not strictly thymomimetic include: augmentation of lymphokine-induced macrophage phagocytosis and activation, augmentation of macrophage and granulocyte motility, and induction of interferon. Similarly, additional features of isoprinosine's in vitro actions which are not strictly thymomimetic include: induction of B-cell differentiation, potentiation of gamma-interferon production by T cells, increase in natural killer cell activity, increased monocyte phagocytosis, potentiation of lymphokine-induced macrophage proliferation and activation, and increased antibody-dependent cytotoxicity by eosinophils.

Table 2. Classification of thymomimetic drugs

Thymomimetic drugs	T-cell induction	Active rosettes	Cell-mediated immunity	T-dependent B-cell response
Class I: Sufur-containing compounds				
Levamisole	+*	+	+	+
Diethyldithiocarbamate	+*	NT	+	+
NPT 16416	NT	+	NT	+
Thiabendazole	+* (with antigen)	NT	+	NT
Cimetidine	NT	+	+	+
Class II: Purine-containing compounds				
Isoprinosine	+	+	+	+
NPT 15392	+	+	+	+
NPT 16416	+	+	NT	+
Transfer factor	+	+	+	+

* Via a serum factor induced in vivo; NT, not tested.

Table 3. In vivo effects of levamisole, isoprinosine and thymic hormones on immune function

Immune function	Levamisole	Isoprinosine	Thymic hormones
T-cell marker induction	+	+	+
T-cell mitogen responses	+	+	+
Lymphokine production and cytotoxicity	+	+	+
Cell-mediated immunity	+	+	+
T-cell-dependent antibody production	+	+	+
Resistance to phatogen challenge	+	+	+
Resistance to tumor recurrence	+	NT	+
Reduction of autoimmunity	+	+	+
Reversal of effects of aging on immune response	+	+	+

NT, Not tested.

Many of the immune functions shown to be affected by levamisole, isoprinosine and the thymic hormones in vitro have been confirmed in vivo following administration to experimental animals and human subjects. The in vivo results in animals and man are summarized qualitatively in Table 3. For the purposes of simplicity, the actions of the various thymic hormone preparations have been grouped collectively to indicate that these are general actions of thymic hormones. This table makes the general point that, to the extent tested, levamisole and isoprinosine share the immunopharmacologic actions of the thymic hormones, as assessed by in vitro parameters, delayed type hypersensitivity, and resistance to viral infection, cancer, and autoimmunity.

Immunopharmacologic Regulation of T-Cell Ontogeny

Most reviews describe the action of the biologicals and drugs on mature T cells. While association of thymic hormones with T-cell differentiation is known, the roles of the endocrine thymus and, for that matter, other possible mediators in the regulation of T-cell ontogeny remain unclear. The successful therapeutic correction of T-cell deficiencies depends upon a more complete understanding of the regulation of T-cell maturation. In order to understand the potential of these substances to reconstitute T-cell number as well as T-cell function, I will review some recent studies on their actions at various levels of T-cell ontogeny.

The first step of T-cell development is determined by the method of Komuro and Boyse (1973). The Komuro-Boyse assay employs prothymocytes obtained from athymic nude mouse spleens in a 2-h incubation with various inducers. The induction of Thy 1 (formerly θ) is assessed as a measure of one of the earliest steps of T-cell differentiation.

A number of thymic hormone preparations are active in the induction of T-cell differentiation in this assay. These include thymosin fraction V, thymosin alpha 1, thymulin, and thymopoietin (Hadden et al. 1986a, b). We have recently found that both natural and recombinant IL2 (2–32 units/ml) (Hadden et al. 1986 a) are active to induce maturation in this assay. We have also found that IL2 regulates the basal proliferation of this cell population. These represent the first observations delineating a functional role for IL2 on prothymocytes and indicate that these cells have IL2 receptors.

It was previously thought by us and others that these prothymocytes were unresponsive to IL1 (Hadden et al. 1986 b); however, our recent studies (Hadden et al. 1988) show that IL1 alone has a small effect to induce proliferation and acts synergistically with IL2. The effect of the combination of recombinant IL1 and IL2 is approximately the effect of a natural mixed lymphokine preparation.

Inosine-like compounds, isoprinosine and NPT 15392, have been previously shown by Ikehara et al. (1981) to induce prothymocyte maturation leading to the description of these compounds as thymomimetic drugs (Hadden 1985). We previously postulated that these drugs act to induce T-cell differentiation via a purine (nonadenosine) receptor, perhaps the same receptor acted on by transfer factor since the latter has been shown to contain inosine (Hadden et al. 1983). Transfer factor prepared by S. S. Chen was found to induce prothymocyte differentiation strengthening the postulate that the action of transfer factor and thymomimetic purines may be related phenomena (Hadden et al. 1986 b). Also active in this system are sera from athymic mice treated with sulfur-containing drugs such as levamisole and diethyldithiocarbamate (DTC) which, according to Renoux, contains a factor derived from liver, termed hepatosin (Renoux et al. 1979; Renoux 1984).

The degree of maturation in the prothymocyte induction assay is small in terms of the degree of receptor expression found on thymocytes and we found that the additional presence in coculture of thymic epithelial cells was necessary to bring out surface marker induction and proliferation manifested by the intrathymic immature T cell (Wiranowska et al. 1987).

The induction of maturation of Thy 1^- cells to Thy 1^+ cells is not known to be associated with the acquisition of any of the functions characteristic of mature T lymphocytes and it has not been shown that any of the aforementioned substances alone can induce function of Thy 1^+ prothymocytes. It therefore becomes important to assess the question as to what are the appropriate inducers of intrathymic maturation for mature phenotype and function.

Another assay used by us in the study of thymocyte ontogeny involves the use of immature cortical thymocytes prepared by peanut agglutination (PNA^+) followed by a 16–24 h incubation with various inducers (Chen et al. 1983). The induction of concanavalin A (Con A) responsiveness is measured by thymidine incorporation after 72 h of culture. Since only PNA^- mature, medullary thymocytes are Con A responsive, this assay measures the maturation of PNA^+ cells to acquire functional traits of PNA^- cells. The receptor correlates of these intrathymic maturation steps have been previously reported by us (Chen et al. 1983). We showed that both recombinant IL2 and IL1 are active on these immature thymocytes to induce proliferation in the absence of Con A and to induce Con A responsiveness; together, their action is markedly synergistic and similar to the effect of a natural mixed lymphokine preparation (Hadden et al. 1986b, 1988). Preincubation experiments confirmed the inductive nature of this IL1/IL2 signal. As expected, the mature thymocytes (PNA^-) show marked Con A responsiveness and both IL1 and IL2 promote the responses, but in a nonsynergistic manner. Thymosin fraction V was inactive in promoting the development of immature T cells in these assays and the thymomimetic drugs were not tested.

As previously noted, the effects of thymic hormones, IL1, IL2, and the thymomimetic drugs on mature T cells have been well studied and documented. Recent emphasis on the central role of IL2 in immunologic orchestration by T helper cells makes it relevant to reemphasize the actions of these agents in this regard. IL1, of course, induces IL2. Thymosin fraction V and the thymomimetic drugs, isoprinosine and NPT 15392 promote IL2 production by mature T cells in the presence of a mitogenic influence (Zatz et al. 1985; Wiranowska et al. 1986).

These collected observations are summarized in Table 4. They indicate that a variety of agents are capable of modulating T-cell development at several different stages. They imply that these agents may be useful singly and collectively in promoting T-cell development and function.

In order to put this prediction to the test we approached the athymic nude mouse model. The athymic mouse (4–8 weeks) has few T cells which bear Thy 1.2 surface markers and respond to Con A (approximately 3%). It is not clear whether the few T cells which develop do so extrathymically or via interaction with thymic epithelial remnants known to exist in the mice (Ikehara et al. 1984, 1987). Previous experiments suggested that thymic hormones, IL2, and thymomimetic drugs could reconstitute functional T cells in these mice (Ikehara et al. 1975; Renoux et al. 1979; Stötter et al. 1980). Our own unpublished experience (manuscript in preparation) is that prolonged treatment of these mice with thymosin fraction V, recombinant IL2 (rIL2), mixed natural lymphokines, isoprinosine and diethyldithiocarbamate yields little effect to induce mature T cells by marker or functional criteria. By 3 weeks of treatment all of these agents were active to double mitogen responses; yet no significant effect on markers were observed. With

Table 4. Immunopharmacologic attributes of various biologicals and drugs

	Pro-thymocyte induction	Immature thymocyte induction	Mature T-cell modulation	IL2 induction
Thymic hormones	+	0	+	+ (with mitogen)
IL2	+	+	+	NA
IL1	+ (synergy with IL2)	+ (synergy with IL2)	+ +	+ +
Isoprinosine and/or related compounds	+	0	+	+ (with mitogen)
Levamisole and/or related compounds	+	ND	+	?

MA, Not available.

longer treatments the effects abated. After 12 weeks of treatment only a thymus graft showed significant effects to restore T cells. We have concluded that variable results may result from variable degrees of thymic remnants; however, immunopharmacologic means to bypass the thymus are ineffective.

As indicated by our own observations (Wiranowska et al. 1987), we shifted to a neonatal model in which a thymic epithelial environment is present; yet functional T cells are not yet present in the periphery. In these experiments, in progress, we have observed marked effects of mixed lymphokines, rIL1, rIL2, and NPT 15392 to promote the development of functional T cells in these neonatal mice. We anticipate that the results of these experiments will help to ascertain which biologicals or thymomimetic drugs or their combinations will be most effective in restoring T-cell number and function. The answers to these questions will allow us to predict which may be most appropriate to use therapeutically in patients with T-cell deficiencies secondary to burns or trauma.

References

Antonacci AC (1986) Immune dysfunction and immunomodulation following trauma. In: Gallin JI, Fauci A (eds) Advances in host defense mechanisms, vol 6. Raven, New York, p 81

Calvano SE (1986) Hormonal mediation of immune dysfunction following thermal and traumatic injury. In: Gallin JI, Fauci A (eds) Advances in host defense mechanisms, vol 6. Raven, New York, p 111

Chen SS, Tung JS, Gillis S, Good RA, Hadden JW (1983) Changes in surface antigens of immature thymocytes under the influence of interleukin II and thymic factors. Proc Natl Acad Sci USA 80:5980

Davis JM, Shires GT (1986) Host defenses in trauma and surgery, vol 6. In: Gallin JI, Fauci A (eds) Advances in host defense mechanisms. Raven, New York

Goldstein A (ed) (1984) Thymic hormones and lymphokines. Plenum, New York

Hadden JW (1985) Thymomimetic drugs. In: Meischer P, Bolis L, Ghione M (eds) Immunopharmacology. Serono Symposium Press, New York, p 183

Hadden JW (1987 a) Current status of the immunotherapy of AIDS and the AIDS-related complex. In: Wormser G, Stahl RE, Bottone EJ (eds) AIDS-acquired immunodeficiency syndrome – and other manifestations of HIV infections. Noyes Publications, Park Ridge, p 992

Hadden JW (1987b) Corrections of secondary T cell immunodeficiencies with biological substances and drugs. Cancer Detect Prev 9:409

Hadden JW (1987c) Neuroendocrine modulation of the thymus-dependent immune system: agonists and mechanisms. NY Acad Sci 496:39

Hadden JW, Cornaglia-Ferraris P, Coffey RG (1983) Purine analogs as immunomodulators. In: Yamamura Y, Tada T (eds) V. Progress in immunology. Academic, Tokyo, p 1393

Hadden J, Specter S, Hadden JW (1986a) Effects of T cell growth factor (interleukin II) and thymic hormones on prothymocytes and immature thymocytes. Lymphokine Res 5:49

Hadden JW, Specter S, Galy A, Touraine J-L, Hadden EM (1986b) Thymic hormones, interleukins, endotoxin and thymomimetic drugs. In: Chedid L, Hadden J, Spreafico F, Dukor P, Willoughby D (eds) III. Immunopharmacology. Pergamon, Oxford, p 487

Hadden EM, Galy A, Chen H, Dinarello C, Hadden JW (1988) Interleukin I and interleukin II are synergistic on the proliferation of immature T cells. Fourth International Conference on Immunopharmacology. Osaka, Japan, May 15–19, 1988 (Abstract) (in press)

Ikehara S, Hamashima Y, Masuda T (1975) Immunological restoration of both thymectomised and athymic nude mice by a thymus factor. Nature 258:335

Ikehara S, Hadden JW, Good RA, Pahwa R (1981) In vitro effects of two immunopotentiators, isoprinosine and NPT 15392 on murine T cell differentiation and function. Thymus 3:97

Ikehara S, Pahwa R, Fernandez G, Hansen C, Good RA (1984) Functional T cells in athymic nude mice. Proc Natl Acad Sci USA 81:886

Ikehara S, Shimizu J, Yasumizu R, Nakamura T, Inaba M, Inoue S, Oyaizu N, Sugiura K, Oo MM, Hamashima Y, Good RA (1987) Thymic sediments are responsible for induction of functional T cells in nu/nu mice. Thymus 10:93

Komuro K, Boyse EA (1973) Induction of T lymphocytes from precursor cells in vitro by a product of the thymus. J Exp Med 138:479

Raulet DH (1985) Expression and function of interleukin-2 receptors on immature thymocytes. Nature 314:101

Renoux G (1984) The mode of action of imuthiol (sodium diethyldithiocarbamate): a new role for the brain neocortex and the endocrine liver in the regulation of the T cell lineage. In: Fenichel R, Chirigos MA (eds) Immune modulation agents and their mechanisms. Dekker, New York, p 607

Renoux G, Renoux M, Guillaumin J-M, Gouzien C (1979) Differentiation and regulation of lymphocyte populations: evidence for immunopotentiator-induced T cell recruitment. J Immunopharmacol 1:415

Stötter H, Rüde E, Wagner H (1980) T cell factor (interleukin 2) allows in vivo induction of T helper cells against heterologous erythrocytes in athymic (nu/nu) mice. Eur J Immunol 10:719

Wiranowska-Stewart M, Hadden JW (1986) Effects of isoprinosine and NPT 15392 on interleukin 2 (IL2) production. Int J Immunopharmacol 8:63

Wiranowska M, Kaido T, Caspritz G, Cook J, Hadden JW (1987) Interleukin 2 and coculture with thymic epithelial cells synergistically induce prothymocyte differentiation and proliferation. Thymus 10:231

Zatz M, Goldstein A (1985) Mechanism of action of thymosin. I. Thymosin fraction 5 increases lymphokine production by mature murine T cells responding in a mixed lymphocyte reaction. J Immunol 134:1032

Immunomodulation as a Potential Therapeutic Approach in Immunodeficiencies

K. Bolla, R. Cappel, J. Duchateau, and E. Faist

Introduction

The term immunomodulation has started to come into use through an increasing number of experiments showing that substances of various origin can stimulate as well as inhibit immune responses induced by a primary stimulus. At the beginning of this decade, it had been generally accepted that the effect of such substances (named as immunomodulators, immune regulators, biological response modifiers, etc.) depends on the dose, route of administration, and treatment regimen as well as on the actual immune status of the subject treated [1–3]. The influence of the dose is easy to understand and even the importance of the actual immune status of the subject treated cannot be declared as surprising. Considering that any immune response is the net result of a series of interactions between different cell populations, the response will necessarily be modified by any change in the proportion or function of the various cells involved. In fact, investigations into the mechanism of action of thymopentin – a pentapeptide segment 32–36 of the thymic hormone thymopoietin [4–6] – showed that the actual immune status is not only one but the most important factor in determining the outcome of the immunomodulation [7]. As to the other factors mentioned, only the dose of the immunomodulator has been shown as being of primary importance; the influence of timing and frequency of drug administration reflect only the importance of the actual immune status [7], while that of the route of administration can be explained by the bioavailability of the pentapeptide [7, 8].

Interpretation of the Phenomenon "Immunomodulation"

Accepting the central role of the actual immune status in the outcome of immunomodulation, three different types of immunomodulatory process can be distinguished depending on timing and/or the presence of the primary immune stimulus. Figure 1 illustrates this consideration. In the absence of a primary immunological stimulus, the effect of an immunomodulator is reversible and physiologically silent (*"silent modulation"* – pathway 4 in Fig. 1). If the administration of the immunomodulator precedes the challenge with the immune stimulus, a modified immune system will react to the stimulus with a modified immune response; the term *"preventive modulation"* has been proposed for this alternative (pathway 3 in Fig. 1). Even an immune system in the process of generating an immune response can be modulated (pathway 2). However, the involvement of various cell

Immune Consequences of
Trauma, Shock and Sepsis
Eds. Faist/Ninnemann/Green

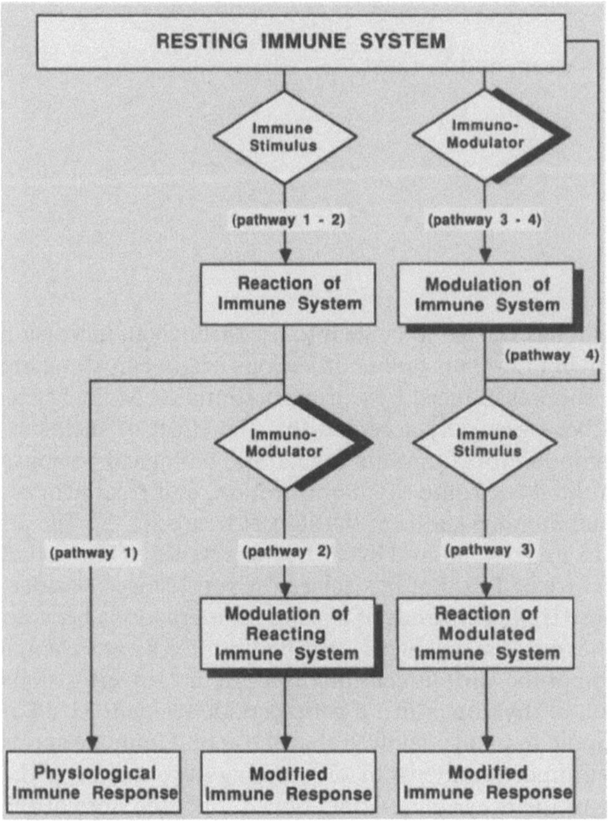

Fig. 1. Simplified flowchart indicating various forms of immunomodulation in the context of immune response. *Pathway 1,* process of physiological immune response; *pathway 2,* regulative immunomodulation; *pathway 3,* preventive immunomodulation; *pathway 4,* silent modulation

populations in an ongoing immune response modifies their availability for being influenced by an immunomodulator. Consequently, the influence of immunomodulation on the immune response should be different from that which can be achieved by preventive modulation. For this type of response modification the term *regulative or therapeutic immunomodulation* has been coined [7].

The introduction of the term "silent modulation" provided a possibility for a new interpretation of the phenomenon of immunomodulation. Accordingly, immunomodulation can be considered as a temporary alert of the immune system without any physiologically obvious immune response. If an additional immunological stimulus turns up during this alert, the result will be a modified immune response; on the other hand, a physiological immune response will be registered if the immunological stimulus occurs after cessation of the alert. Accepting this interpretation, the basic mechanism of immunomodulation can best be understood by investigation into the phenomenon of silent modulation.

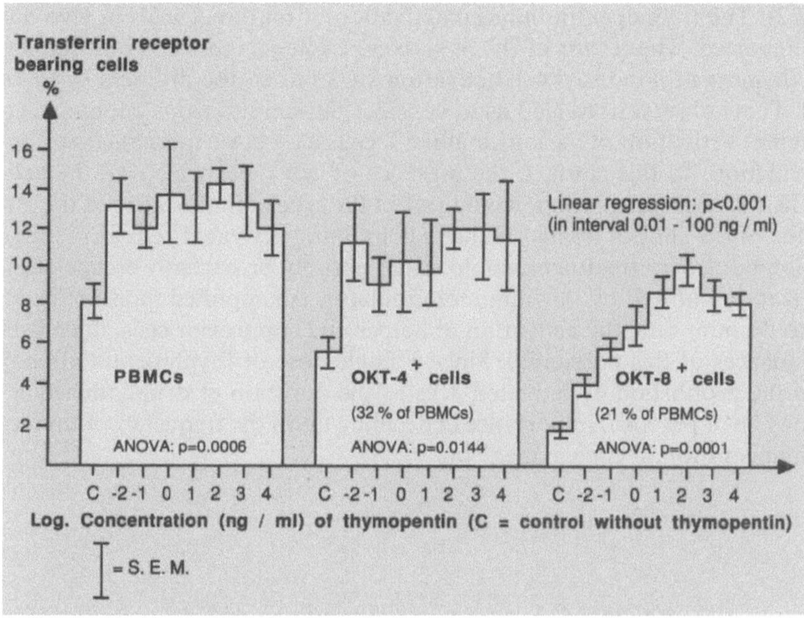

Fig. 2. Effect of thymopentin on the induction of transferrin receptor-bearing cells in various populations of peripheral blood mononuclear cells (PBMCs) of healthy blood donors; $n=8$ (from Ref. 9)

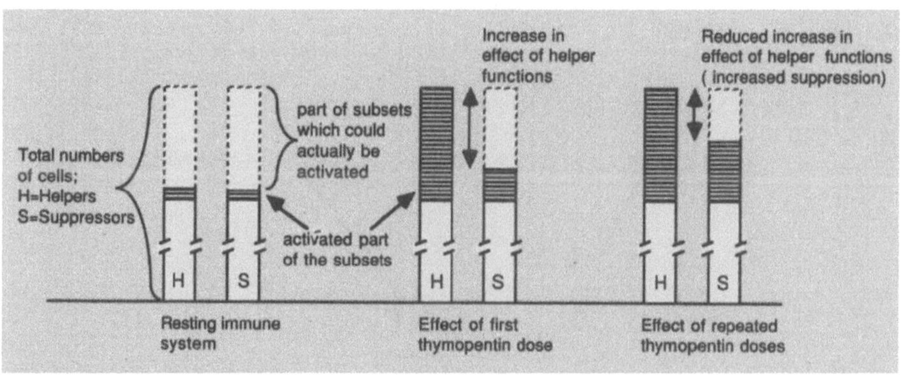

Fig. 3. Simplified model to explain the effect of repeated doses of thymopentin on helper and suppressor functions

Assuming that the early stage of activation of T cells may represent a type of temporary alert of the immune system, we assessed the percentage of transferrin receptor-bearing OKT-4- and OKT-8-positive cells in the presence of various thymopentin concentrations [9]. The results of this in vitro experiment clearly showed that thymopentin simultaneously activated helper and suppressor T cells. Moreover, it also showed that the ratio of the activated (transferrin receptor-bearing) OKT-4- and OKT-8-positive cells depends on the concentration of the drug (Fig. 2). The thymopentin-induced activation of mature T cells in vivo has also been reported. The results of the in vivo experiments indicated that the duration of thymopentin-induced cell activation varies as to the different types of T cells [9]. These observations lead us to consider the simultaneous but quantitatively different activation of various mature T cells as a basic mechanism of immunomodulation. In this context, the presence of cell types which can be activated at all, and their proportion, would reflect the crucial importance of the immune status of the subject treated. Subsets containing activated cells at the time of immunomodulatory treatment would either entirely or partially escape additional activation induced by the immunomodulator. A simplified model (Fig. 3), taking into account only the activation of helper and suppressor cells, illustrates the consequences of this possibility. Since a single dose of thymopentin already induces in the proportion of activated T cells, the duration of drug-induced activation may be of practical importance in deciding upon the frequency of thymopentin administration in clinical medicine.

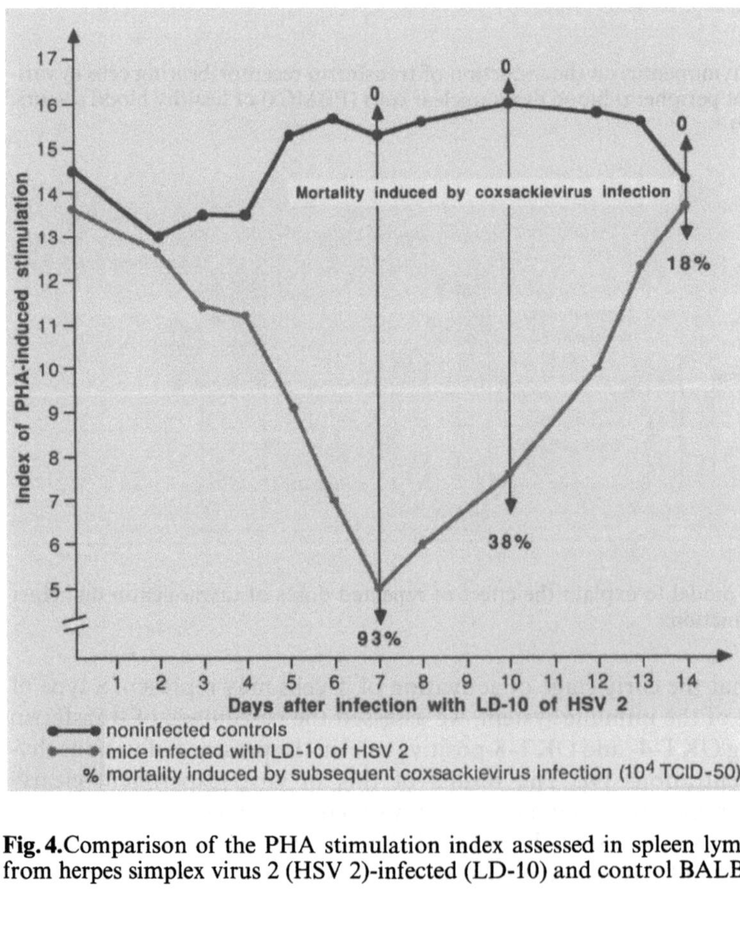

Fig. 4. Comparison of the PHA stimulation index assessed in spleen lymphocyte cultures from herpes simplex virus 2 (HSV 2)-infected (LD-10) and control BALB/c mice

Immunomodulation in Temporary Immune Depression (an Experimental Approach)

As with the unwanted effect of immune depressive therapy, temporary immune depression induced by infections or trauma is also known to increase the risk of opportunistic infections [10–12]. The theoretical considerations discussed above suggest that both preventive and regulative immunomodulation could be used for reducing the grade of induced immune depression and the risk of secondary infections. To check this possibility a series of experiments has been performed in mice. In these experiments, herpes simplex virus 2 (LD-10), thymopentin, and coxsackie B-5 virus were used as immunodepressive agent, immunomodulator, and pathogen for secondary infection, respectively.

In the first experiment, the PHA stimulation index was assessed daily or on every 2nd day in cultures of pooled spleen lymphocytes (five mice/assessment) up to 14 days after HSV 2 infection. In the second, 40 mice/group were infected with 10^4 TCID-50 coxsackie B 5 virus 7 days after the HSV 2 infection and the cumulative mortality was recorded. One group of mice was treated intraperitoneally

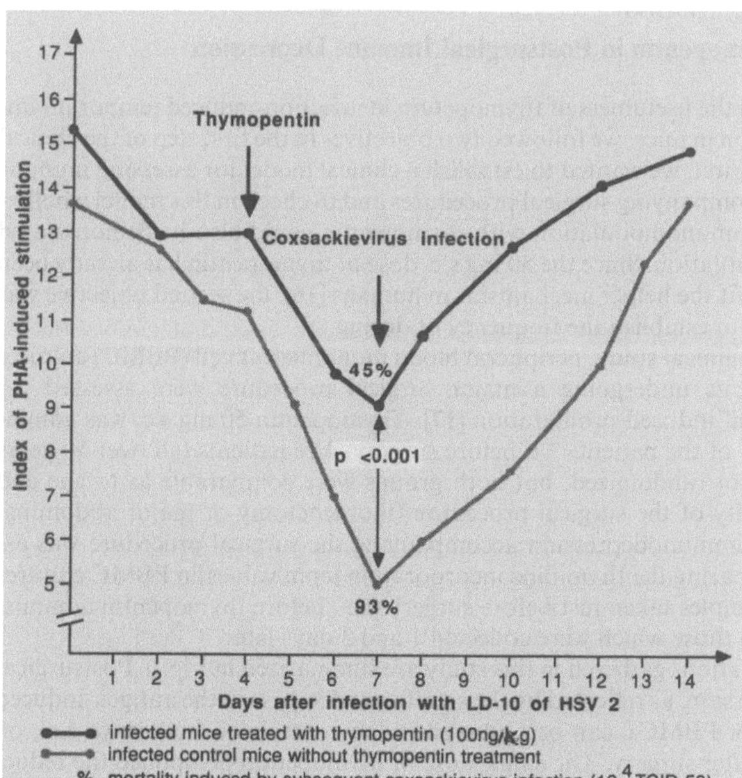

Fig. 5. The effect of thymopentin on HSV 2-induced reduction of the PHA stimulation index assessed in spleen lymphocyte cultures from BALB/c mice

(i.p.) with thymopentin, 100 ng/kg body weight, in both experiments 4 days after the HSV 2 infection. Mice not infected with HSV 2 were used as controls. The results of these experiments are summarized in Figs. 4 and 5.

Figure 4 shows that the infection with LD-10 of HSV 2 resulted in a temporary (about 2 weeks duration) immune depression. It progressively developed during the 1st week and was restored during the 2nd week after the infection. The sensitivity against a secondary infection (coxsackie virus) developed parallel with the grade of the immune depression.

Secondary infection on day 7 after the HSV 2 challenge resulted in a mortality rate of over 90%, while only 38% of the mice died if the coxsackie infection had been administered on day 10. The same dose of coxsackie virus did not induce mortality in the group which had not been infected with HSV 2. Figure 5 shows the effect of the immunomodulation with thymopentin. The HSV 2-induced immunodepression as well as the sensitivity against the secondary infection was significantly reduced compared with the mice not treated with thymopentin. Thymopentin has also been reported to be able to improve the function of leukocytes and macrophages in burned animals [13, 14] and to reduce the mortality in a guinea pig burn-wound sepsis model [15].

Effect of Thymopentin in Postsurgical Immune Depression

Having proved the usefulness of thymopentin in infection-induced temporary immune depression in mice, we followed two objectives in the first step of the clinical development. First, we wanted to establish a clinical model for assessing immune depression accompanying surgical procedures and to check in this model whether the effect of immunomodulation with thymopentin could also be demonstrated in the clinical situation. Since the 50 mg s.c. dose of thymopentin has already been shown to benefit the helper mechanisms in humans [16], the second objective was to collect data to establish the frequency of dosing.

In the first clinical study, peripheral blood mononuclear cell (PBMC) cultures from 18 patients undergoing a major surgical procedure were assessed for antigen-cocktail-induced proliferation [17]. Thymopentin 50 mg s.c. was administered to 50% of the patients 2 h before surgery. The patients (all over 50 years of age) were not randomized, but both groups were comparable as to age and grade of severity of the surgical procedure (thoracoctomy or major abdominal surgery). The immunodepression accompanying the surgical procedure was assessed by comparing the thymidine incorporation (cpm values)in PBMC cultures from blood samples taken just before surgery (i.e., before thymopentin administration) and in those which were collected 1 and 3 days later.

The observations gathered in this study are summarized in Fig. 6. Postsurgical immune depression, as reflected by the significant decrease in the antigen-induced proliferation of PBMCs, can be observed in the controls on both days, i.e., on days 1 and 3 after surgery. The single dose of thymopentin postponed the reduction of the antigen-induced proliferation by at least 1 day; a significant reduction in the thymidine incorporation was recorded only in the assessments on the third postoperative day.

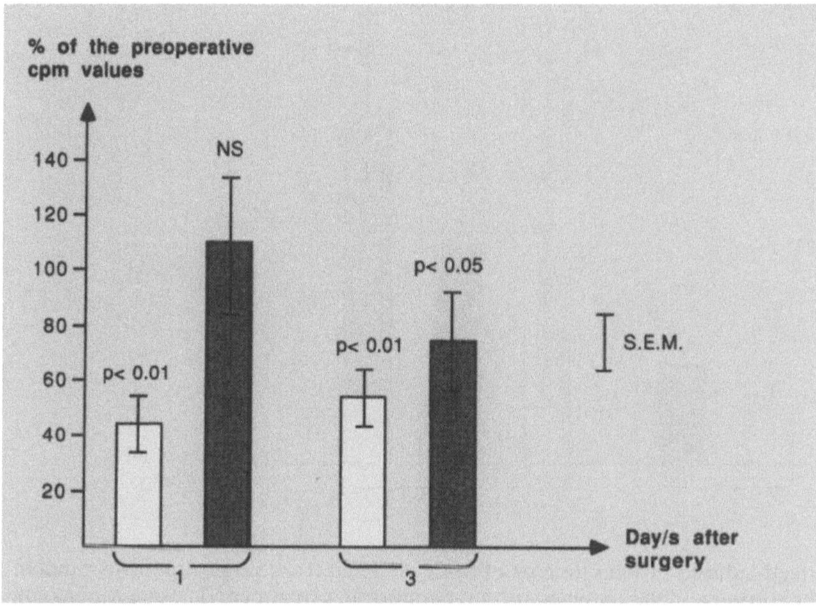

Fig. 6. Antigen-induced proliferation of peripheral blood mononuclear cells (PBMCs) obtained from surgical patients. Nine patients without thymopentin treatment (□) were used as controls; nine patients (■) were treated with thymopentin 50 mg s.c. 2 h before surgery (Ref. 17)

These observations seemed to confirm our assumption that preventive immunomodulation could be used in the treatment of temporary immunodeficiency in the clinical situation. In addition they suggested that the treatment should be continued with a second dose on day 2 after surgery. Accordingly, the second study had the objective of comparing the effect of two different thymopentin treatment regimens with each other and against placebo. In this randomized single-blind study nine patients were treated with a single dose of thymopentin 50 mg s.c. 2 h before and eight patients 2 h before as well as 2 days after surgery; eight patients were used as controls treated with placebo corresponding to the thymopentin treatment regimens. All the patients underwent cardiac surgery necessitating extracorporeal circulation.

The three groups were comparable as to age and severity of the surgical procedure. The antigen-induced proliferation was assessed in PBMC cultures from blood samples taken 2 h before, as well as 1 and 7 days after, surgery. The thymidine incorporation assessed after surgery is expressed as a percentage of the baseline cpm values for each individual. In addition, delayed-type hypersensitivity was assessed with the Mérieux multitest before and 1 week after surgery.

Preliminary results from this study (Figs. 7, 8) show a significant difference in favor of the treatment with two doses of thymopentin compared with placebo with regard to the values assessed 1 week after surgery. The values assessed in the group treated only with a single dose of the drug had a mean between the two

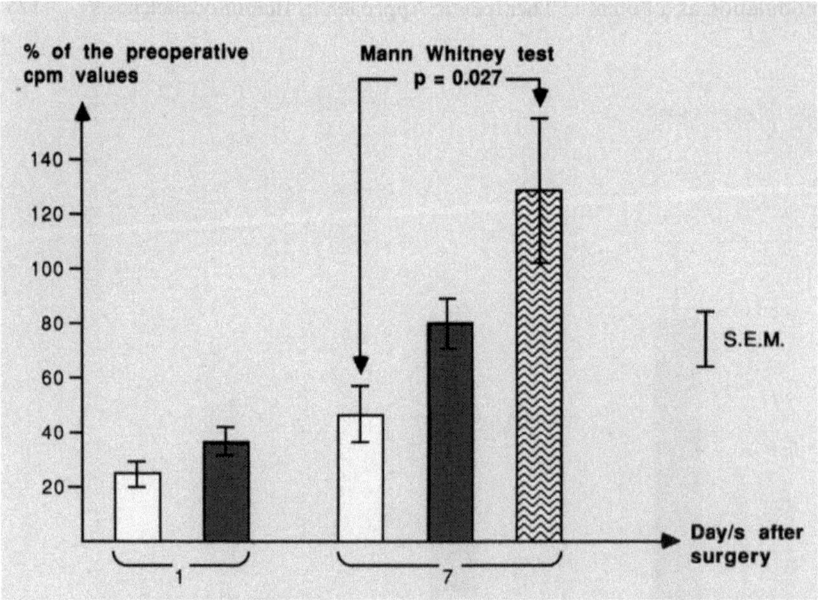

Fig. 7. Antigen-induced proliferation of PBMCs obtained from surgical patients randomized into three groups. Eight patients without thymopentin treatment (□) were used as controls, nine patients were treated with thymopentin 50 mg s.c. 2 h before surgery (■), and eight patients were treated with thymopentin 50 mg s.c. 2 h before and 2 days after surgery (▤). The values from the thymopentin-treated groups assessed on day 1 are pooled

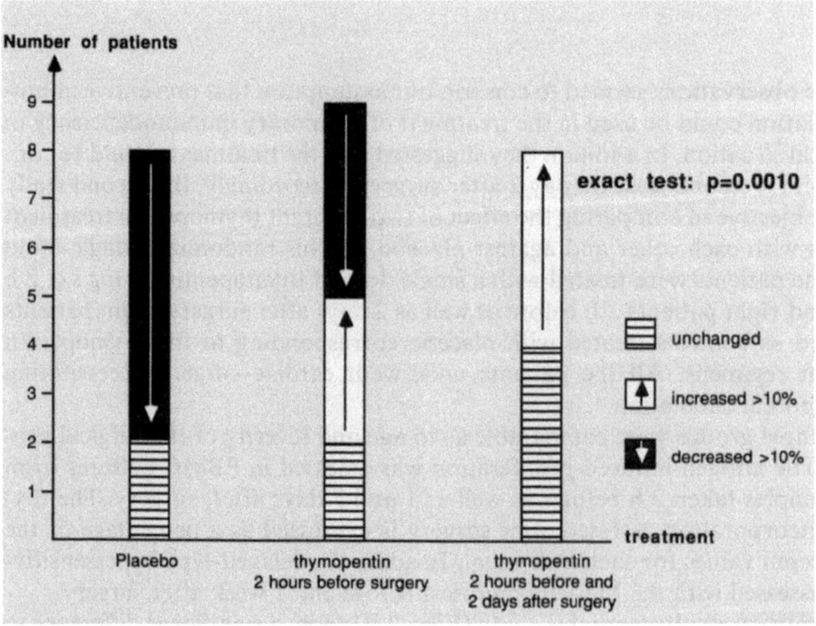

Fig. 8. Distribution of surgical patients according to postoperative changes in Mérieux multitest scores assessed 1 week after surgery versus those which were assessed during the week before surgery

other groups. In contrast to the first study thymopentin was not able to prevent the reduction in the thymidine incorporation on the first postoperative day. The lack of this effect in this second study may be only an apparent contradiction.

It should be realized that in the second study all patients underwent extracorporeal circulation, while no patients did so in the first study. Thus the blood of the patients in the second study was at least partly exchanged some hours after

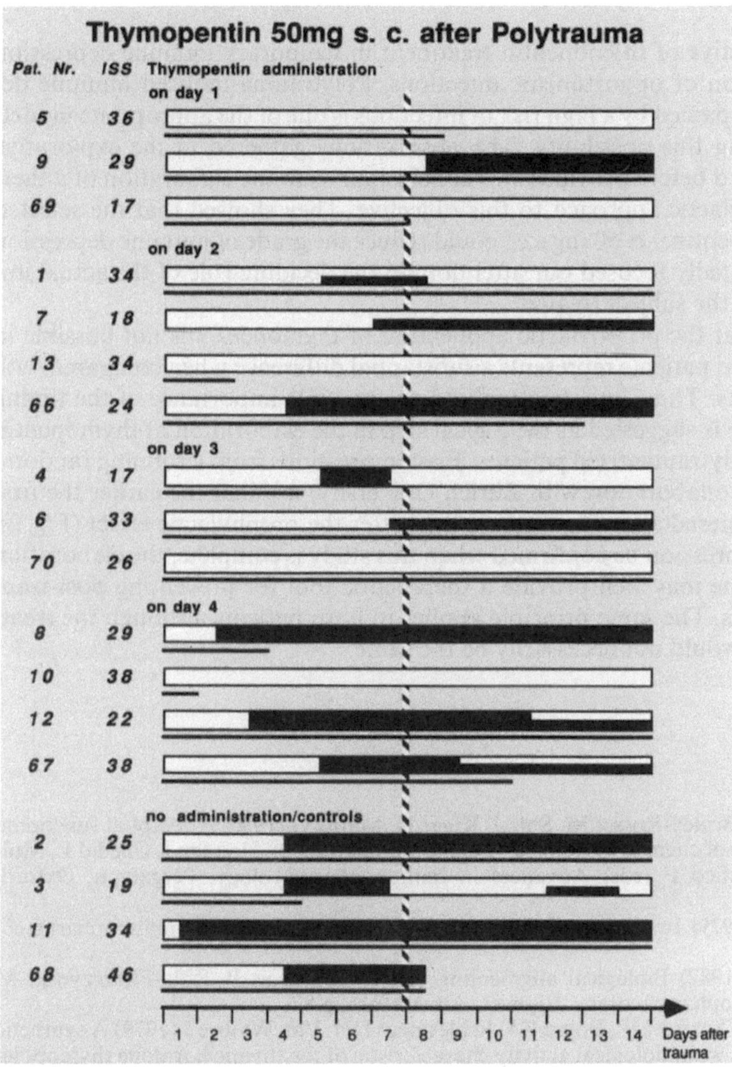

Fig. 9. Frequency and duration of infections during the first 2 weeks after multiple trauma (preliminary results of collaboration with Zurich University). The patients were randomized into five groups. Thymopentin was administered as a single dose. No infection, ▭; definitive infection, ■; suspicion of infection treated with antibiotics, ▬; duration of intubation, —; ISS, injury severity score

the first dose of thymopentin and the remaining cells became influenced by the extracorporeal circulation. Considering the importance of the immune system in determining the outcome of immunomodulation, it would be very surprising if the same reaction to the first dose of thymopentin had been observed in both studies.

Perspectives

The final objective of thymopentin treatment in temporary immune depression is the prevention of opportunistic infections. Polytrauma-induced immune depression accompanied by a high risk of infections is one of the appropriate models for investigating this possibility. The observations gathered in the explorative studies discussed before provided two conclusions as to the elaboration of a therapeutic/prophylactic approach to this objective. They showed that the selected dose of thymopentin, i.e. 50 mg s.c., could reduce the grade of immune depression and have repeatedly focused our attention on the deciding role of the actual immune status of the subject treated.

The fact that the prophylactic application of thymopentin is not possible in polytraumatized patients represents a substantial difference when compared with surgical patients. Thus, investigation into the possible importance of the timing of the first dose is suggested as the logical step in the elaboration of thymopentin treatment in polytraumatized patients. First impressions from a running randomized study (in collaboration with Zürich University) are that the earlier the first dose is administered after the trauma, the better the prophylactic effect (Fig. 9). Should this impression be confirmed when this study is complete, the elaboration of a dose regime may well provide a therapeutic tool for preventing post-traumatic infections. The same principle applies in burn patients although the treatment regimen would not necessarily be the same.

References

1. Florentin I, Bruley-Rosset M, Sulz J, Kiger N, Mathe G (1980) Attempt at functional classification of chemically defined immunomodulators. In: Hadden J, Chedid L, Mullen P, Spreafico F (eds) Advances in immunopharmacology. Pergamon, Oxford, p 311
2. Hadden J (1979) Immunopharmacology of mice and men. Int J Immunopharmacol 1:5
3. Renoux G (1982) Biological augmenting agents. In: Sirois P, Rola-Pleszczynski M (eds) Immunopharmacology. Elsevier, Amsterdam, p 87
4. Goldstein G, Scheid MP, Boyse EA, Schlesinger DH, Van Wauwe J (1979) A synthetic pentapeptide with biological activity characteristic of the thymic hormone thymopoietin. Science 204:1309–1310
5. Schlesinger DH, Goldstein G (1975) The amino acid sequence of thymopoietin II. Cell 5:361–365
6. Audhya T, Schlesinger DH, Goldstein G (1981) Complete amino acid sequences of bovine thymopoietins I, II and III: closely homologous polypeptides. Biochemistry 20:6195–6200

7. Bolla K, Duchateau J, Cappel R (1987) Strategical aspects of immunomodulation based on the influence of thymopentin on immune responses. In: Immune regulation by characterized polypeptides. Liss, New York, p 61
8. Audhya T, Goldstein G (1985) Thymopentin: stability considerations and potency by various routes of administration. Surv Immunol Res 4(1):17
9. Bolla K, Cappel R, Duchateau J (1987) Activation of peripheral blood lymphocytes as a potential basic mechanism of immunomodulation. Int J Immunotherapy 3:71
10. Howard RJ (1979) Effect of burn injury, mechanical trauma and operation on immune defenses. Surg Clin North Am 59:199
11. Miller SE, Miller CL, Trunkey DD (1982) The immune consequences of trauma. Surg Clin North Am 62:167
12. Baker CC, Miller CL, Trunkey DD (1979) Identity of mononuclear cells which compromise the resistance of trauma patients. J Surg Res 26:478
13. Waymack JP, Gonce SJ, Miskell P, Alexander JW (1985) Mechanisms of action of two new immunomodulators. Arch Surg 120:43
14. Waymack JP, Metz J, Garnet D, Sax H, Alexander JW (1985) Effect of immunomodulators on macrophage function in burned animals. Surg Forum 36:110
15. Waymack JP, Miskell P, Gonce S, Alexander JW (1984) Immunomodulators in the treatment of peritonitis in burned malnourished animals. Surgery 96:336
16. Bolla K, Duchateau J, Delespesse G, Servais G (1984) Immunomodulation with thymopentin in humans. Int J Clin Pharm Res 6:431
17. Faist E, Riedel A, Bolla K (1987) Influence of thymopentin on postsurgical immune deficiency, a clinic pilot study. Int J Clin Pharm Res 7:83–87

Perioperative Immunomodulation in Patients with Major Surgical Trauma

E. Faist

Introduction

Perioperative immunomodulatory therapy is designed to give immunoprotective support to those patients in whom iatrogenic mechanical trauma may give rise to a high susceptibility to infection, especially when other risk factors (e.g., malnourishment, age, malignancy) are present [12].

When the posttraumatic immunologic changes on a cellular level were studied in patients with burns or accidental mechanical or elective surgical trauma, it was found [9–11, 13, 36, 40] that the impairment of the monocyte/T-cell interaction results mainly from two functional aberrations (Fig. 1):

1. The lack of functionally intact CD4+ helper/inducer cells
2. The overrepresentation of negative regulatory active suppressor monocytes (Mø) mediated through the cytokine prostaglandin E_2 (PGE_2).

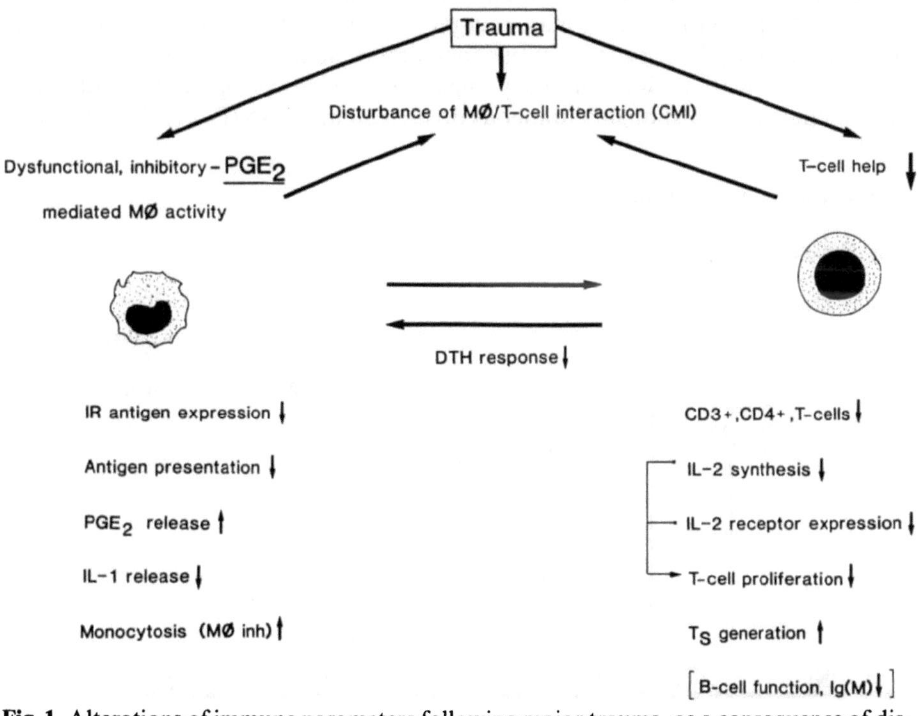

Fig. 1. Alterations of immune parameters following major trauma, as a consequence of disturbed Mø/T-cell interaction

Immune Consequences of
Trauma, Shock and Sepsis
Eds. Faist/Ninnemann/Green

Study Designs

Several synthetic immunomodulatory agents that may help to restore the altered immunologic parameters and to counteract the action of active suppressor cells have recently been investigated in animal models. One of these compounds, thymopentin (TP-5), a synthetic pentapeptide with the five amino acids ARG–LYS–ASP–VAL–TYR corresponding to the amino acids 32–36 of thymopoietin, possesses the biological activities of this naturally occurring polypeptide hormone [17, 30]. The immunoregulatory effects of TP-5 on peripheral T-cells are mediated via elevated intracellular cyclic GMP (cGMP). This thymomimetic substance is characterized by an ability selectively to induce rapid T-cell differentiation and to normalize immune dysbalances in a number of model systems [42].

Patients who preoperatively lack adequate immunoreactivity are deemed to be anergic or relatively anergic; they run a 1:3 chance of major sepsis compared to 1:20 in controls if they undergo major surgery without correction of suppressed host defense mechanisms [6]. In the course of preliminary studies, we found that the subcutaneous administration of 50 mg TP-5 in elderly, mostly hyporesponsive or anergic, patients resulted in a considerable elevation of their in vitro lymphocyte proliferation capacity 2 h after treatment [14]. In further studies it was therefore our objective to determine if perioperative treatment with TP-5 could significantly enhance in vivo and in vitro parameters of cell-mediated immunity (CMI) in patients after major surgery. To this end, in a placebo-controlled randomized study [15], patients with congenital or acquired heart disease undergoing surgery with cardiopulmonary bypass were each perioperatively administered a single or two-shot subcutaneous dose of 50 mg TP-5 (P_{TP-5}) (Fig. 2). CMI

group A: n=9; 1x50 mg TP-5 s.c. d 0

group B: n=8; 2x50 mg TP-5 s.c. d0/ d2

group C: n=8; Placebo d 0/d 2

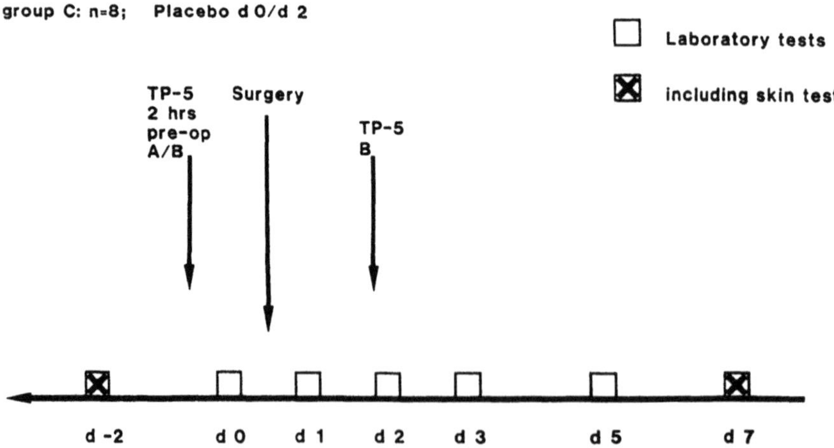

Fig. 2. The experimental protocol, showing time of TP-5 administration and frequency of laboratory tests

parameters assessed were the in vivo delayed type hypersensitivity (DTH) response [preoperatively on day (D) 0 and on D7 postoperatively] to a seven recall antigen skin test battery (Multitest Mérieux), the antigen cocktail induced in vitro lymphocyte proliferation (LP) of peripheral blood mononuclear cells (PBMCs), and in vitro interleukin 2 (IL-2) synthesis.

In a further series of human in vivo studies we evaluated the efficacy of a prostaglandin synthetase inhibitor in correcting postoperative abnormalities of CMI and in preventing infectious morbidity and mortality [16]. Elevated levels of prostaglandins of the E series (PGE) have long been postulated to represent one of the major trigger mechanisms of posttraumatic immunosuppression, thus contributing substantially to the ensuing high risk of opportunistic infection in injured people [37]. Increased release of PGE_2 in the trauma victim from macrophages (Mø) and skin cells occurs after injury. A wide array of abnormalities of immunoregulation have been attributed to excessive PGE_2 activity [18], such as decreased T-cell blastogenesis [10, 27], IL-2 synthesis [11, 52], depressed cytolysis by activated T-cells [31], suppression of antibody formation [19], and impairment of neutrophil migration [51]. Nonsteroidal antiinflammatory drugs (NSAIDS), by inhibiting PGE_2 production, also modulate immune responses in vitro and in vivo [2, 20]. A number of laboratories have found evidence that immunoreactive PGE_2 is to be identified as the common link in the malfunction of the Mø/T-cell interactive network after trauma [28, 37]. PGE_2-mediated suppression of cellular immunity has furthermore been characterized as a reproducible in vitro abnormality in patients with melanoma, head and neck carcinoma, lung carcinoma, and Hodgkin's lymphoma [3, 4, 26, 27]. It was also in hyporesponsive patients with Hodgkin's disease that Goodwin et al., over a decade ago, successfully demonstrated the in vivo efficacy of prostaglandin synthetase inhibitors in restoring impaired immune responses [21].

Use of the cyclooxygenase blocker indomethacin to enhance posttraumatic immune responses in vivo has been attempted in murine models of burn injury. Hansbrough et al. noted an enhancement of depressed hypersensitivity after NSAIDS injection [29], while Kupper et al. noted that defects of antigen presen-

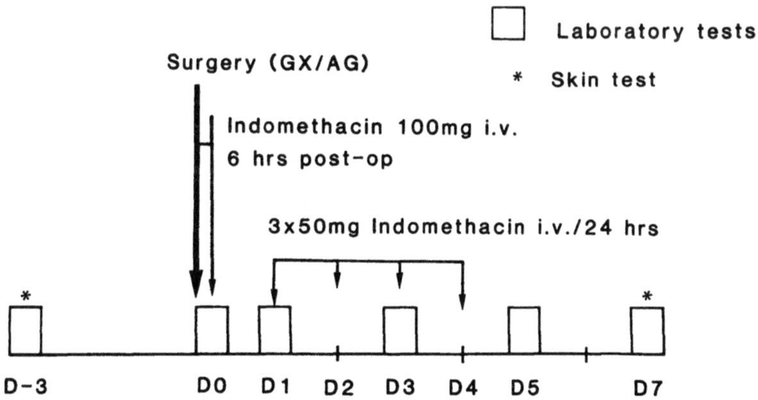

Fig. 3. The experimental protocol, showing time of indomethacin administration and frequency of laboratory tests

tation and induction of T-cell blastogenesis in splenic macrophages from burned mice could be reversed with NSAIDS [33].

Two groups of patients who had undergone gastrectomy (GX) or reconstruction of the abdominal aorta (AG) comprised the study population for in vivo experiments with the cyclooxygenase inhibitor indomethacin (Fig. 3). Following randomization, patients in the treated group (P_{Indo}) received 100 mg indomethacin i.v. 6 h postoperatively, and 3 × 50 mg indomethacin i.v. over 24 h on the postoperative days 1, 2, 3, and 4. The number and type of infectious complications was recorded. CMI parameters studied in vivo and in vitro included DTH skin response to recall antigens, PBMC phenotyping, mitogen-induced lymphoproliferation, and IL-2 synthesis.

Results

PBMC Proliferation

The baseline values of PBMC proliferation (lymphocyte transformation test) in all three patient groups of the TP-5 study were very similar (Fig. 4). On D1 postoperatively, the proliferative responses were depressed to 22 ± 8% (group C, un-

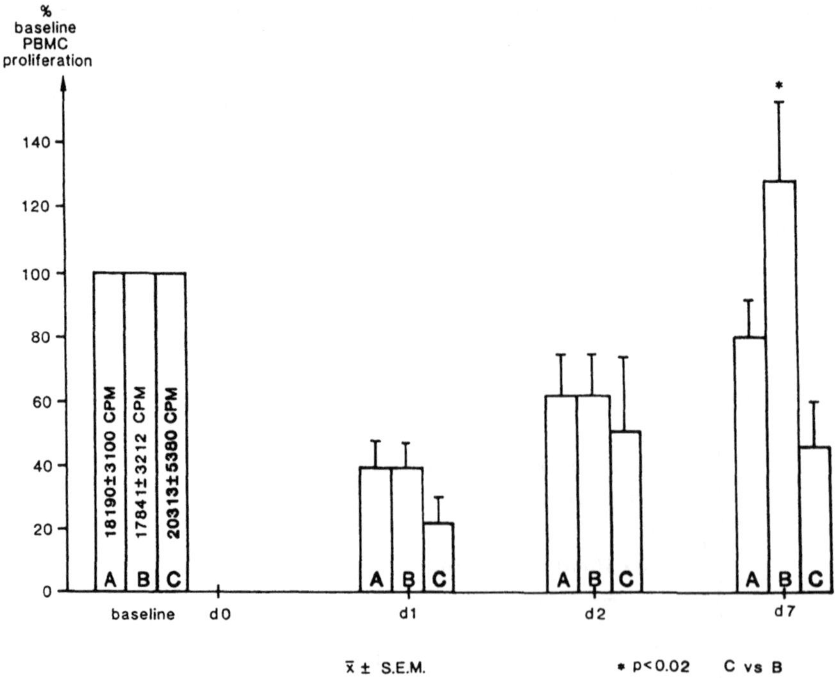

Fig. 4. The lymphocyte proliferation capacity (LTT) of in vitro PBMC cultures on different days following surgery. The results are expressed as percentage changes compared to the baseline values (d0) for all three patient groups (mean ± SEM). *p«0.02 compared to group C

treated) and to 39±8% (groups A+B, treated) of the corresponding baseline values. On D2 postoperatively, proliferation mounted to 51±23% (group C) and to 62±13% (groups A+B). On D7, it remained significantly suppressed (46±14%) in the untreated patients (group C), but had increased to 80±12% in group A (single dose) and to 129±25% in group B (double dose). There is a significant difference ($p < 0.02$, Mann–Whitney test) in proliferation on D7 between the placebo-treated group C patients and those who were administered a double dose of TP-5.

Lymphocyte proliferation in the indomethacin protocol was carried out with two stimulators, the lectin PHA and an antigen cocktail. The PBMCs of control patients (P_C) in the AG and GX group showed considerable depression of their proliferative responses on D3 and D5 (Fig. 5). The impairment of proliferation, compared to the corresponding baseline values, was more profound in cultures using the antigen cocktail, proliferative responses being 49%–57% of baseline values compared to an average suppression of 25% in the PHA cultures. The profile of P_C in the GX group is also shown. In contrast to P_C, the PBMCs of P_{Indo} following aortic grafting did not show any significant alteration of the proliferative responses during the whole observation period. Especially on D3, there was a tendency for values to be above baseline. PBMC proliferation for P_{Indo} in the GX group was within the normal range until D5 in PHA cultures. In antigen cocktail cultures of P_{Indo}, there was considerably less depression of proliferation on all days postoperatively, compared to P_C.

DTH Responses

Within the indomethacin study, in P_C both types of operative procedures resulted in a massive decrease in the quality and quantity of the skin responses (Fig. 6). In comparison, calculation of the average number and diameter of the skin responses postoperatively in P_{Indo} revealed that cyclooxygenase therapy could apparently preserve the preoperative CMI status in these patients. The average number of positive antigen responses (1.9±0.4 for AG and 0.75±0.3 for GX) and the average diameter of the antigen responses (8.5±2.5 for AG and 3.1±1.5 for GX) were reduced in AG P_C to 55%/56% and in GX P_C to 60%/23%. Postoperatively, the number of DTH responses was increased in P_{Indo} to 160% (AG) and 148% (GX) of the corresponding baseline values, while in P_{Indo} of the AG group no essential reduction of DTH responses was seen postoperatively. Of the P_C, 20% became anergic. It was interesting to see that two preoperatively anergic P_{Indo} showed normal DTH responses postoperatively, while all preoperatively anergic P_C remained so after surgery.

There was a deterioration in DTH reactivity in 50% of the normergic P_C (GX), while only 22% of the P_{Indo} patients had impaired immune reactivity postoperatively. Of all GX patients, 53% were anergic preoperatively. Of the previously anergic P_{Indo}, 22% had a normal skin response postoperatively, while one P_{Indo} became anergic following surgery.

The evaluation of the DTH skin responses in the TP-5 study did not show any significant differences between the patient groups before surgery (Fig. 7). On D7

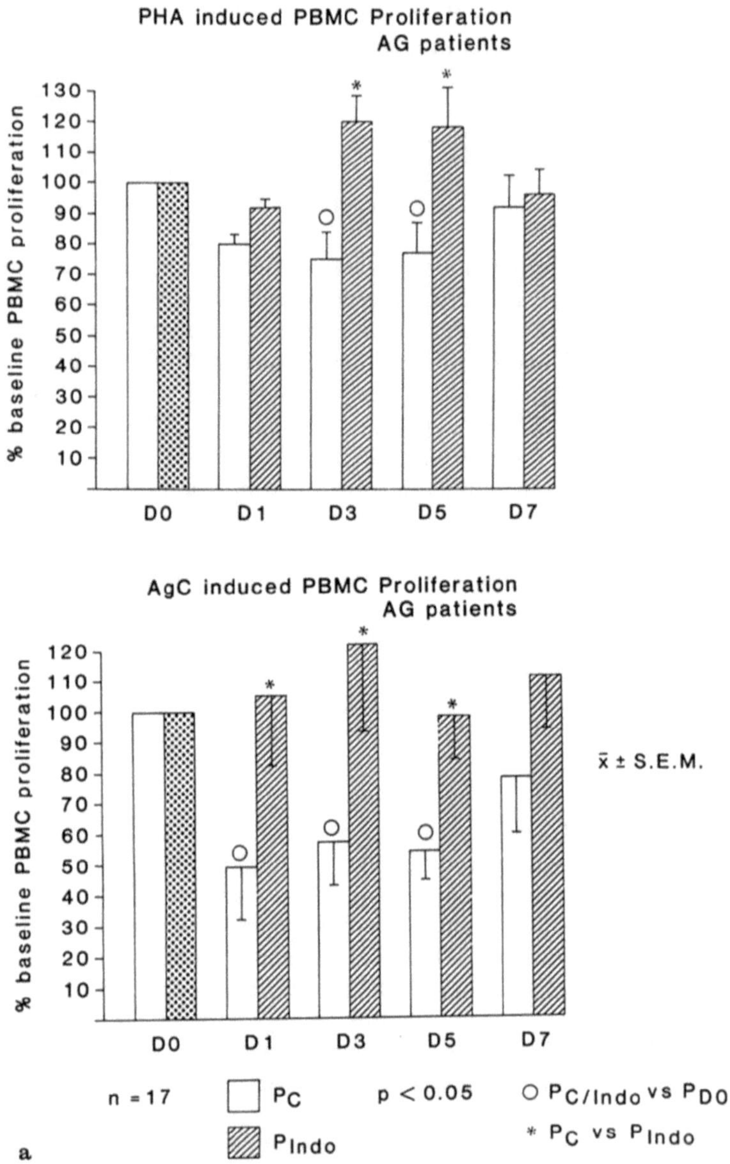

Fig. 5 a, b. PHA and antigen cocktail responses in PBMCs of P_{Indo} and P_C on consecutive days following gastrectomy (**b** GX) or implantation of an aortic graft (**a** AG). Responses are shown as mean percentages of baseline responses. * Significant difference ($p \ll 0.05$) between P_C and P_{Indo}

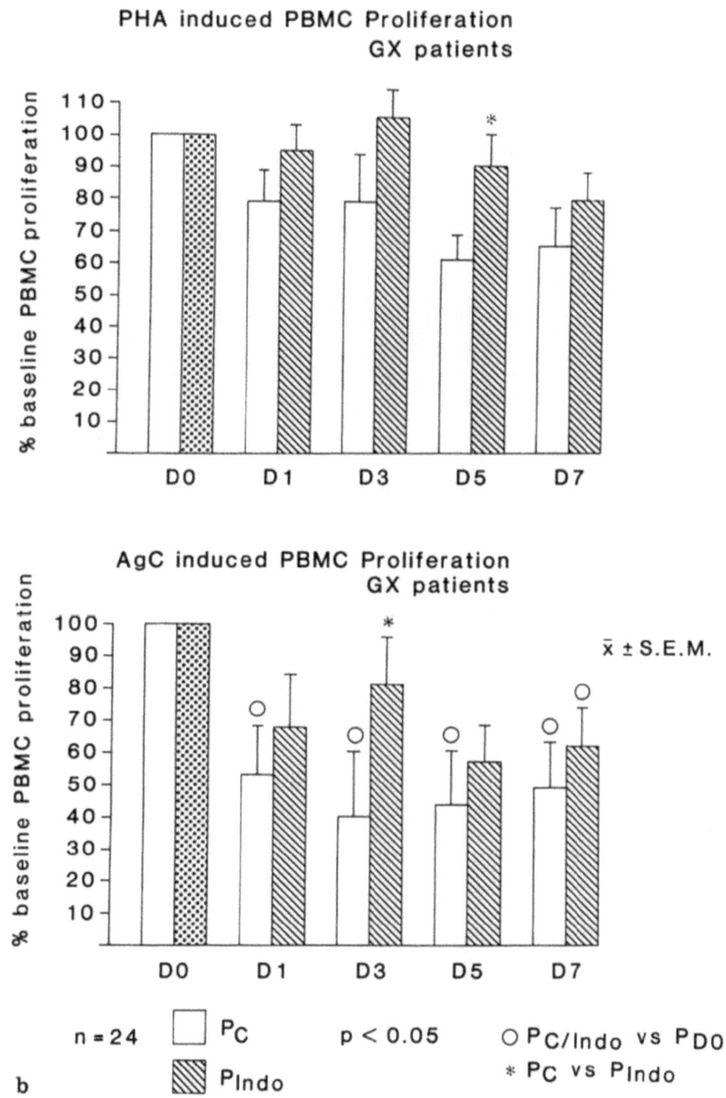

b

Fig. 5b

postoperatively, a significant depression of both measures was noted for the placebo-treated patients in group C ($p<0.05$). The number of positive reactions dropped from 2.4 ± 0.6 to 1.8 ± 0.5 ($p<0.05$), and the sum of diameters was reduced to half of the baseline value, from 12 ± 3 to 6 ± 2 mm ($p<0.05$). In the TP-5-treated patients the number of positive reactions changed from 2.6 ± 0.4 on D0 to 2.1 ± 0.5 on D7 (group A), and from 2.4 ± 0.9 to 2.6 ± 3.8 (group B). The sum of diameters fell slightly in group A patients from 10 ± 2 to 8 ± 2, while in group B it changed from 11 ± 4 to 12 ± 4. The intergroup comparison showed a significant difference between the controls and patients treated twice with TP-5 (group C vs group B) for the number of positive reactions ($p<0.05$) and the sum of mean diameters ($p<0.01$).

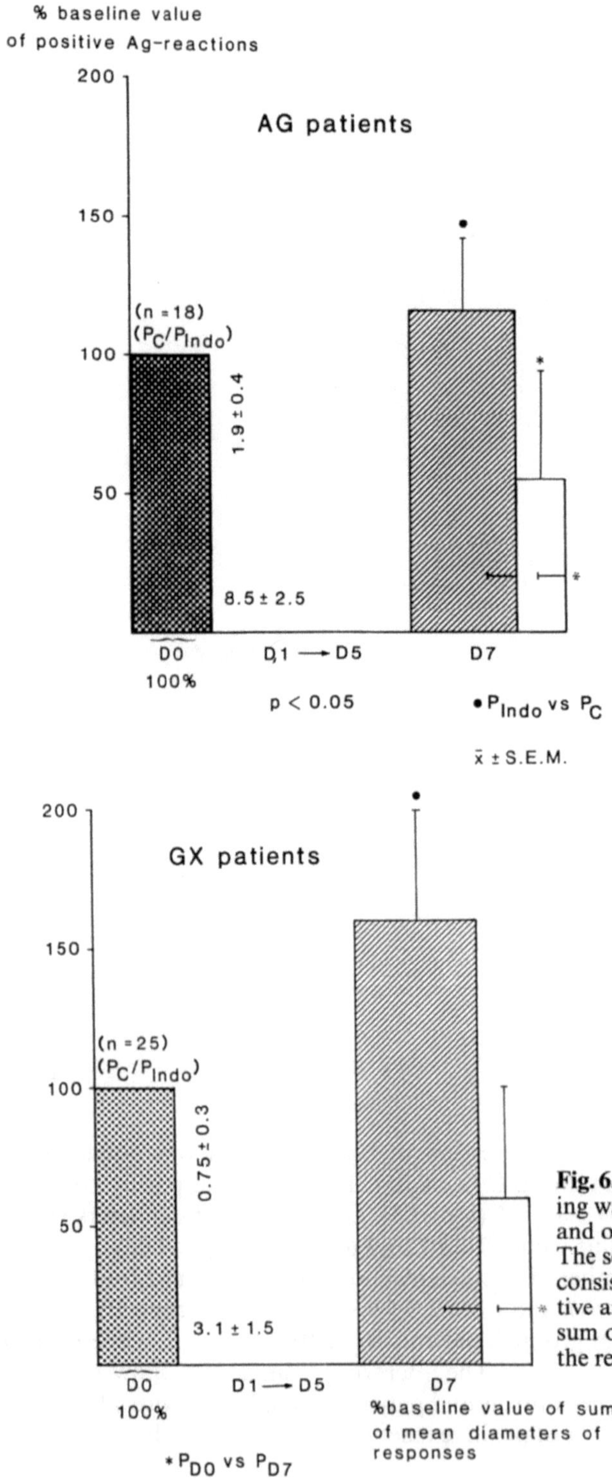

Fig. 6. DTH response skin testing was done preoperatively and on D 7 postoperatively. The score of the DTH response consists of the number of positive antigen reactions and the sum of the mean diameters of the responses

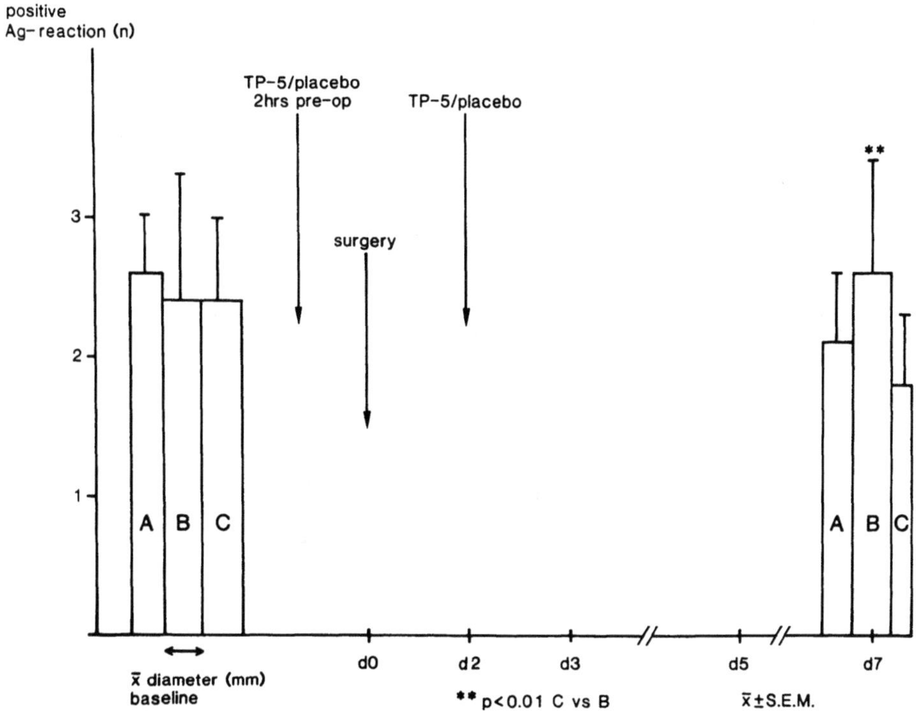

Fig. 7. DTH response skin testing was done preoperatively and on D 7 postoperatively. The score of the DTH response consists of the number of positive antigen reactions and sum of the mean diameter of the responses. ** $p \ll 0.01$ compared to group C for the sum of diameters

PBMC Phenotyping

While TP-5 treatment in our studies did not cause any essential change in the PBMC subpopulations compared to untreated control patients, postoperative administration of cyclooxygenase inhibitors resulted in most remarkable changes of the capacity of T-lymphocytes to express receptor sites.

A considerable reduction, compared to baseline levels, of cell surface receptor expression for the CD3+, CD4+, and IL-2R+ subpopulations following AG and GX, was observed in P_C (Fig. 8). The reduction of CD3+, CD4+ and IL-2R+ PBMCs varied between 30% and 70% of baseline until D5, with a tendency towards recovery on D7, especially in the GX group. The PBMCs of P_{Indo} were significantly less depleted of these T-cell receptors than the P_C group. CD3+ and CD4+ subpopulations never fell below 82% (CD3+) and 75% (CD4+) of the corresponding baseline values. On the majority of days, the baseline values were either reached or even slightly exceeded. There was also a considerable indomethacin-induced protective effect for IL-2R expression. In P_C of the GX group, the number of IL-2R+ cells was consistently suppressed to 60% of baseline values (53 ± 4% of PBMCs) on all days postoperatively. In P_{Indo} the number of IL-2R+ PBMCs never dropped below baseline values until D5 postoperatively.

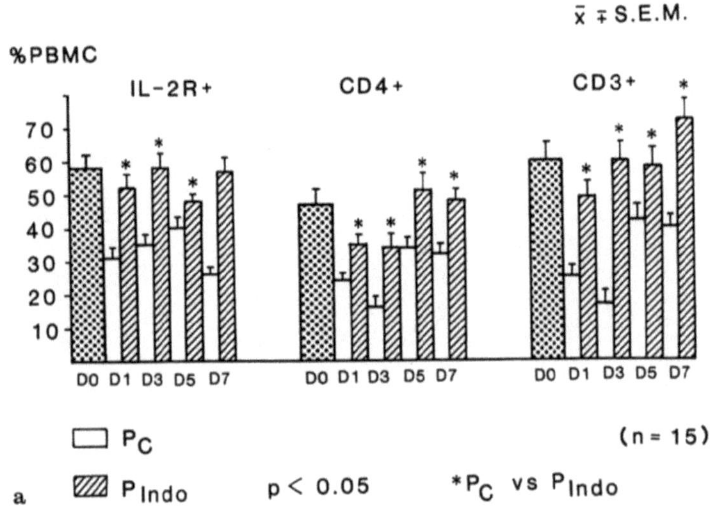

a

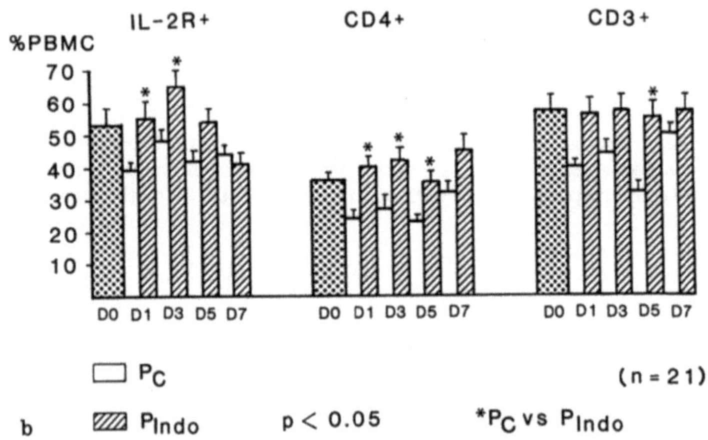

b

Fig. 8 a, b. Phenotyping of CD3+, CD4+ and IL−2R+ PBMC subpopulations of **a** AG and **b** GX P_C and P_{Indo}. *Asterisks* on consecutive days following GX and AG indicate values that are significantly different ($p \ll 0.05$) between P_C and P_{Indo}

The trauma-induced monocytosis in all patients after surgery was expressed through a considerable elevation of LeuM3+ PBMCs (Fig. 9). The Mø baseline levels of 20 ± 2% (GX) or 21 ± 2% of PBMCs (AG) were exceeded. P_{Indo}, in contrast, developed a significantly less pronounced monocytosis, numbers remaining within the range of baseline values during the observation period in the majority of patients.

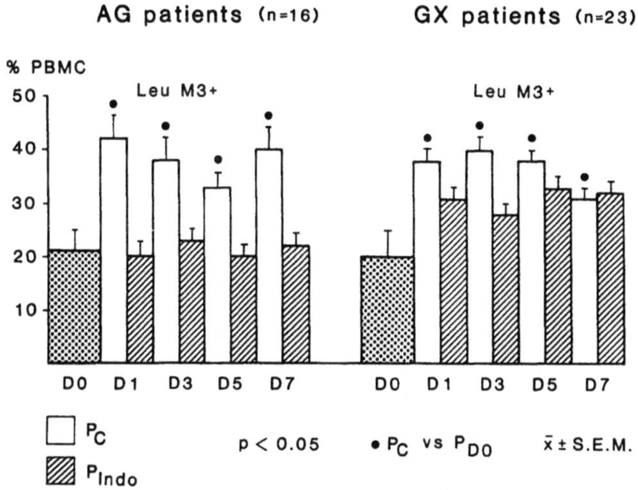

Fig. 9. Phenotyping of LeuM3+ mononuclear leukocytes of P_C and P_{Indo} on consecutive days following surgery. Values that are significantly different ($p \ll 0.05$) from baseline data on D0 are dotted

In Vitro IL-2 Synthesis

The capacity of PBMC cultures to produce IL-2-containing supernatants following 48 h stimulation with PHA was evaluated in both study protocols. Compared to preoperative values, IL-2 synthesis was massively suppressed postoperatively ($p<0.05$) in almost all PBMC cultures of patients undergoing cardiac surgery (Fig. 10). Although there was a clear difference in baseline levels between TP-5-treated patients (groups A and B pooled, $n=17$) and controls (group C; $n=7$), with 0.7 ± 0.1 U/ml versus 1.1 ± 0.1 U/ml, due most likely to the small number of placebo-treated patients assessed, the absolute quantity of IL-2 synthesis postoperatively was not essentially different between the groups. In TP-5-treated patients there was a persistent suppression to 0.3 U/ml on all days documented, while in group C patients the IL-2 output varied between 0.3 and 0.5 U/ml. Thus, there was a uniform average suppression of $\geqq 50\%$ for both groups. The addition of the PGE_2 inhibitor indomethacin to the PBMC cultures resulted in a postoperative elevation of 57% in the TP-5-treated patients, compared to 18% in group C. Between D1 and D7 postoperatively, indomethacin consistently increased IL-2 synthesis in both groups by between 100% and 130%, compared to the corresponding native PHA-stimulated cultures. This resulted in a virtually complete restoration to the levels of preoperative synthesis in patients treated with TP-5.

Compared to the patients undergoing cardiac surgery in the TP-5 study, in whom preoperative IL-2 synthesis was clearly at a level similar to that in young healthy control persons (0.95 ± 0.01 U/ml), the average preoperative values for in vitro IL-2 synthesis in AG and GX patients (0.48 ± 0.008 U/ml) were considerably lower (Fig. 11). As the baseline values in the GX and AG group did not differ significantly, the analysis of postoperative changes of lymphokine synthesis was

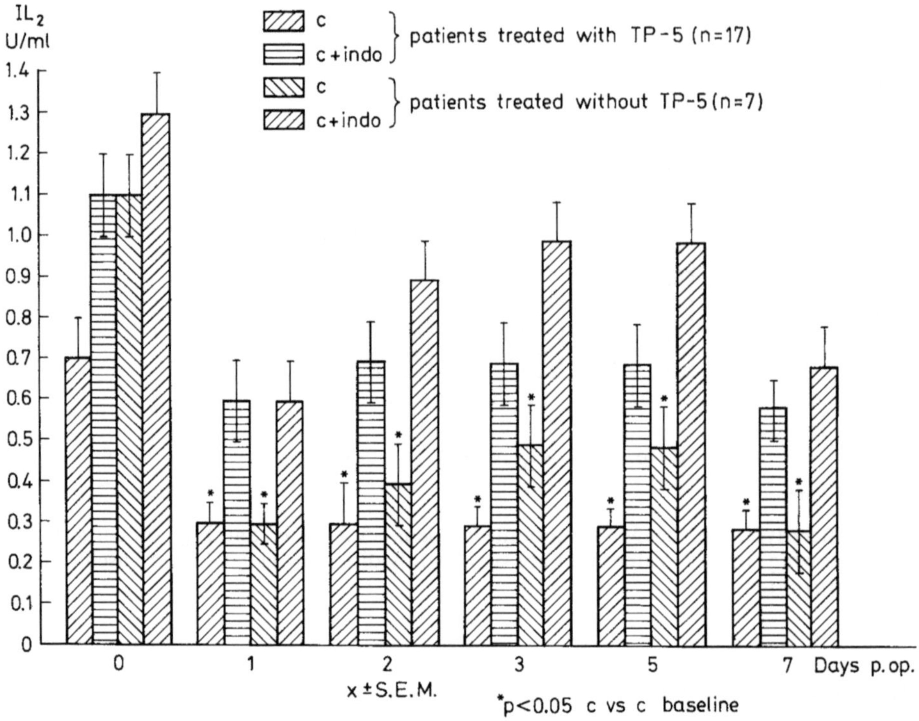

Fig. 10. In vitro IL-2 synthesis on various days following surgery in patients treated with and without TP-5. *c*, IL-2 synthesis from native, PHA-stimulated cultures; *c+indo*, IL-2 synthesis following addition of indomethacin to the cell cultures

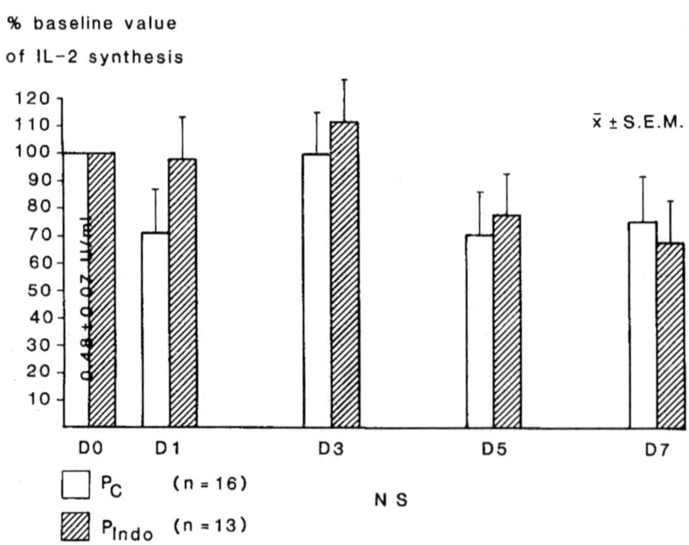

Fig. 11. IL-2 synthesis of PBMC cultures of P_C and P_{Indo} on various days following major surgery (GX or AG). IL-2 output is expressed as percentage of the baseline value (0.48 ± 0.07 U/ml = 100%) on consecutive days after surgery

carried out from the pooled data for both operative procedures. In vitro IL-2 synthesis in 16 P_C was compared with that in 13 P_{Indo}. IL-2 synthesis of P_C fell to 71% of the baseline values on D1 with complete recovery on D3, then dropped back to 71% (D5) and 76% (D7). PBMCs of the P_{Indo} group showed practically unaltered IL-2 synthesis until D3 (D1 98%, D3 112%), which was then reduced to 78% on D5 and 68% on D7. Also, there is no significant suppression of IL-2 synthesis in the P_C group until D3, while the reduction of IL-2 synthesis on D5 (78%) and D7 (68%) was comparable to that in the P_{Indo} group. No statistical differences were found in the intergroup comparison. Analysis of the individual profiles of IL-2 synthesis of P_C and P_{Indo} patients revealed that there was apparently no essential protective effect of cyclooxygenase inhibition for this particular cell function, as 46% of P_{Indo} (6/13) showed suppressed lymphokine synthesis compared to 56% (9/16) in the P_C group.

Discussion

From the analysis of the immunomodulatory studies presented above, it can be concluded that postoperative impairment of the in vivo DTH response and in vitro lymphocyte proliferation can be effectively counteracted by perioperative subcutaneous administration of TP-5 and postoperative administration of the cyclooxygenase inhibitor indomethacin. Repeated treatment with TP-5 for 2 days postoperatively was superior to a single preoperative administration.

In contrast to TP-5 treatment, which in our experience did not result in any reproducible change of receptor expression capacity, postoperative indomethacin therapy had a considerable effect on T-cell receptor expression. Compared to the significant decrease of CD3+, CD4+ and IL-2R+ T-cells following surgery in P_C, the inhibition of prostaglandin synthesis did indeed have a pronounced protective effect for these receptor sites. Also, P_{Indo} developed a significantly lower degree of monocytosis than P_C.

In parallel with the IL-2R protection [44], it might be expected that the depression of IL-2 synthesis in PBMC cultures of traumatized individuals would be counterbalanced following blockage of the cAMP pathway. Such an IL-2 synthesis protective effect has been demonstrated by Rodrick et al., who administered ibuprofen, another cyclooxygenase inhibitor, prior to endotoxin infusion in young volunteers [41]. In our study, the in vitro synthesis of IL-2 was equally depressed postoperatively in almost all patients, independent of whether they were undergoing perioperative TP-5 treatment, postoperative indomethacin therapy, or no treatment.

Following our in vivo studies, we have the impression that, according to all possible measures of T-cell function, IL-2 synthesis response is highly sensitive to even slight changes of systemic conditions. There is a rapid reduction of IL-2 output following any disturbance; conversely, however, it is most difficult to achieve consistent increases with immunomodulatory interventions in vivo.

The in vitro addition of indomethacin (1 mg/ml) to PBMC cultures from P_C, P_{Indo}, and TP-5-treated patients resulted, as previously reported by several authors from other experiments, in a dramatic enhancement of IL-2 synthesis [11,

40]. Additional in vitro studies have demonstrated that TP-5 can only increase IL-2 synthesis in antigen-stimulated cultures, and only at certain concentrations when used in the preculture period [1].

As both P_C and P_{Indo} PBMC cultures responded equally well to PGE_2 inhibition, we must assume that the in vivo stimulus with indomethacin at the concentrations used in this study is too weak, or it undergoes some process of inactivation for it to result in a measurable, lasting effect in terms of enhanced lymphokine synthesis. Perhaps by looking at the intracellular concentrations of cAMP or cGMP in PBMCs one might be able to get sufficient evidence on a molecular basis for an effect of in vivo cyclooxygenase administration on immunocompetent cells [32].

Our studies investigating the efficacy of TP-5 as a perioperative immunopotentiating agent have been preceeded by a number of animal studies. Waymack et al. demonstrated that TP-5 treatment could prevent the onset of septic complications in immunocompromised animals and thus resulted in significantly improved survival time [48]. Investigating the mechanisms of action, the authors observed an increase in neutrophil bactericidal function as well as an enhanced ability of macrophages to phagocytose and kill bacteria [49]. Stinnet et al. found that TP-5 was beneficial in terms of preventing *Pseudomonas aeruginosa* infection in burned guinea pigs [43]. Greenhalgh et al. tested the effect of TP-5 on macrophage function during wound healing in burned mice, but could not find any stimulatory effect [22]. Cell mediated immune function in burned guinea pigs following TP-5 injections was measured by Magsudi and Miller, using the in vitro antibody forming cell assay [34]. They demonstrated a significant improvement of splenocytes in producing a secondary immune response to sheep red blood cells in animals treated with TP-5 compared to untreated animals. The failure of TP-5, however, to completely restore the depressed antibody forming cell response was postulated to result from involvement of the PGE_2-mediated suppressor activity of macrophages. Almost complete restoration of depressed secondary immune responses was found by these authors when TP-5 therapy was combined with indomethacin.

The in vivo effect of indomethacin in subjects with depressed cellular immunity has been demonstrated previously in patients with adult combined immunodeficiency by J. Goodwin. Gross et al. evaluated the effect of administration of the NSAID and niflumic acid in vivo [23]. In their study, the suppressive effect of burn serum on mixed lymphocyte (MLC) and PHA cultures was reduced slightly, but administration of NSAID to patients did not make any difference to clinical outcome. Robinson and coworkers reported as early as 1968 that pretreatment of mice with indomethacin enhanced their ability to resist infection, but this result aroused little attention, presumably because the mechanisms of action of indomethacin were not known at that time [39].

The evaluation of the clinical course in our patients also suggests a beneficial effect of indomethacin treatment in terms of reducing the rate of postoperative infectious complications. Although there were too few patients in this study to show a statistically significant benefit, cyclooxygenase inhibition seems to protect the organism, especially from early opportunistic infection (Table 1). In all P_{Indo} we just saw one case (K.E.) of an early infectious episode of pneumonia and soft

Table 1. Data of postoperative course in patients

	Patient population		P_{Indo}		P_C	
	n	%	*n*	%	*n*	%
GX	25	100	13		12	
Infectious complication	10	40	4/13	31	6/12	50
Uneventful	15	60	9/13	69	6/12	50
AG	18	100	10		8	
Infectious complication	2	11	–/	0	2/ 8	25
Uneventful	16	89	10/10	100	6/ 8	75

Table 2. Postoperative infections

Patient	Age (years)	Sex	P_C/P_{Indo}	Surgery	Site of infection	Severity of infection	Re-intervention	Manifestation of infection ≦D5	Manifestation of infection >D5	Death
N. A.	69	m	P_C	GX	Abd.	Major	+	+	–	–
F. I.	60	f	P_C	GX	ST/UT	Minor	–	+	–	–
R. E.	65	m	P_C	GX	P	Minor	–	+	–	–
S. J.	84	f	P_C	GX	ST/P	Major	+	+	–	–
A. D.	45	m	P_C	GX	P	Minor	–	+	–	–
G. J.	54	m	P_C	GX	ST	Minor	–	+	–	–
B. N.	67	m	P_{Indo}	GX	P	Minor	–	–	+	–
K. E.	66	f	P_{Indo}	GX	Abd.	Major	–	+	–	†
M. W.	56	m	P_{Indo}	GX	ST/P	Major	+	+	–	–
M. J.	64	m	P_{Indo}	GX	P	Major	–	–	+	–
S. A.	48	m	P_C	AG	P	Minor	–	+	–	–
H. M.	60	m	P_C	AG	P	Minor	–	+	–	–

Site of infection: P, pulmonary; ST, soft tissue; UT, urinary tract; Abd., intraabdominal

tissue infection (Table 2). In two other P_{Indo} pneumonia appeared, on D7 and D8 postoperatively. The onset was preceeded in both cases by depression of the immune response, which was normal until D5 under indomethacin treatment. From this clinical observation and the analysis of other laboratory data in a number of patients, we had the impression that the immunoprotective effect of indomethacin decreased immediately after administration was stopped. Thus, we believe that the cyclooxygenase inhibitor treatment should be continued at least up to 7 days posttrauma.

The use of indomethacin at the optimal dosage of 2 mg/kg bodyweight per day was not accompanied by negative side effects like gastroduodenal ulcers, acute tubular necrosis, inhibition of platelet activity, or bronchospasm. Posttraumatic immunologic perturbations are certainly not based solely on immunoreactive PGE_2 activity, but rather, especially in older patients, they are associated with a disturbance of quantitatively and qualitatively inadequate T-cell recruitment. Thus, attempts at therapeutic immunorestoration should aim at a combination of immunopotentiating agents that complement each other functionally. We would assume that the combination of a cyclooxygenase inhibitor with thymomimetic drugs should be the basic therapy to accomplish effective upregulation of CMI in surgical patients at risk. Besides TP-5, isoprinosine (inosine-pranobax-inosiplex), a thymomimetic purine, has been shown in vitro and in vivo to augment various functions of mature T-lymphocytes. It can restore depressed immune responses in both animals and men [24, 25]. Incubation of peripheral blood lymphocytes from patients with acquired immune deficiency syndrome (AIDS) resulted in significant increases or normalization of mitogen-induced lymphocyte proliferative responses. Restoration to normal and supranormal values of lymphocyte proliferation with isoprinosine could also be achieved in patients with multiple injuries, as demonstrated in our own experiments. Incubation of PBMCs with isoprinosine also led to a significant increase in the percentage and number of T helper lymphocytes and resulted in an increase of IL-1 synthesis by monocytes from both normals and patients; depressed production of IL-2 by lymphocytes from AIDS patients was nearly normalized in the presence of isoprinosine. Finally, it could increase the expression of IL-2R on the CD8+ T-lymphocytes as well [45–47].

Instead of using thymomimetic immune response-modifying agents, the administration of IL-2, alone or combined with interferon-γ (both lymphokines being administered in low doses in order to avoid toxic side effects), might be the most pragmatic way of reconstituting or preserving host resistance mechanisms. Intraperitoneal administration of IL-2 has been shown to protect mice from a lethal intraperitoneal challenge of gram-negative bacteria by inducing an influx of polymorphonuclear cells (PMN), whereby the degree of PMN influx into the peritoneal cavity is proportional to the intensity of the inflammatory stimulus [5, 35].

While, as demonstrated, perioperative subcutaneous administration of TP-5 proved to be a most effective immunopotentiating regimen, studies of Waymack et al., evaluating its efficacy in correcting postburn immunologic abnormalities and preventing infectious morbidity and mortality in 24 burn patients, did not show any comparable effect [50]. There were no differences noted between treated and untreated patients in terms of patient mortality, infectious complications or antibiotic use. In contrast, there was even a decreased lymphocyte blastogenic response in the TP-5 treated group 2 weeks after injury, and no difference in CD4/CD8 ratios. However, the authors found a lesser degree of leukopenia during the first week after injury in patients treated with TP-5. The different findings in our studies and the study with burn patients following TP-5 treatment might be considered to reflect the sensitivity of the delicately balanced immune system to manipulation. From a number of experiments it is known that subcutaneous administration of TP-5 in low doses represents the least aggressive immune stimulus, and is thus optimally adaptive [7, 8]. From all that has been understood so far, daily repetition of 50 mg TP-5, via the intravenous route, results in clear overstimulation of the system, adding up to undesired downregulation, as reflected by decreased lymphocyte proliferation in the burn study.

From this last example, we can conclude that successful immunomodulatory intervention is most dependent on long-term evaluation of the dosage, the timing, and the route of administration. Successful immune response modification should optimally avoid stimulating active suppressor cells, should increase helper cell activity, and should be characterized by rapid activity and minimal side effects [38].

In summary, our in vivo studies confirmed a number of in vitro experiments showing that administration of thymomimetic drugs such as indomethacin and prostaglandin synthetase inhibitors could restore the trauma-induced impairment of cell mediated immune responses. Further in vivo work appears warranted to clarify a number of unresolved points before preventive or interventive immunomodulatory therapy can become firmly established. This would include obtaining more information on optimal timing of therapy, patient selection, compatibility following complete derangement of homeostasis (e.g., hemorrhagic shock, onset of septic states), and possible autoimmune side effects.

In spite of all our progress, knowledge about the delicate balance of the immune system is still fragmentary. Further studies must proceed with great caution so as not to give rise to unjustified expectations that the magic bullet for posttraumatic immunorestoration might lie within easy reach.

References

1. Antonacci AC, Chiao J, Reid A et al. (1986) Effect of thymopentin (TP-5) on interleukin-2 production by normal peripheral blood mononuclear cells. J Cell Biochem 81:10A
2. Bacon PA (1984) Nonsteroidal anti-inflammatory drugs and immunologic function – overview of the European experience. The American College of Medicine, October 15, pp 26–31
3. Balch CM, Dougherty PA, Cloud GA et al. (1984) Prostaglandin E_2-mediated suppression of cellular immunity in colon cancer patients. Surgery 95:71–76
4. Balch CM (1986) Immune responses to tumor antigens and their clinical applications. Surgery 100:562–571
5. Chong K (1987) Prophylactic administration of interleukin-2 protects mice from lethal challenge with gram-negative bacteria. Infect Immunol 55:668–673
6. Christou NV (1983) Anergy testing in surgical patients. Infect Surg 10:692
7. Duchateau J, Servais G, Cooman R et al. (1985) In vitro influence of thymopentin on proliferative responses and PHA induced interleukin 2 production in normal human lymphocyte cultures. Surv Immunol Res 1:116
8. Duchateau J, Servais G, Vreyens R et al. (1985) Modulation of immune response in aged humans through different administration modes of thymopentin. Surv Immunol Res 1:116
9. Ertel W, Faist E, Salmen B et al. (in press) Influence of cyclooxygenase inhibition on interleukin-2 receptor (IL-2R) expression after major trauma. Harwood, Surg Res Comm
10. Faist E, Kupper S, Baker CC et al. (1986) Depression of cellular immunity after major injury. Arch Surg 121:1000–1005
11. Faist E, Mewes A, Baker CC et al. (1987) Prostaglandin E_2 (PGE_2)-dependent suppression of interleukin-2 (IL-2) production in patients with major trauma. J Trauma 27:837–848
12. Faist E, Ertel W, Salmen B et al. (in press) The immune enhancing effect of perioperative thymopentin administration in elderly patients undergoing major surgery. Arch Surg

13. Faist E, Mewes A, Strasser Th et al. (1988) Alteration of monocyte (Mø) function following major injury. Arch Surg 123,3:287
14. Faist E, Riedel A, Bolla K (1987) Influence of thymopentin on postsurgical immune deficiency: a clinical pilot study. Int J Clin Pharm Res 7:83
15. Faist E, Baue AE, Dittmer H et al. (1983) Multiple organ failure in polytrauma patients. J Trauma 23:775–787
16. Faist E, Ertel W, Cohnert T et al. (in press) Immunoprotective effects of cyclooxygenase inhibition in patients with major surgical trauma. J Trauma
17. Goldstein G, Audhya TK (1985) Thymopoietin to thymopentin: experimental studies. Surv Immunol Res 4:1
18. Goodwin JS, Webb DR (1980) Regulation of the immune response by prostaglandins. Clin Immunol Immunopathol 15:106–122
19. Goodwin JS, Ceuppens JL (1983) Effect of nonsteroidal antiinflammatory drugs on immune function. Semin Arthritis Rheum 13:134–143
20. Goodwin JS (1980) Prostaglandin synthetase inhibitors as immunoadjuvants in the treatment of cancer. J Immunopharmacol 2:397
21. Goodwin JS, Selinger DS, Messner RP et al. (1978) Effect of indomethacin in vivo on humoral and cellular immunity in humans. Infect Immun 19:430–433
22. Greenhalger D, Garnelli L (1987) Immunomodulators and wound healing. J Trauma 27:510
23. Gros P, Laurent P, Marichy J (1987) The effect of a nonsteroidal antiinflammatory agent on lymphocyte activity after burn (Abstract). Geneva international congress on burn injury
24. Hadden JW (1987) The action of immunopotentiators in vitro on lymphocyte and macrophage activation. In: Werner GH, Loh F (eds) The pharmacology of immunoregulation. Academic, London, p 369
25. Hadden JW (1985) Thymomimetic drugs. In: Miescher PA, Bolis L, Ghione M (eds) Immunopharmacology. Serono Symposia Publications, vol 23. Raven, New York, pp 183–192
26. Han T, Takita H (1980) Indomethacin-mediated enhancement of lymphocyte response to mitogens in healthy subjects and lung cancer patients. Cancer 46:2416–2420
27. Han T, Winnicki MS (1980) Indomethacin-mediated enhancement of lymphocyte response to mitogens. NY State J Med 80:1070–1075
28. Hansbrough JF, Peterson V, Kortz E et al. (1983) Postburn immunosuppression in an animal model: monocyte dysfunction induced by burned tissue. Surgery 93:415–423
29. Hansbrough J, Peterson V, Zapata-Sirvent R et al. (1984) Post burn immunosuppression in an animal model: II. Restoration of cell mediated immunity by immunomodulating drugs. Surgery 95:290–294
30. Heavner GA (1985) Thymopentin structure and relation of thymic factors. Surv Immunol Res 4:11
31. Henney CS, Bourne HR, Lichtenstein LM (1972) The role of cyclic-3′,5′-adenosine monophosphate in the specific cytolytic activity of lymphocytes. J Immunol 108:1526–1534
32. Kammer GM The adenylate cyclase –cAMP – protein kinase A pathway and regulation of the immune response. Immunol Today 9:222–229
33. Kupper TS, Green DR, Baker CC (1985) Defective antigen presentation to a closed T helper cell by macrophages from burned mice can be restored with interleukin-1. Surgery 98:199–206
34. Maghsudi M, Miller CL (1984) The immunomodulating effect of TP5 and indomethacin in burn induced hypoimmunity. J Surg Res 37:133
35. Maddaus MA, Simmons RL (1988) Intraperitoneal administration of recombinant interleukin-2 protects against lethal IP gram-negative sepsis by induction of a neutrophil influx. Am Coll Surg Surg Forum 39:105
36. McLoughlin GA, Wu AV, Saporoschetz et al. (1979) Correlation between anergy and a circulating immunosuppressive factor following major surgical trauma. Ann Surg 190:297
37. Miller-Graziano CL, Fink M, Wu JY et al. (1988) Mechanisms of altered monocyte prostaglandin E_2 production in severely injured patients. Arch Surg 123:293–299

38. Munster AM (1983) Immunologic manipulation of the injured patient–looking into the future. In: Ninnemann JL (ed) Traumatic injury infection and other immunologic sequelae. University Park Press, Baltimore, p 231
39. Robinson HJ, Phares HF, Graessle OE (1968) Effects of indomethacin on acute, subacute, and latent infections in mice and rats. J Bacteriol 96:6–13
40. Rodrick ML, Wood JJ, Grbic JT et al. (1986) Defective IL-2 production in patients with severe burns and sepsis. Lymphokine Res 5:75–80
41. Rodrick ML, Michie HR, Moss NM et al. (in press) In vivo infusion of a single dose of endotoxin in healthy humans causes in vitro alterations of both t cell and adherent cell functions. Proceedings, 1st International congress or immune consequences of trauma, shock and sepsis. Springer, Berlin Heidelberg New York
42. Sundal E, Bolla K (1986) Therapy with thymopentin – a clinical overview. In: Goldstein G, Bach JF (eds) Immune regulation by characterized polypeptides. Alan R. Liss, New York, p 121 (UCLA symposia on molecular and cellular biology, new series)
43. Stinnett JD, Loose LD, Miskell P et al. (1983) Synthetic immunomodulators for prevention of fatal infections in a burned guinea pig model. Ann Surg 198:53
44. Teodorczyk-Injeyan JA, Sparkes BG, Mulls GB et al. (1987) Impaired expression of interleukin-2 receptor (IL-2R) in the immunosuppressed burned patient: reversal by exogenous IL-2. J Trauma 27:180
45. Tsang KY, Fudenberg HH, Donnelly RP (1984)In vitro augmentation of interleukin-2 production and lymphocytes with the tac antigen marker in patients with AIDS. New Engl J Med 310:987
46. Tsang KY, Fudenberg HH, Galbraith GMP et al. (1985) Partial restoration of impaired interleukin-2 production and tac antigen (putative interleukin-2 receptor) expression in patients with acquired immune deficiency syndrome by isoprinosine treatment in vitro. J Clin Invest 75:1538
47. Tsang KY, Donelly RP, Gilbraith PM, Fudenberg HH (1986) Isoprinosine effects on interleukin-1 production in acquired immune deficiency syndrome (AIDS). Int J Immunopharmacol 8:437
48. Waymack JP, Miskell P, Gonce SJ et al. (1984) Immunomodulators in the treatment of peritonitis in burned and malnourished animals. Surgery 96:308
49. Waymack JP, Gonce SJ, Miskell P et al. (1985) Mechanisms of action of two new immunomodulators. Arch Surg 120:23
50. Waymack JP, Jenkins M, Warden GD et al. (1987) A prospective study of thymopentin in severely burned patients. Surg Gynecol Obstet 164:423–430
51. Waymack JP, Yurt RW (in press) The effect of prostaglandin E on immune function in multiple animal models. Arch Surg
52. Wood JJ, Grbic JT, Rodrick ML et al. (1987) Suppression of interleukin 2 production in an animal model of thermal injury is related to prostaglandin synthesis. Arch Surg 122:179–184

Effect of Therapeutic Gamma-Interferon Administration on Wound Infection After Resuscitated Hemorrhagic Shock

D. H. Livingston and M. A. Malangoni

Introduction

Infection remains the leading cause of late morbidity and mortality after injury. Despite the common use of antibiotic prophylaxis in the trauma patient, over two-thirds of patients who die after the initial 48 h after injury do so secondary to sepsis [1]. Our previous work has demonstrated that the use of conventional antibiotic prophylaxis failed to prevent wound infection following hemorrhagic shock and resuscitation [2].

Multiple immunologic derangements have been reported following hemorrhagic shock that may contribute to an increase in susceptibility to infection. Neutrophil, macrophage, and lymphocyte functions have all been shown to be depressed following shock and major injury [3, 4]. Specifically, interferon-gamma (IFN-γ) production has been shown to be depressed following hemorrhagic shock and major injury [5].

Interferon-γ is a glycoprotein produced by lymphocytes exposed to bacteria, viruses, and other antigens. IFN-γ possesses pluripotential immunostimulatory effects on macrophages [6]. Recently, IFN-γ has been shown to increase intracellular killing of bacteria by neutrophils [7]. We investigated the use of IFN-γ, given after bacterial contamination, both alone and combined with antibiotic prophylaxis in a model of infection following hemorrhagic shock.

Materials and Methods

Adult female Sprague-Dawley rats were anesthetized with intraperitoneal ketamine and xylazine. After heparin (1 000 u/kg) was given intravenously, animals were subjected to hemorrhagic shock by bleeding to a mean arterial pressure (MAP) of 45 mmHg for 45 min and then were resuscitated to preshock MAP by infusion of shed blood and 1.5 volumes of normal saline. The mortality of this shock preparation was 15%. All deaths occurred within 24 h following shock and these animals were excluded from analysis. The mean volume of blood withdrawn was 2.9% $\pm$0.2% of body weight or approximately 40% of blood volume. Animals undergoing sham procedure had only their vessels exposed.

The dorsal fur was clipped and five separate inocula of 1×10^8 *Staphylococcus aureus* (0.25 ml) were injected subcutaneously on the back 1 h following shock or sham procedure. Rats were divided into four treatment groups: (1) Control, no treatment, (2) IFN-γ recombinant rat IFN-γ (Amgen Biologicals) 7 500 u given

Immune Consequences of
Trauma, Shock and Sepsis
Eds. Faist/Ninnemann/Green

subcutaneously 30 min *after* inoculation and daily for 3 days, (3) MAN-cefamandole nafate 30 mg/kg, given intraperitoneally 30 min *before* and 4 h *after* inoculation, and (4) MAN+IFN-γ as in (2) and (3). Animals were killed on day 7 and abscess number, diameter, and weight were measured.

Statistical comparisons of abscess diameter and weight were performed using a prior analysis of variance with Tukey HSD multiple comparisons of means. Comparisons between abscess number were performed using Fisher's exact test. Significance was set at $P<0.05$.

Results

Results are summarized in Table 1. In unshocked animals, MAN significantly reduced abscess number, diameter, and weight. Following hemorrhagic shock, the beneficial effect of MAN was no longer demonstrable.

Interferon-γ alone did not alter any of the parameters measured in either shocked or unshocked animals. After hemorrhagic shock, MAN+IFN-γ decreased abscess diameter and weight compared with control, IFN-γ, or MAN alone; however, abscess number was unchanged.

The correlation between the bacterial inoculum and the ultimate size and weight of the abscess formed was determined in a separate study. In 89 abscesses, there were significant correlations between the bacterial inoculum and abscess diameter ($r=0.915$, $r^2=0.837$, $P<0.01$). Furthermore, there was a demonstrable relationship between abscess diameter and weight which was strongest when the abscess diameter was less than 15 mm ($r=0.839$, $r^2=0.690$, $P<0.01$). These correlations indicate that changes in abscess diameter and weight accurately reflect the success or failure of an animal's ability to combat the bacterial challenge. The mean tissue levels for MAN were 15.4 ± 3.7 µg/g and there were no significant differences between groups. The minimal inhibitory concentration (MIC) for the *S. aureus* used was less than 0.3 µg/ml and the tissue half-life was 70 min.

Discussion

In a model of incisional wound infection, we previously demonstrated that hemorrhagic shock markedly increased the susceptibility to infection despite resuscitation [2]. Our present results further confirm that observation using a subcutaneous abscess model and demonstrate that shock permits local bacterial proliferation by either direct impairment of local cellular or humoral factors or indirectly by stimulating the production of immunosuppressive substances which impair host defense.

The efficacy of antibiotics to prevent infection is based on experimental work that demonstrated antibiotics given prior to or shortly after bacterial challenge effectively diminished the liklihood of infection [8, 9]. While it is impractical to administer an antibiotic prior to injury, antibiotics given within the decisive period after contamination should prevent infection. A recent study has shown that administration of a 1-day course of antibiotics to patients who had intraabdomi-

Table 1. Effect of hemorrhagic shock, cefamandole, and IFN-γ on *S. aureus* abscess formation

	No shock				Shock			
	Control	IFN-γ	MAN	MAN+IFN-γ	Control	IFN-γ	MAN	MAN+IFN-γ
Abscess no. ($N=20$)	20	20	11*	8*	20	20	20	20
Abscess diameter (mm)	11.7 ± 2.8	14.6 ± 3.8	4.6 ± 3.8*	2.7 ± 3.2*	13.4 ± 1.9	13.8 ± 1.7	13.0 ± 1.9	8.1 ± 1.8*, **
Abscess weight (mg)	600 ± 199	711 ± 214	103 ± 97*	49 ± 60*	504 ± 124	769 ± 212	491 ± 152	252 ± 132*, **

* $P < 0.05$ vs. control and IFN-γ alone; ** $P < 0.05$ vs. MAN alone.

nal contamination due to penetrating trauma was as effective as a 5-day course [10]. Thus, we chose an antimicrobial that was effective against the bacterium used and gave the drug for a short period. MAN significantly reduced abscess number, diameter, and weight in unshocked animals; however, MAN was ineffective following shock despite resuscitation and tissue antibiotic concentrations 30–50 times the MIC for the *S. aureus* used. This implies that these observations are not from a lack of antibiotic delivery to the site of infection.

A multitude of adjuvants have been used to enhance host defenses against bacterial infection; however, most must be given prior to bacterial inoculation but within the decisive period of infection when the interaction between host defenses and bacteria can be influenced by antibiotics. IFN-γ has been shown to augment macrophage function and exert a protective effect against bacterial and protozoan infections [11]. Hypoopsonemia has been implicated as a cause of posttraumatic infection and the phagocytosis of nonopsonized bacteria by mouse peritoneal macrophages has been enhanced by treatment with IFN-γ [12].

In unshocked animals, IFN-γ produced lesions that were larger than in control rats and showed increased necrosis of the overlying skin. This would suggest that IFN-γ is not directly bactericidal to *S. aureus* and may enhance the local inflammatory response to infection.

The combination of IFN-γ and MAN significantly reduced lesion diameter and weight following hemorrhagic shock and resuscitation. In unshocked animals, MAN + IFN-γ resulted in a decrease of abscess number and size compared with MAN alone. While we could not demonstrate statistical significance in this treatment group, the effect of IFN-γ may be obscured by the presence of a type II statistical error. It is unlikely that IFN-γ alters antibiotic activity but it may augment or restore local bacterial defenses and enhance the killing of *S. aureus*.

In conclusion, this experiment demonstrates that despite resuscitation from shock there is a persistent increased susceptibility to *S. aureus* infection. MAN effectively reduced the risk of infection in unshocked animals. However, this ability was lost following shock despite resuscitation and the presence of effective tissue antibiotic concentrations. The combination of IFN-γ plus an antibiotic appears to restore bactericidal capability after shock. The restoration of antibiotic efficacy is likely due to an improvement of systemic host defenses rather than changes in antibiotic efficacy. IFN-γ alone was ineffective in combating infection in both shocked and unshocked animals. Stimulation of host defense following hemorrhagic shock can effectively decrease infection.

References

1. Baker CC, Oppenheimer L, Stephens B, Lewis FR, Trunkey DD (1980) Epidemiology of trauma deaths. Am J Surg 140:141
2. Livingston DH, Malangoni MA (1987) Prolonged susceptibility to infection exists after hemorrhagic shock despite resuscitation and antibiotics. Surg Forum 38:64
3. Davis JM, Stevens JM, Peitzman A, Corbett WA, Illner H, Shires GT III, Shires GT (1983) Neutrophil migratory activity in severe hemorrhagic shock. Circ Shock 10:199
4. Polk HC Jr, George C, Wellhausen SR, Cost K, Davidson PF, Regan MP, Borzotta AP (1986) A systematic study of host defense processes in badly injured patients. Ann Surg 204:282

5. Faist E, Mewes A, Baker CC, Strasser T, Alkan S, Rieber P, Heberer G (1987) Prostaglandin E_2 (PGE_2)-dependent suppression of interleukin (IL-2) production in patients with major trauma. J Trauma 27:837
6. De-Maeyer-Guignard J, De-Maeyer E (1985) Immunomodulation by interferons: recent developments. Interferon 6:69
7. Shalaby MR, Aggarwal BB, Rinderknecht E, Svedersky LP, Finkle BS, Palladino MA (1985) Activation of human polymorphonuclear neutrophil functions by interferon-γ and tumor necrosis factors. J Immunol 135:2069
8. Burke JF (1961) The effective period of preventive antibiotic action in experimental incisions and dermal lesions. Surgery 50:161
9. Alexander JW, Altemeier WA (1965) Penicillin prophylaxis of experimental staphylococcal wound infections. Surg Gynecol Obstet 120:243
10. Dellinger EP, Wertz MJ, Lennard S, Oreskovich MR (1986) Efficacy of short-course antibiotic prophylaxis after penetrating intestinal injury: a prospective randomized trial. Arch Surg 121:23
11. Sonnenfeld G, Gould CL, Kierszenbaum F, Degee ALW, Mansfield JM (1986) Interferon in resistance to bacterial and protozoan infections. In: Stewart WE II, Schellekens H (eds) The biology of the interferon system. Elsevier, Amsterdam, p 291
12. Rollag H, Degre M (1981) Effect of interferon preparations on the uptake of non-opsonized *Escherichia coli* by mouse peritoneal macrophages. Acta Pathol Microbiol Immunol Scand 89:153

Subject Index

MIX
Papier aus verantwortungsvollen Quellen
Paper from responsible sources
FSC® C105338

If you have any concerns about our products,
you can contact us on
ProductSafety@springernature.com

In case Publisher is established outside the EU,
the EU authorized representative is:
Springer Nature Customer Service Center GmbH
Europaplatz 3, 69115 Heidelberg, Germany

Printed by Libri Plureos GmbH
in Hamburg, Germany